Trisha Minium

ANATOMICAL DIRECTIONS

Directional Terms	Definition	Example of Usage
Left	To the left of body (not *your* left, the subject's)	The stomach is to the *left* of the liver.
Right	To the right of the body or structure being studied	The *right* kidney is damaged.
Lateral	Toward the side; away from the midsagittal plane	The eyes are *lateral* to the nose.
Medial	Toward the midsagittal plane; away from the side	The eyes are *medial* to the ears.
Anterior	Toward the front of the body	The nose is on the *anterior* of the head.
Posterior	Toward the back (rear)	The heel is *posterior* to the head.
Superior	Toward the top of the body	The shoulders are *superior* to the hips.
Inferior	Toward the bottom of the body	The stomach is *inferior* to the heart.
Dorsal	Along (or toward) the vertebral surface of the body	Her scar is along the *dorsal* surface.
Ventral	Along (toward) the belly surface of the body	The navel is on the *ventral* surface.
Caudad (caudal)	Toward the tail	The neck is *caudad* to the skull.
Cephalad	Toward the head	The neck is *cephalad* to the tail.
Proximal	Toward the trunk (describes relative position in a limb or other appendage)	The joint is *proximal* to the toenail.
Distal	Away from the trunk or point of attachment	The hand is *distal* to the elbow.
Visceral	Toward an internal organ; away from the outer wall (describes positions inside a body cavity)	This organ is covered with the *visceral* layer of the membrane.
Parietal	Toward the wall; away from the internal structures	The abdominal cavity is lined with the *parietal* peritoneal membrane.
Deep	Toward the inside of a part; away from the surface	The thigh muscles are *deep* to the skin.
Superficial	Toward the surface of a part; away from the inside	The skin is a *superficial* organ.
Medullary	Refers to an inner region, or medulla	The *medullary* portion contains nerve tissue.
Cortical	Refers to an outer region, or cortex	The *cortical* area produces hormones.

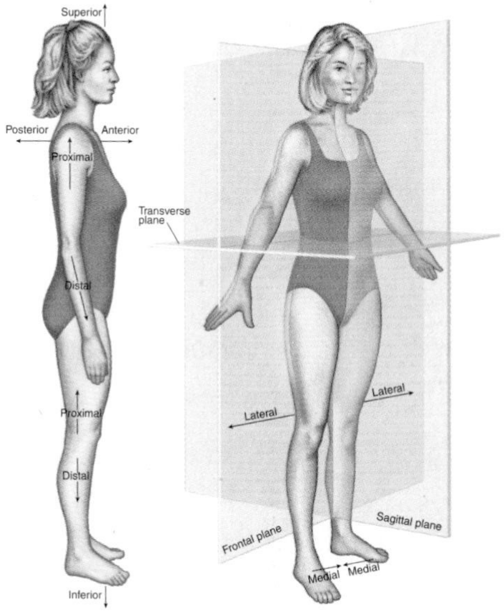

To make the reading of anatomical figures a little easier, an anatomical compass is used throughout this book. On many figures, you will notice a small compass rosette similar to those on geographical maps. Rather than being labeled N, S, E, and W, the anatomical rosette is labeled with abbreviated anatomical directions.

A = Anterior
D = Distal
I = Inferior
L (opposite R) = Left
L (opposite M) = Lateral
M = Medial
P (opposite A) = Posterior
P (opposite D) = Proximal
R = Right
S = Superior

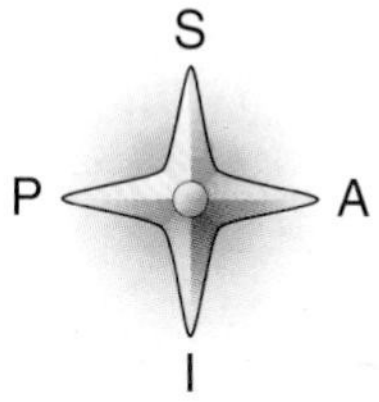

Structure & Function of the Body

12th Edition

GARY A. THIBODEAU, PhD
Chancellor Emeritus and Professor Emeritus of Biology
University of Wisconsin–River Falls
River Falls, Wisconsin

KEVIN T. PATTON, PhD
Professor, Department of Life Sciences
Saint Charles Community College
Saint Peters, Missouri
Adjunct Assistant Professor of Physiology
Saint Louis University Medical School
Saint Louis, Missouri

Mosby
An Affiliate of Elsevier

11830 Westline Industrial Drive
St. Louis, Missouri 63146

STRUCTURE & FUNCTION OF THE BODY, TWELFTH EDITION 0-323-02242-1

Library of Congress Cataloging in Publication Data

Thibodeau, Gary A.
Structure & function of the body/Gary A. Thibodeau, Kevin T. Patton.—12th ed.
p. cm.
Includes bibliographical references and index.
ISBN 0-323-02242-1 — ISBN 0-323-02241-3
1. Human physiology. 2. Human anatomy. I. Title: Structure & function of the body.
II. Patton, Kevin T. III. Title.

QP34.5.T5 2004
612—dc22

2003062235

Executive Vice President, Nursing & Health Professions: Sally Schrefer
Executive Publisher: Robin Carter
Senior Editor: Tom Wilhelm
Senior Developmental Editor: Jeff Downing
Publishing Services Manager: Deborah L. Vogel
Senior Project Manager: Ann E. Rogers
Senior Book Designers: Mark Oberkrom, Kathi Gosche

Printed in the United States of America.

Last digit is the print number: 9 8 7 6 5 4 3 2

In loving memory of our son

Douglas J. Thibodeau
July 23, 1965 – November 21, 2002

He left a legacy of treasured memories, love, and courage.

Gary A. Thibodeau
Emogene J. Thibodeau

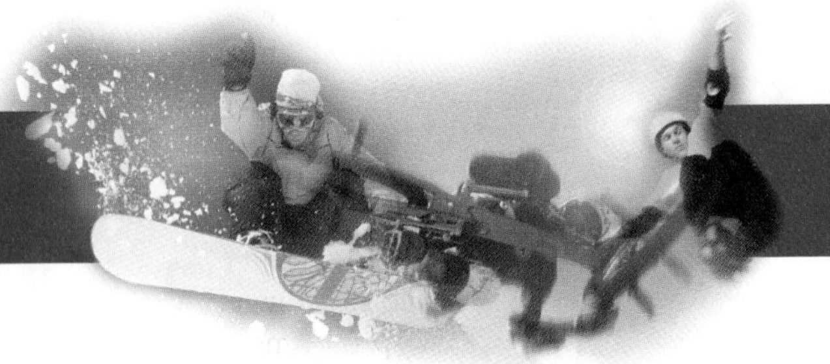

Preface

The true quality of a textbook is best measured by how well it supports, promotes, and encourages both good teaching and effective learning. The twelfth edition of *Structure & Function of the Body* is a new text with a long tradition of excellence. It is based on profound respect for both the teacher and the student. That respect is coupled with an excitement for the subject matter honed during decades of teaching anatomy and physiology by both authors. We have listened carefully to input from users of previous editions. We know that teachers use different techniques to convey ideas, esent difficult concepts, or explain how applica- of principles of anatomy and physiology can or example, health, diverse personal inter- di dents in the class, or other areas of biol- for s, of course, learn in different ways, at text; and for different reasons. Success rely h y predicated on readability of the learn b cepts. A e visual in their learning and accommodent illustrations; still others both teache by verbal review of con- flexible enough to help se differing needs of

Now that we have begun a new century of discovery, success in both teaching and learning is, in many ways, determined by how effective we are in transforming information into knowledge. This is especially true in anatomy and physiology, where both student and teacher are now being confronted with an enormous accumulation of factual information. *Structure & Function of the Body* is intended to help transform that information into a coherent knowledge base. It was written at an appropriate level to help students with divergent needs and learning styles to unify information, stimulate critical thinking, and hopefully acquire a taste for knowledge about the wonders of the human body. The new edition is designed for ease of use and will encourage students to explore, question, and look for relationships not only between related facts in a single discipline but also among fields of academic inquiry and personal experience.

This twelfth edition of *Structure & Function of the Body* retains many features that have proved successful in several decades of classroom use; yet as a new text it presents a wealth of carefully selected new content in both anatomy and physiology, as well as pedagogical enhancements that will better serve the needs of today's instructors and students. The writing style and depth of coverage

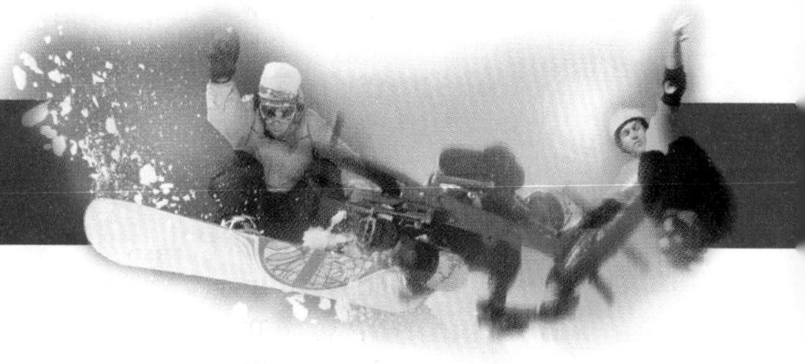

Preface

The true quality of a textbook is best measured by how well it supports, promotes, and encourages both good teaching and effective learning. The twelfth edition of *Structure & Function of the Body* is a new text with a long tradition of excellence. It is based on profound respect for both the teacher and the student. That respect is coupled with an excitement for the subject matter honed during decades of teaching anatomy and physiology by both authors. We have listened carefully to input from users of previous editions. We know that teachers use different techniques to convey ideas, present difficult concepts, or explain how applications of principles of anatomy and physiology can affect, for example, health, diverse personal interests of students in the class, or other areas of biology. Students, of course, learn in different ways, at different paces, and for different reasons. Success for some is largely predicated on readability of the text; others are more visual in their learning and rely heavily on excellent illustrations; still others learn best in groups and by verbal review of concepts. A good text must be flexible enough to help accommodate, not hinder, these differing needs of both teacher and student.

Now that we have begun a new century of discovery, success in both teaching and learning is, in many ways, determined by how effective we are in transforming information into knowledge. This is especially true in anatomy and physiology, where both student and teacher are now being confronted with an enormous accumulation of factual information. *Structure & Function of the Body* is intended to help transform that information into a coherent knowledge base. It was written at an appropriate level to help students with divergent needs and learning styles to unify information, stimulate critical thinking, and hopefully acquire a taste for knowledge about the wonders of the human body. The new edition is designed for ease of use and will encourage students to explore, question, and look for relationships not only between related facts in a single discipline but also among fields of academic inquiry and personal experience.

This twelfth edition of *Structure & Function of the Body* retains many features that have proved successful in several decades of classroom use; yet as a new text it presents a wealth of carefully selected new content in both anatomy and physiology, as well as pedagogical enhancements that will better serve the needs of today's instructors and students. The writing style and depth of coverage

In loving memory of our son

Douglas J. Thibodeau
July 23, 1965 – November 21, 2002

He left a legacy of treasured memories, love, and courage.

Gary A. Thibodeau
Emogene J. Thibodeau

are intended to challenge, reward, and reinforce introductory students as they grasp and assimilate important concepts.

During the revision of this text, each change in content and organization was evaluated by anatomy and physiology teachers working in the field—teachers currently assisting students to learn about human structure and function for the first time. The result is a text that students will read—one designed to help the teacher teach and the student learn. It is particularly suited to introductory anatomy and physiology courses in nursing and allied health–related programs. Emphasis is on material required for entry into more advanced courses, completion of professional licensing examinations, and successful application of information in a practical, work-related environment.

Special Features

Unifying Themes

Structure & Function of the Body is dominated by two major unifying themes. First, structure and function complement one another in the normal, healthy human body. Second, nearly all structure and function in the body can be explained in terms of keeping conditions in the internal environment relatively constant—in homeostasis. Repeated emphasis of these principles encourages students to integrate otherwise isolated factual information into a cohesive and understandable whole. As a result, anatomy and physiology emerge as living and dynamic topics of personal interest and importance to the student.

Presentation of Clinical, Wellness, Research, and Science Applications

Carefully selected clinical examples are included in each chapter of the book to help students understand that the disease process is a disruption in homeostasis and a breakdown of the normal integration of form and function. We use clinical examples to reinforce the concepts of how disease affects normal function and how therapies can restore normal function. We have found in our own teaching that such examples stimulate student interest. Boxed information highlighting health and wellness issues likewise reinforces the basic concepts of human structure and function by applying them in practical ways to current problems in public health, athletics, and fitness. A few select boxed essays on issues and trends in research and medicine will spark an interest in the dynamic fields of science, technology, and ethics that underlie the modern arena of human biology. New to this edition is a collection of Science Applications that feature possible career paths that use the concepts taught in this text. These career paths are mentioned in the context of the work of an important figure in the history of scientific endeavor. Such information will further motivate learning by illustrating its practical applications and will stimulate students to think about their own career choices.

Also new to this edition is Appendix A: Body Mass Index, which provides a BMI diagram along with instructions for assessing an individual's risk for health problems related to obesity.

Organization and Content

The 21 chapters of *Structure & Function of the Body* present the core material of anatomy and physiology most important for introductory students. The selection of appropriate information in both disciplines eliminates the confusing mix of nonessential and overly specialized material that unfortunately accompanies basic information in many introductory textbooks. Information is presented in a way that makes it easy for students to know and understand what is important. Further, pedagogical aids in each chapter identify learning objectives and then reinforce successful mastery of this clearly identified core material. The sequencing of chapters in the book follows a course organization most commonly used in teaching at the undergraduate level. But because each chapter is self-contained, instructors have the flexibility to alter the sequence of material to fit personal teaching preferences or the special content or time constraints of their courses or students.

For the first time in this edition, we have included material on biological chemistry as the second chapter of the text rather than as a separate appendix at the back of the book. We made this change at the request of many of the users of previous editions of the book. As with any chapter in this text, teachers and students may skip over the chapter if they already have sufficient background in chemistry. We trust that this new organization of material will make it even easier for students to march into the central concepts of human structure and function with a valuable knowledge of basic chemical principles.

At every level of organization, both within and among chapters, care has been taken to couple structural information with important functional concepts. In each chapter of the text, appropriate physiological content balances the anatomical information that is presented. As a result, the student has a more integrated understanding of human structure and function. Throughout the text, examples that stress the complementarity of structure and function have been consciously selected to emphasize the importance of homeostasis as a unifying concept.

Acquiring and using the terms so necessary for any study of anatomy and physiology can be difficult for many students. To assist students in this area, new terms are introduced, defined, and incorporated into a working vocabulary. Every chapter also utilizes skillfully designed visuals to reinforce written information with sensory input. The style of presentation of material in this text and its readability, accuracy, and level of coverage have been carefully developed to meet the needs of undergraduate students taking an introductory course in anatomy and physiology. *Structure & Function of the Body* remains an introductory textbook—a teaching book rather than a reference text. No textbook can replace the direction and stimulation provided by an enthusiastic teacher to a curious and involved student. A good textbook, however, can and should be enjoyable to read and helpful to both.

Pedagogical Features

Structure & Function of the Body is a student-oriented text. Written in a very readable style, it has numerous pedagogical aids that maintain interest and motivation. Every chapter contains the following elements that facilitate learning and the retention of information in the most effective manner.

Chapter outline: An overview outline introduces each chapter and enables the student to preview the content and direction of the chapter at the major concept level before the detailed reading.

Chapter objectives: The opening page of each chapter contains several measurable objectives for the student. Each objective clearly identifies for the student, before he or she reads the chapter, what the key goals should be and what information should be mastered.

Key terms and pronunciation guide: Key terms, when introduced and defined in the text body, are identified in boldface to highlight their importance. A pronunciation guide follows each new term that students may find difficult to pronounce correctly. A listing of these new terms is recapped at the end of each chapter.

Quick Check questions: New to this edition, the Quick Check feature provides a way for students to check their basic reading comprehension at the end of each passage that they have read. Each Quick Check consists of a few questions scattered at appropriate points throughout the text of each chapter. The questions are very simple, meant only to check to see if the student read and understood the main points of each passage.

Boxed inserts and essays: Boxed information appears in every chapter. In this edition, we have grouped these boxed features into four categories: Health & Well-Being; Clinical Application; Research, Issues, & Trends; and (new to this edition) Science Applications. The boxed features increase student interest. They also help students apply information learned in the course to help them develop critical thinking skills.

Outline summaries: Extensive and detailed end-of-chapter summaries in outline format provide excellent guides for students as they review the text materials when preparing for examinations. Many students also find these detailed guides useful as a chapter preview in conjunction with the chapter outline.

Review questions: Subjective review questions at the end of each chapter allow students to use a narrative format to discuss concepts and synthesize important chapter information for review by the instructor. The answers to these review questions are available in the Instructor's Resource Manual that accompanies the text.

Critical thinking questions: Review questions that encourage students to use critical thinking skills are highlighted at the end of each chapter. Answers to these questions are also found in the Instructor's Resource Manual.

Chapter tests: Objective-type chapter test questions are included at the end of each chapter. They serve as quick checks for the recall and mastery of important subject matter. They are also designed as aids to increase the retention of information. Answers to all chapter test questions are provided at the end of the text.

Study tips: Each chapter includes a list of specific tips and hints on how to most effectively study the concepts of that chapter. Prepared by veteran teacher Ed Calcaterra, these tips are a unique and useful feature that make this text even more "student friendly."

Body mass index (BMI) appendix: A brief overview of the body mass index and how it is used to assess risk for weight-related health conditions is included as a separate appendix that can be used in the introduction to the body in Chapter 1, the study of tissues in Chapter 3, the study of nutrition and metabolism in Chapter 16, or anywhere else the student or teacher finds it useful.

Additional learning and study aids at the end of the text include Common Medical Abbreviations, Prefixes, and Suffixes; an extensive Glossary of Terms to assist students in mastering the vocabulary of anatomy and physiology; and a detailed Index that serves as a ready reference for locating information.

Illustrations

A major strength of *Structure & Function of the Body* is the exceptional quality, accuracy, and beauty of the illustration program. The truest test of any illustration is how effectively it can complement and strengthen written information found in the text and how successfully it can be used by the student as a learning tool. Extensive use has been made of full-color illustrations, micrographs, and dissection photographs throughout the text. Each illustration is carefully referred to in the text and is designed to support the text discussion. For example, the new Figure 21-7 on page 524 shows not only the details of early prenatal development but also integrates the concept of risk of birth defects at various stages of embryonic development.

Continuing in this edition of *Structure & Function of the Body* is the careful use of anatomical rosettes in all anatomical illustrations (see the first page of the Front Matter for an illustration of this useful element). These rosettes, like the compass rosettes found on all modern maps, orient the user to the "direction" or "orientation" of the figure by pointing which way is left and which way is right—directions that in anatomy may appear "backwards" to the beginning student. As with map users, the need for these rosettes will diminish as one becomes more and more familiar with "the territory" of the human body.

Supplements

The supplements package has been carefully planned and developed to assist instructors and to enhance their use of the text. Each supplement, including the test items and Study Guide, has been thoroughly reviewed by many of the same instructors who reviewed the text.

Instructor's Resource Manual and Test Bank

The Instructor's Resource Manual and Test Bank, prepared by Judith Diehl of Pensacola Junior College, provides text adopters with substantial support in teaching from the text.

Mosby's Electronic Image Collection

Includes nearly 300 anatomy and physiology images to enhance your lectures.

Study Guide

Written by Linda Swisher of Sarasota County Technical Institute, this guide provides students with additional self-study aids, including chapter overviews, topic reviews, application and labeling exercises (including matching, crossword puzzles, fill in the blank, and multiple choice), as well as answers to the questions in the Study Guide.

Panorama of Anatomy & Physiology/Body Spectrum CD-ROM

This exciting CD-ROM combines two of our most popular interactive programs. The Panorama of Anatomy & Physiology provides students with a multitude of exercises, quizzes, and activities that cover essential anatomy and physiology content. The Body Spectrum: Mosby's Electronic Anatomy Coloring Book offers 80 detailed anatomy illustrations that the student can color online or print out to color and study offline.

EVOLVE

EVOLVE is an interactive website with content updates, student resources, and WebLinks. WebLinks provide students with access to hundreds of important sites simply by clicking on a subject in the book's table of contents. EVOLVE is a virtual library of information at your fingertips.

A Word of Thanks

Many people have contributed to the development and success of *Structure & Function of the Body*. We extend our thanks and deep appreciation to the various students and classroom instructors who have provided us with helpful suggestions following their use of earlier editions of this text.

A special "thank you" to Ed Calcaterra for his many previous contributions to this text. A specific "thank you" goes to the following clinicians, researchers, and instructors who critiqued in detail the previous editions of this text or various drafts of the revision. Their invaluable comments were instrumental in the development of this new edition.

JOAN I. BARBER, PhD
Delaware Technical & Community College
Newark, Delaware

DONNA J. BURLESON, RN, MS, MSN
Cisco Junior College
Abilene, Texas

ED CALCATERRA, BS, MEd
Instructor, DeSmet Jesuit High School
Creve Coeur, Missouri

SUSAN M. CALEY, MS
Illinois Valley Community College
Oglesby, Illinois

LINDA C. COLE, MA, MSN, RN, CS, FNP
Saint Charles Community College
Saint Charles, Missouri

KATHLEEN REILLY DOLIN
Northampton Community College
Bethlehem, Pennsylvania

MELANIE S. MacNEIL, MS, PhD
Brock University
St. Catharines, Ontario, Canada

HENRY M. SEIDEL, MD
The Johns Hopkins University School of Medicine
Baltimore, Maryland

KATHLEEN STOCKMAN
Delaware Technical & Community College
Newark, Delaware

PATRICIA LAING-ARIE
Meridian Technology Center
Stillwater, Oklahoma

BERT ATSMA
Union County College
Cranford, New Jersey

ETHEL J. AVERY
Trenholm State Technical College
Montgomery, Alabama

BARBARA BARGER
Clarion County Career Center
Shippenville, Pennsylvania

LYDIA R. CHAVANA
South Texas Vo-Tech Institute
McAllen, Texas

MARIA CONN
Mayo State Vo-Tech School
Pikeville, Kentucky

JOSEPH DEVINE
Allied Health Careers
Austin, Texas

EDNA M. DILMORE
Bessemer State Technical College
Bessemer, Alabama

SALLY FLESCH
Black Hawk College
Moline, Illinois

DENISE L. KAMPFHENKEL
Schreiner College
Kerrville, Texas

ANNE LILLY
Santa Rosa Junior College
Santa Rosa, California

RICHARD E. McKEEBY
Union County College
Cranford, New Jersey

KEITH R. ORLOFF
California Paramedical and Technical College
Long Beach, California

CHRISTINE PAYNE
Sarasota County Technical Institute
Sarasota, Florida

ANN SENISI SCOTT
Nassau Tech VOCES
Westbury, New York

ANNA M. STRAND
Gogebic Community College
Ironwood, Michigan

EUGENE R. VOLZ
Sacramento City College
Sacramento, California

IRIS WILKELHAKE
Southeast Community College
Lincoln, Nebraska

At Mosby, Inc., thanks are due all who have worked with us on this new edition. We wish especially to acknowledge the support and efforts of Sally Schrefer, Executive Vice President, Nursing & Health Professions; Robin Carter, Executive Publisher; Tom Wilhelm, Senior Editor; Jeff Downing, Senior Developmental Editor; Ann Rogers, Senior Project Manager; and Mark Oberkrom and Kathi Gosche, Senior Book Designers; all of whom were instrumental in bringing this edition to successful completion.

GARY A. THIBODEAU
KEVIN T. PATTON

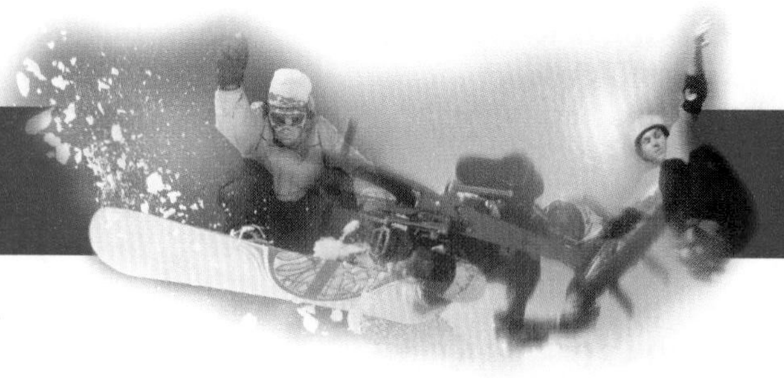

Contents

1 An Introduction to the Structure and Function of the Body

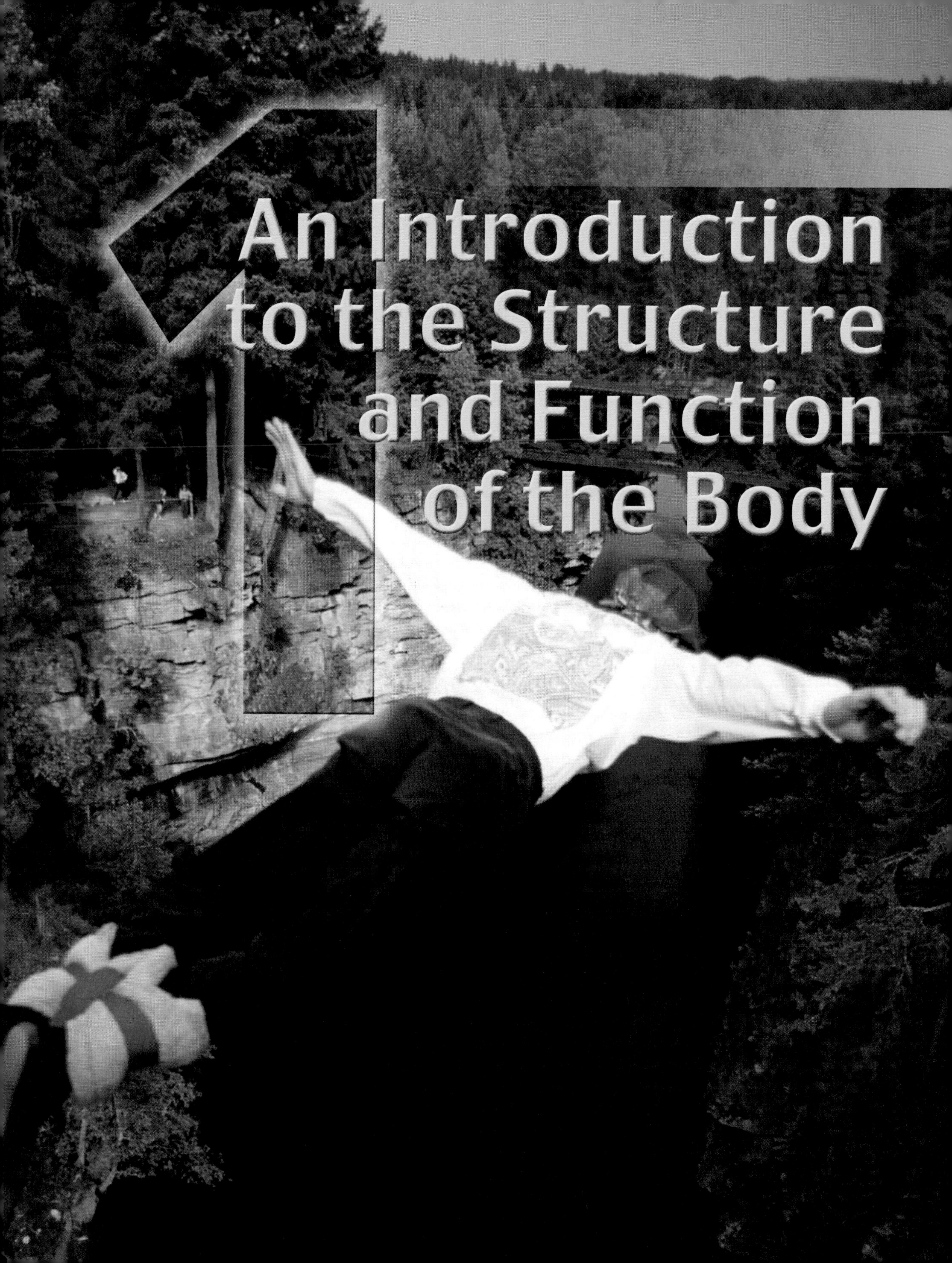

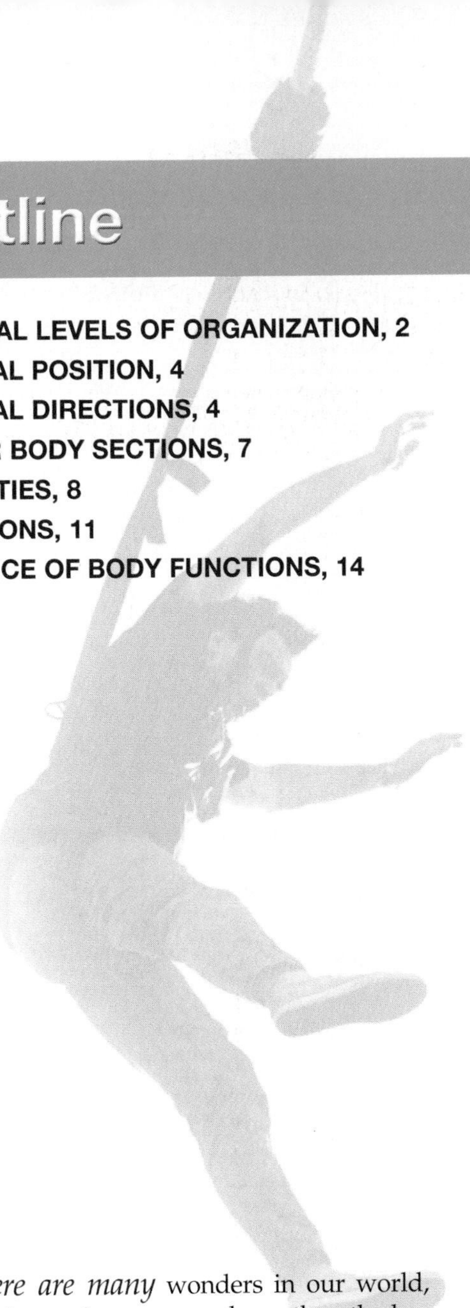

Outline

Objectives

AFTER YOU HAVE COMPLETED THIS CHAPTER, YOU SHOULD BE ABLE TO:

1. Define the terms *anatomy* and *physiology*.
2. List and discuss in order of increasing complexity the levels of organization of the body.
3. Define the term *anatomical position*.
4. List and define the principal directional terms and sections (planes) used in describing the body and the relationship of body parts to one another.
5. List the nine abdominopelvic regions and the abdominopelvic quadrants.
6. List the major cavities of the body and the subdivisions of each.
7. Discuss and contrast the axial and the appendicular subdivisions of the body. Identify a number of specific anatomical regions in each area.
8. Explain the meaning of the term *homeostasis* and give an example of a typical homeostatic mechanism.

T*here are many* wonders in our world, but none is more wondrous than the human body. This is a textbook about that incomparable structure. It deals with two very distinct and yet interrelated sciences: **anatomy** and **physiology.** As a science, anatomy is often defined as the study of the structure of an organism and the relationships of its parts. The word *anatomy* is derived from two Greek words that mean "a cutting up." Anatomists learn about the structure of the human body by cutting it apart. This process, called **dissection,** is still the principal technique used to isolate and study the structural components or parts of the human body. Physiology is the study of the functions of living organisms and their parts. It is a dynamic science that requires active experimentation. In the chapters that follow, you will see again and again that anatomical structures seem designed to perform specific functions. Each has a particular size, shape, form, or position in the body related directly to its ability to perform a unique and specialized activity.

Science Applications

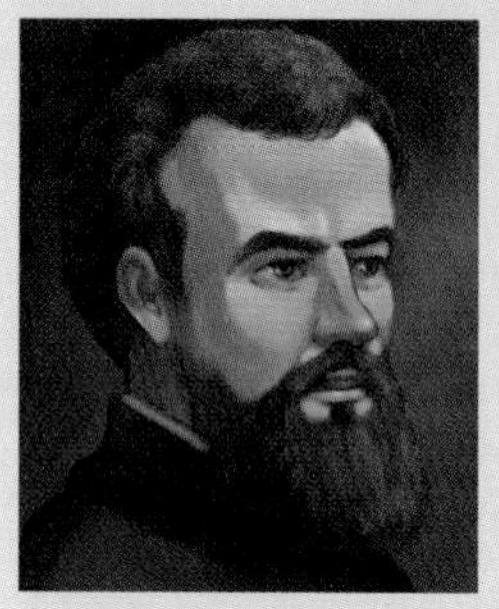

Modern Anatomy

Andreas Vesalius (1514-1564).

Anatomists study the structure of the human body. Modern anatomy started during the Renaissance in Europe with the Flemish scientist Andreas Vesalius (left) and his contemporaries. Vesalius was the first to apply a scientific method (see the box on p. 5) to the study of the human body. Most anatomists still dissect *cadavers* (preserved human remains). However, today many anatomists also use imaging technologies such as x-rays, computerized scans, and even digitized photographs of thin slices of the body as you can see in the figure below from the National Library of Medicine's Visible Human Project. Such digitized images can be reconstructed into dissectible, three-dimensional body views by computers.

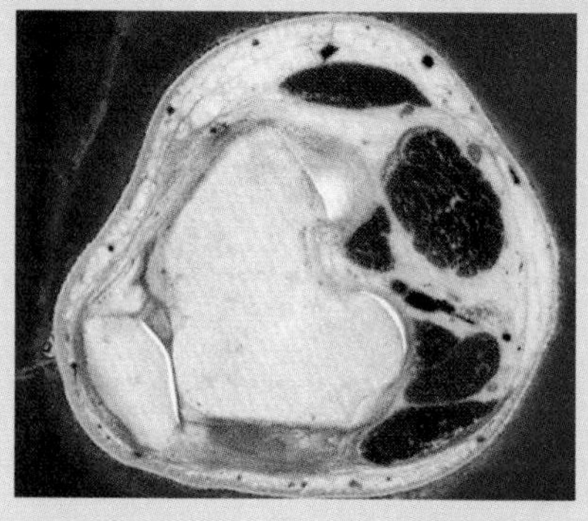

Horizontal section of the human arm.

Modern anatomy also finds applications in the fields of forensic science, anthropology, medicine and allied health professions, sports and athletics, dance, and even art and computerized animation.

STRUCTURAL LEVELS OF ORGANIZATION

Before you begin the study of the structure and function of the human body and its many parts, it is important to think about how those parts are organized and how they might logically fit together into a functioning whole. Examine Figure 1-1. It illustrates the differing levels of organization that influence body structure and function. Note that the levels of organization progress from the least complex (chemical level) to the most complex (body as a whole).

Organization is one of the most important characteristics of body structure. Even the word *organism*, used to denote a living thing, implies organization.

Although the body is a single structure, it is made up of trillions of smaller structures. Atoms and molecules are often referred to as the **chemical level** of organization. The existence of life depends on the proper levels and proportions of

FIGURE 1-1

Structural levels of organization in the body (opposite). Atoms, molecules, and cells can ordinarily only be seen with a microscope, but the gross (large) structures of tissues, organs, systems, and the whole organism can be seen easily with the unaided eye.

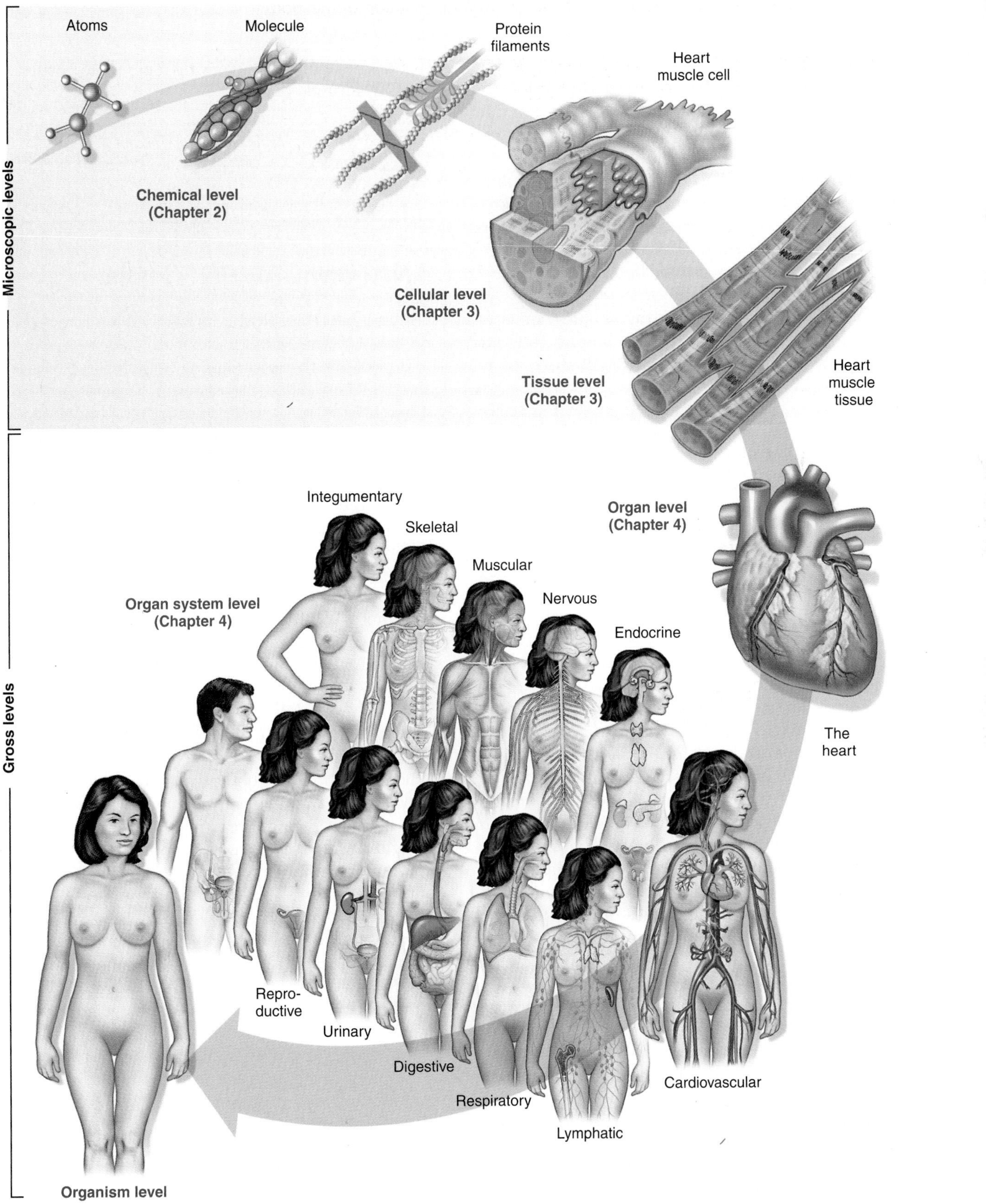
Microscopic levels
Atoms
Molecule
Protein filaments
Heart muscle cell
Chemical level (Chapter 2)
Cellular level (Chapter 3)
Tissue level (Chapter 3)
Heart muscle tissue
Gross levels
Organ level (Chapter 4)
The heart
Organ system level (Chapter 4)
Integumentary
Skeletal
Muscular
Nervous
Endocrine
Cardiovascular
Lymphatic
Respiratory
Digestive
Urinary
Reproductive
Organism level

many chemical substances in the cells of the body. Many of the physical and chemical phenomena that play important roles in the life process will be reviewed in Chapter 2. Such information provides an understanding of the physical basis for life and for the study of the next levels of organization so important in the study of anatomy and physiology—cells, tissues, organs, and systems.

Cells are considered to be the smallest "living" units of structure and function in our body. Although long recognized as the simplest units of living matter, cells are far from simple. They are extremely complex, a fact you will discover in Chapter 3.

Tissues are somewhat more complex than cells. By definition a tissue is an organization of many similar cells that act together to perform a common function. Cells are held together and surrounded by varying amounts and varieties of gluelike, nonliving intercellular substances.

Organs are larger and more complex than tissues. An organ is a group of several different kinds of tissues arranged so that they can together act as a unit to perform a special function. For instance, the heart shown in Figure 1-1 is an example of organization at the organ level. Unlike microscopic molecules and cells, some tissues and most organs are gross (large) structures that can be seen easily without a microscope.

Systems are the most complex units that make up the body. A system is an organization of varying numbers and kinds of organs arranged so that they can together perform complex functions for the body. The organs of the cardiovascular system shown in Figure 1-1 all allow blood to carry nutrients, oxygen, and wastes to and from the tissues of the body. The heart and each of the blood vessels are the organs that pump blood and carry it through the body as it carries out its functions.

The **body as a whole** is all the atoms, molecules, cells, tissues, organs, and systems that you will study in subsequent chapters of this text. Although capable of being dissected or broken down into many parts, the body is a unified and complex assembly of structurally and functionally interactive components, each working together to ensure healthy survival.

Quick
1. What is *anatomy*? What is *physiology*?
2. What are the major levels of organization in the body?
3. How is a tissue different than an organ?

ANATOMICAL POSITION

Discussions about the body, the way it moves, its posture, or the relationship of one area to another assume that the body as a whole is in a specific position called the **anatomical position.** In this reference position (Figure 1-2) the body is in an erect or standing posture with the arms at the sides and palms turned forward. The head and feet also point forward. The anatomical position is a reference position that gives meaning to the directional terms used to describe the body parts and regions.

Supine and **prone** are terms used to describe the position of the body when it is not in the anatomical position. In the supine position the body is lying face upward, and in the prone position the body is lying face downward.

ANATOMICAL DIRECTIONS

When studying the body, it is often helpful to know where an organ is in relation to other structures. The following directional terms are used in describing relative positions of body parts. To help you understand them better, they are listed in sets of opposite pairs:

1. **Superior** and **inferior** (Figure 1-3)—*superior* means "toward the head," and *inferior* means "toward the feet." *Superior* also means "upper" or "above," and *inferior* means "lower" or "below." For example, the lungs are located superior to the diaphragm, whereas the stomach is located inferior to it (check Figure 1-7 if you are not sure where these organs are).
2. **Anterior** and **posterior** (Figure 1-3)—*anterior* means "front" or "in front of"; *posterior* means

Research, Issues & Trends

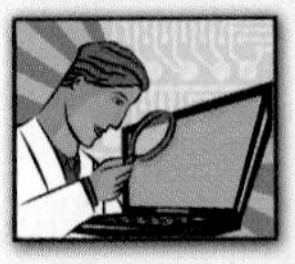

The Scientific Method

What we call the **scientific method** is merely a systematic approach to discovery. Although there is no single method for scientific discovery, many scientists follow the steps outlined here (see the figure) to discover the concepts of human biology discussed in this textbook.

First, one makes a tentative explanation, called a **hypothesis.** A hypothesis is a reasonable guess based on previous informal observations or on previously tested explanations.

After a hypothesis has been proposed, it must be tested—a process called **experimentation.** Scientific experiments are designed to be as simple as possible, to avoid the possibility of errors. Often, **experimental controls** are used to ensure that the test situation itself is not affecting the results. For example, if a new cancer drug is being tested, half the test subjects will get the drug and half the subjects will be given a harmless substitute. The group getting the drug is called the *test group,* and the group getting the substitute is called the *control group*. If both groups improve, or if only the control group improves, the drug's effectiveness hasn't been proven. If the test group improves, but the control group doesn't, the hypothesis that the drug works is tentatively accepted as true. Experimentation requires accurate measurement and recording of data.

If the results of experimentation support the original hypothesis, it is tentatively accepted as true, and the researcher moves on to the next step. If the data do not support the hypothesis, the researcher tentatively rejects the hypothesis. Knowing which hypotheses are untrue is as valuable as knowing which hypotheses are true.

Initial experimental results are published in scientific journals so that other researchers can benefit from them and verify them. If experimental results cannot be reproduced by other scientists, then the hypothesis is not widely accepted. If a hypothesis withstands this rigorous retesting, the level of confidence in the hypothesis increases. A hypothesis that has gained a high level of confidence is called a **theory** or **law.**

The facts presented in this textbook are among the latest theories of how the body is built and how it functions. As methods of imaging the body and measuring functional processes improve, we find new data that cause us to replace old theories with newer ones.

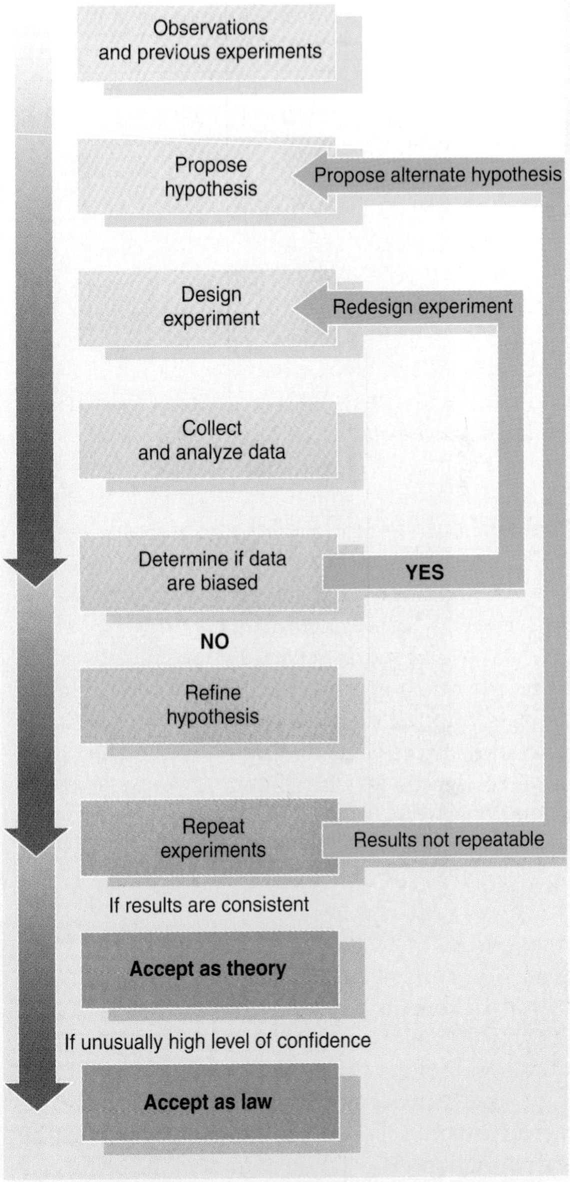

The scientific method. In this classic example, initial observations or results from other experiments may lead to formation of a new hypothesis. As more testing is done, eliminating outside influences or biases and ensuring consistent results, scientists begin to have more confidence in the principle and call it a theory or law.

FIGURE 1-2

Anatomical position. The body is in an erect or standing posture with the arms at the sides and the palms forward. The head and feet also point forward. The anatomical compass rosette is explained at the bottom of the second column on this page.

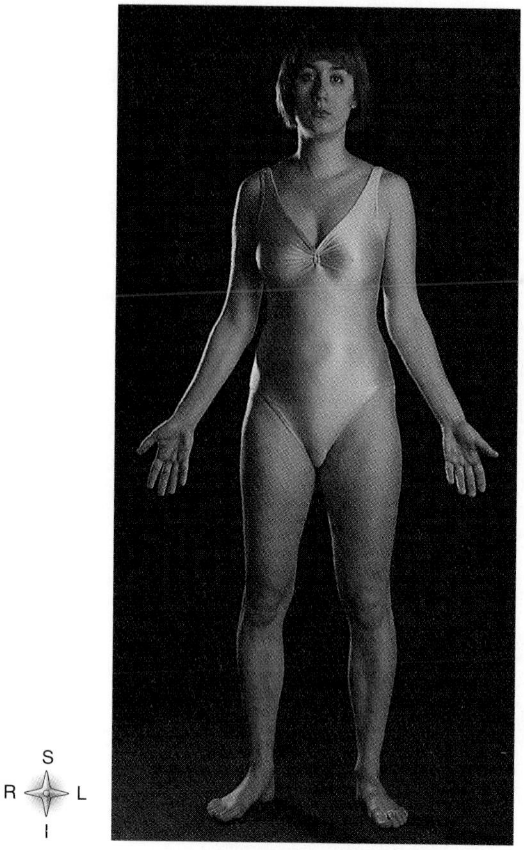

"back" or "in back of." In humans, who walk in an upright position, *ventral* (toward the belly) can be used in place of anterior, and *dorsal* (toward the back) can be used for posterior. For example, the nose is on the anterior surface of the body, and the shoulder blades are on its posterior surface.

3. **Medial** and **lateral** (Figure 1-3)—*medial* means "toward the midline of the body"; *lateral* means "toward the side of the body or away from its midline." For example, the great toe is at the medial side of the foot, and the little toe is at its lateral side. The heart lies medial to the lungs, and the lungs lie lateral to the heart.
4. **Proximal** and **distal** (Figure 1-3)—*proximal* means "toward or nearest the trunk of the body, or nearest the point of origin of one of its parts"; *distal* means "away from or farthest from the trunk or the point of origin of a body part." For example, the elbow lies at the proximal end of the lower arm, whereas the hand lies at its distal end.
5. **Superficial** and **deep**—*superficial* means nearer the surface; *deep* means farther away from the body surface. For example, the skin of the arm is superficial to the muscles below it, and the bone of the upper arm is deep to the muscles that surround and cover it.

To make the reading of anatomical figures a little easier for you, we have used an anatomical compass rosette throughout this book. On many figures, you will see a small compass rosette like you might see on a geographical map. Instead of being labeled **N, S, E,** or **W,** the anatomical rosette is labeled with abbreviated anatomical directions. For example, in Figure 1-2, the rosette is labeled **S** (for superior) on top and **I** (for inferior) on the bottom. Notice that in Figure 1-2 the rosette shows **R** (right) on the subject's right—not your right. Here are the directional abbreviations used with the rosettes in this book:

A = Anterior
D = Distal
I = Inferior
L (opposite M) = Lateral
L (opposite R) = Left
M = Medial
P (opposite A) = Posterior
P (opposite D) = Proximal
R = Right
S = Superior

Quick Check

1. What is the *anatomical position*?
2. Why are the anatomical directions listed in pairs?

FIGURE 1-3

Directions and planes of the body.

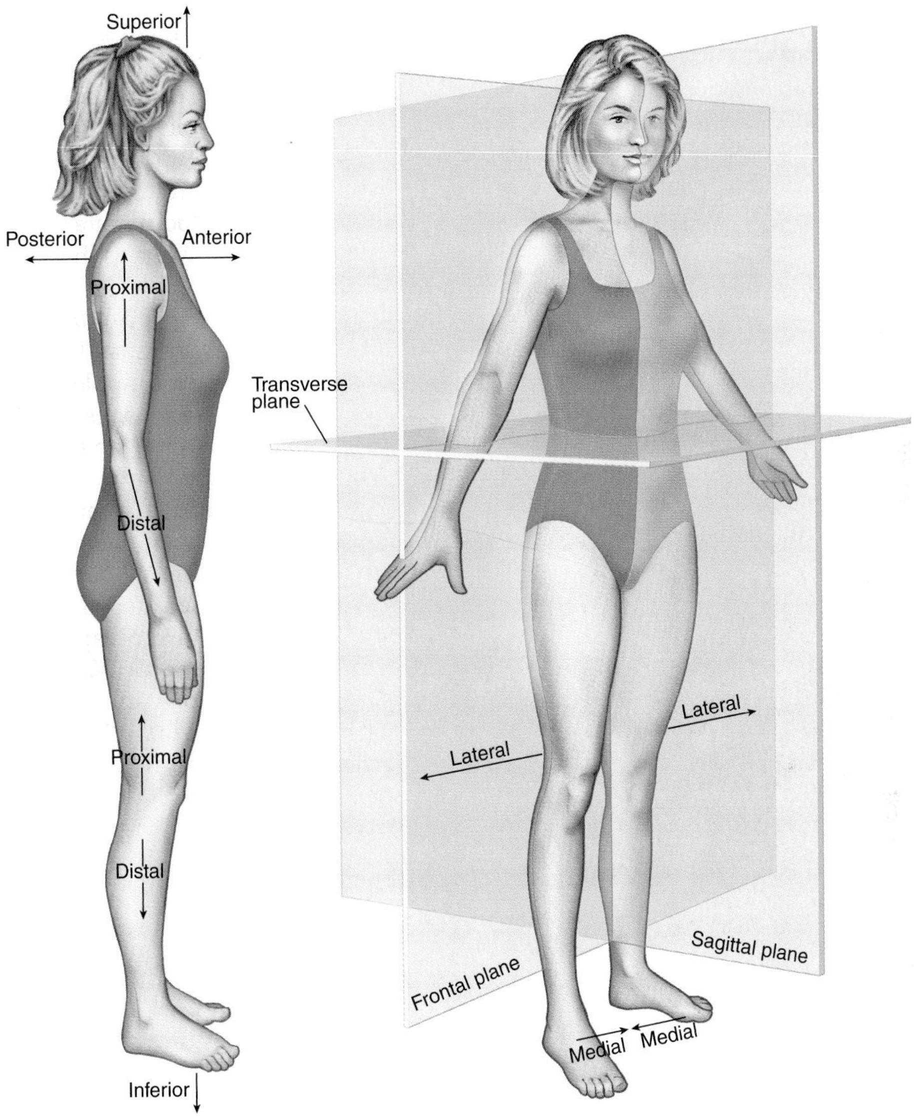

PLANES OR BODY SECTIONS

To facilitate the study of individual organs or the body as a whole, it is often useful to subdivide or "cut" it into smaller segments. To do this, body planes or sections have been identified by special names. Read the following definitions and identify each term in Figure 1-3.

1. **Sagittal**—a sagittal cut or section is a lengthwise plane running from front to back. It divides the body or any of its parts into right and left sides. The sagittal plane shown in Figure 1-3

divides the body into two *equal halves.* This unique type of sagittal plane is called a **midsagittal plane.**

2. **Frontal**—a frontal *(coronal)* plane is a lengthwise plane running from side to side. As you can see in Figure 1-3, a frontal plane divides the body or any of its parts into anterior and posterior (front and back) portions.
3. **Transverse**—a transverse plane is a horizontal or crosswise plane. Such a plane (Figure 1-3) divides the body or any of its parts into upper and lower portions.

BODY CAVITIES

Contrary to its external appearance, the body is not a solid structure. It is made up of open spaces or cavities that in turn contain compact, well-ordered arrangements of internal organs. The two major body cavities are called the **ventral** and **dorsal body cavities.** The location and outlines of the body cavities are illustrated in Figure 1-4. The upper part of the ventral cavity includes the **thoracic cavity,** a space that you may think of as your chest cavity. Its midportion is a subdivision of the thoracic cavity, called the **mediastinum;** its other subdivisions are called the right and left **pleural cavities.** The lower part of the ventral cavity in Figure 1-4 includes an **abdominal cavity** and a **pelvic cavity.** Actually, they form only one cavity, the **abdominopelvic cavity,** because no physical partition separates them. In Figure 1-4 a dotted line shows the approximate point of separation between the abdominal and pelvic subdivisions. Notice, however, that an actual physical partition, represented in the figure as a wide band, separates the thoracic cavity from the abdominal cavity. This muscular partition is the **diaphragm.** It is dome-shaped and is the most important muscle for breathing.

To make it easier to locate organs in the large abdominopelvic cavity, anatomists have divided

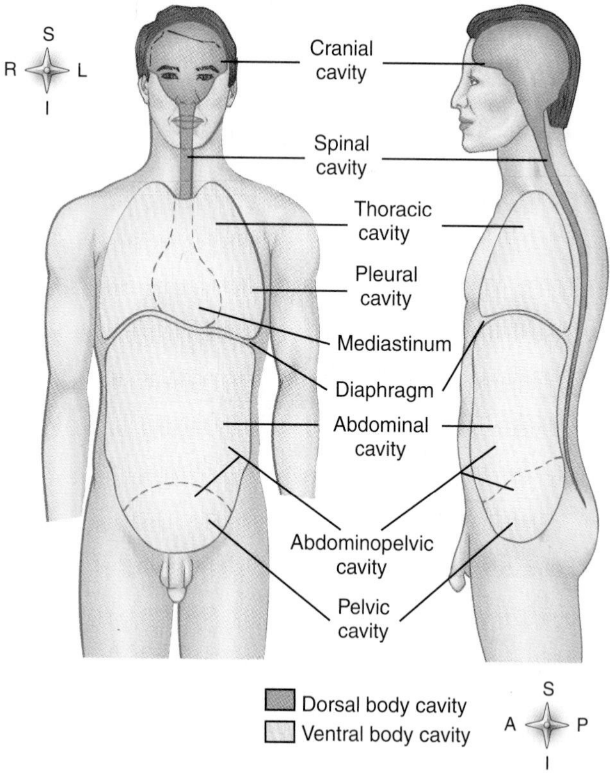

FIGURE 1-4

Body cavities. Location and subdivisions of the dorsal and ventral body cavities as viewed from the front (anterior) and from the side (lateral).

the abdominopelvic cavity into the nine regions shown in Figure 1-5 and defined them as follows:

1. Upper abdominopelvic regions—the **right** and **left hypochondriac regions** and the **epigastric region** lie above an imaginary line across the abdomen at the level of the ninth rib cartilages.
2. Middle regions—the **right** and **left lumbar regions** and the **umbilical region** lie below an imaginary line across the abdomen at the level of the ninth rib cartilages and above an imaginary line across the abdomen at the top of the hip bones.
3. Lower regions—the **right** and **left iliac** (or **inguinal**) **regions** and the **hypogastric region** lie below an imaginary line across the abdomen at the level of the top of the hip bones.

Another, perhaps easier, way to divide the abdominopelvic cavity is shown in Figure 1-6. This

FIGURE 1-5

The nine regions of the abdominopelvic cavity. The most superficial organs are shown. Look at Figure 1-7 (p. 10). Can you identify the deeper structures in each region?

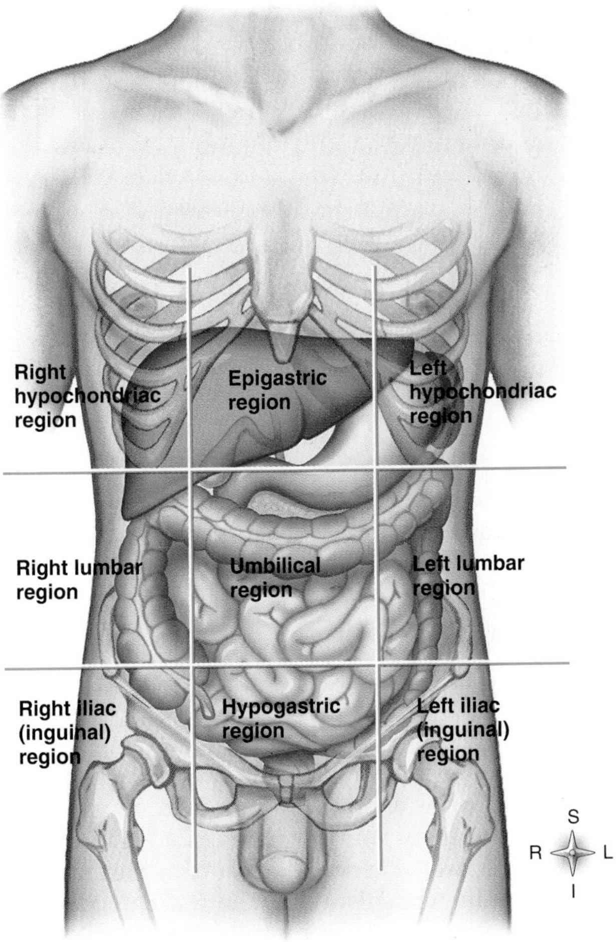

FIGURE 1-6

Division of the abdominopelvic cavity into four quadrants. Diagram showing relationship of internal organs to the four abdominal quadrants.

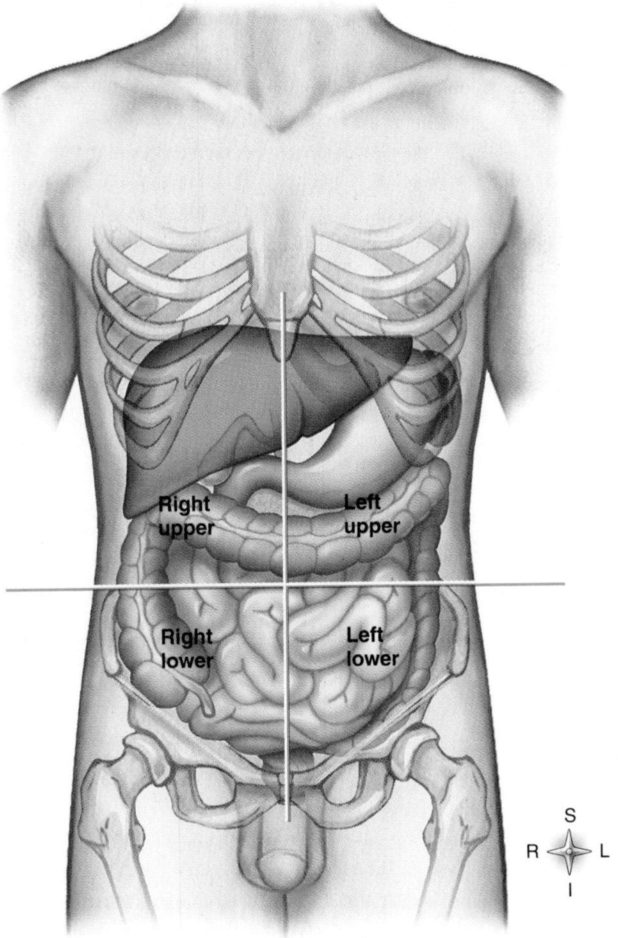

FIGURE 1-7

Organs of the major body cavities. A view from the front.

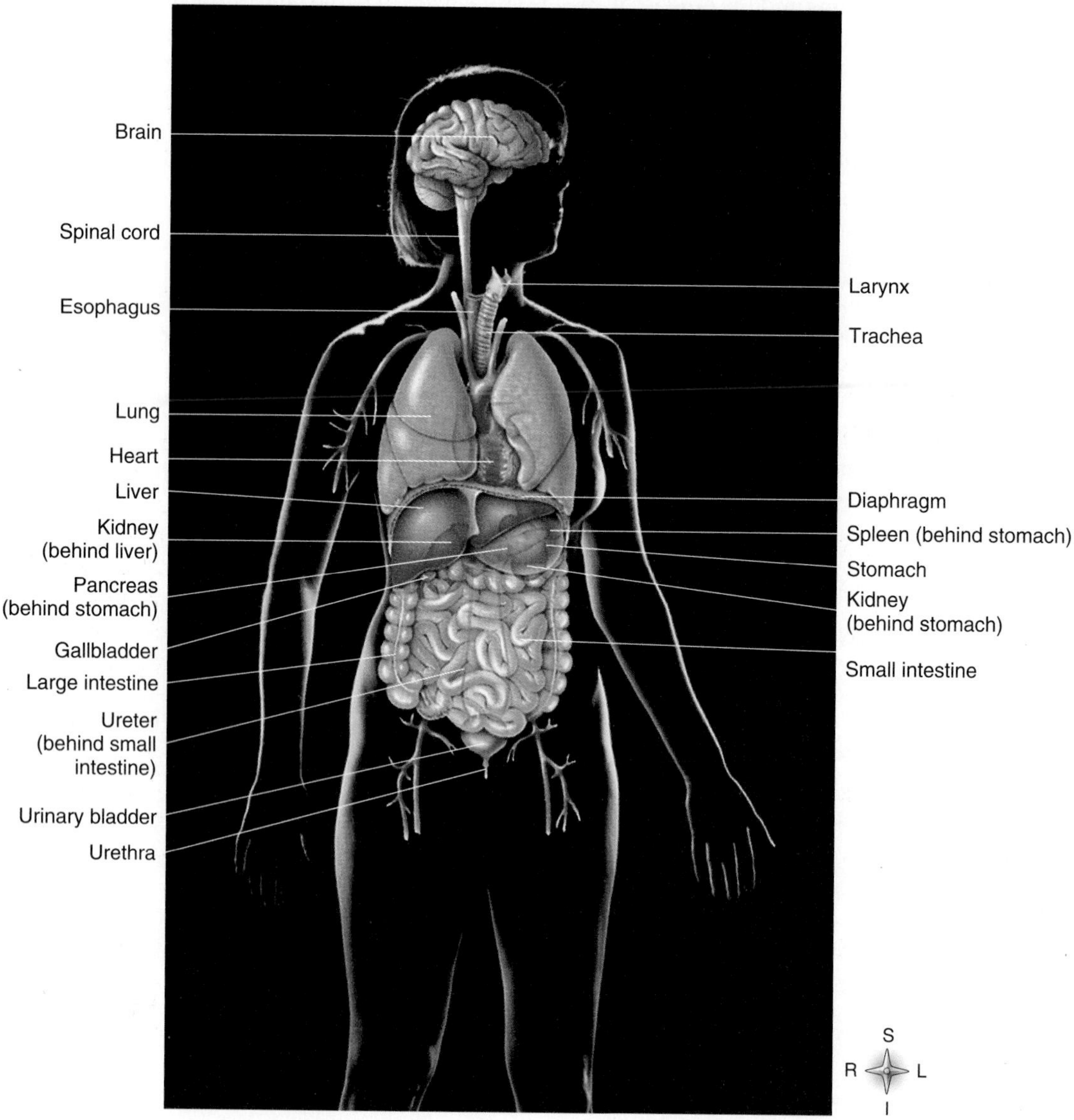

method is frequently used by health professionals and is useful for locating pain or describing the location of a tumor. As you can see in Figure 1-6, the midsagittal and transverse planes, which were described in the previous section, pass through the navel (umbilicus) and divide the abdominopelvic region into the following **four quadrants:** right upper or superior, right lower or inferior, left upper or superior, and left lower or inferior.

The dorsal cavity shown in Figure 1-4 includes the space inside the skull that contains the brain; it is called the **cranial cavity.** The space inside the spinal column is called the **spinal cavity;** it contains the spinal cord. The cranial and spinal cavi-

TABLE 1-1

Body Cavities

BODY CAVITY	ORGAN(S)
VENTRAL BODY CAVITY	
Thoracic cavity	
Mediastinum	Trachea, heart, blood vessels
Pleural cavities	Lungs
Abdominopelvic cavity	
Abdominal cavity	Liver, gallbladder, stomach, spleen, pancreas, small intestine, parts of large intestine
Pelvic cavity	Lower (sigmoid) colon, rectum, urinary bladder, reproductive organs
DORSAL BODY CAVITY	
Cranial cavity	Brain
Spinal cavity	Spinal cord

ties are **dorsal cavities,** whereas the thoracic and abdominopelvic cavities are **ventral cavities.**

Some of the organs in the largest body cavities are visible in Figure 1-7 and are listed in Table 1-1. Find each body cavity in a model of the human body if you have access to one. Try to identify the organs in each cavity, and try to visualize their locations in your own body. Study Figures 1-4 and 1-7.

Quick

1. What is meant by a *section* of the body?
2. What are the two major cavities of the body?
3. What is the difference between the *abdominal cavity* and the *abdominopelvic cavity*?

BODY REGIONS

To recognize an object, you usually first notice its overall structure and form. For example, a car is recognized as a car before the specific details of its tires, grill, or wheel covers are noted. Recognition of the human form also occurs as you first identify overall shape and basic outline. However, for more specific identification to occur, details of size, shape, and appearance of individual body areas must be described. Individuals differ in overall appearance because specific body areas such as the face or torso have unique identifying characteristics. Detailed descriptions of the human form require that specific regions be identified and appropriate terms be used to describe them.

The ability to identify and correctly describe specific body areas is particularly important in the health sciences. For a patient to complain of pain in the head is not as specific and therefore not as useful to a physician or nurse as a more specific and localized description. Saying that the pain is facial provides additional information and helps to more specifically identify the area of pain. By using correct anatomical terms such as forehead, cheek, or chin to describe the area of pain, attention can be focused even more quickly on the specific anatomical area that may need attention. Familiarize yourself with the more common terms used to describe specific body regions identified in Figure 1-8 and listed in Table 1-2.

The body as a whole can be subdivided into two major portions or components: **axial** and **appendicular.** The axial portion of the body consists of the head, neck, and torso or trunk; the appendicular portion consists of the upper and lower extremities. Each major area is subdivided as shown in Figure 1-8. Note, for example, that the torso is composed of thoracic, abdominal, and pelvic areas, and the upper extremity is divided into arm, forearm, wrist, and hand components. Although most terms used to describe gross body regions are well understood, misuse is common. The word *leg* is a good example: it refers to the area of the lower extremity between the knee and ankle and not to the entire lower extremity.

The structure of the body changes in many ways and at varying rates during a lifetime. Before young adulthood, the body develops and grows; after young adulthood, it gradually undergoes degenerative changes. With advancing age, there is a generalized decrease in size or a wasting away of many body organs and tissues that affects the structure and function of many body areas. This degenera-

FIGURE 1-8

Axial and appendicular divisions of the body. Specific body regions are labeled. Notice how the axial and appendicular regions of the body frame are distinguished by contrasting colors.

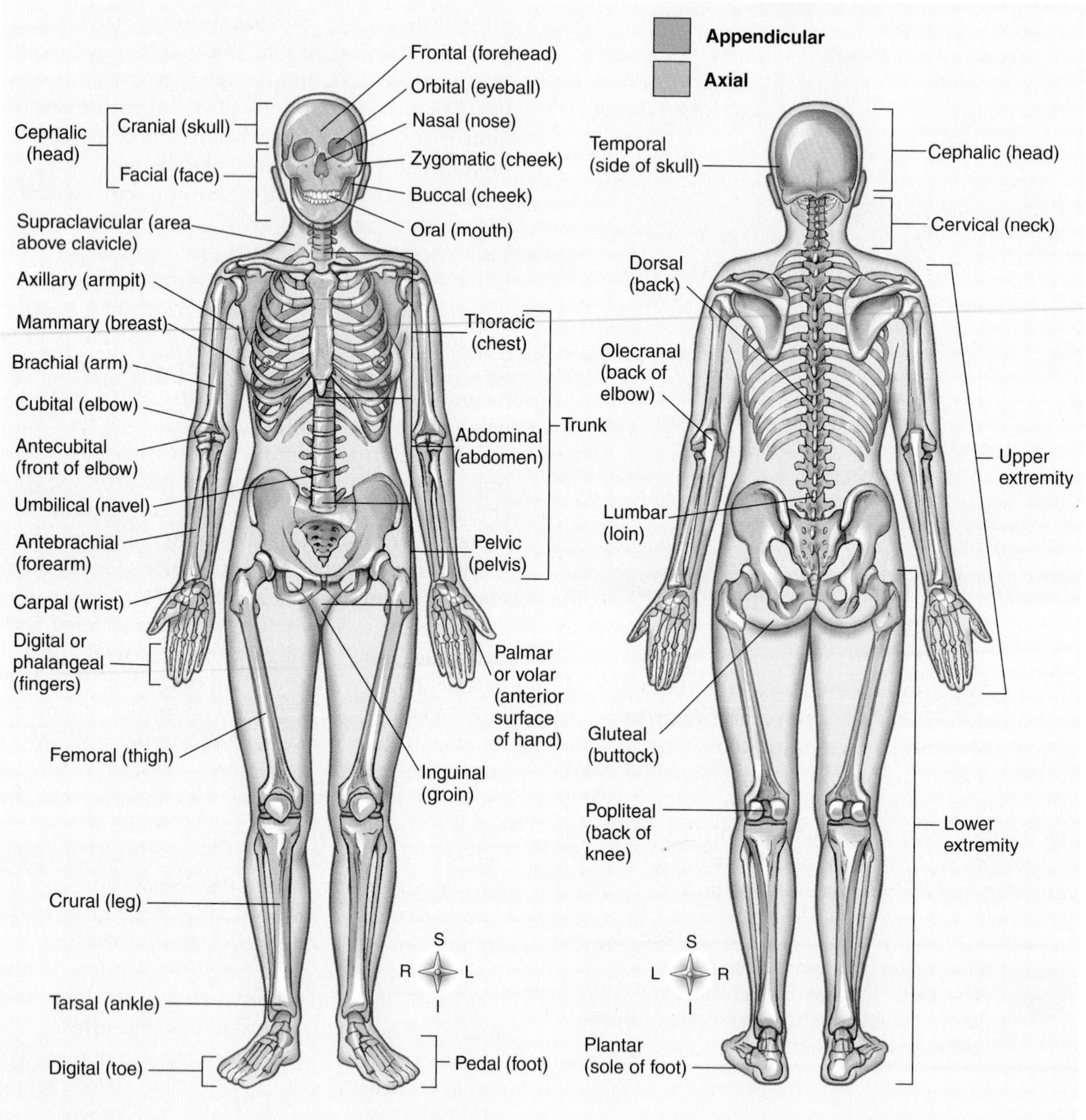

TABLE 1-2

Descriptive Terms for Body Regions

AREA OR BODY REGION	EXAMPLE
Abdominal (ab-DOM-in-al)	Anterior torso below diaphragm
Antebrachial (an-tee-BRAY-kee-al)	Forearm
Antecubital (an-tee-KYOO-bi-tal)	Depressed area just in front of elbow
Axillary (AK-si-lair-ee)	Armpit
Brachial (BRAY-kee-al)	Arm
Buccal (BUK-al)	Cheek
Carpal (KAR-pal)	Wrist
Cephalic (se-FAL-ik)	Head
Cervical (SER-vi-kal)	Neck
Cranial (KRAY-nee-al)	Skull
Crural (KROOR-al)	Leg
Cubital (KYOO-bi-tal)	Elbow
Cutaneous (kyoo-TANE-ee-us)	Skin (or body surface)
Digital (DIJ-i- tal)	Fingers or toes
Dorsal (DOR-sal)	Back
Facial (FAY-shal)	Face
Frontal (FRON-tal)	Forehead
Nasal (NAY-zal)	Nose
Oral (OR-al)	Mouth
Orbital (OR-bi-tal) or **ophthalmic** (op-THAL-mik)	Eyes
Zygomatic (zye-go-MAT-ik)	Upper cheek
Femoral (FEM-or-al)	Thigh
Gluteal (GLOO-tee-al)	Buttock
Inguinal (ING-gwi-nal)	Groin
Lumbar (LUM-bar)	Lower back between ribs and pelvis
Mammary (MAM-er-ee)	Breast
Occipital (ok-SIP-i-tal)	Back of lower skull
Olecranal (oh-LEK-kra-nal)	Back of elbow
Palmar (PAHL-mar)	Palm of hand
Pedal (PED-al)	Foot
Pelvic (PEL-vik)	Lower portion of torso
Perineal (pair-i-NEE-al)	Area (perineum) between anus and genitals
Plantar (PLAN-tar)	Sole of foot
Popliteal (pop-li-TEE-al)	Area behind knee
Supraclavicular (soo-pra-kla-VIK-yoo-lar)	Area above clavicle
Tarsal (TAR-sal)	Ankle
Temporal (TEM-por-al)	Side of skull
Thoracic (tho-RAS-ik)	Chest
Umbilical (um-BILL-ih-kal)	Area around navel or umbilicus
Volar (VO-lar)	Palm or sole

tive process is called **atrophy.** Nearly every chapter of this book will refer to a few of these changes.

Quick Check

1. What is the difference between the *axial* portion of the body and the *appendicular* portion of the body?
2. What are some of the regions of the upper extremity and lower extremity?

THE BALANCE OF BODY FUNCTIONS

Although they may have very different structures, all living organisms maintain mechanisms that ensure survival of the body and success in propagating its genes through its offspring. Survival depends on the body maintaining relatively constant conditions within the body. **Homeostasis** is what physiologists call the relative constancy of the internal environment. The cells of the body live in an internal environment made up mostly of water combined with salts and other dissolved substances. Like fish in a fishbowl, the cells are able to survive only if the conditions of their watery environment remain stable. The temperature, salt content, acid level (pH), fluid volume and pressure, oxygen concentration, and other vital conditions must remain within acceptable limits. To maintain constant water conditions in a fishbowl, one may add a heater, an air pump, and filters. Likewise, the body has mechanisms that act as heaters, air pumps, and the like, to maintain conditions of its internal fluid environment.

Because the activities of cells and external disturbances are always threatening internal stability, or homeostasis, the body must constantly work to maintain or restore that stability. To accomplish this self-regulation, a highly complex and integrated communication control system is required. The basic type of control system in the body is called a **feedback loop.** The idea of a feedback loop is borrowed from engineering. Figure 1-9, *A*, shows how an engineer would describe the feedback loop that maintains stability of temperature in a building. Cold winds outside a building may cause a decrease in building temperature below normal. A **sensor,** in this case a thermometer, detects the change in temperature. Information from the sensor *feeds back* to a **control center**—a thermostat in this example—that compares the actual temperature with the normal temperature and responds by activating the building's furnace. The furnace is called an **effector** because it has an effect on the controlled condition (temperature). Because the sensor continually feeds information back to the control center, the furnace will be automatically shut off when the temperature has returned to normal.

As you can see in Figure 1-9, *B*, the body uses a similar feedback loop in restoring body temperature when we become chilled. Nerve endings that act as temperature sensors feed information to a control center in the brain that compares actual body temperature to normal body temperature. In response to a chill, the brain sends nerve signals to muscles that shiver. Shivering produces heat that increases our body temperature. We stop shivering when feedback information tells the brain that body temperature has increased to normal.

Feedback loops such as those shown in Figure 1-9 are called **negative feedback loops** because they oppose, or negate, a change in a controlled condition. Most homeostatic control loops in the body involve negative feedback because reversing changes back toward a normal value tends to stabilize conditions—exactly what homeostasis is all about. An example of a negative feedback loop occurs when decreasing blood oxygen concentration caused by muscles using oxygen during exercise is counteracted by an increase in breathing to bring the blood oxygen level back up to normal. Another example is the excretion of larger than usual volumes of urine when the volume of fluid in the body is greater than the normal, ideal amount.

Although not common, **positive feedback loops** exist in the body and are involved in normal function. Positive feedback control loops are stimulatory. Instead of opposing a change in the internal environment and causing a "return to normal," positive feedback loops temporarily amplify the change that is occurring. This type of feedback loop causes an ever-increasing rate of events to occur until something stops the process. An example of a positive feedback loop includes the events that cause rapid increases in uterine contractions

FIGURE 1-9

Negative feedback loops. A, An engineer's diagram showing how a relatively constant room temperature (*controlled condition*) can be maintained. A thermostat (*control center*) receives feedback information from a thermometer (*sensor*) and responds by counteracting a change from normal by activating a furnace (*effector*). **B,** A physiologist's diagram showing how a relatively constant body temperature (*controlled condition*) can be maintained. The brain (*control center*) receives feedback information from nerve endings called cold receptors (*sensors*) and responds by counteracting a change from normal by activating shivering by muscles (*effectors*).

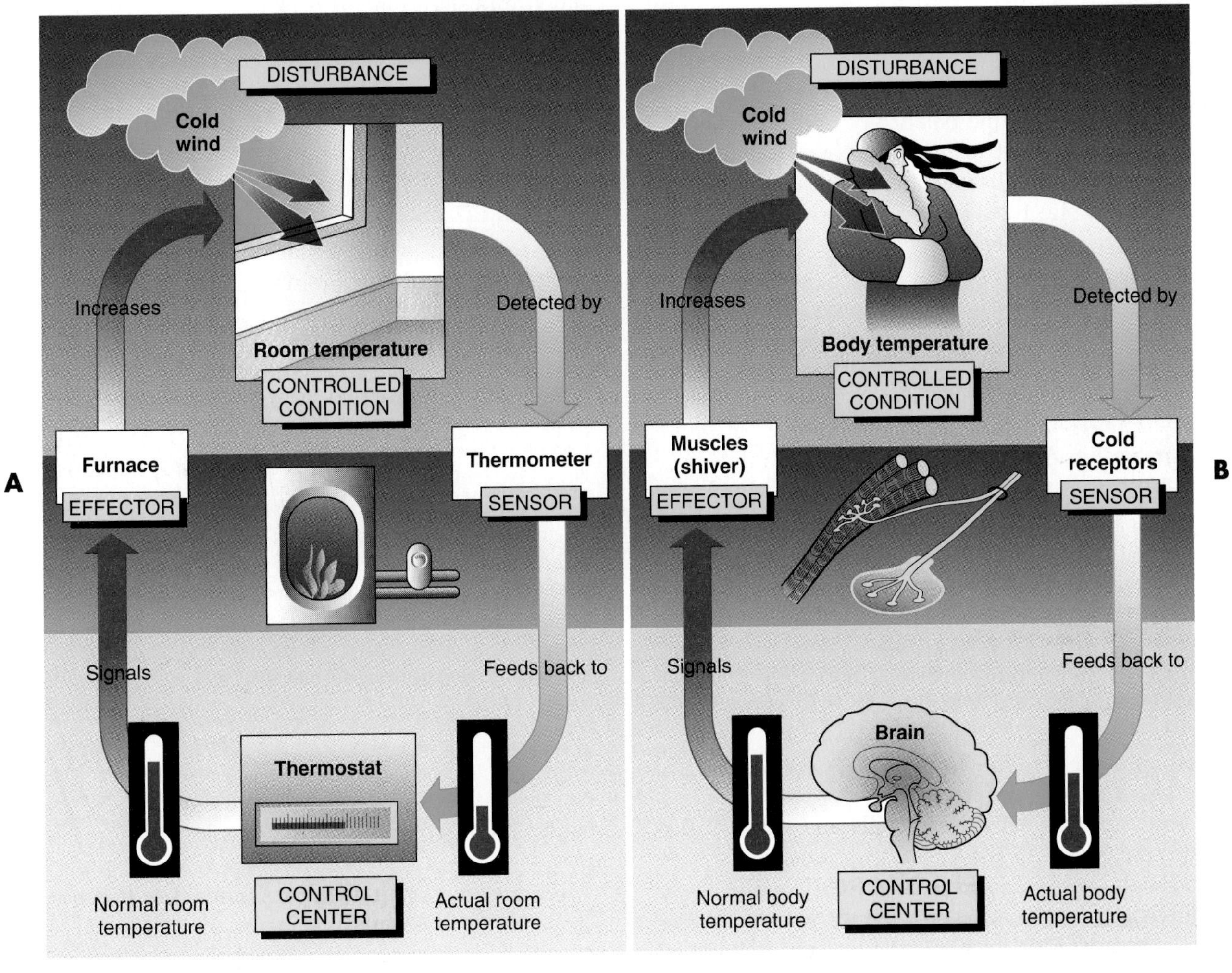

before the birth of a baby. Another example is the increasingly rapid sticking together of blood cells called *platelets* to form a plug that begins formation of a blood clot. In each of these cases, the process increases rapidly until the positive feedback loop is stopped suddenly by the birth of a baby or the formation of a clot. In the long run, such normal positive feedback events also help maintain constancy of the internal environment.

It is important to realize that homeostatic control mechanisms can only maintain a *relative* constancy. All homeostatically controlled conditions in the body do not remain absolutely constant. Rather, conditions normally fluctuate near a normal, ideal value. Thus body temperature, for example, rarely remains exactly the same for very long; it usually fluctuates up and down near a person's normal body temperature.

Because all organs function to help maintain homeostatic balance, we will be discussing negative and positive feedback mechanisms often throughout the remaining chapters of this book.

Before leaving this brief introduction to physiology, we must pause to state the important principle that maintaining the balance of body functions is related to age. During childhood, homeostatic functions gradually become more and more efficient and effective. They operate with maximum efficiency and effectiveness during young adulthood. During late adulthood and old age, they gradually become less and less efficient and effective. Changes and functions occurring during the early years are called *developmental processes;* those occurring after young adulthood are called *aging processes.* In general, developmental processes improve efficiency of functions; aging processes usually diminish it.

Quick

1. Why is *homeostasis* also called "balance" of body function?
2. What is a *feedback loop* and how does it work?
3. How does *negative feedback* differ from *positive feedback?*

Health & Well-Being

Exercise Physiology

Exercise physiologists study the effects of exercise on the body organ systems. They are especially interested in the complex control mechanisms that preserve or restore homeostasis during or immediately after periods of strenuous physical activity. Exercise, defined as any significant use of skeletal muscles, is a normal activity with beneficial results. However, exercise disrupts homeostasis. For example, when muscles are worked, the core body temperature rises and carbon dioxide levels in the blood increase. These and many other body functions quickly deviate from "normal ranges" that exist at rest. Complex control mechanisms must then "kick in" to restore homeostasis.

As a scientific discipline, exercise physiology attempts to explain many body processes in terms of how they maintain homeostasis. Exercise physiology has many practical applications in therapy and rehabilitation, athletics, occupational health, and general wellness. This specialty concerns itself with the function of the whole body, not just one or two body systems.

Outline Summary

STRUCTURAL LEVELS OF ORGANIZATION (FIGURE 1-1)

A. Organization is an outstanding characteristic of body structure

B. The body is a unit constructed of the following smaller units:

1. Cells—the smallest structural units; organizations of various chemicals
2. Tissues—organizations of similar cells
3. Organs—organizations of different kinds of tissues
4. Systems—organizations of many different kinds of organs

ANATOMICAL POSITION (FIGURE 1-2)

Standing erect with the arms at the sides and palms turned forward

ANATOMICAL DIRECTIONS

A. Superior—toward the head, upper, above
Inferior—toward the feet, lower, below

Outline Summary—*cont'd*

B. Anterior—front, in front of (same as ventral in humans)
Posterior—back, in back of (same as dorsal in humans)
C. Medial—toward the midline of a structure
Lateral—away from the midline or toward the side of a structure
D. Proximal—toward or nearest the trunk, or nearest the point of origin of a structure
Distal—away from or farthest from the trunk, or farthest from a structure's point of origin
E. Superficial—nearer the body surface
Deep—farther away from the body surface

PLANES OR BODY SECTIONS (FIGURE 1-3)

A. Sagittal plane—lengthwise plane that divides a structure into right and left sections
B. Midsagittal—sagittal plane that divides the body into two equal halves
C. Frontal (coronal) plane—lengthwise plane that divides a structure into anterior and posterior sections
D. Transverse plane—horizontal plane that divides a structure into upper and lower sections

BODY CAVITIES (FIGURE 1-4)

A. Ventral cavity
  1. Thoracic cavity
    a. Mediastinum—midportion of thoracic cavity; heart and trachea are located in mediastinum
    b. Pleural cavities—right lung located in right pleural cavity, left lung is in left pleural cavity
  2. Abdominopelvic cavity
    a. Abdominal cavity contains stomach, intestines, liver, gallbladder, pancreas, and spleen
    b. Pelvic cavity contains reproductive organs, urinary bladder, and lowest part of intestine
    c. Abdominopelvic regions (Figures 1-5 and 1-6)
      (1) Nine regions
      (2) Four quadrants
B. Dorsal cavity
  1. Cranial cavity contains brain
  2. Spinal cavity contains spinal cord

BODY REGIONS (FIGURE 1-8)

A. Axial region—head, neck, and torso or trunk
B. Appendicular region—upper and lower extremities

THE BALANCE OF BODY FUNCTIONS

A. Survival of the individual and of the genes is the body's most important business
B. Survival depends on the maintenance or restoration of homeostasis (relative constancy of the internal environment; Figure 1-9); the body uses negative feedback loops and, less often, positive feedback loops to maintain or restore homeostasis
C. All organs function to maintain homeostasis
D. Body functions are related to age; peak efficiency is during young adulthood, diminishing efficiency occurs after young adulthood

NEW WORDS

abdominopelvic quadrants (4)
abdominopelvic regions (9)
anatomical position
anatomy
atrophy
cavities
  abdominal
  cranial
  pelvic
  pleural
  spinal
  thoracic
control center

Continued

NEW WORDS—*cont'd*

directional terms
- superior
- inferior
- anterior
- posterior
- ventral
- dorsal
- medial
- lateral
- proximal
- distal
- superficial
- deep

effector loop
experimentation
feedback
homeostasis
hypothesis
mediastinum
negative feedback
organization (structural levels)
- chemical
- cellular
- tissue
- organ
- system

physiology
planes of section
- sagittal
- midsagittal
- frontal
- transverse

positive feedback
prone
sensor
supine
theory

REVIEW QUESTIONS

1. Define *anatomy* and *physiology*.
2. List and explain the levels of organization in a living thing.
3. Describe the *anatomical position*.
4. Name and explain the three planes or sections of the body.
5. List two organs of the mediastinum, two organs of the abdominal cavity, and two organs of the pelvic cavity.
6. From the upper left to the lower right, list the nine regions of the abdominopelvic cavity.
7. Name the two subdivisions of the dorsal cavity. What structures does each contain?
8. Explain the difference between the terms *lower extremity*, *thigh*, and *leg*.
9. List four conditions in the cell that must be kept in homeostatic balance.
10. List the three parts of a negative feedback loop and give the function of each.

CRITICAL THINKING

11. Name a structure that is inferior to the heart, superior to the heart, anterior to the heart, posterior to the heart, and lateral to the heart.
12. The maintenance of body temperature and the birth of a baby are two body functions that are regulated by feedback loops. Explain the different feedback loops that regulate each process.
13. If a person complained of a pain in the epigastric region, what organs could be involved?

* CHAPTER TEST Due Wed. 24, 2005, Aug

1. Anatomy is a term derived from two Greek words meaning "cutting up."
2. Physiology means the study of the function of living organisms and their parts.
3. Atoms, molecules, cells, tissues, and organs are the five organizational levels of a living thing.
4. supine and prone are terms used to describe the body position when it is not in anatomical position.
5. A transverse section cuts the body or any of its parts into upper and lower portions.
6. A frontal section cuts the body or any of its parts into front and back portions.

CHAPTER TEST

7. A sagittal section cuts the body or any of its parts into left and right portions.
8. If the body is cut into equal right and left sides, the cut is called a midsagittal section or plane.
9. The body portion that consists of the head, neck, and torso is called the __________ portion.
10. The body portion that consists of the upper and lower extremities is the __________ portion.
11. The two major cavities of the body are the:
    a. thoracic and abdominal
    b. abdominal and pelvic
    c. dorsal and ventral
    d. anterior and posterior
12. The structure that divides the thoracic cavity from the abdominal cavity is the:
    a. mediastinum
    b. diaphragm
    c. lungs
    d. stomach
13. The epigastric region of the abdominopelvic cavity:
    a. is inferior to the umbilical region
    b. is lateral to the umbilical region
    c. is medial to the umbilical region
    d. none of the above
14. The hypogastric region of the abdominopelvic cavity:
    a. is inferior to the umbilical region
    b. is lateral to the left iliac region
    c. is medial to the right iliac region
    d. both a and c
15. The following is an example of a positive feedback loop:
    a. maintaining a constant body temperature
    b. contractions of the uterus during childbirth
    c. maintaining a constant volume of water in the body
    d. both a and c

Match the directional terms in Column B with its opposite term in Column A.

COLUMN A	COLUMN B
16. E superior	a. posterior
17. D distal	b. superficial
18. A anterior	c. medial
19. C lateral	d. proximal
20. B deep	e. inferior

STUDY TIPS

There are a number of topics introduced in the chapter that will be important throughout the rest of the course. The most important one is probably homeostasis. The word itself tells you what it means: *homeo* means "the same," *stasis* means "staying." Homeostasis is the balance the body tries to maintain by keeping its internal environment "staying the same." Make sure you understand this concept. Become familiar with the directional terms. You will see them in almost every diagram in the text and in the names of several body structures (for example, superior vena cava, distal convoluted tubule). They are easier to learn because they are in opposite pairs, so if you know one term you almost automatically know its opposite. Flash cards will help in learning them. Table 1-2 and Appendix B are helpful resources to keep in mind when you see an unfamiliar term. The chapter also introduces you to levels of organization. This organizational structure should help you with the big picture as you go through the rest of the text.

In your study groups try to come up with examples of negative feedback loops that help maintain a balance. Be creative; don't just use the furnace example. Go over your directional flash cards or photocopy Figure 1-3 and blacken out the terms and use it to quiz each other. Go over the questions in the back of the chapter and discuss possible test questions.

2 Chemistry of Life

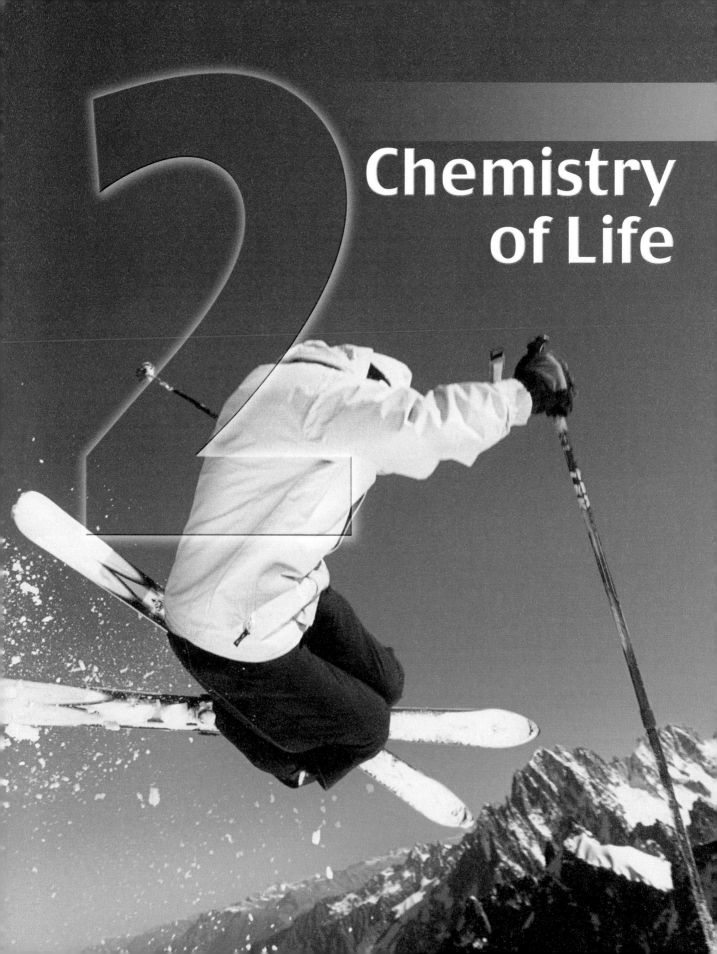

Outline

Objectives

AFTER YOU HAVE COMPLETED THIS CHAPTER, YOU SHOULD BE ABLE TO:

1. Define the terms *atom, element, molecule,* and *compound.*
2. Describe the structure of an atom.
3. Compare and contrast ionic and covalent types of chemical bonding.
4. Distinguish between *organic* and *inorganic* chemical compounds.
5. Discuss the chemical characteristics of water.
6. Explain the concept of pH.
7. Discuss the structure and function of the following types of organic molecules: *carbohydrate, lipid, protein,* and *nucleic acid.*

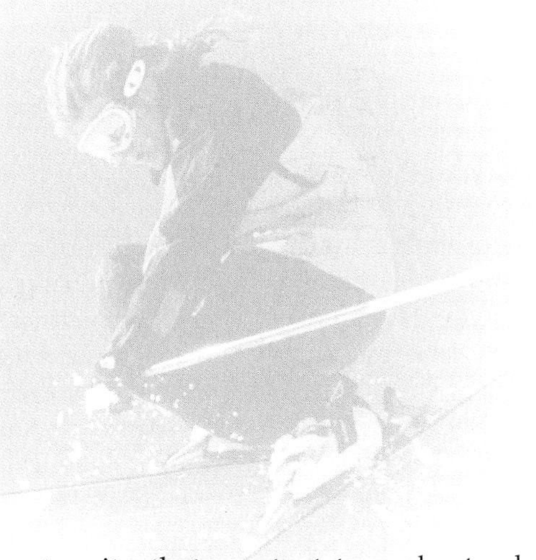

Life is chemistry. It's not quite that simple, but the more we learn about human structure and function, the more we realize that it all boils down to interactions among chemicals. The digestion of food, the formation of bone tissue, and the contraction of a muscle are all chemical processes. Thus the basic principles of anatomy and physiology are ultimately based on principles of chemistry. A whole field of science, **biochemistry,** is devoted to studying the chemical aspects of life. To truly understand the human body, it is important to understand a few basic facts about biochemistry, the chemistry of life.

LEVELS OF CHEMICAL ORGANIZATION

Matter is anything that occupies space and has mass. Biochemists classify matter into several levels of organization for easier study. In the body, most chemicals are in the form of **molecules.** Molecules are particles of matter that are composed of one or more smaller units called **atoms.** Atoms in turn are composed of several kinds of *subatomic particles*: **protons, electrons,** and **neutrons.**

Atoms

Atoms are units that until recently could not be seen by scientists. New instruments, including *tunneling microscopes* and *atomic force microscopes*, produce pictures of atoms that confirm current models of how atoms are put together. At the core of each atom is a **nucleus** composed of positively charged protons and uncharged neutrons. The number of protons in the nucleus is an atom's **atomic number.** The number of protons and neutrons combined is the atom's **atomic mass.**

Negatively charged electrons surround the nucleus at a distance. In an electrically neutral atom, there is one electron for every proton. Electrons move about within certain limits called **orbitals.** Each orbital can hold two electrons. Orbitals are arranged into **energy levels** (shells), depending on their distance from the nucleus. The farther an orbital extends from the nucleus, the higher its energy level. The energy level closest to the nucleus has one orbital, so it can hold two electrons. The next energy level has up to four orbitals, so it can hold eight electrons. Figure 2-1 shows a carbon (C) atom. Notice that the first energy level (the innermost shell) contains two electrons and the outer energy level contains four electrons. The outer energy level of a carbon atom could hold up to four more electrons (for a total of eight). The number of electrons in the outer energy level of an atom determines how it behaves chemically (that is, how it may unite with other atoms). This behavior, called *chemical bonding*, will be discussed later in this chapter.

FIGURE 2-1

A model of the atom. The nucleus—protons (+) and neutrons—is at the core. Electrons inhabit outer regions called *energy levels*. This is a carbon atom, a fact that is determined by the number of its protons. All carbon atoms (and only carbon atoms) have six protons. (One proton in the nucleus is not visible in this illustration.)

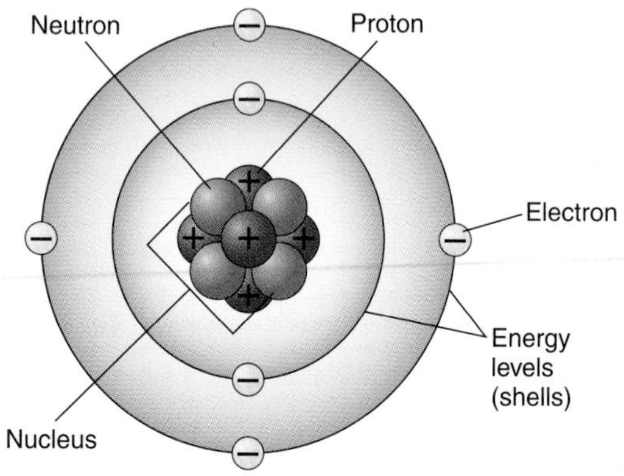

Elements, Molecules, and Compounds

Substances can be classified as **elements** or **compounds.** Elements are pure substances, composed of only one of more than a hundred types of atoms that exist in nature. Four kinds of atoms (**oxygen, carbon, hydrogen,** and **nitrogen**) make up about 96% of the human body, but there are traces of about 20 other elements in the body. Table 2-1 lists some of the elements in the body. Table 2-1 also gives for each element its universal chemical *symbol*—the abbreviation used by chemists worldwide.

Atoms usually unite with each other to form larger chemical units called **molecules.** Some molecules are made of several atoms of the same element. *Compounds* are substances whose molecules have more than one element in them. The *formula* for a compound contains symbols for the elements in each molecule. The number of atoms of each element in the molecule is expressed as a subscript after the elemental symbol. For example, each molecule of the compound **carbon dioxide** has one carbon (C) atom and two oxygen (O) atoms; thus its molecular formula is CO_2.

Quick Check

1. Of what kinds of particles is matter made up?
2. What is a compound? An element?
3. Describe an energy level.

TABLE 2-1

Important Elements in the Human Body

ELEMENT	SYMBOL	NUMBER OF ELECTRONS IN OUTER SHELL*
MAJOR ELEMENTS (GREATER THAN 96% OF BODY WEIGHT)		
Oxygen	O	6
Carbon	C	4
Hydrogen	H	1
Nitrogen	N	5
TRACE ELEMENTS (EXAMPLES OF MORE THAN 20 TRACE ELEMENTS FOUND IN THE BODY)		
Calcium	Ca	2
Phosphorus	P	5
Sodium (Latin *natrium*)	Na	1
Potassium (Latin *kalium*)	K	1
Chlorine	Cl	7
Iodine	I	7

*Maximum is eight, except for hydrogen. The maximum for that element is two.

CHEMICAL BONDING

Chemical bonds form to make atoms more stable. An atom is said to be chemically stable when its outer energy level is "full" (that is, when its energy shells have the maximum number of electrons they can hold). All but a handful of atoms have room for more electrons in their outermost energy level. A basic chemical principle states that atoms react with one another in ways to make their outermost energy level full. To do this, atoms can share, donate, or borrow electrons.

For example, a hydrogen atom has one electron and one proton. Its single energy shell has one electron but can hold two—so it's not full. If two hydrogen atoms "share" their single electrons with each other, then both will have full energy shells, making them more stable as a molecule than either would be as an atom. This is one example of how atoms **bond** to form molecules. Other atoms may donate or borrow electrons until the outermost energy level is full.

Ionic Bonds

One common way in which atoms make their outermost energy level full is to form **ionic bonds** with other atoms. Such a bond forms between an atom that has only one or two electrons in the outermost level (that would normally hold eight) and an atom that needs only one or two electrons to fill its outer level. The atom with one or two electrons simply "donates" its outer shell electrons to the one that needs one or two.

For example, as you can see in Table 2-1, the sodium (Na) atom has one electron in its outer level and the chlorine (Cl) atom has seven. Both need to have eight electrons in their outer shell. Figure 2-2 shows how sodium and chlorine form an ionic bond when sodium "donates" the electron in its outer shell to chlorine. Now both atoms have full outer shells (although sodium's outer shell is now one energy level lower). Because the sodium atom lost an electron, it now has one more proton than it has electrons. This makes it a positive **ion**, an electrically charged atom. Chlorine has "borrowed" an electron to become a negative ion called the *chloride* ion. Because oppositely charged particles attract one another, the sodium and chloride ions are drawn together to form a sodium chloride (NaCl) molecule—common table salt. The molecule is held together by an *ionic bond.*

Ionic molecules usually dissolve easily in water because water molecules wedge between the ions and force them apart. When this happens, we say the molecules **dissociate** (dis-SO-see-ayt) to form free ions. Molecules that form ions when dissolved in water are called **electrolytes** (el-EK-tro-lites). Chapter 18 describes mechanisms that maintain the homeostasis of electrolytes in the

FIGURE 2-2

Ionic bonding. The sodium atom donates the single electron in its outer energy level to a chlorine atom having seven electrons in its outer level. Now both have eight electrons in their outer shells. Because the electron/proton ratio changes, the sodium atom becomes a positive sodium ion. The chlorine atom becomes a negative chloride ion. The positive-negative attraction between these oppositely charged ions is called an *ionic bond*.

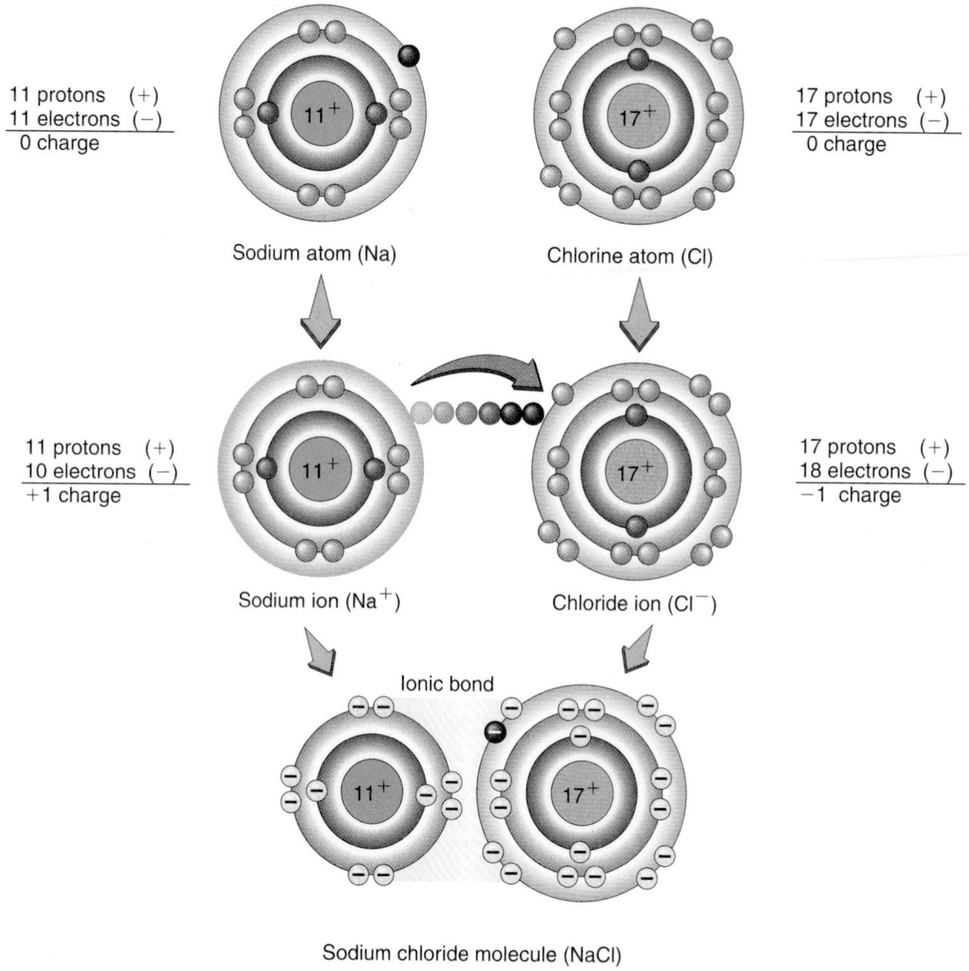

body. Table 2-2 lists some of the more important ions present in body fluids.

The formula of an ion always shows its charge by a superscript after the chemical symbol. Thus the sodium ion is Na^+, and the chloride ion is Cl^-. Calcium (Ca) atoms lose two electrons when they form ions, so the calcium ion formula is Ca^{++}.

Covalent Bonds

Atoms may also fill their energy levels by sharing electrons rather than donating or receiving them. When atoms share electrons, a **covalent** (ko-VAY-lent) **bond** forms. For example, Figure 2-3 shows how two hydrogen atoms may move together closely so that their energy levels overlap. Each

TABLE 2-2

Important Ions in Human Body Fluids

NAME	SYMBOL
Sodium	Na^+
Chloride	Cl^-
Potassium (Latin *kalium*)	K^+
Calcium	Ca^{++}
Hydrogen	H^+
Magnesium	Mg^{++}
Hydroxide	OH^-
Phosphate	$PO_4^=$
Bicarbonate	HCO_3^-

FIGURE 2-3

Covalent bonding. Two hydrogen atoms move together, overlapping their energy levels. Although neither gains nor loses an electron, the atoms share the electrons, forming a covalent bond.

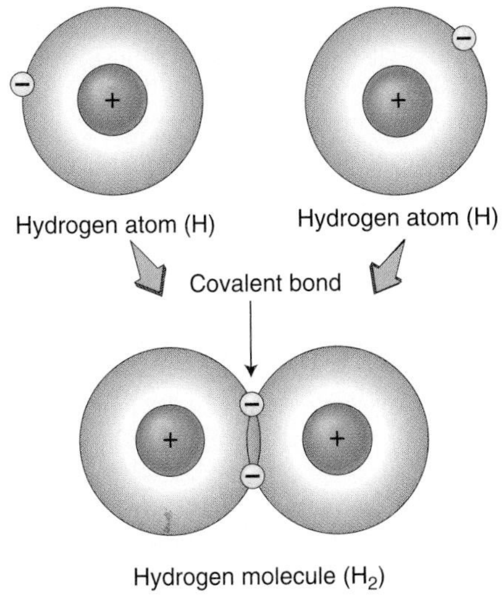

energy level contributes its one electron to the sharing relationship. This way, both outer levels have access to both electrons. Because atoms involved in a covalent bond must stay close to each other, it is not surprising that covalent bonds are not easily broken. Covalent bonds normally do not break apart in water.

Quick
1. How is an ion formed?
2. What is meant by an electrolyte *dissociating* in water?
3. What is covalent chemical bonding?

INORGANIC CHEMISTRY

In living organisms, there are two kinds of compounds: **organic** and **inorganic.** Organic compounds are composed of molecules that contain carbon-carbon (C-C) covalent bonds or carbon-hydrogen (C-H) covalent bonds—or both kinds of bonds. Few inorganic compounds have carbon atoms in them and none have C-C or C-H bonds. Organic molecules are generally larger and more complex than inorganic molecules. The human body has both kinds of compounds because both are equally important to the chemistry of life. We will discuss the chemistry of inorganic compounds first, and then move on to some of the important types of organic compounds.

Water

One of the compounds that is most essential to life—water—is an inorganic compound. Water is the most abundant compound in the body, found in and around each cell. It is the **solvent** in which most other compounds or **solutes** are dissolved. When water is the solvent for a *mixture* (a blend of two or more kinds of molecules), the mixture is called an **aqueous solution.** An aqueous solution containing common salt (NaCl) and other molecules forms the "internal sea" of the body. Water molecules not only compose the basic internal environment of the body, but they also participate in many important *chemical reactions.* Chemical reactions are interactions among molecules in which atoms regroup into new combinations.

A common type of chemical reaction in the body is **dehydration synthesis.** In any kind of synthesis reaction, the **reactants** combine to form a larger **product.** In dehydration synthesis, reactants combine only after hydrogen (H) and oxygen (O) atoms are removed. These leftover H and O atoms come together, forming H_2O, or water. As Figure 2-4 shows, the result is both the large product molecule and a water molecule. Just as dehydration of a cell is a loss of water from the cell and dehydration of the body is loss of fluid from the entire internal environment, dehydration synthesis is a reaction in which water is lost from the reactants.

Another common reaction in the body, **hydrolysis** (hye-DROL-i-sis), also involves water. In this reaction, water (*hydro-*) disrupts the bonds in large molecules, causing them to be broken down into smaller molecules (*lysis*). Hydrolysis is virtually the reverse of dehydration synthesis, as Figure 2-4 shows.

Chemical reactions always involve energy transfers. Energy is required to build the molecules. Some of that energy is stored as potential energy in the chemical bonds. The stored energy can then be released when the chemical bonds in the molecule are later broken apart. For example, a molecule called **adenosine triphosphate (ATP)** breaks apart in the muscle cells to yield the energy needed for muscle contraction (see Figure 16-2).

Chemists often use a *chemical equation* to represent a chemical reaction. In a chemical equation, the reactants are separated from the products by an arrow (→) showing the "direction" of the reaction. Reactants are separated from each other and products are separated from each other by addition signs (+). Thus the reaction *potassium and chloride combine to form potassium chloride* can be expressed as the equation:

$$K^+ + Cl^- \rightarrow KCl$$

The single arrow (→) is used for equations that occur in only one direction. For example, when hydrochloric acid (HCl) is dissolved in water, all of it dissociates to form H^+ and $Cl^=$.

$$HCl \rightarrow H^+ + Cl^-$$

The double arrow ($\rightleftarrows$) is used for reactions that happen in "both directions" at the same time. When carbonic acid (H_2CO_3) dissolves in water, some of it dissociates into H^+ (hydrogen ion) and HCO_3^- (bicarbonate), but not all of it. As additional

FIGURE 2-4

Water-based chemistry. Dehydration synthesis (on the left) is a reaction in which small molecules are assembled into large molecules by removing water (H and O atoms). Hydrolysis (on the right) operates in the reverse direction; H and O from water are added as large molecules are broken down into small molecules.

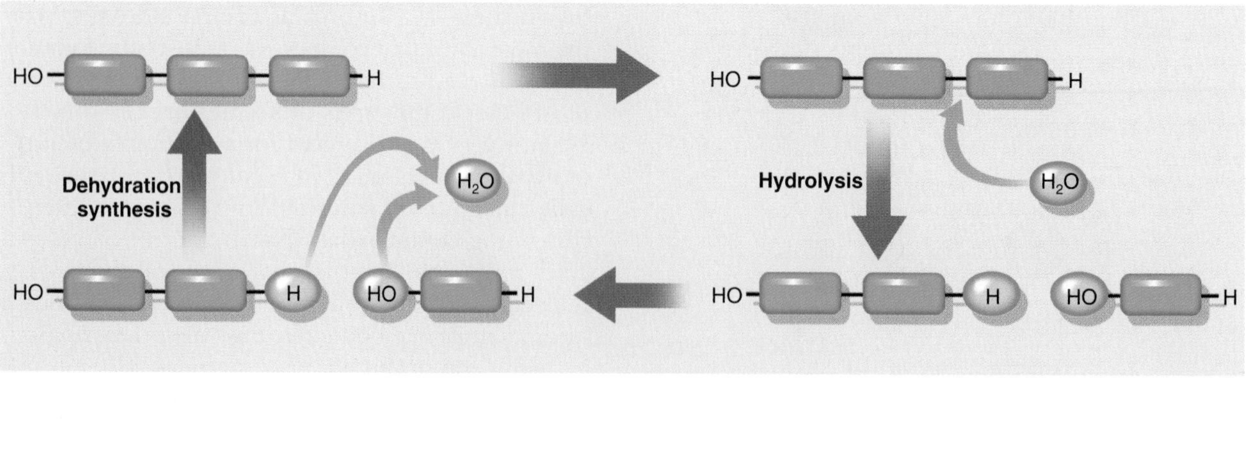

ions dissociate, previously dissociated ions bond together again, forming H_2CO_3.

$$H_2CO_3 \rightleftarrows H^+ \; HCO_3^-$$

In short, the double arrow indicates that at any instant in time both reactants and products are present in the solution at the same time.

Acids, Bases, and Salts

Besides water, many other inorganic compounds are important in the chemistry of life. For example, acids and bases are compounds that profoundly affect chemical reactions in the body. As explained in more detail at the beginning of Chapter 19, a few water molecules dissociate to form the H^+ ion and the OH^- (hydroxide) ion:

$$\mathbf{H_2O \rightleftarrows H^+ + OH^-}$$

In pure water, the balance between these two ions is equal. However, when an acid such as hydrochloric acid (HCl) dissociates into H^+ and Cl^-, it shifts this balance in favor of excess H^+ ions. In the blood, carbon dioxide (CO_2) forms carbonic acid (H_2CO_3) when it dissolves in water. Some of the carbonic acid then dissociates to form H^+ ions and HCO_3^- (bicarbonate) ions, producing an excess of H^+ ions in the blood. Thus high CO_2 levels in the blood make the blood more acidic.

Bases or **alkaline** compounds, on the other hand, shift the balance in the opposite direction. For example, sodium hydroxide (NaOH) is a base that forms OH^- ions but no H^+ ions. In short, acids are compounds that produce an excess of H^+ ions, and bases are compounds that produce an excess of OH^- ions (or a decrease in H^+).

The relative H^+ concentration is a measure of how acidic or basic a solution is. The H^+ concentration is usually expressed in units of **pH.** The formula used to calculate pH units gives a value of 7 to pure water. A higher pH value indicates a low relative concentration of H^+—a base. A lower pH value indicates a higher H^+ concentration—an acid. Figure 2-5 shows a scale of pH from 0 to 14.

FIGURE 2-5

The pH scale. The H^+ concentration is balanced with the OH^- concentration at pH 7. At values above 7 (low H^+), the scale tips in the basic direction. At values below 7 (high H^+), the scale tips toward the acid side.

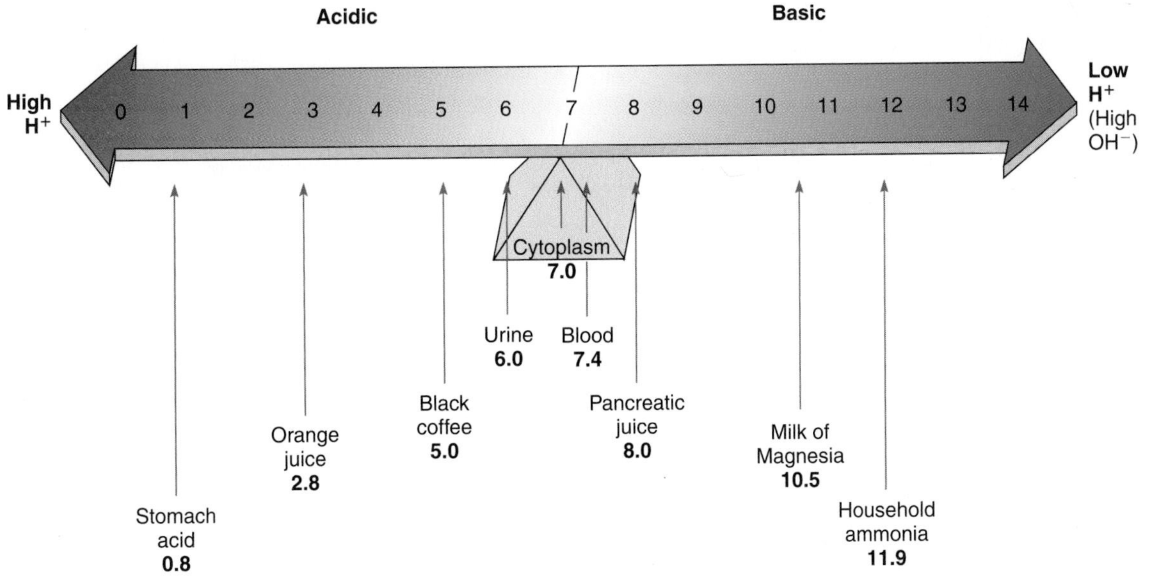

Notice that when the pH of a solution is less than 7, the scale "tips" toward the side marked "high H^+." When the pH is more than 7, the scale "tips" toward the side marked "low H^+." pH units increase or decrease by factors of 10. Thus a pH 5 solution has ten times the H^+ concentration of a pH 6 solution. A pH 4 solution has a hundred times the H^+ concentration of a pH 6 solution.

A *strong acid* is an acid that completely, or almost completely, dissociates to form H^+ ions. A *weak acid*, on the other hand, dissociates very little and therefore produces few excess H^+ ions in solution.

When a strong acid and a strong base mix, excess H^+ ions may combine with the excess OH^- ions to form water. That is, they may neutralize each other. The remaining ions usually form neutral ionic compounds called *salts*. For example:

$$\underset{\text{acid}}{HCl} + \underset{\text{base}}{NaOH} \rightarrow H^+ + Cl^- + NA^+ + OH^- \rightarrow \underset{\text{water}}{H_2O} + \underset{\text{salt}}{NaCl}$$

The pH of body fluids affects body chemistry so greatly that normal body function can be maintained only within a narrow range of pH. The body can remove excess H^+ ions by excreting

Clinical Application

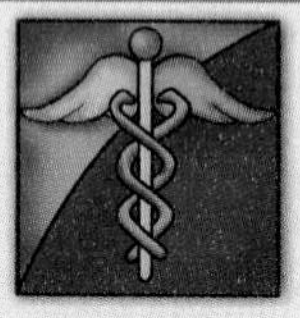

Radioactive Isotopes

Each element is unique because of the number of protons it has. In short, each element has its own *atomic number*. However, atoms of the same element can have different numbers of neutrons. Two atoms that have the same atomic number but different atomic masses are **isotopes** of the same element. An example is hydrogen. Hydrogen has three isotopes: ^1H (the most common isotope), ^2H, and ^3H. The figure shows that each different isotope has only one proton but different numbers of neutrons.

Some isotopes have unstable nuclei that radiate (give off) particles. Radiation particles include protons, neutrons, electrons, and altered versions of these normal subatomic particles. An isotope that emits radiation is called a **radioactive isotope**.

Radioactive isotopes of common elements are sometimes used to evaluate the function of body parts. Radioactive iodine (^{125}I) put into the body and taken up by the thyroid gland gives off radiation that can be easily measured. Thus the rate of thyroid activity can be determined. Images of internal organs can be formed by radiation scanners that plot out the location of injected or ingested radioactive isotopes. For example, radioactive technetium (^{99}Tc) is commonly used to image the liver and spleen. The radioactive isotopes ^{13}N, ^{15}O, and ^{11}C are often used to study the brain in a technique called the *PET scan*.

Radiation can damage cells. Exposure to high levels of radiation may cause cells to develop into cancer cells. Higher levels of radiation completely destroy tissues, causing *radiation sickness*. Low doses of radioactive substances are sometimes given to cancer patients to destroy cancer cells. The side effects of these treatments result from the unavoidable destruction of normal cells with the cancer cells.

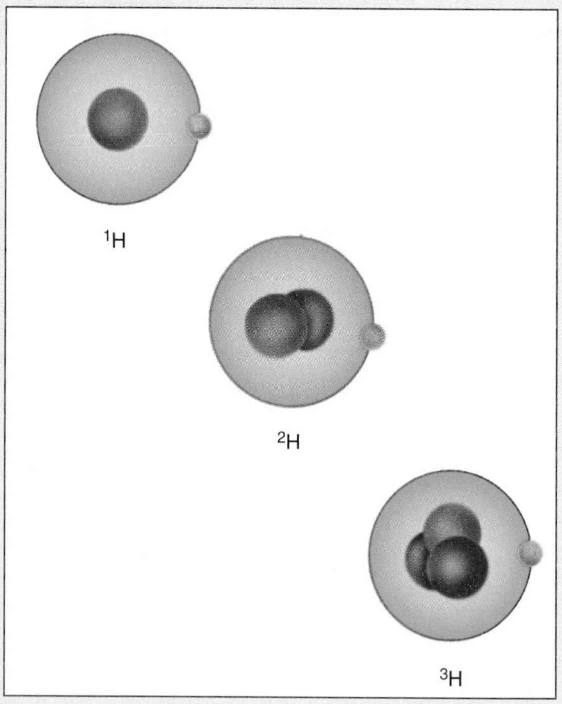

them in the urine (see Chapter 17). Another way to remove acid is by increasing the loss of CO_2 (an acid) by the respiratory system (see Chapter 14). A third way to adjust the body's pH is the use of buffers—chemicals in the blood that maintain pH. Buffers maintain pH balance by preventing sudden changes in the H^+ ion concentration. Buffers do this by forming a chemical system that neutralizes acids and bases as they are added to a solution. The mechanisms by which the body maintains pH homeostasis, or acid-base balance, are discussed further in Chapter 19.

Quick Check

1. Define an organic compound.
2. What is the difference between dehydration synthesis and hydrolysis?
3. Does an acid have a low pH or a high pH? A base?

Research, Issues & Trends

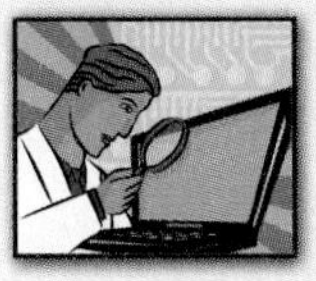

Metric System

Scientists, many government agencies, and increasing numbers of American industries are using or moving toward the conversion of our system of English measurements to the metric system. The metric system is a decimal system in which measurement of length is based on the *meter* (39.37 inches) and weight or mass is based on the *gram* (about 454 grams equal a pound).

A micrometer is one millionth of a meter. (*Micron* is another name for micrometer.) In the metric systems the units of length are as follows:

1 meter (m) = 39.37 inches
1 centimeter (cm) = 1/100 m
1 millimeter (mm) = 1/1,000 m
1 micrometer (μm) or micron (μ) = 1/1,000,000 m
1 nanometer (nm) = 1/1,000,000,000 m
1 Angstrom (Å) = 1/10,000,000,000 m
Approximately equal to 1 inch:
25 cm
250 mm
25,000 μm
25,000,000 nm

ORGANIC CHEMISTRY

Organic compounds are much more complex than inorganic compounds. In this section, we will describe the basic structure and function of each major type of organic compound found in the body: **carbohydrates, lipids** (fats), **proteins,** and **nucleic acids.** Table 2-3 summarizes the structure and the function of each type. Refer to this table as you read through the descriptions that follow.

Carbohydrates

The name *carbohydrate* literally means "carbon (C) and water (H_2O)," signifying the types of atoms that form carbohydrate molecules. The basic unit of carbohydrate molecules is called a *monosaccharide* (mah-no-SAK-ah-ride) (Figure 2-6). Glucose (dextrose) is an important monosaccharide in the body; cells use it as their primary source of energy (see Chapter 16). A molecule made of two saccharide units is a double sugar or *disaccharide.* The disaccharides sucrose (table sugar) and lactose (milk sugar) are important dietary carbohydrates. After they are eaten, the body digests them to form monosaccharides that can be used as cellular fuel. Many saccharide units joined together form *polysaccharides.* Examples of polysaccharides are **glycogen** (GLY-ko-jen) and *starch.* Each glycogen molecule is a chain of glucose molecules joined together. Liver cells and muscle cells form glycogen when there is an excess of glucose in the blood, thus putting them into "storage" for later use.

Carbohydrates have potential energy stored in their bonds. When the bonds are broken in cells, the energy is released and then trapped by the cell's chemistry to do work. Chapter 16 explains more about the process by which the body extracts energy from carbohydrates and other food molecules.

Lipids

Lipids are fats and oils. Fats are lipids that are solid at room temperature, such as the fat in butter and lard. Oils, such as corn oil and olive oil, are liquid at room temperature. There are several important types of lipids in the body:

TABLE 2-3

Major Types of Organic Compounds

EXAMPLE	COMPONENTS	FUNCTIONS
CARBOHYDRATE		
Monosaccharide (glucose, galactose, fructose)	Single monosaccharide unit	Used as a source of energy; used to build other carbohydrates
Disaccharide (sucrose, lactose, maltose)	Two monosaccharide units	Can be broken into monosaccharides
Polysaccharide (glycogen, starch)	Many monosaccharide units	Used to store monosaccharides (thus to store energy)
LIPID		
Triglyceride	One glycerol, three fatty acids	Stores energy
Phospholipid	Phosphorus-containing unit, two fatty acids	Forms cell membranes
Cholesterol	Four carbon rings at core	Transports lipids; is basis of steroid hormones
PROTEIN		
Structural proteins	Amino acids	Form structures of the body (fibers)
Functional proteins (enzymes, hormones)	Amino acids	Facilitate chemical reactions; send signals; regulate functions
NUCLEIC ACID		
Deoxyribonucleic acid (DNA)	Nucleotides (contain deoxyribose)	Contains information (genetic code) for making proteins
Ribonucleic acid (RNA)	Nucleotides (contain ribose)	Serves as a copy of a portion of the genetic code

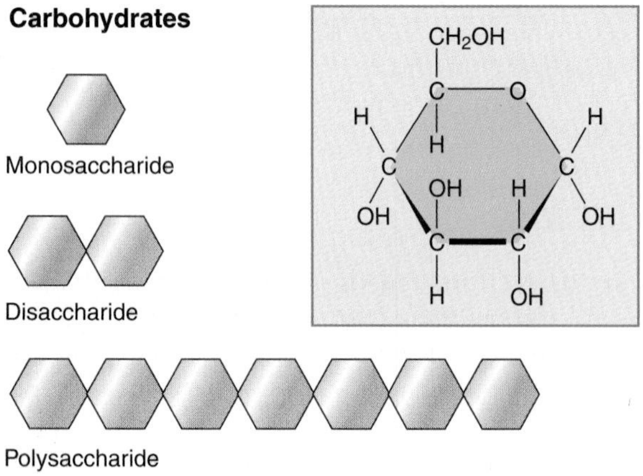

FIGURE 2-6

Carbohydrates. Monosaccharides are single carbohydrate units joined by dehydration synthesis to form disaccharides and polysaccharides. The detailed chemical structure of the monosaccharide glucose is shown in the inset.

1. **Triglycerides** (try-GLIS-er-ides) are lipid molecules formed by a *glycerol* unit joined to three *fatty acids* (Figure 2-7). Like carbohydrates, their bonds can be broken apart to yield energy (see Chapter 16). Thus triglycerides are useful in storing energy in cells for later use.
2. **Phospholipids** are similar to triglycerides but, as their name implies, have phosphorus-containing units in them. The phosphorus-containing unit in each molecule forms a "head" that attracts water. Two fatty acid "tails" repel water. Figure 2-8, *A*, shows the head and tail of the phospholipid molecule. This structure allows them to form a stable *bilayer* in water that forms the foundation for the cell membrane. In Figure 2-8, *B*, the water-attracting heads face the water and the water-repelling tails face away from the water (and toward each other).
3. **Cholesterol** is a *steroid* lipid (a multiple ring structure) that performs several important functions in the body. It combines with phospholipids in the cell membrane to help stabilize its bilayer structure. The body also uses cholesterol as a starting point in making steroid hormones such as estrogen, testosterone, and cortisone (see Chapter 10).

FIGURE 2-7

Triglyceride. Each triglyceride is composed of three fatty acid units attached to a glycerol unit.

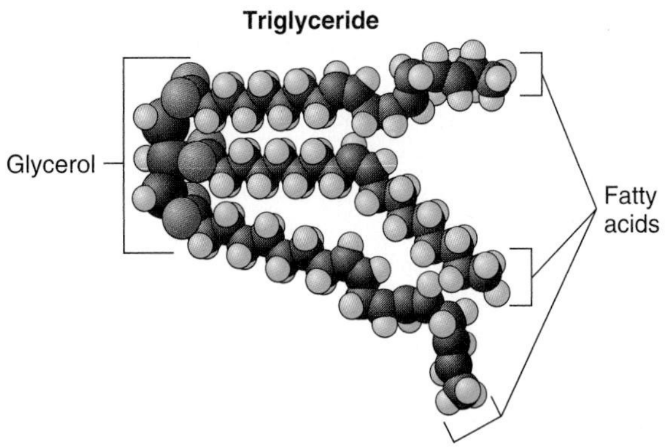

FIGURE 2-8

Phospholipids. A, Each phospholipid molecule has a phosphorus-containing "head" that attracts water and a lipid "tail" that repels water. **B,** Because the tails repel water, phospholipid molecules often arrange themselves so that their tails face away from water. The stable structure that results is a bilayer sheet forming a small bubble.

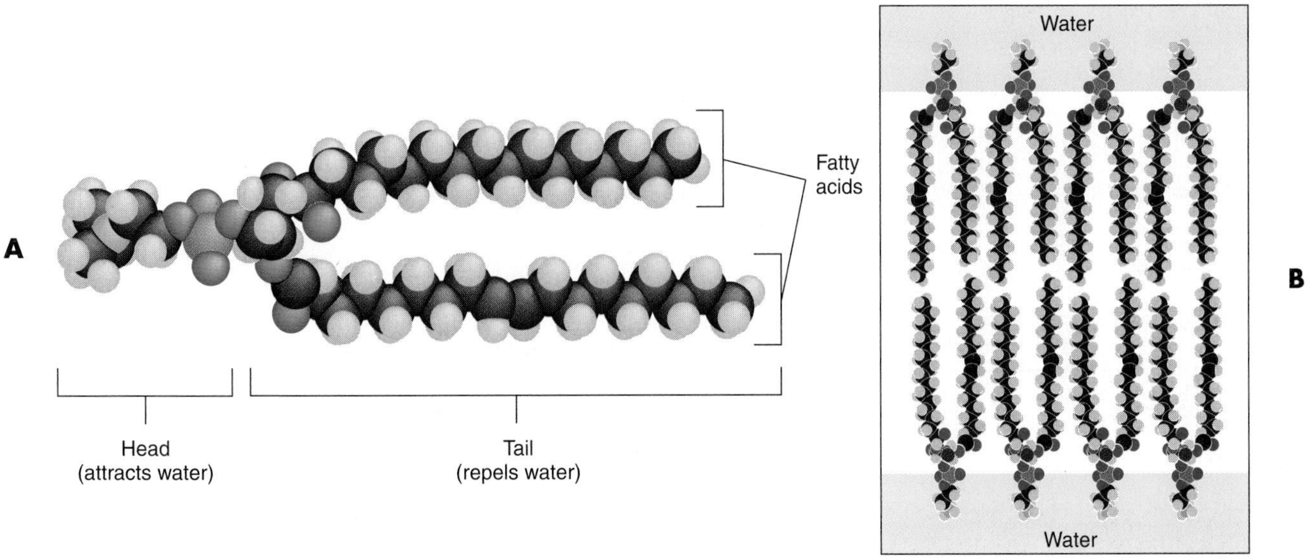

Proteins

Proteins are very large molecules composed of basic units called **amino acids.** In addition to carbon, hydrogen, and oxygen, amino acids contain nitrogen (N). By means of a process described fully in Chapter 3, a particular sequence of amino acids is strung together and held by **peptide bonds.** Positive-negative attractions between different atoms in the long amino acid strand cause it to coil on itself and maintain its shape. The complex, three-dimensional molecule that results is a protein molecule (Figure 2-9).

The shape of a protein molecule determines its role in body chemistry. **Structural proteins** are shaped in ways that allow them to form essential structures of the body. Collagen, a protein with a fiber shape, holds most of the body tissues together. Keratin, another structural protein, forms a network of waterproof fibers in the outer layer of the skin. **Functional proteins** participate in chemical processes of the body. Functional proteins include some of the hormones, growth factors, cell membrane channels and receptors, and enzymes.

Enzymes are chemical catalysts. This means that they help a chemical reaction occur but are not reactants or products themselves. They participate in chemical reactions but are not changed by the reactions. Enzymes are vital to body chemistry. No reaction in the body occurs fast enough unless the specific enzymes needed for that reaction are present.

Figure 2-10 illustrates how shape is important to the function of enzyme molecules. Each enzyme has a shape that "fits" the specific molecules it works on much as a key fits specific locks. This explanation of enzyme action is sometimes called the **lock-and-key model.**

FIGURE 2-9

Protein. Protein molecules are large, complex molecules formed by a twisted and folded strand of amino acids. Each amino acid is connected to the next amino acid by covalent peptide bonds.

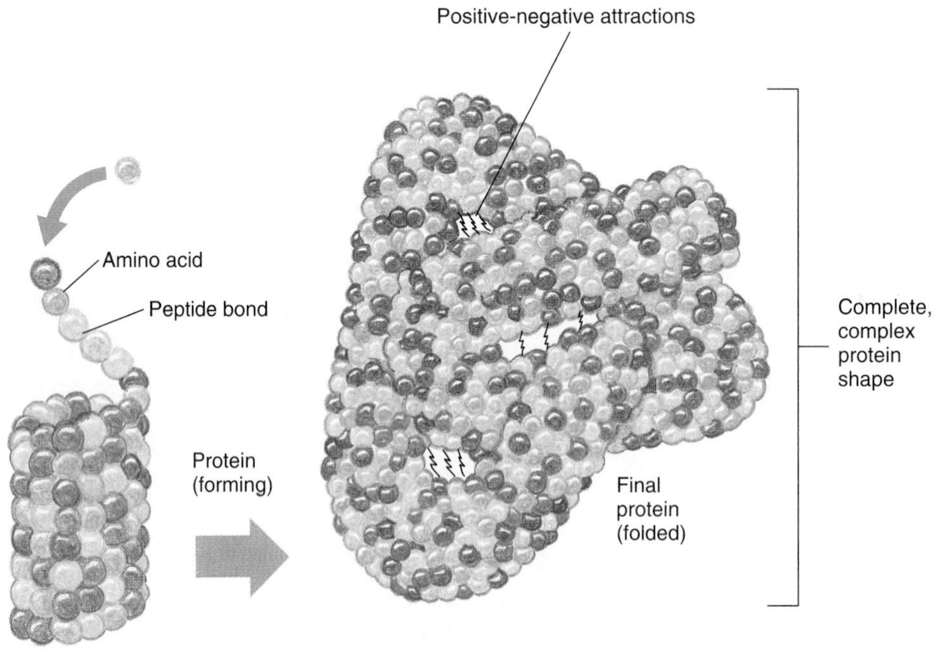

Proteins can bond with other organic compounds and form "mixed" molecules. For example, *glycoproteins* are proteins with sugars attached. *Lipoproteins* are lipid-protein combinations.

Nucleic Acids

The two forms of nucleic acid are **deoxyribonucleic acid (DNA)** and **ribonucleic acid (RNA).** As outlined in Chapter 3, the basic building blocks of nucleic acids are called **nucleotides**. Each nucleotide consists of a *phosphate unit,* a sugar (*ribose* or *deoxyribose*), and a *nitrogen base.* DNA nucleotide bases include **adenine, thymine, guanine,** and **cytosine.** RNA uses the same set of bases, except for the substitution of **uracil** for thymine. See Table 2-4.

FIGURE 2-10

Enzyme action. Enzymes are functional proteins whose molecular shape allows them to catalyze chemical reactions. Molecules *A* and *B* are brought together by the enzyme to form a larger molecule, *AB*.

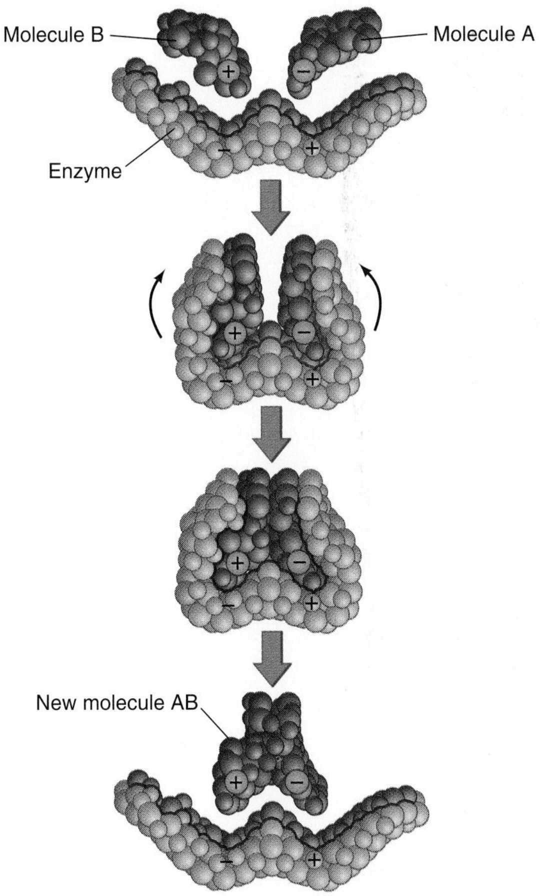

Clinical Application

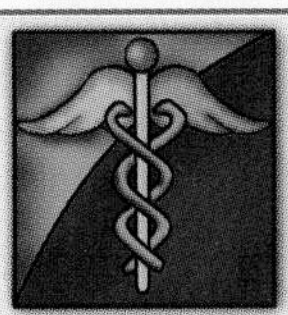

Blood Lipoproteins

A lipid such as cholesterol can travel in the blood only after it has attached to a protein molecule—forming a lipoprotein. Some of these molecules are called *high-density lipoproteins (HDLs)* because they have a high density of protein (more protein than lipid). Another type of molecule contains less protein (and more lipid), so it is called *low-density lipoprotein (LDL).*

The cholesterol in LDLs is often called "bad" cholesterol because high blood levels of LDL are associated with **atherosclerosis,** a life-threatening blockage of arteries. LDLs carry cholesterol to *cells*, including the cells that line blood vessels. HDLs, on the other hand, carry so-called "good" cholesterol *away from cells* and toward the liver for elimination from the body. A high proportion of HDL in the blood is associated with a low risk of developing atherosclerosis. Factors such as cigarette smoking decrease HDL levels and thus contribute to risk of atherosclerosis. Factors such as exercise increase HDL levels and thus decrease the risk of atherosclerosis.

TABLE 2-4

Components of Nucleotides

NUCLEOTIDE	DNA	RNA
Sugar	Deoxyribose	Ribose
Phosphate	Phosphate	Phosphate
Nitrogen base	Cytosine	Cytosine
	Guanine	Guanine
	Adenine	Adenine
	Thymine	Uracil

Nucleotides bind to one another to form strands or other structures. In the DNA molecule, nucleotides are arranged in a twisted, double strand called a **double helix** (Figure 2-11).

The sequence of different nucleotides along the DNA double helix is the "master code" for assembling proteins and other nucleic acids. *Messenger RNA (mRNA)* molecules have a sequence that forms a temporary "working copy" of a portion of the DNA code called a *gene*. The code in nucleic acids ultimately directs the entire symphony of living chemistry.

Quick

1. Which category of organic chemical is made up of monosaccharides? Of fatty acids? Of amino acids? Of nucleotides?
2. Why is the structure of protein molecules important?
3. What is the role of DNA in the body?

FIGURE 2-11

DNA. Deoxyribonucleic acid (DNA), like all nucleic acids, is composed of units called *nucleotides*. Each nucleotide has a phosphate, a sugar, and a nitrogen base. In DNA, the nucleotides are arranged in a double helix formation.

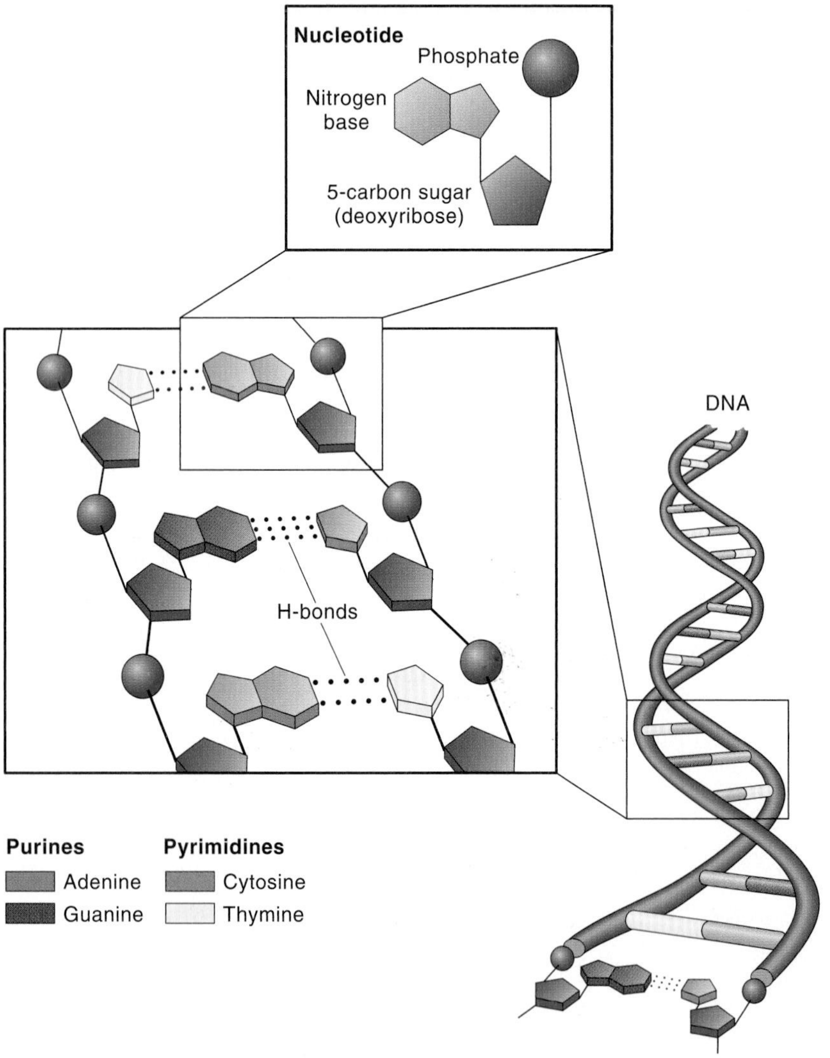

Science Applications

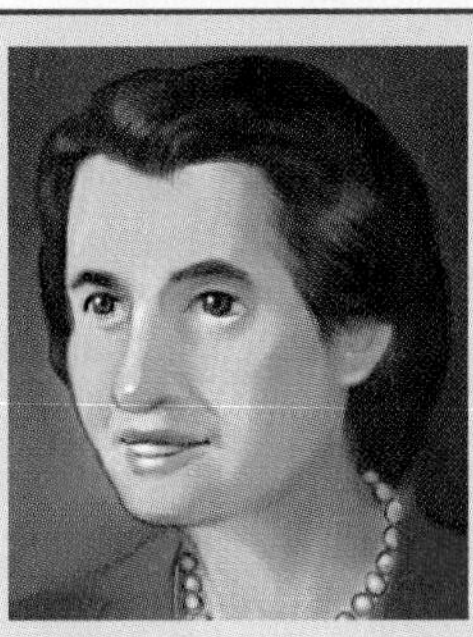

Biochemistry

Rosalind Franklin

British scientist Rosalind Franklin (1920-1958) was one of the leading biochemists of the modern age. Franklin used x-rays to cast shadows through DNA to analyze its structure. When she was only 32 years old, she discovered the unusual helical (spiral) structure of the DNA molecule and how the sugars and phosphates form an outer backbone to the molecule (see Figure 2-11). Her breakthrough helped James Watson, Francis Crick, and Maurice Wilkins to finally work out the structure and function of DNA in 1953 and thus crack the "code of life." The three men received a Nobel Prize for their achievement in 1962 but Franklin's early death from cancer in 1958 prevented her from sharing in the credit for one of the greatest discoveries of all time.

Biochemists continue to make important discoveries that increase our understanding of human structure and function. Aided by laboratory technicians and assistants, biochemists also find ways to help other professionals apply biochemistry to solve everyday problems. For example, clinical laboratory professionals analyze samples from the bodies of patients for signs of health or disease. Others who use biochemistry as a basis for their work include pharmacists and pharmacy technicians, dietitians, forensic investigators, genetic counselors, and even science journalists.

OUTLINE SUMMARY

LEVELS OF CHEMICAL ORGANIZATION

A. Atoms
- **1.** Nucleus—central core of atom
  - **a.** Proton—positively charged particle in nucleus
  - **b.** Neutron—non-charged particle in nucleus
  - **c.** Atomic mass—number of protons in the nucleus; determines the type of atom
- **2.** Energy levels—regions surrounding atomic nucleus that contain electrons
  - **a.** Electron—negatively charged particle
  - **b.** May contain up to eight electrons in each level
  - **c.** Energy increases with distance from nucleus

B. Elements, molecules, and compounds
- **1.** Element—a pure substance; made up of only one kind of atom
- **2.** Molecule—a group of atoms bound together in a group
- **3.** Compound—substances whose molecules have more than one kind of atom

CHEMICAL BONDING

A. Chemical bonds form to make atoms more stable
- **1.** Outermost energy level of each atom is full
- **2.** Atoms may share electrons, or donate or borrow them to become stable

B. Ionic bonds
- **1.** Ions form when an atom gains or loses electrons in its outer energy level to become stable
  - **a.** Positive ion—has lost electrons; indicated by superscript positive sign(s), as in Na^+ or Ca^{++}
  - **b.** Negative ion—has gained electrons; indicated by superscript negative sign(s), as in Cl^-
- **2.** Ionic bonds form when positive and negative ions attract each other because of electrical attraction
- **3.** Electrolyte—molecule that dissociates (breaks apart) in water to form individual ions; an ionic compound

Continued

OUTLINE SUMMARY—cont'd

C. Covalent bonds
   1. Covalent bonds form when atoms shared their outer energy to fill up and thus become stable
   2. Covalent bonds do not ordinarily easily dissociate in water

INORGANIC CHEMISTRY

A. *Organic* molecules contain carbon-carbon covalent bonds or carbon-hydrogen covalent bonds; *inorganic* molecules do not

B. Examples of inorganic molecules: water and some acids, bases, and salts

C. Water
   1. Water is a solvent (liquid into which solutes are dissolved), forming aqueous solutions in the body
   2. Water is involved in chemical reactions
      a. Dehydration synthesis—chemical reaction in which water is removed from small molecules so they can be strung together to form a larger molecule
      b. Hydrolysis—chemical reaction in which water is added to the subunits of a large molecule to break it apart into smaller molecules
      c. Chemical reactions always involve energy transfers, as when energy is used to build ATP molecules
      d. Chemical equations show how reactants interact to form products; arrows separate the reactants from the products

D. Acids, bases, and salts
   1. Water molecules dissociate to form equal amounts of H^+ (hydrogen ion) and OH^- (hydroxide ion)
   2. Acid—substance that shifts the H^+/OH^- balance in favor of H^+; opposite of base
   3. Base—substance that shifts the H^+/OH^- balance against H^+; also known as an alkaline; opposite of acid
   4. pH—mathematical expression of relative H^+ concentration in an aqueous solution
      a. 7 is neutral (neither acid nor base)
      b. pH values above 7 are basic; pH values below 7 are acidic
   5. Neutralization occurs when acids and bases mix and form salts
   6. Buffers are chemical systems that absorb excess acids or bases and thus maintain a relatively stable pH

ORGANIC CHEMISTRY

A. Carbohydrates—sugars and complex carbohydrates
   1. Contain carbon (C), hydrogen (H), oxygen (O)
   2. Made up of six-carbon subunits called monosaccharides or single sugars (e.g., glucose)
   3. Disaccharide—double sugar made up of two monosaccharide units (e.g., sucrose, lactose)
   4. Polysaccharide—complex carbohydrate made up of many monosaccharide units (e.g., glycogen made up of many glucose units)
   5. Function of carbohydrates is to store energy for later use

B. Lipids—fats and oils
   1. Triglycerides
      a. Made up of one glycerol unit and three fatty acids
      b. Store energy for later use
   2. Phospholipids
      a. Similar to triglyceride structure, except with only two fatty acids, and with a phosphorus-containing group attached to glycerol
      b. The head attracts water and the double tail does not, thus forming stable double layers (bilayers) in water
      c. Form membranes of cells

OUTLINE SUMMARY—cont'd

3. Cholesterol
   a. Molecules have a steroid structure made up of multiple rings
   b. Cholesterol stabilizes the phospholipid tails in cellular membranes and is also converted into steroid hormones by the body

C. Proteins
1. Very large molecules made up of amino acids held together in long, folded chains by peptide bonds
2. Structural proteins
   a. Form structures of the body
   b. Collagen is a fibrous protein that holds many tissues together
   c. Keratin forms tough, waterproof fibers in the outer layer of the skin
3. Functional proteins
   a. Participate in chemical processes
   b. Examples: hormones, cell membrane channels and receptors, enzymes
   c. Enzymes
      (1) Catalysts—help chemical reactions occur
      (2) Lock-and-key model—each enzyme fits a particular molecule that it acts on as a key fits into a lock
4. Proteins can combine with other organic molecules to form glycoproteins or lipoproteins

D. Nucleic acids
1. Made up of nucleotide units
2. Sugar (ribose or deoxyribose)
3. Phosphate
   a. Nitrogen base (adenine, thymine or uracil, guanine, cytosine)
4. DNA (deoxyribonucleic acid)
   a. Used as the cell's "master code" for assembling proteins
   b. Uses deoxyribose as the sugar and A, T (not U), C, and G as bases
   c. Forms a double helix shape
5. RNA (ribonucleic acid)
   a. Used as a temporary "working copy" of a gene (portion of the DNA code)
   b. Uses ribose as the sugar and A, U (not T), C, and G as bases
6. By directing the formation of structural and functional proteins, nucleic acids ultimately direct overall body structure and function

NEW WORDS

acid
alkaline
aqueous solution
atom
atomic mass
atomic number
base
carbohydrate
compound
covalent
dehydration
dissociation
double helix
electrolyte
electron
element
energy level
enzyme
glycogen
hydrolysis
inorganic compound
ionic bond
lipid
matter
molecule
neutron
nucleic acid
nucleus
organic compound
peptide bond
pH
product
protein
proton
reactant
solute
solvent

REVIEW QUESTIONS

1. Define the following terms: *element, compound, atom, molecule.*
2. Name and define three kinds of particles within an atom.
3. What is an energy level?
4. What is a chemical bond?
5. What is an electrolyte? An ion?
6. Define the terms *organic compound* and *inorganic compound.*
7. What is a solvent? A solute?
8. Explain the concept of pH.
9. What is an acid? A base?
10. Briefly describe the structure of each of these: *protein, lipid, carbohydrate, nucleic acid.*
11. Briefly state the principle functions of each of these: *carbohydrate, protein, lipid, nucleic acid.*

CRITICAL THINKING

12. Compare and contrast how ionic bonds and chemical bonds solve the problem of achieving stability in atoms.
13. A certain protein molecule is hydrolyzed by an enzyme. How would you explain that statement to someone unfamiliar with chemical terminology?
14. Your blood normally has a pH of around 7.4—is your blood alkaline, acid, or neutral?
15. A newly discovered protein is found to regulate how hormones influence the functions of cells in the body. Is this protein a structural protein or a functional protein?
16. What mechanism does DNA use to regulate all of the body's structures and function?
17. How would you explain the difference between ^{1}H, ^{2}H, and ^{3}H?

CHAPTER TEST

1. __________ is anything that occupies space and has mass.
2. Molecules are made up of particles called __________.
3. Positively charged particles within the nucleus of an atom are called __________.
4. Electrons inhabit regions of the atoms called __________ levels.
5. Substances with molecules having more than one kind of atom are called __________.
6. A(n) __________ chemical bond occurs when atoms share electrons.
7. The symbol K^{+} represents the potassium __________.
8. A compound that dissociates in water to form ions is called a(n) __________.
9. Molecules that have a carbon-carbon bond in them are classified as __________ compounds.
10. In saltwater, salt is the solute and water is the __________.
11. When water is used to build up small molecules into larger molecules, we call the process __________.
12. __________ are solutions that have an excess of hydrogen ions.
13. The blood contains chemicals called __________ that maintain a stable pH.

Match each type of compound in Column B with the example given in Column A.

COLUMN A	COLUMN B
14. ____ glycogen	a. salt
15. ____ collagen	b. acid
16. ____ RNA	c. base
17. ____ cholesterol	d. carbohydrate
18. ____ NaCl	e. lipid
19. ____ NaOH	f. protein
20. ____ HCl	g. nucleic acid

CHAPTER TEST—*cont'd*

21. An ion is formed when
  a. electrons are shared
  b. electrons remain in place
  c. electrons are gained or lost
  d. neutrons are added to the nucleus

22. In the equation $H_2O + CO_2 \rightarrow H^+ + HCO_3^-$, which of these is a reactant?
  a. CO_2
  b. HCO_3^-
  c. O_2
  d. $\rightarrow$

23. Which of these chemical subunits is found in DNA?
  a. uracil
  b. ribose
  c. amino acid
  d. deoxyribose

24. Which of these represents an acid?
  a. pH 7.5
  b. pH 6.1
  c. pH 9.0
  d. pH 7.0

25. Steroid hormones are
  a. carbohydrates
  b. proteins
  c. lipids
  d. nucleic acids

STUDY TIPS

This chapter introduces you to some basic chemical concepts that will used later to describe structures and functions of the body. First of all, it's important that you can read a handful of important chemical symbols and equations. Practice by putting the chemical symbols found in Tables 2-1 and 2-2 on flash cards and then quiz each other on what they stand for. Also practice by identifying whether each one is an ion or not an ion.

If your instructor will require you to know the parts of the atom, make your own labeled diagram or a model out of household items such as marshmallows, toothpicks, and string. Using multiple senses will help you learn and remember. The concept of pH is also important for later discussions. Practice identifying whether a pH value is neutral, acid, or base, by making a simple "wheel of fortune" with a paper and a paper clip. On the various spokes of the wheel, print different pH values. Spin the paperclip and identify whether the value it lands on is acid, base, or neutral.

Table 2-3 summarizes some important concepts of the structure and function of the major organic compounds that you will be using later in the course. Make your own version of the table on a poster-sized piece of paper and add simple pictures of the different molecules. Then make flash cards and practice identifying which category different molecules belong to: protein, carbohydrate, lipid, or nucleic acid. Then practice by telling which function each performs.

3 Cells and Tissues

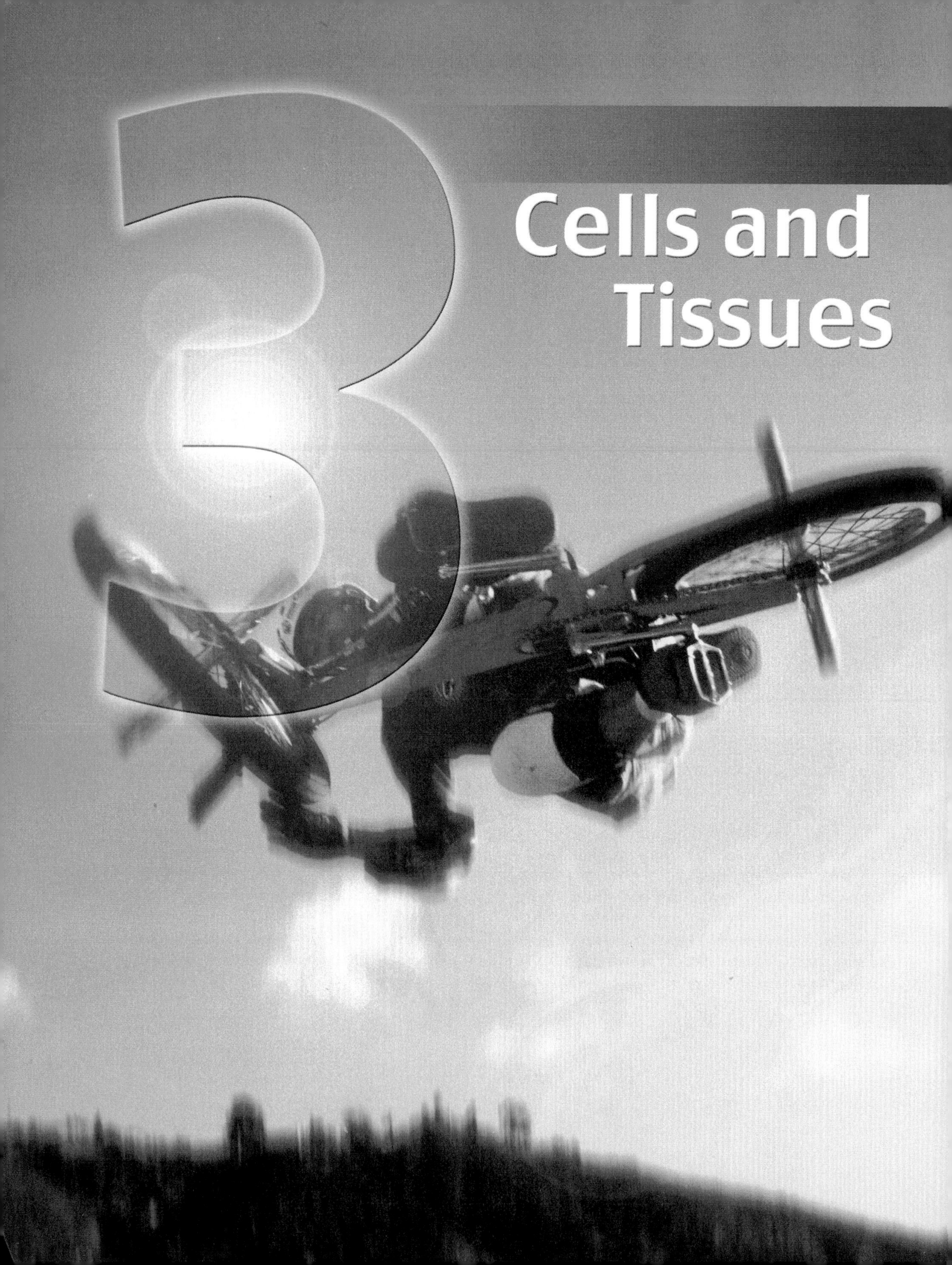

Outline

Objectives

AFTER YOU HAVE COMPLETED THIS CHAPTER, YOU SHOULD BE ABLE TO:

1. Identify and discuss the basic structure and function of the three major components of a cell.
2. List and briefly discuss the functions of the primary cellular organelles.
3. Compare the major passive and active transport processes that act to move substances through cell membranes.
4. Compare and discuss DNA and RNA and their function in protein synthesis.
5. Discuss the stages of mitosis and explain the importance of cellular reproduction.
6. Explain how epithelial tissue is grouped according to shape and arrangement of cells.
7. List and briefly discuss the major types of connective and muscle tissue.
8. List the three structural components of a neuron.

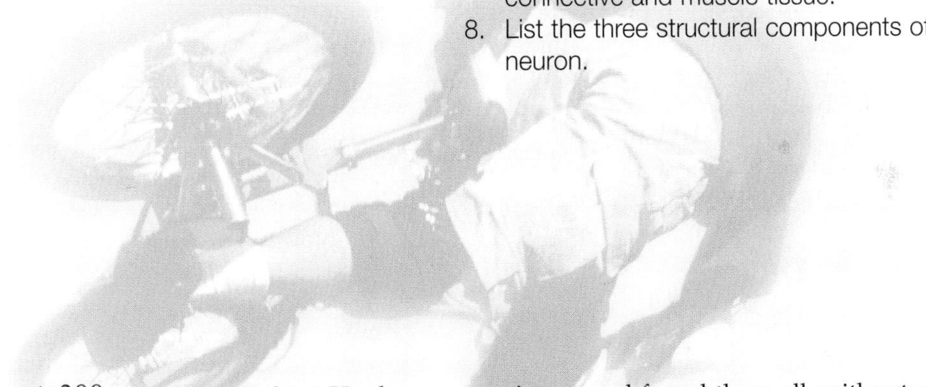

A*bout 300 years* ago Robert Hooke looked through his microscope—one of the very early, somewhat primitive ones—at some plant material. What he saw must have surprised him. Instead of a single magnified piece of plant material, he saw many small pieces. Because they reminded him of miniature monastery cells, that is what he called them: cells. Since Hooke's time, thousands of individuals have examined thousands of plant and animal specimens and found them all, without exception, to be composed of cells. This fact, that cells are the smallest structural units of living things, has become the foundation of modern biology. Many living things are so simple that they consist of just one cell. The human body, however, is so complex that it consists not of a few thousand or millions or even billions of cells but of many trillions of them. This chapter discusses cells first and then groups of similar cells, which are called tissues.

CELLS

Size and Shape

Human cells are microscopic in size; that is, they can be seen only when magnified by a microscope. However, they vary considerably in size. An ovum (female sex cell), for example, has a diameter of about 150 micrometers, whereas red blood cells have a diameter of only 7.5 micrometers. Cells differ even more notably in shape than in size. Some are flat, some are brick shaped, some are threadlike, and some have irregular shapes.

Composition

Cells contain **cytoplasm** (SI-to-plazm), or "living matter," a substance that exists only in cells. The term cyto- is a Greek combining form and denotes a relationship to a cell. Each cell in the body is surrounded by a thin membrane, the **plasma membrane.** This membrane separates the cell contents from the dilute salt water solution called **interstitial** (in-ter-STISH-al) **fluid,** or simply **tissue fluid,** which bathes every cell in the body. Numerous specialized structures called **organelles** (or-gan-ELZ), which will be described in subsequent sections, are contained within the cytoplasm of each cell. A small, circular body called the **nucleus** (NOO-kle-us) is also inside the cell.

Parts of the Cell

The three main parts of a cell are:

1. Plasma membrane
2. Cytoplasm
3. Nucleus

The plasma membrane surrounds the entire cell, forming its outer boundary. The cytoplasm is all the living material inside the cell (except the nucleus). The nucleus is a large, membrane-bound structure in most cells that contains the genetic code.

Plasma Membrane

As the name suggests, the **plasma membrane** is the membrane that encloses the cytoplasm and forms the outer boundary of the cell. It is an incredibly delicate structure—only about 7 nm (nanometers) or 3/10,000,000 of an inch thick! Yet it has a precise, orderly structure (Figure 3-1). Two layers of phosphate-containing fat molecules called **phospholipids** form a fluid framework for the plasma membrane. Another kind of fat molecule called *cholesterol* is also a component of the plasma membrane. Cholesterol helps stabilize the phospholipid molecules to prevent breakage of the plasma membrane. Note in Figure 3-1 that protein molecules dot the surfaces of the membrane and extend all the way through the phospholipid framework.

Despite its seeming fragility, the plasma membrane is strong enough to keep the cell whole and intact. It also performs other life-preserving functions for the cell. It serves as a well-guarded gateway between the fluid inside the cell and the fluid around it. Certain substances move through it, but it bars the passage of others. The plasma membrane even functions as a communication device. How? Some proteins on the membrane's outer surface serve as receptors for certain other molecules when these other molecules contact the proteins. In other words, certain molecules bind to certain receptor proteins. For example, some hormones (chemicals secreted into blood from ductless glands) bind to membrane receptors, and a change in cell functions follows. We might therefore think of such hormones as chemical messages, communicated to cells by binding to their cytoplasmic membrane receptors.

The plasma membrane also identifies a cell as coming from one particular individual. Its surface proteins serve as positive identification tags because they occur only in the cells of that individual. A practical application of this fact is made in *tissue typing*, a procedure performed before an organ from one individual is transplanted into another. Carbohydrate chains attached to the surface of cells often play a role in the identification of cell types.

Cytoplasm

Cytoplasm is the internal living material of cells. It lies between the plasma membrane and the nucleus, which can be seen in Figure 3-2 as a round or spherical structure in the center of the cell. Nu-

FIGURE 3-1

Structure of the plasma membrane. Note that protein molecules may penetrate completely through the two layers of phospholipid molecules.

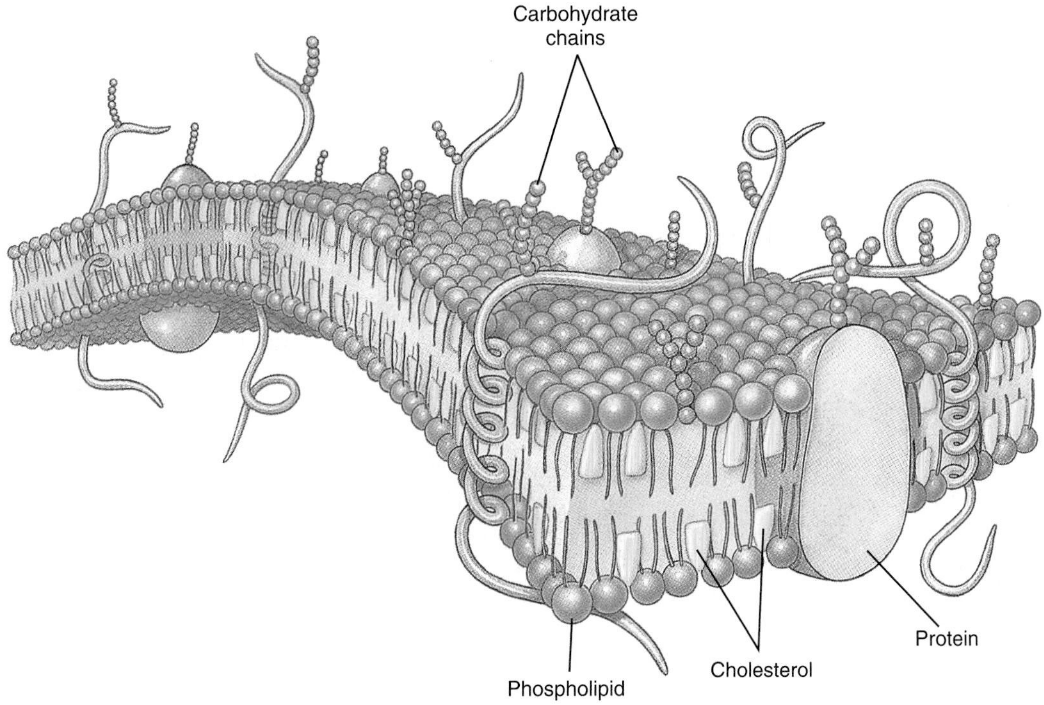

merous small structures are part of the cytoplasm, along with the fluid that serves as the interior environment of each cell. As a group, the small structures that make up much of the cytoplasm are called **organelles**. This name means "little organs," an appropriate name because they function just as organs function for the body.

Look again at Figure 3-2. Notice how many different kinds of structures you can see in the cytoplasm of this cell. A little more than a generation ago, almost all of these organelles were unknown. They are so small that they are invisible even when magnified 1000 times by a light microscope. Electron microscopes brought them into view by magnifying them many thousands of times. We shall briefly discuss the following organelles, which are found in cytoplasm (see also Table 3-1):

1. Ribosomes
2. Endoplasmic reticulum
3. Golgi apparatus
4. Mitochondria
5. Lysosomes
6. Centrioles
7. Cilia
8. Flagella

Ribosomes. Organelles called **ribosomes** (RI-bo-sohms), shown as dots in Figure 3-2, are very tiny particles found throughout the cell. They are each made up of two tiny subunits constructed mostly of a special kind of RNA called *ribosomal RNA (rRNA)*. Some ribosomes are found temporarily attached to a network of membranous canals called *endoplasmic reticulum (ER)*—another type of organelle described in the next paragraph. Ribosomes may also be free in the cytoplasm. Ribosomes perform a very complex function; they make enzymes and other protein compounds.

FIGURE 3-2

General characteristics of the cell. Artist's interpretation of cell structure.

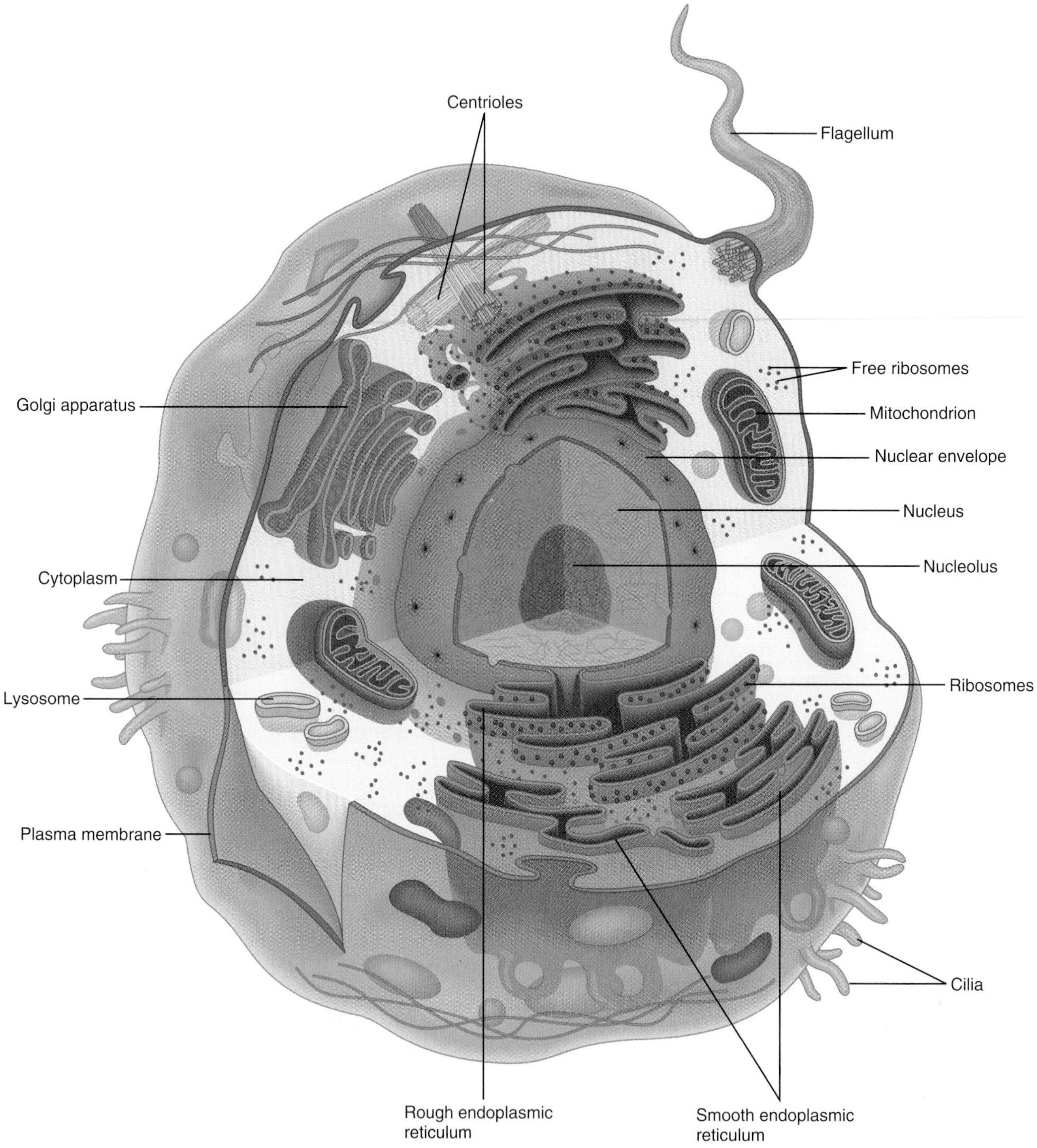

TABLE 3-1

Structure and Function of Some Major Cell Parts

CELL PART	STRUCTURE	FUNCTION(S)
Plasma membrane	Phospholipid bilayer studded with proteins	Serves as the boundary of the cell; protein and carbohydrate molecules on the outer surface of plasma membrane perform various functions; for example, they serve as markers that identify cells of each individual or as receptor molecules for certain hormones
Ribosomes	Tiny particles each made up of rRNA subunits	Synthesize proteins; a cell's "protein factories"
Endoplasmic reticulum (ER)	Membranous network of inter-connectedcanals and sacs, some with ribosomes attached (rough ER) and some without attachments (smooth ER)	Rough ER receives and transports reticulum (ER) synthesized proteins (from ribosomes); smooth ER synthesizes lipids and (rough ER) and some certain carbohydrates
Golgi apparatus	Stack of flattened, membranous sacs	Chemically processes, then packages substances from the ER
Mitochondria	Membranous capsule containing a large, folded membrane encrusted with enzymes	ATP synthesis; a cell's "powerhouses"
Lysosomes	"Bubble" of enzymes encased by membrane	A cell's "digestive system"
Centrioles	Pair of hollow cylinders, each made up of tiny tubules	Function in cell reproduction
Cilia	Short, hairlike extensions on a surface of some cells	Move substances over surface of the cell
Flagella	Single and much longer projection of some cells	The only example in humans is the "tail" of a sperm cell, propelling the sperm through fluids
Nucleus	Double-membraned, spherical envelope containing DNA strands	Dictates protein synthesis, thereby playing an essential role in other cell activities, namely active transport, metabolism, growth, and heredity
Nucleoli	Dense region of the nucleus	Play an essential role in the formation of ribosomes

Their nickname, "protein factories," indicates this function.

Endoplasmic reticulum. An **endoplasmic reticulum** (en-doe-PLAZ-mik ree-TIK-yoo-lum) (ER) is a system of membranes forming a network of connecting sacs and canals that wind back and forth through a cell's cytoplasm, all the way from the nucleus and almost to the plasma membrane. The tubular passageways or canals in the ER carry proteins and other substances through the cytoplasm of the cell from one area to another. There are two types of ER: *rough* and *smooth*. Rough ER gets its name from the fact that many ribosomes are attached to its outer surface, giving it a rough texture similar to sandpaper. As ribosomes make their proteins, they may attach to the rough ER and drop the protein into the interior of the ER. The ER then transports the proteins to areas where chemical processing takes place. These areas of the ER are so full that ribosomes do not attach to pass their proteins, giving this type of ER a smooth texture. Fats, carbohydrates, and proteins that make up cellular membrane material are manufactured in smooth ER. Thus the smooth ER makes new membrane for the cell. To sum up: rough ER receives and transports newly made proteins and smooth ER makes new membrane.

Golgi apparatus. The **Golgi** (GOL-jee) **apparatus** consists of tiny, flattened sacs stacked on one another near the nucleus. Little bubbles, or sacs, break off the smooth ER and carry new proteins and other compounds to the sacs of the Golgi apparatus. These little sacs, also called **vesicles,** fuse with the Golgi sacs and allow the contents of both to mingle. The Golgi apparatus chemically processes the molecules from the ER, and then packages them into little vesicles that break away from the Golgi apparatus and move slowly outward to the plasma membrane. Each vesicle fuses with the plasma membrane, opens to the outside of the cell, and releases its contents. An example of a Golgi apparatus product is the slippery substance called mucus. If we wanted to nickname the Golgi apparatus, we might call it the cell's "chemical processing and packaging center."

Mitochondria. **Mitochondria** (my-toe-KON-dree-ah) are another kind of organelle in all cells. Mitochondria are so tiny that a lineup of 15,000 or more of them would fill a space only about 2.5 cm or 1 inch long. Two membranous sacs, one inside the other, compose a mitochondrion. The inner membrane forms folds that look like miniature incomplete partitions. Within a mitochondrion's fragile walls, complex, energy-releasing chemical reactions occur continuously. Because these reactions supply most of the power for cellular work, mitochondria have been nicknamed the cell's "power plants." The survival of cells and therefore of the body depends on mitochondrial chemical reactions. Enzymes (molecules that promote specific chemical reactions), which are found in mitochondrial walls and inner substance, use oxygen to break down glucose and other nutrients to release energy required for cellular work. The process is called *aerobic* or *cellular respiration*. Each mitochondrion has its own DNA molecule, sometimes called a mitochondrial chromosome, which contains information for building and running the mitochondrion.

Lysosomes. The **lysosomes** (LYE-so-sohms) are membranous-walled organelles that in their active stage look like small sacs, often with tiny particles in them (see Figure 3-2). Because lysosomes contain enzymes that can digest food compounds, they have the nickname "digestive bags." Lysosomal enzymes can also digest substances other than foods. For example, they can digest and thereby destroy microbes that invade the cell. Thus lysosomes can protect cells against destruction by microbes. Formerly, scientists thought lysosomes were involved in programmed cell death. However, a different set of mechanisms has been found to be responsible for "cell suicide" or **apoptosis** (ap-oh-TOE-sis) that clears space for newer cells.

Centrioles. The **centrioles** (SEN-tree-olz) are paired organelles. Two of these rod-shaped structures exist in every cell. They are arranged so that they lie at right angles to each other (see Figure 3-2). Each centriole is composed of fine tubules that play an important role during cell division.

Cilia. **Cilia** (SIL-ee-ah) are extremely fine, almost hairlike extensions on the exposed or free surfaces of some cells. Cilia are organelles capable of movement. One cell may have a hundred or more cilia capable of moving together in a wavelike fashion over the surface of a cell. They often have highly specialized functions. For example, by moving as a group in one direction, they propel mucus upward over the cells that line the respiratory tract.

Flagella. A **flagellum** (flah-JEL-um) is a single projection extending from the cell surface. Flagella are much larger than cilia. In the human, the only example of a flagellum is the "tail" of the male sperm cell. Propulsive movements of the flagellum make it possible for sperm to "swim" or move toward the ovum after they are deposited in the female reproductive tract (Figure 3-3).

Nucleus

Viewed under a light microscope, the **nucleus** of a cell looks like a very simple structure—just a small sphere in the central portion of the cell. However, its simple appearance belies the complex and critical role it plays in cell function. The nucleus ultimately controls every organelle in the cytoplasm. It also controls the complex process of cell reproduction. In other words, the nucleus must function properly for a cell to accomplish its normal activities and be able to duplicate itself.

Note that the cell nucleus in Figure 3-2 is surrounded by a **nuclear envelope.** The envelope, made up of two separate membranes, encloses a special type of cell material in the nucleus called **nucleoplasm.** Nucleoplasm contains a number of specialized structures; two of the most important are shown in Figure 3-2. They are the **nucleolus** (noo-KLEE-oh-lus) and the **chromatin** (KRO-mah-tin) **granules.**

FIGURE 3-3

Human sperm. Note the tail-like flagellum on each sperm cell. The flagella are so long that they do not fit into the photograph at this magnification.

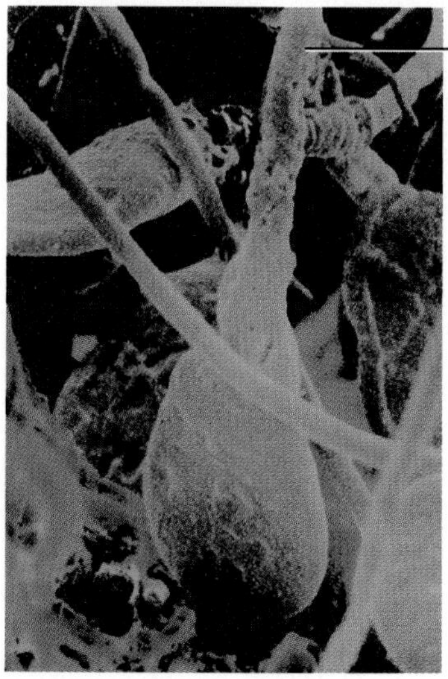

Nucleolus. The nucleolus is a dense region of the nuclear material that is critical in protein formation because it "programs" the formation of ribosomes in the nucleus. The ribosomes then migrate through the nuclear envelope into the cytoplasm of the cell and produce proteins.

Chromatin and chromosomes. Chromatin granules in the nucleus are threadlike structures made of proteins and hereditary molecules called **DNA** or **deoxyribonucleic** (dee-OK-see-rye-bo-noo-KLEE-ik) **acid.** DNA is the genetic material often described as the chemical "cookbook" of the body. Because it contains the code for building both structural proteins and functional proteins, DNA determines everything from gender and metabolism to body build and hair color in every human being. During cell division, DNA molecules become tightly coiled. They then look like short, compact structures and are called **chromosomes.** Each cell of the body contains a total of 46 different DNA molecules in its nucleus and one copy of a 47th DNA molecule in each of its mitochondria. The importance and function of DNA will be explained in greater detail in the section on cell reproduction later in this chapter.

Relationship of Cell Structure and Function

Every human cell performs certain functions; some maintain the cell's survival, and others help maintain the body's survival. In many instances, the number and type of organelles allow cells to differ dramatically in terms of their specialized functions. For example, cells that contain large numbers of mitochondria, such as heart muscle cells, are capable of sustained work. Why? Because the numerous mitochondria found in these cells supply the necessary energy required for rhythmic and ongoing contractions. Movement of the flagellum of a sperm cell is another example of the way a specialized organelle has a specialized function. The sperm's flagellum propels it through the reproductive tract of the female, thus increasing the chances of successful fertilization. This is how and why organizational structure at the cellular level is so important for function in living organisms. There are examples in every chapter of the text to illustrate how structure and function are intimately related at every level of body organization.

Quick Check

1. What is molecular structure of the plasma membrane of the cell?
2. What is cytoplasm? What does it contain?
3. List five major structures of the cell and briefly describe their function.
4. Which two kinds of cell structures contain DNA?

MOVEMENT OF SUBSTANCES THROUGH CELL MEMBRANES

The plasma membrane in every healthy cell separates the contents of the cell from the tissue fluid that surrounds it. At the same time the membrane must permit certain substances to enter the cell and allow others to leave. Heavy traffic moves continuously in both directions through cell membranes. Molecules of water, foods, gases, wastes, and many other substances stream in and out of all cells in endless procession. A number of processes allow this mass movement of substances into and out of cells. These transport processes are classified under two general headings:

1. Passive transport processes
2. Active transport processes

As implied by their name, active transport processes require the expenditure of energy by the cell, and

Science Applications

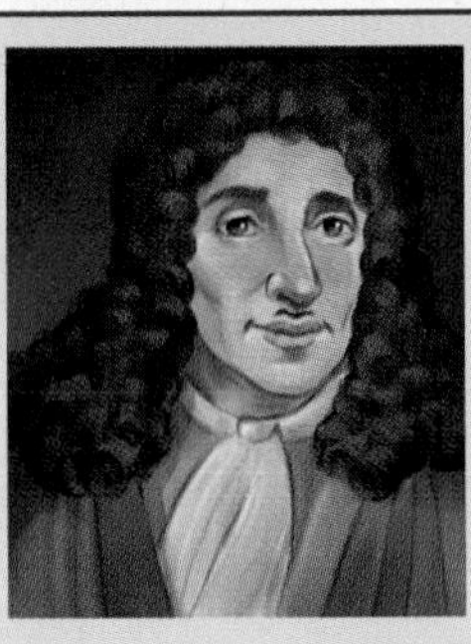

Microscopy

Antoni van Leeuwenhoek (1632–1723).

Until the very hour of his death in 1723, the Dutch drapery merchant Antoni van Leeuwenhoek (left) spent most of his 91 years pursuing adventures with the hundreds of microscopes he had built or collected. Using what were, even then, very simple lenses or combinations of lenses, van Leeuwenhoek discovered a whole world of tiny structures he called "animalcules" in body fluids. Although scientists a century later would declare that all living organisms are made up of cells, van Leeuwenhoek was the first to see and describe human blood cells (see Figure 3-18), human sperm cells (see Figure 3-3), and many other cells and tissues of the body. He was also the first to observe many microscopic organisms that live on or in the human body—many of which are capable of producing disease.

Today, many scientists use more advanced light microscopes (see figure) than van Leewenhoek did. Some modern microscopes called *electron microscopes* use electron beams instead of light to produce images of very high magnification (see Figure 3-13). Both cell biologists and *histologists* (tissue biologists) use microscopes to research the fine structure and function of the human body.

Many different professionals also use microscopy in a variety of practical applications. For example, clinical laboratory technicians and pathologists frequently use microscopes to assess the health of human cells and tissues. Most health professionals use microscopes, or at least images produced with microscopes, to perform routine duties. Even outside of the health sciences, professionals such as law enforcement investigators, archaeologists, anthropologists, paleontologists, and others often use microscopes to study human and animal tissues.

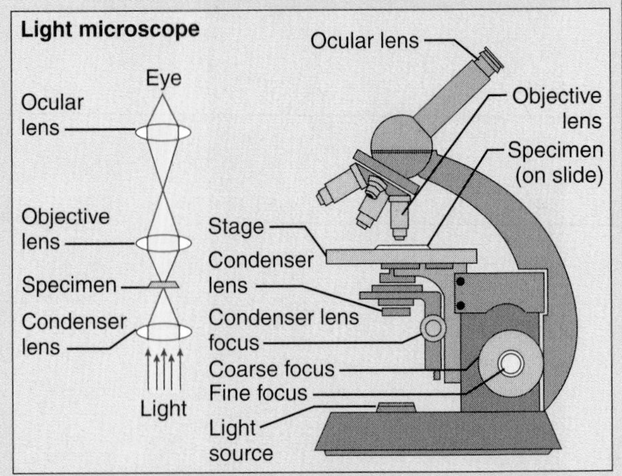

Modern compound light microscope.

passive transport processes do not. The energy required for active transport processes is obtained from a very important chemical substance called **adenosine triphosphate** (ah-DEN-o-sen tri-FOS-fate) or **ATP.** ATP is produced in the mitochondria using energy from nutrients and is capable of releasing that energy to do work in the cell. For active transport processes to occur, the breakdown of ATP and the use of the released energy are required.

The details of active and passive transport of substances across cell membranes are much easier to understand if you keep in mind the following two key facts: (1) in passive transport processes, no cellular energy is required to move substances from a high concentration to a low concentration; and (2) in active transport processes, cellular energy is required to move substances from a low concentration to a high concentration.

Passive Transport Processes

The primary passive transport processes that move substances through the cell membranes include the following:

1. Diffusion
   a. Osmosis
   b. Dialysis
2. Filtration

Scientists describe the movement of substances in passive systems as going "down a concentration gradient." This means that substances in passive systems move from a region of high concentration to a region of low concentration until they reach equal proportions on both sides of the membrane. As you read the next few paragraphs, refer to Table 3-2, which summarizes important information about passive transport processes.

TABLE 3-2

Passive Transport Processes

PROCESS	DESCRIPTION		EXAMPLES
Diffusion	Movement of particles through a membrane from an area of high concentration to an area of low concentration—that is, down the concentration gradient	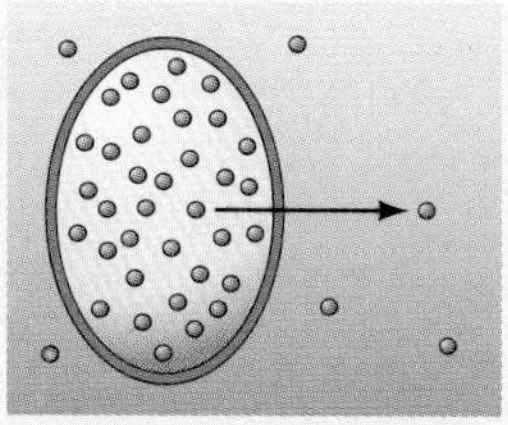	Movement of carbon dioxide out of all cells; movement of sodium ions into nerve cells as they conduct an impulse
Osmosis	Diffusion of water through a selectively permeable membrane in the presence of at least one impermeant solute	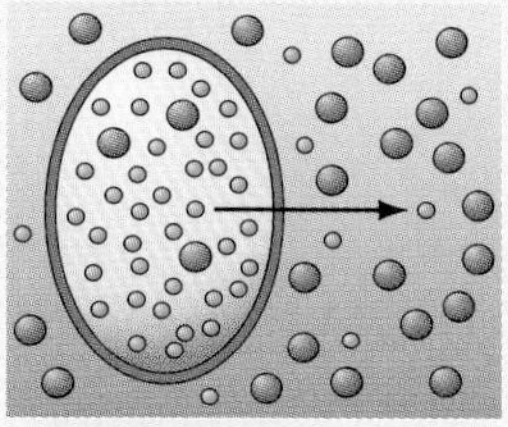	Diffusion of water molecules into and out of cells to correct imbalances in water concentration
Filtration	Movement of water and small solute particles, but not larger particles, through a filtration membrane; movement occurs from area of high pressure to area of low pressure	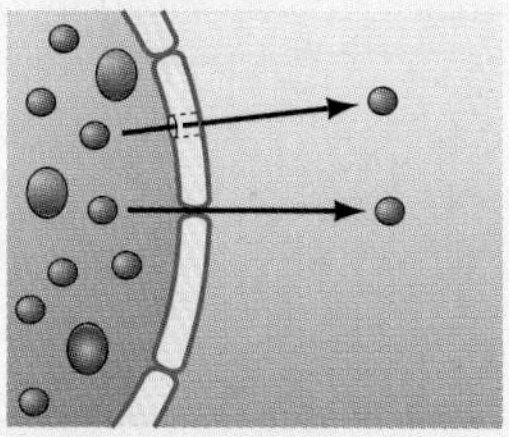	In the kidney, movement of water and small solutes from blood vessels but lack of movement by blood proteins and blood cells; begins the formation of urine

Diffusion

Diffusion is a good example of a passive transport process. Diffusion is the process by which substances scatter themselves evenly throughout an available space. The system does not require additional energy for this movement. To demonstrate diffusion of particles throughout a fluid, perform this simple experiment the next time you pour yourself a cup of coffee or tea. Place a cube of sugar on a teaspoon and lower it gently to the bottom of the cup. Let it stand for 2 or 3 minutes, and then, holding the cup steady, take a sip off the top. It will taste sweet. Why? Because some of the sugar molecules will have diffused from the area of high concentration near the sugar cube at the bottom of the cup to the area of low concentration at the top of the cup.

The process of diffusion is shown in Figure 3-4. Note that both substances diffuse rapidly through the membrane in both directions. However, as indicated by the green arrows, more glucose moves out of the 20% solution, where the concentration is higher, into the 10% solution, where the concentration is lower, than in the opposite direction. This is an example of movement down a concentration gradient. Simultaneously, more water moves from the 10% solution, where there are more water molecules, into the 20% solution, where there are fewer water molecules. This is also an example of movement down a concentration gradient. Water moves from high to low concentration. The result? Equilibration (balancing) of the concentrations of the two solutions after an interval of time. From then on, equal amounts of glucose will diffuse in both directions, as will equal amounts of water.

Osmosis and dialysis. **Osmosis** (os-MO-sis) and **dialysis** (dye-AL-i-sis) are specialized examples of diffusion. In both cases, diffusion occurs across a selectively permeable membrane. The plasma membrane of a cell is said to be selectively permeable because it permits the passage of certain substances but not others. This is a necessary property if the cell is to permit some substances, such as nutrients, to gain entrance to the cell while excluding others. Osmosis is the diffusion of *water* across a selectively permeable membrane when some of the **solutes** (substances dissolved in the water) cannot cross the membrane. However, in the case of dialysis, solutes do move across a selectively permeable membrane by diffusion.

FIGURE 3-4

Diffusion. Note that the membrane is permeable to glucose and water and that it separates a 10% glucose solution from a 20% glucose solution. The container on the left shows the two solutions separated by the membrane at the start of diffusion. The container on the right shows the result of diffusion over time.

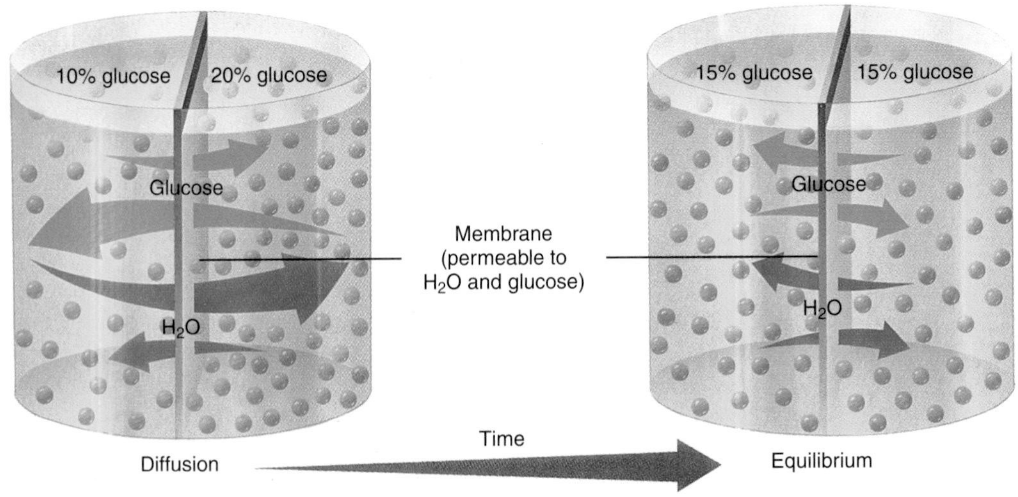

Filtration

Filtration is the movement of water and solutes through a membrane because of a greater pushing force on one side of the membrane than on the other side. The force is called *hydrostatic pressure,* which is simply the force or weight of a fluid pushing against some surface (e.g., blood pressure). A principle about filtration that is of great physiological importance is that it always occurs *down* a hydrostatic pressure gradient. This means that when two fluids have unequal hydrostatic pressures and are separated by a membrane, water and diffusible solutes or particles (those to which the membrane is permeable) filter out of the solution that has the higher hydrostatic pressure into the solution that has the lower hydrostatic pressure. Filtration is the process responsible for urine formation in the kidney; wastes are filtered out of the blood into the kidney tubules because of a difference in hydrostatic pressure.

Active Transport Processes

Active transport is the uphill movement of a substance through a living cell membrane. *Uphill* means "up a concentration gradient" (that is, from a lower to a higher concentration). The energy required for this movement is obtained from ATP. Because the formation and breakdown of ATP require complex cellular activity, active transport mechanisms can take place only through living membranes. Table 3-3 summarizes active transport processes.

Ion Pumps

A specialized cellular component called the *ion pump* makes possible a number of active transport mechanisms. An ion pump is a protein structure in the cell membrane called a *carrier*. The ion pump uses energy from ATP to actively move ions across cell membranes *against* their concentration gradients. "Pump" is an appropriate term because it

Clinical Application

Tonicity

A salt (NaCl) solution is said to be **isotonic** (*iso* = equal) if it contains the same concentration of salt normally found in a living red blood cell. A 0.9% NaCl solution is isotonic; that is, it contains the same level of NaCl as found in red cells. Salt particles (Na^+ and Cl^- ions) do not cross the plasma membrane easily, so salt solutions that differ in concentrations from the cell's fluid will promote the osmosis of water one way or the other. A solution that contains a higher level of salt than the cell does (above 0.9%) is said to be **hypertonic** (*hyper* = above) to the cell and one containing less salt (below 0.9%) is **hypotonic** (*hypo* = below) to the cell. With what you now know about filtration, diffusion, and osmosis, can you predict what would occur if red blood cells were placed in isotonic, hypotonic, and hypertonic solutions?

Examine the figures. Note that red blood cells placed in isotonic solution remain unchanged because there is no effective difference in salt or water concentrations. The movement of water into and out of the cells is about equal. This is not the case with red cells placed in hypertonic salt solution; they immediately lose water from their cytoplasm into the surrounding salty solution, and they shrink. This process is called **crenation.**

The opposite occurs if red cells are placed in a hypotonic solution; they swell as water enters the cell from the surrounding dilute solution. Eventually the cells break or **lyse,** and the hemoglobin they contain is released into the solution.

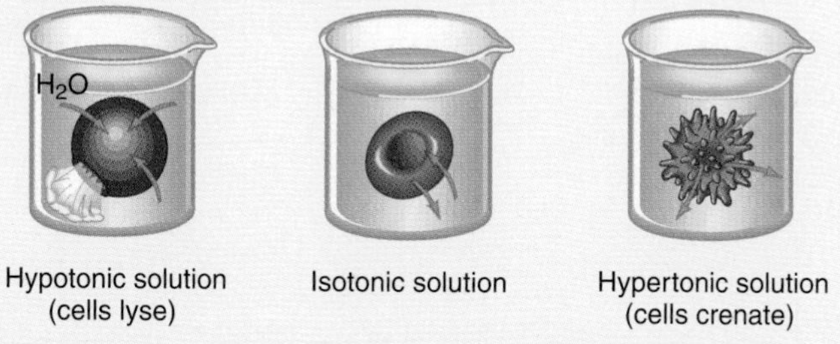

Hypotonic solution (cells lyse) | Isotonic solution | Hypertonic solution (cells crenate)

suggests that active transport moves a substance in an uphill direction just as a water pump, for example, moves water uphill.

Ion pumps are very specific, and different ion pumps are required to move different types of ions. For example, sodium pumps move sodium ions only. Likewise, calcium pumps move calcium ions, and potassium pumps move potassium ions.

Some ion pumps are "coupled" to one another so that two or more different substances may be moved through the cell membrane at one time. For example, the **sodium-potassium pump** shown in Figure 3-5 is an ion pump that pumps sodium ions out of a cell while it pumps potassium ions into the cell. Because both ions are moved against their concentration gradients, this pump creates a high sodium concentration outside the cell and a high potassium concentration inside the cell. Such a pump is required to remove sodium from the inside of a nerve cell after it has rushed in as a result of the passage of a nerve impulse. Some ion pumps are coupled with other specific carriers that transport glucose, amino acids, and other substances.

Phagocytosis and Pinocytosis

Phagocytosis (fag-o-sye-TOE-sis) is another example of how a cell can use its active transport mechanism to move an object or substance through the plasma membrane and into the cytoplasm. The term *phagocytosis* comes from a Greek word meaning "to eat." The word is appropriate because the phagocytosis process permits a cell to engulf and literally "eat" foreign material. Certain white blood cells destroy bacteria in the body by phagocytosis. During this process the cell membrane forms a pocket around the material to be moved

TABLE 3-3

Active Transport Processes

PROCESS	DESCRIPTION		EXAMPLES
Ion pump	Movement of solute particles from an area of low concentration to an area of high concentration (up the concentration gradient) by means of a carrier protein structure	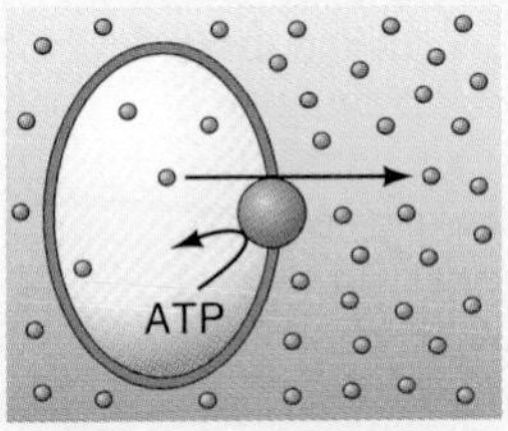	In muscle cells, pumping of nearly all calcium ions to special compartments—or out of the cell
Phagocytosis	Movement of cells or other large particles into cell by trapping it in a section of plasma membrane that pinches off inside the cell	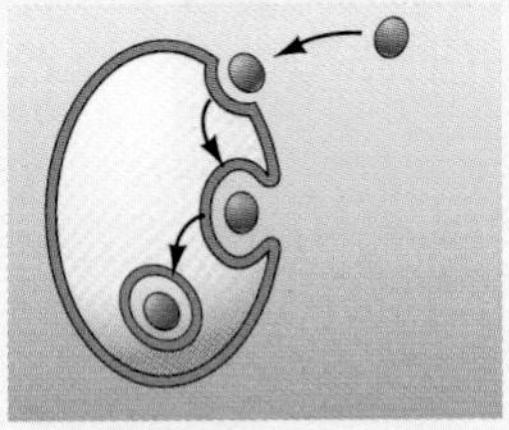	Trapping of bacterial cells by phagocytic white blood cells
Pinocytosis	Movement of fluid and dissolved molecules into a cell by trapping them in a section of plasma membrane that pinches off inside the cell	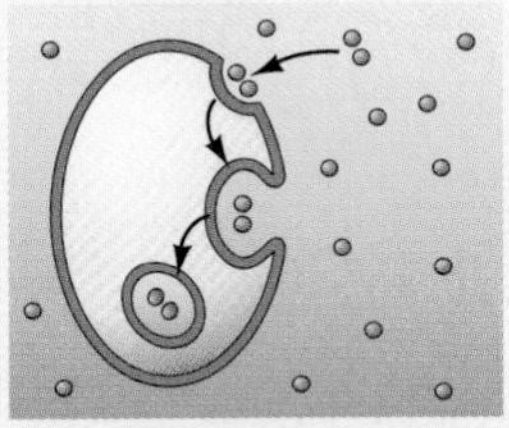	Trapping of large protein molecules by some body cells

into the cell and, by expenditure of energy from ATP, the object is moved to the interior of the cell. Once inside the cytoplasm, the bacterium fuses with a lysosome and is destroyed.

Pinocytosis (pin-o-sye-TOE-sis) is an active transport mechanism used to incorporate fluids or dissolved substances into cells by trapping them in a pocket of plasma membrane that pinches off inside the cell. Again, the term is appropriate because the word part *pino-* comes from the Greek word meaning "drink."

Quick CHECK

1. What is the difference between a passive transport process and an active transport process?
2. What is osmosis?
3. How does an ion pump work? Is it active or passive?
4. Can you describe the process of phagocytosis?

FIGURE 3-5

Sodium-potassium pump. Three sodium ions (Na^+) are pumped out of the cell and two potassium ions (K^+) are pumped into the cell during one pumping cycle of this carrier molecule. ATP is broken down in the process so that the energy freed from ATP can be used to pump the ions.

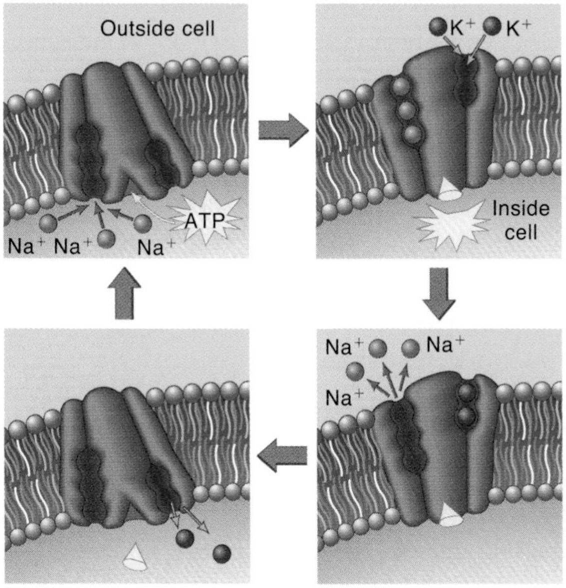

CELL REPRODUCTION AND HEREDITY

All human cells that reproduce do so by a process called **mitosis** (my-TOE-sis). During this process a cell divides to multiply; one cell divides to form two cells. Cell reproduction and, ultimately, the transfer of heritable traits is closely tied to the production of proteins. Two *nucleic acids*, **ribonucleic acid** or **RNA** in the cytoplasm and **deoxyribonucleic acid** or **DNA** in the nucleus play crucial roles in protein synthesis.

DNA Molecule and Genetic Information

Chromosomes, which are composed largely of DNA, make heredity possible. The "genetic information" contained in DNA molecules ultimately determines the transmission and expression of heritable traits such as skin color and blood group from each generation of parents to their children.

Structurally, the DNA molecule resembles a long, narrow ladder made of a pliable material. It is twisted round and round its axis, taking on the shape of a double helix. Each DNA molecule is made of many smaller units, namely, a sugar, bases, and phosphate units (Table 3-4). The bases are adenine, thymine, guanine, and cytosine. These nitrogen-containing chemicals are called bases because

TABLE 3-4

Components of Nucleotides

NUCLEOTIDE	DNA	RNA
Sugar	Deoxyribose	Ribose
Phosphate	Phosphate	Phosphate
Nitrogen base	Cytosine	Cytosine
	Guanine	Guanine
	Adenine	Adenine
	Thymine	Uracil

FIGURE 3-6

Protein synthesis. A, The DNA molecule contains a sequence of base pairs, or gene, that represents a sequence of amino acids. **B,** During transcription, the DNA code is "transcribed" as an mRNA molecule forms. **C,** During translation, the mRNA code is "translated" at the ribosome and the proper sequence of amino acids is assembled. The amino acid strand coils or folds as it is formed. **D,** The coiled amino acid strand folds again to form a protein molecule with a specific, complex shape.

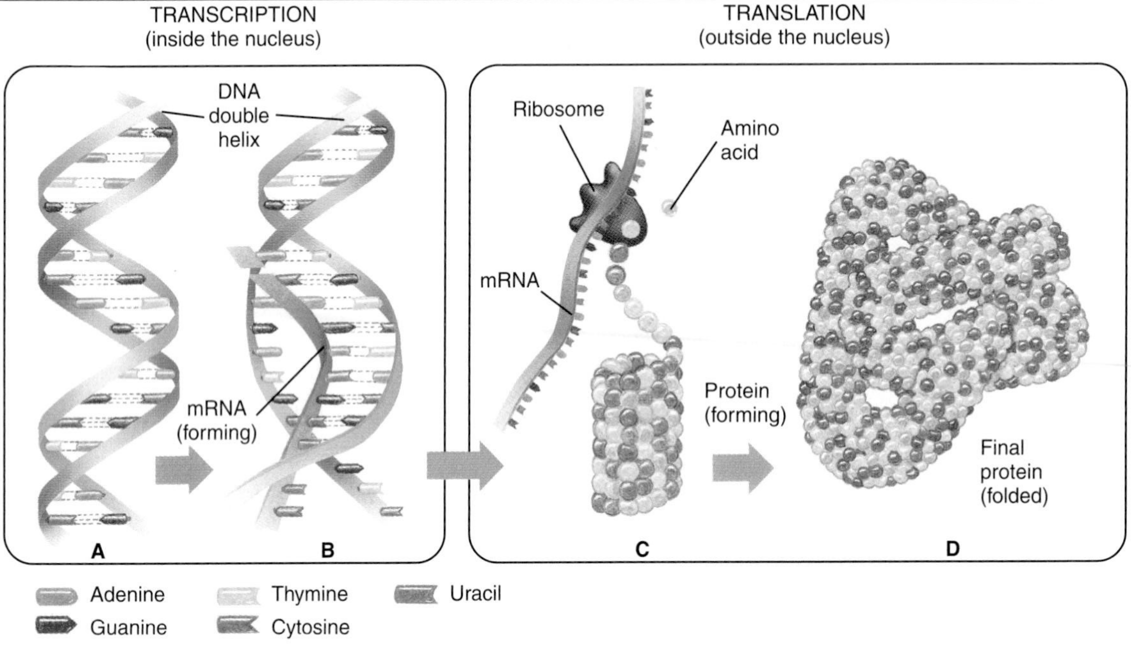

by themselves they have a high pH and chemicals with a high pH are called "bases" (see p. 27 for a discussion of acids and bases). As you can see in Figure 3-6, *A*, each step in the DNA ladder consists of a pair of bases. Only two combinations of bases occur, and the same two bases invariably pair off with each other in a DNA molecule. Adenine always binds to thymine, and cytosine always binds to guanine. This characteristic of DNA structure is called **complementary base pairing.**

A **gene** is a specific segment of base pairs in a chromosome. Although the types of base pairs in all chromosomes are the same, the order or *sequence* of base pairs is not the same. This fact has tremendous functional importance because it is the sequence of base pairs in each gene of each chromosome that determines heredity. Each gene directs the synthesis of one kind of protein molecule that may function, for example, as an enzyme, a structural component of a cell, or a specific hormone. In humans having 46 chromosomes in each body cell, the nuclear DNA has a content of genetic information totaling more than *3 billion* base pairs in 80,000 or so genes. This means that each parent contributes about one and half billion bits of genetic information in the 23 chromosomes he or she provides for the original cell of each offspring. Is it any wonder, then, with all of this genetic information packed into each of our cells, that no two of us inherit exactly the same traits?

Genetic Code

How do genes bring about heredity? There is, of course, no short and easy answer to that question. We know that the genetic information contained in each gene is capable of "directing" the synthesis of a specific protein. The unique sequence of a thousand or so base pairs in a gene determines the sequence of specific building blocks required to form a particular protein. This store of information in each gene is called the *genetic code*. In summary, the coded information in genes controls protein and enzyme production, enzymes facilitate cellular chemical reactions, and cellular chemical reactions determine cell structure and function and therefore heredity.

RNA Molecules and Protein Synthesis

DNA, with its genetic code that dictates directions for protein synthesis, is contained in the nucleus of the cell. The actual process of protein synthesis, however, occurs in ribosomes and on ER. Another specialized nucleic acid, ribonucleic acid or RNA, transfers this genetic information from the nucleus to the cytoplasm. (*Note:* If you are not familiar with the chemical structure of proteins or nucleic acids, you may want to review Chapter 2, Chemistry of Life, before reading further.)

Both RNA and DNA are composed of four bases, a sugar, and phosphate. RNA, however, is a single-stranded rather than a double-stranded molecule, and it contains a different sugar and base component. The base uracil replaces thymine.

The process of transferring genetic information from the nucleus into the cytoplasm, where proteins are actually produced, requires completion of two specialized steps called **transcription** and **translation.**

Transcription. During transcription the double-stranded DNA molecule separates or unwinds, and a special type of RNA called **messenger RNA** or **mRNA** is formed (Figure 3-6, *B*). Each strand of mRNA is a duplicate or copy of a particular gene sequence along one of the newly separated DNA spirals. The messenger RNA is said to have been "transcribed" or copied from its DNA mold or template. The mRNA molecules pass from the nucleus to the cytoplasm to direct protein synthesis in the ribosomes and ER.

Translation. *Translation* is the synthesis of a protein by ribosomes, which use the information contained in an mRNA molecule to direct the choice and sequencing of the appropriate chemical building blocks called *amino acids* (Figure 3-6, *C*). As amino acids are assembled into their proper sequence by a ribosome, a protein strand forms. This strand then folds on itself and perhaps even combines with another strand to form a complete protein molecule. The specific, complex shape of each type of protein molecule allows the molecule to perform specific functions in the cell. It is clear that because DNA directs the shape of each protein, DNA also directs the function of each protein in a cell.

Research, Issues & Trends

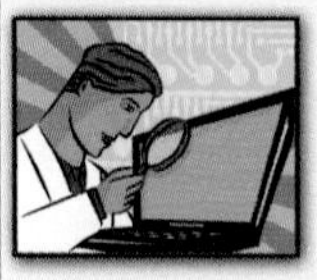

Human Genome

All of the DNA in each cell of the body is called the **genome** (JEE-nome). An intense, coordinated effort recently mapped all the gene locations in the human genome. Efforts at reading the different genetic codes possible at each location are still underway. Much of the work of mapping the human genome was done as part of the Human Genome Project (HGP), which was started in 1990. Besides producing a complete human genetic map and developing tools of genetic mapping, a field called *genomics*, HGP also addresses the ethical, legal, and social issues that may arise—a notable first for such a massive scientific research effort. HGP is sponsored by the Department of Energy (DOE) and the National Institutes of Health (NIH), and its first director was James Watson, one of the scientists credited with originally discovering the structure of the DNA molecule in 1953. With the human genome already mapped, many scientists are working to fill in the details of the many genes and gene variants found in the human genome. Many are also working in the emerging field of *proteomics*—the study of all the proteins encoded by each of the genes of the human genome.

Cell Division

The process of cell reproduction involves the division of the nucleus (mitosis) and the cytoplasm. After the process is complete, two daughter cells result; both have the same genetic material as the cell that preceded them. As you can see in Figure 3-7, the specific and visible stages of cell division are preceded by a period called **interphase** (IN-ter-faze). During interphase the cell is said to be "resting." However, it is resting only from the standpoint of active cell division. In all other aspects it is exceedingly active. During interphase and just before mitosis begins, the DNA of each chromosome replicates itself.

DNA Replication

DNA molecules possess a unique ability that no other molecules in the world have. They can make copies of themselves, a process called **DNA replication.** Before a cell divides to form two new cells, each DNA molecule in its nucleus forms another DNA molecule just like itself. When a DNA molecule is not replicating, it has the shape of a tightly coiled double helix. As it begins replication, short segments of the DNA molecule uncoil and the two strands of the molecule pull apart between their base pairs. The separated strands therefore contain unpaired bases. Each unpaired base in each of the two separated strands attracts its complementary base (in the nucleoplasm) and binds to it. Specifically, each adenine attracts and binds to a thymine, and each cytosine attracts and binds to a guanine. These steps are repeated over and over throughout the length of the DNA molecule. Thus each half of a DNA molecule becomes a whole DNA molecule identical to the original DNA molecule. After DNA replication is complete, the cell continues to grow until it is ready for the first phase of mitosis.

FIGURE 3-7

Mitosis. For simplicity, only four chromosomes are shown in the diagram.

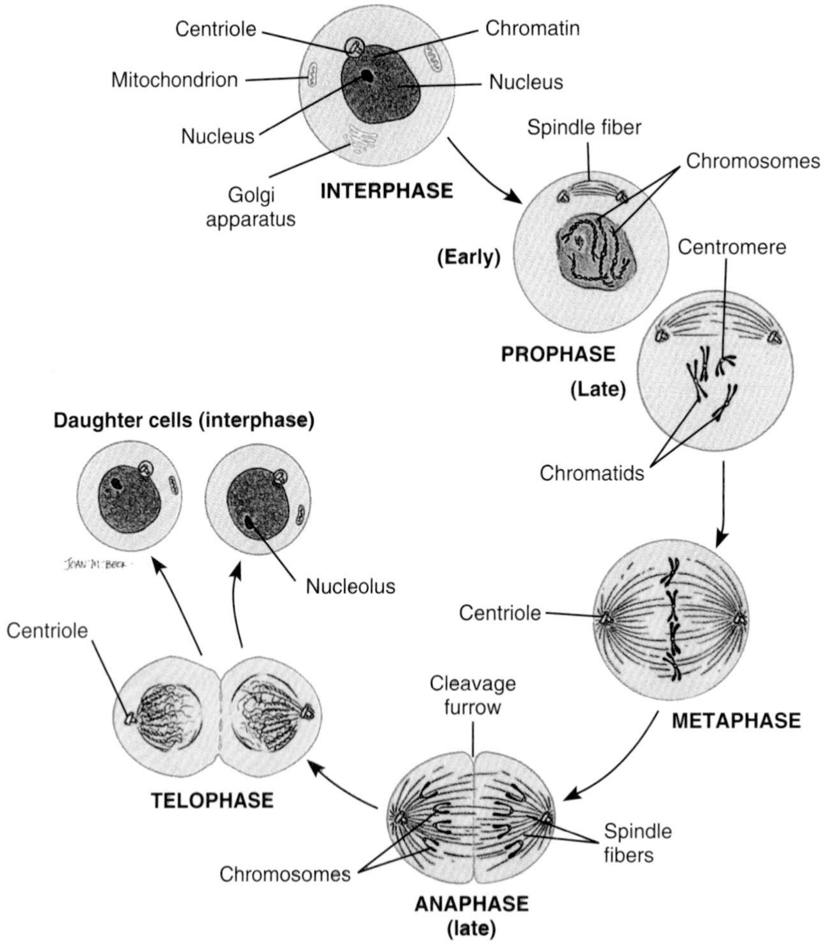

Prophase

Look at Figure 3-7 and note the changes that identify the first stage of mitosis, prophase (PRO-faze). The chromatin becomes "organized." Chromosomes in the nucleus have formed two strands called **chromatids** (KRO-mah-tids). Note that the two chromatids are held together by a beadlike structure called the **centromere** (SEN-tro-meer). In the cytoplasm the centrioles are moving away from each other as a network of tubules called **spindle fibers** forms between them. These spindle fibers serve as "guidewires" and assist the chromosomes to move toward opposite ends of the cell later in mitosis.

Metaphase

By the time metaphase (MET-ah-faze) begins, the nuclear envelope and nucleolus have disappeared. Note in Figure 3-7 the chromosomes have aligned themselves across the center of the cell. Also, the centrioles have migrated to opposite ends of the cell, and spindle fibers are attached to each chromatid.

Anaphase

As anaphase (AN-ah-faze) begins, the beadlike centromeres, which were holding the paired chromatids together, break apart. As a result, the individual chromatids, identified once again as chromosomes, move away from the center of the cell. Movement of chromosomes occurs along spindle fibers toward the centrioles. Note in Figure 3-7 that chromosomes are being pulled to opposite ends of the cell. A **cleavage furrow** that begins to divide the cell into two daughter cells can be seen for the first time at the end of anaphase.

Telophase

During telophase (TEL-o-faze) cell division is completed. Two nuclei appear, and chromosomes become less distinct and appear to break up. As the nuclear envelope forms around the chromatin, the cleavage furrow completely divides the cell into two parts. Before division is complete, each nucleus is surrounded by cytoplasm in which organelles have been equally distributed. By the end of telophase, two separate daughter cells, each having identical genetic characteristics, are formed. Each cell is fully functional and will perhaps itself undergo mitosis in the future.

Results of Cell Division

Mitosis results in the production of identical new cells. In the adult, mitosis replaces cells that have become less functional with age or have been damaged or destroyed by illness or injury. During periods of body growth, mitosis allows groups of similar cells to differentiate, or develop into different **tissues.**

If the body loses its ability to control mitosis, an abnormal mass of proliferating cells develops. This mass is a **neoplasm** (NEE-o-plazm). Neoplasms may be relatively harmless growths called *benign* (be-NINE) *tumors* or dangerous and *malignant* (mah-LIG-nant) cancerous growths. The stages of mitosis are listed in Table 3-5 with descriptions of changes that occur during each stage.

TABLE 3-5

Stages of Cell Division

STAGE	CHARACTERISTICS
Prophase	The chromatin condenses into visible chromosomes Chromatids become attached at the centromere Spindle fibers appear The nucleolus and nuclear envelope disappear
Metaphase	Spindle fibers attach to each chromatid Chromosomes align across the center of the cell
Anaphase	Centromeres break apart Chromosomes move away from the center of the cell The cleavage furrow appears
Telophase	The nuclear envelope and both nuclei appear The cytoplasm and organelles divide equally The process of cell division is completed

Quick

1. How do genes determine the structure and function of the body?
2. Where in the cell is genetic information stored?
3. What are the main steps to making a protein in the cell?
4. What are the four phases of mitotic cell division?

TISSUES

The four main kinds of tissues that compose the body's many organs follow:

1. Epithelial tissue
2. Connective tissue
3. Muscle tissue
4. Nervous tissue

Tissues differ from each other in the size and shape of their cells, in the amount and kind of material between the cells, and in the special functions they perform to help maintain the body's survival. In Tables 3-6 through 3-8, you will find a listing of the four major tissues and the various subtypes of each. The tables also include the structure of each subtype along with examples of the location of the tissues and a primary function of each tissue type.

Epithelial Tissue

Epithelial (ep-i-THEE-lee-al) **tissue** covers the body and many of its parts. It also lines various parts of the body. Because epithelial cells are packed close together with little or no intercellular material between them, they form continuous sheets that contain no blood vessels. Examine Figure 3-8. It illustrates how this large group of tissues can be subdivided according to the **shape** and **arrangement** of the cells found in each type.

TABLE 3-6

Epithelial Tissues

TISSUE	STRUCTURE	LOCATION(S)	FUNCTION(S)
Simple squamous	Single layer of flattened cells	Alveoli of lungs	Diffusion of respiratory gases between alveolar air and blood
		Lining of blood and lymphatic vessels	Diffusion, filtration, and osmosis
Stratified squamous	Many layers; outermost layer(s) are flattened cells	Surface of lining of mouth and esophagus	Protection
		Surface of skin (epidermis)	Protection
Simple columnar	Single layer of tall, narrow cells	Surface layer of lining of stomach, intestines, parts of respiratory tract	Protection, secretion, transport (absorption)
Stratified	Many layers of varying transitional shapes, capable of stretching	Urinary bladder	Protection
Pseudostratified	Single layer of tall cells that wedge together to appear as if there are two or more layers	Surface of lining of trachea	Protection
Simple cuboidal	Single layer of cells that are as tall as they are wide	Glands, kidney tubules	Secretion, absorption

Shape of Cells

If classified according to shape, epithelial cells are:

1. Squamous (flat and scalelike)
2. Cuboidal (cube shaped)
3. Columnar (higher than they are wide)
4. Transitional (varying shapes that can stretch)

Arrangement of Cells

If categorized according to arrangement of cells, epithelial tissue can be classified as the following:

1. Simple (a single layer of cells of the same shape)
2. Stratified (many layers of cells; named for the shape of cells in the outer layer)

Several types of epithelium are described in the paragraphs that follow and are illustrated in Figures 3-9 to 3-12.

Simple Squamous Epithelium

Simple squamous (SKWAY-mus) **epithelium** consists of a single layer of very thin and irregularly shaped cells. Because of its structure, substances can readily pass through simple squamous epithelial tissue, making transport its special function. Absorption of oxygen into the blood, for example, takes place through the simple squamous epithelium that forms the tiny air sacs in the lungs (Figure 3-9).

Stratified Squamous Epithelium

Stratified squamous epithelium (Figure 3-10) consists of several layers of closely packed cells, an arrangement that makes this tissue a specialist at protection. For instance, stratified squamous epithelial tissue protects the body against invasion

TABLE 3-7

Connective Tissues

TISSUE	STRUCTURE	LOCATION(S)	FUNCTION(S)
Areolar	Loose arrangement of fibers and cells	Area between other tissues and organs	Connection
Adipose (fat)	Cells contain large fat compartments	Area under skin Padding at various points	Protection Insulation, support, nutrient reserve
Dense fibrous	Dense arrangement of collagen fiber bundles	Tendons, ligaments, fascia, scar tissue	Flexible but strong connection
Bone	Hard, calcified matrix arranged in osteons	Skeleton	Support, protection
Cartilage	Hard but flexible matrix with imbedded chondrocytes	Part of nasal septum, area covering articular surfaces of bones, larynx, rings in trachea and bronchi Disks between vertebrae External ear	Firm but flexible support Withstand pressure Flexible support
Blood	Liquid matrix with flowing red and white cells	Blood vessels	Transportation
Hemopoietic	Liquid matrix with dense arrangement of blood cell–producing cells	Red bone marrow	Blood cell formation

TABLE 3-8

Muscle and Nervous Tissue

TISSUE	STRUCTURE	LOCATION(S)	FUNCTION(S)
MUSCLE			
Skeletal (striated voluntary)	Long, threadlike cells with multiple nuclei and striations	Muscles that attach to bones	Maintenance of posture, movement of bones
		Eyeball muscles	Eye movements
		Upper third of esophagus	First part of swallowing
Cardiac (striated involuntary)	Branching, interconnected cylinders with faint striations	Wall of heart	Contraction of heart
Smooth (nonstriated involuntary or visceral)	Threadlike cells with single nuclei and no striations	Walls of tubular viscera of digestive, respiratory, and genitourinary tracts	Movement of substances along respective tracts
		Walls of blood vessels and large lymphatic vessels	Changing of diameter of vessels
		Ducts of glands	Movement of substances along ducts
		Intrinsic eye muscles (iris and ciliary body)	Changing of diameter of pupils and shape of lens
		Arrector muscles of hairs	Erection of hairs (goose pimples)
NERVOUS			
	Nerve cells with large cell bodies and thin fiberlike extensions; supportive glial cells also present	Brain, spinal cord, nerves	Irritability, conduction

by microorganisms. Most microbes cannot work their way through a barrier of stratified squamous tissue such as that which composes the surface of skin and of mucous membranes.

One way of preventing infections, therefore, is to take good care of your skin. Don't let it become cracked from chapping, and guard against cuts and scratches.

Simple Columnar Epithelium

Simple columnar epithelium can be found lining the inner surface of the stomach, intestines, and some areas of the respiratory and reproductive tracts. In Figure 3-11 the simple columnar cells are arranged in a single layer lining the inner surface of the colon or large intestine. These epithelial cells are higher than they are wide, and the nuclei are located toward the bottom of each cell. The "open spaces" among the cells are specialized **goblet cells** that produce mucus. The regular columnar-shaped cells specialize in absorption.

Stratified Transitional Epithelium

Stratified transitional epithelium is typically found in body areas subjected to stress and must be able to stretch; an example would be the wall of

FIGURE 3-8

Classification of epithelial tissues. The tissues are classified according to the shape and arrangement of cells.

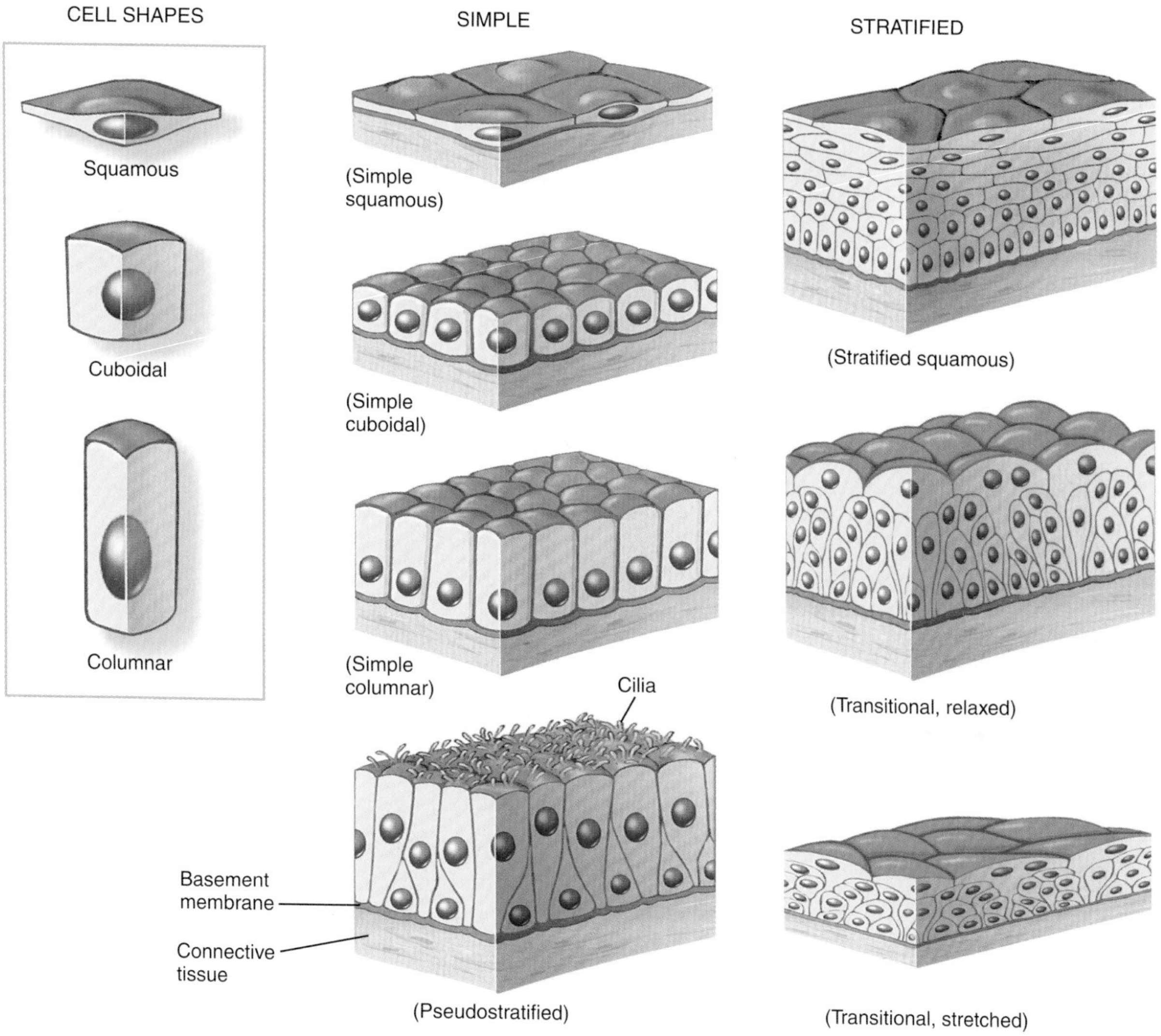

the urinary bladder. In many instances, up to 10 layers of differently shaped cells of varying sizes are present in the absence of stretching. When stretching occurs, the epithelial sheet expands, the number of cell layers decreases, and cell shape changes from roughly cuboidal to nearly squamous (flat) in appearance. The fact that transitional epithelium has this ability keeps the bladder wall from tearing under the pressures of stretching. Stratified transitional epithelium is shown in Figures 3-8 and 3-12.

Pseudostratified Epithelium

Pseudostratified epithelium, illustrated in Figure 3-8, is typical of that which lines the trachea or windpipe. Look carefully at the illustration.

FIGURE 3-9

Simple squamous and simple cuboidal epithelium. A, Photomicrograph shows thin simple squamous epithelium forming some tubules (arrows) and simple cuboidal epithelium forming the walls of other tubules. **B,** Sketch of photomicrograph.

A

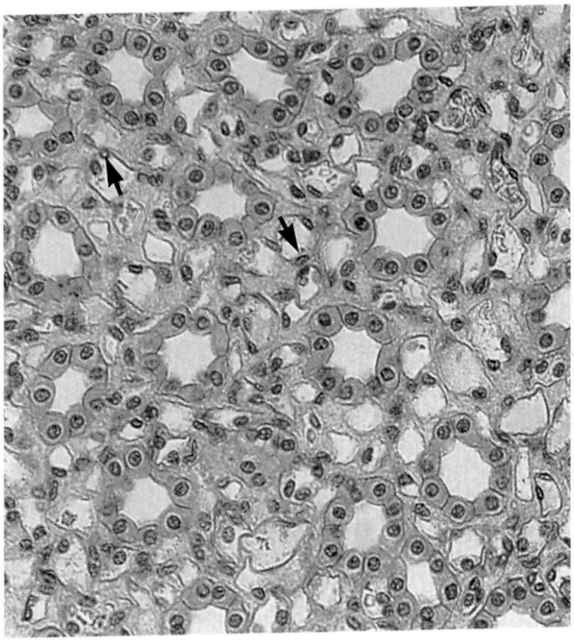

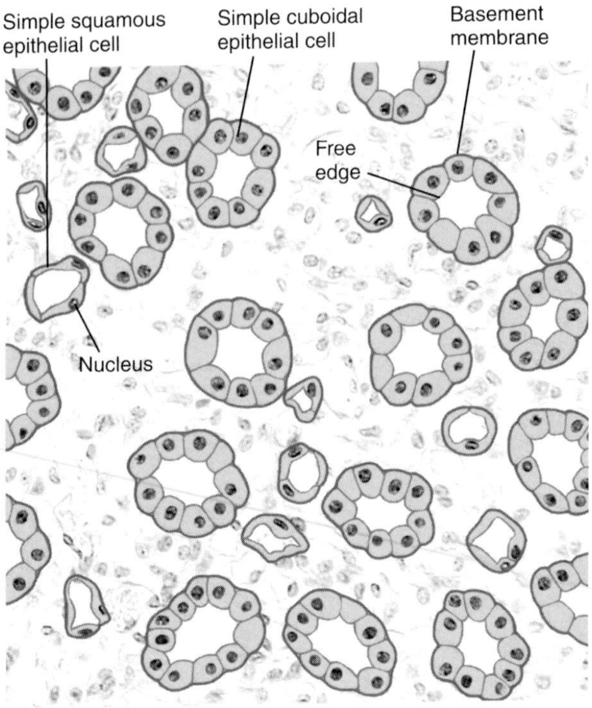

B

Note that each cell actually touches the gluelike **basement membrane** that lies under all epithelial tissues. Although the epithelium in Figure 3-8 (pseudostratified) appears to be two cell layers thick, it is not—which is why it is called *pseudo* (or false) stratified epithelium. The cilia that extend from the cells are capable of moving in unison. In doing so, they move mucus along the lining surface of the trachea, thus affording protection against entry of dust or foreign particles into the lungs.

Cuboidal Epithelium

Simple cuboidal epithelium does not form protective coverings but instead forms tubules or other groupings specialized for secretory activity (Figure 3-13). Secretory cuboidal cells usually function in clusters or tubes of secretory cells commonly called glands. Glands of the body may be classified as exocrine if they release their secretion through a duct or as endocrine if they release their secretion directly into the bloodstream. Examples of glandular secretions include saliva produced by the salivary glands, digestive juices, sweat or perspiration, and hormones such as those secreted by the pituitary or thyroid glands. Simple cuboidal epithelium also forms the tubules that form urine in the kidneys.

Connective Tissue

Connective tissue is the most abundant and widely distributed tissue in the body. It also exists in more varied forms than any of the other

FIGURE 3-10

Stratified squamous epithelium. A, Photomicrograph. **B,** Sketch of the photomicrograph. Note the many layers of epithelial cells and the flattened (squamous) cells in the outer layers.

A

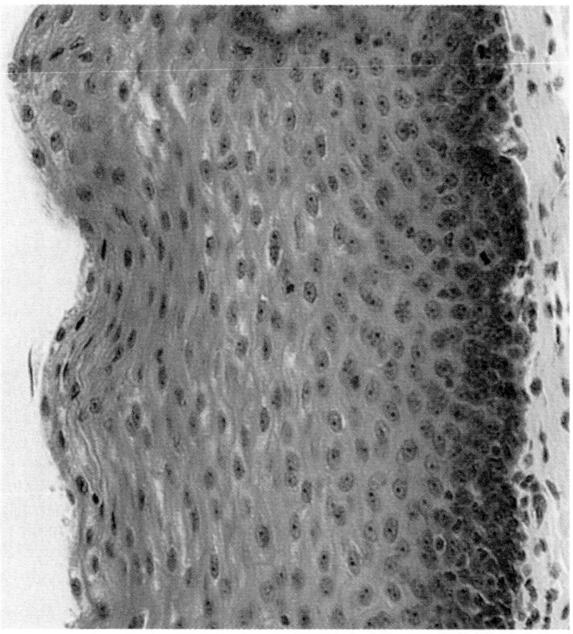

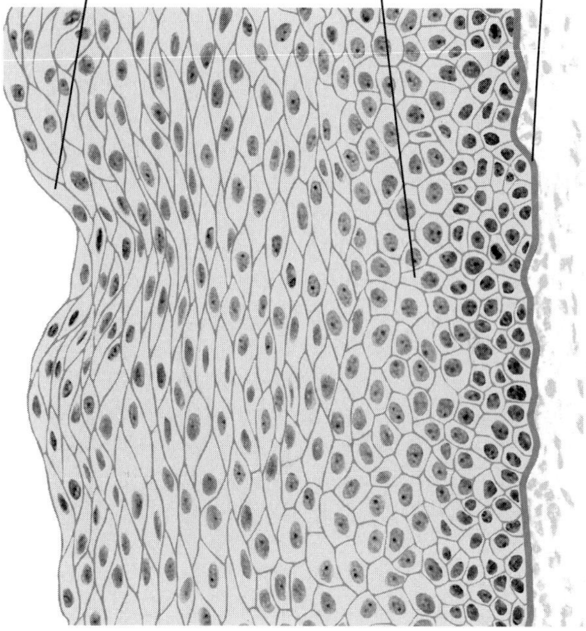

B

tissue types. It is found in skin, membranes, muscles, bones, nerves, and all internal organs. Connective tissue exists as delicate, paper-thin webs that hold internal organs together and give them shape. It also exists as strong and tough cords, rigid bones, and even in the form of a fluid—blood.

The functions of connective tissue are as varied as its structure and appearance. It connects tissues to each other and forms a supporting framework for the body as a whole and for its individual organs. As blood, it transports substances throughout the body. Several other kinds of connective tissue function to defend us against microbes and other invaders.

Connective tissue differs from epithelial tissue in the arrangement and variety of its cells and in the amount and kinds of intercellular material, called matrix, found between its cells. In addition to the relatively few cells embedded in the matrix of most types of connective tissue, varying numbers and kinds of fibers are also present. The structural quality and appearance of the matrix and fibers determine the qualities of each type of connective tissue. The matrix of blood, for example, is a liquid, but other types of connective tissue, such as cartilage, have the consistency of firm rubber. The matrix of bone is hard and rigid, although the matrix of connective tissues such as tendons and ligaments is strong and flexible.

The following list identifies a number of the major types of connective tissue in the body. Photomicrographs of several are also shown.

FIGURE 3-11

Simple columnar epithelium. A, Photomicrograph. **B,** Sketch of the photomicrograph. Note the oblong nuclei in all the cells and the goblet or mucus-producing cells that are present.

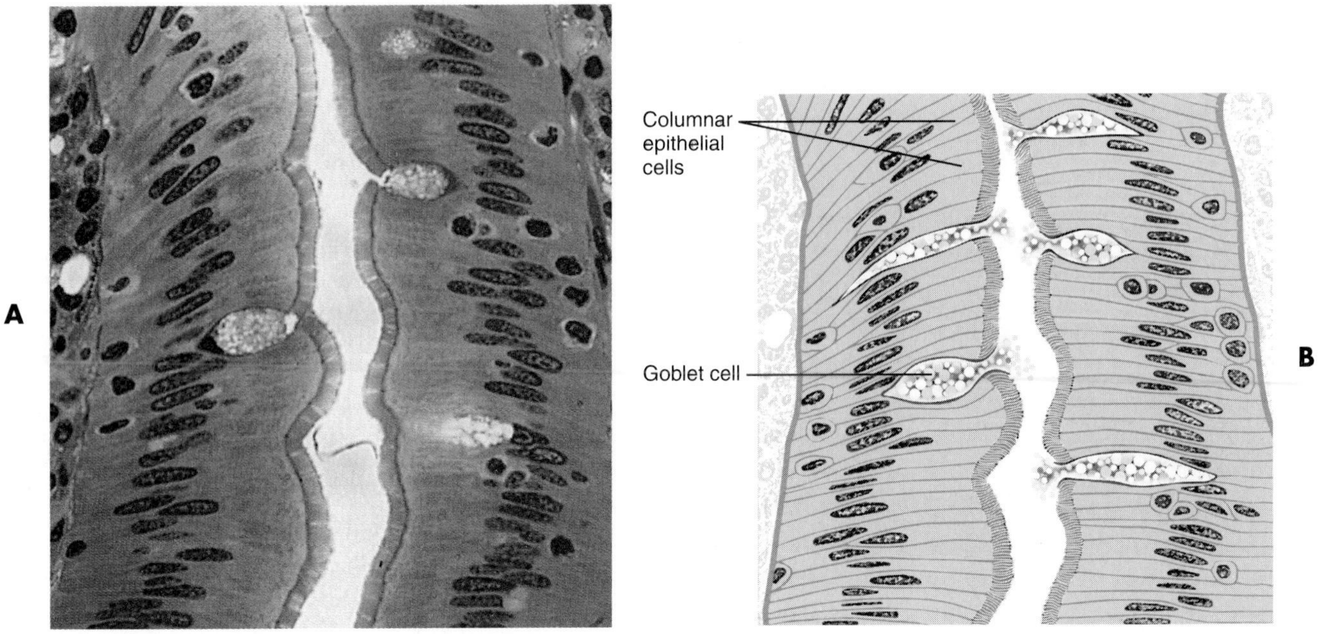

1. Areolar connective tissue
2. Adipose or fat tissue
3. Fibrous connective tissue
4. Bone
5. Cartilage
6. Blood
7. Hemopoietic tissue

Areolar and Adipose Connective Tissue

Areolar (ah-REE-o-lar) **connective tissue** is the most widely distributed of all connective tissue types. It is the "glue" that gives form to the internal organs. It consists of delicate webs of fibers and of a variety of cells embedded in a loose matrix of soft, sticky gel.

Adipose (AD-i-pose), or **fat tissue,** is specialized to store lipids. In Figure 3-14, numerous spaces have formed in the tissue so that large quantities of fat can accumulate inside cells.

Fibrous Connective Tissue

Fibrous connective tissue (Figure 3-15) consists mainly of bundles of strong, white **collagen** fibers arranged in parallel rows. This type of connective tissue composes tendons. It provides great strength and flexibility but it does not stretch. Such characteristics are ideal for these structures that anchor our muscles to our bones.

Bone and Cartilage

Bone is one of the most highly specialized forms of connective tissue. The matrix of bone is hard and calcified. It forms numerous structural building blocks called **osteons** (AHS-tee-onz), or *Haversian* (ha-VER-shan) *systems*. When bone is viewed under a microscope, we can see these circular arrangements of calcified matrix and cells that give bone its characteristic appearance (Figure 3-16). Bones are a

FIGURE 3-12

Stratified transitional epithelium. A, Photomicrograph of tissue lining the urinary bladder wall. **B,** Sketch of the photomicrograph. Note the many layers of epithelial cells of various shapes.

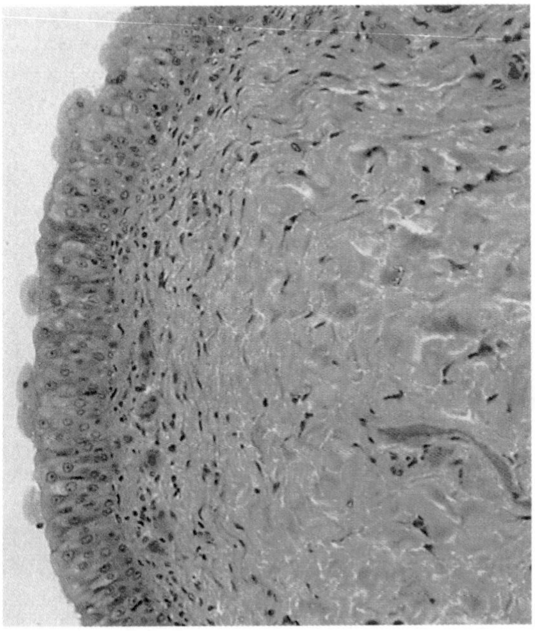

A

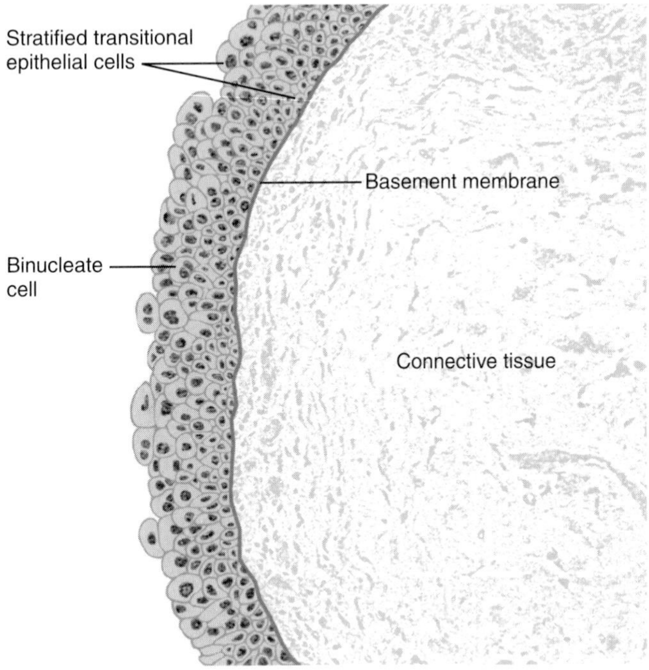

B

storage area for calcium and provide support and protection for the body.

Cartilage differs from bone in that its matrix is the consistency of a firm plastic or a gristlelike gel. Cartilage cells, which are called **chondrocytes** (KON-dro-sites), are located in many tiny spaces distributed throughout the matrix (Figure 3-17).

Blood and Hemopoietic Tissue

Because its matrix is liquid, **blood** is perhaps the most unusual form of connective tissue. It has transportational and protective functions in the body. Red and white blood cells are the cell types common to blood (Figure 3-18).

Hemopoietic (hee-mo-poy-ET-ik) **tissue** is the bloodlike connective tissue found in the red marrow cavities of bones and in organs such as the spleen, tonsils, and lymph nodes. This type of tissue is responsible for the formation of blood cells and lymphatic system cells important in our defense against disease (Table 3-7).

Muscle Tissue

Muscle cells are the movement specialists of the body. They have a higher degree of contractility (ability to shorten or contract) than any other tissue cells. Unfortunately, injured muscle cells are often slow to heal and are frequently replaced by scar tissue if injured. There are three kinds of muscle tissue: **skeletal, cardiac,** and **smooth.**

Skeletal Muscle Tissue

Skeletal or striated muscle is called voluntary because willed or *voluntary* control of skeletal muscle contractions is possible. Note in Figure 3-19 that, when viewed under a microscope, skeletal muscle is characterized by many cross striations and many

FIGURE 3-13

Simple cuboidal epithelium. This scanning electron micrograph shows how a single layer of cuboidal cells can form glands. The secreting cells arrange themselves into single or branched tubules that open onto a surface—the lining of the stomach in this case.

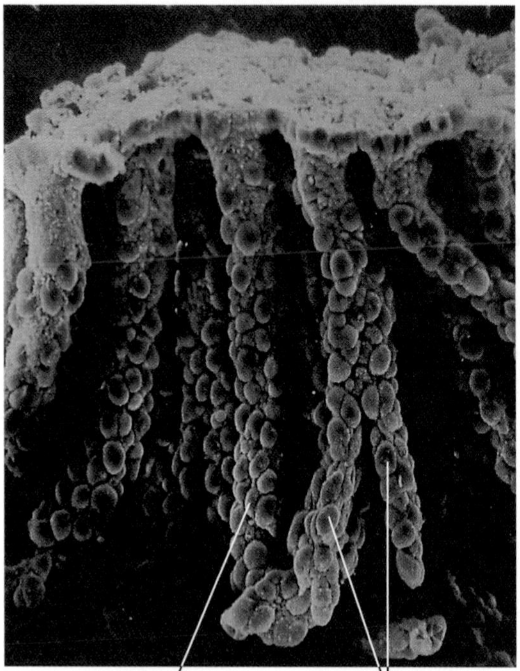

FIGURE 3-14

Adipose tissue. Photomicrograph showing the large storage spaces for fat inside the adipose tissue cells.

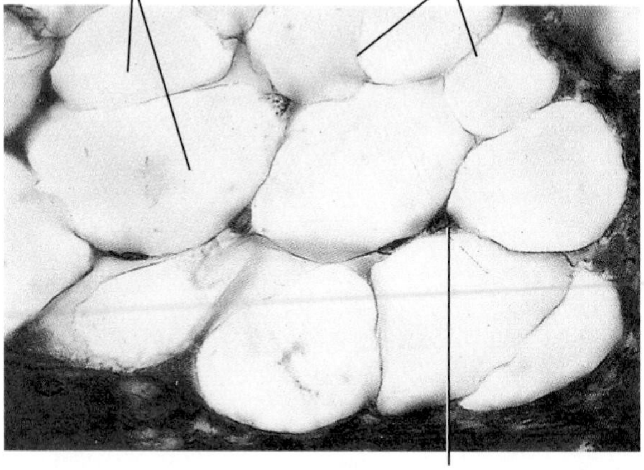

FIGURE 3-15

Dense fibrous connective tissue. Photomicrograph of tissue in the tendon. Note the multiple bundles of collagenous fibers (stained red) in a parallel arrangement.

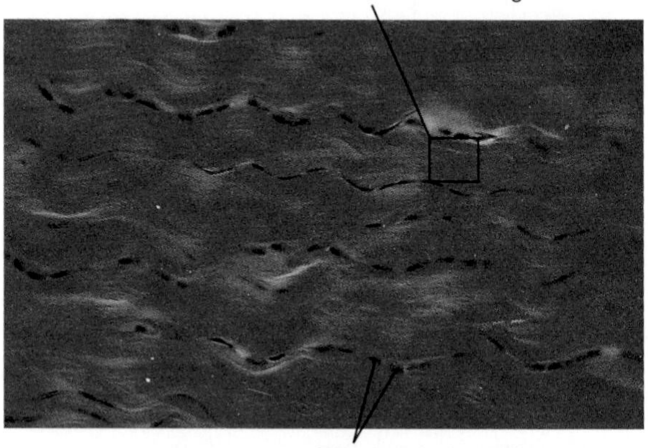

nuclei per cell. Individual cells are long and threadlike and are often called *fibers*. Skeletal muscles are attached to bones and when contracted produce voluntary and controlled body movements.

Cardiac Muscle Tissue

Cardiac muscle forms the walls of the heart, and the regular but involuntary contractions of cardiac muscle produce the heartbeat. Under the light microscope (Figure 3-20), cardiac muscle fibers have faint cross striations (as in skeletal muscle) and thicker dark bands called *intercalated disks*. Cardiac muscle fibers branch and reform to produce an interlocking mass of contractile tissue.

Smooth Muscle Tissue

Smooth (visceral) muscle is said to be involuntary because it is not under conscious or willful control. Under a microscope (Figure 3-21), smooth muscle cells are seen as long, narrow fibers but not nearly as long as skeletal or striated fibers. Individual

FIGURE 3-16

Bone tissue. Photomicrograph of dried, ground bone. A wheel-like structural unit of bone, known as an osteon (Haversian system), is apparent in this section.

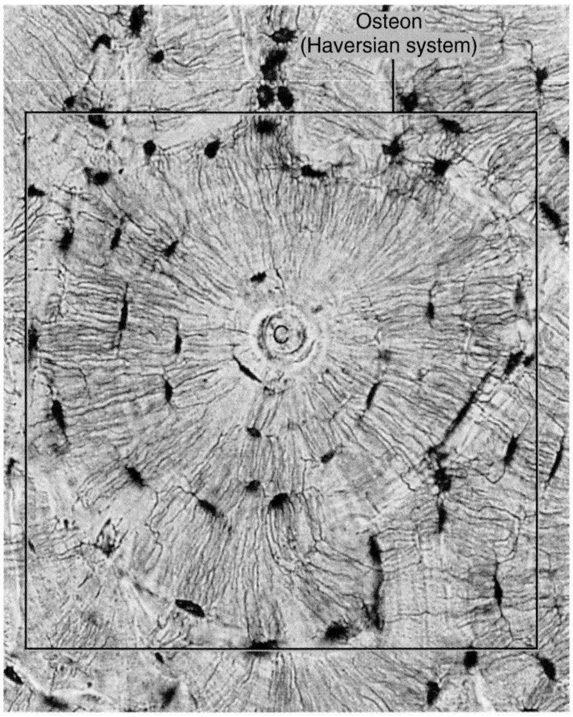

FIGURE 3-17

Cartilage. Photomicrograph showing the chondrocytes distributed throughout the gel-like matrix.

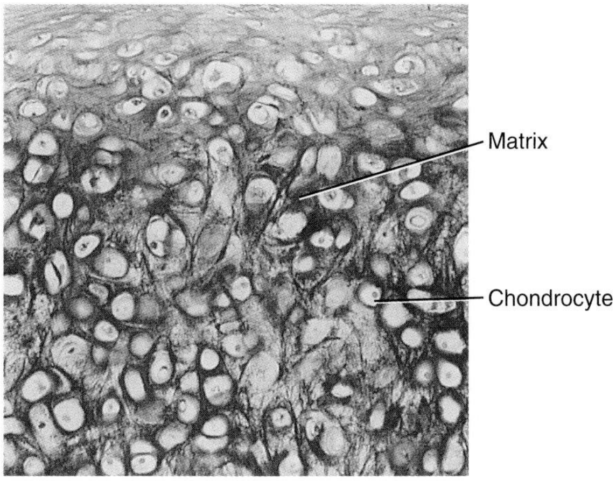

FIGURE 3-18

Blood. Photomicrograph of a human blood smear. This smear shows two white blood cells surrounded by a number of smaller red blood cells. The liquid matrix of this tissue is also called plasma.

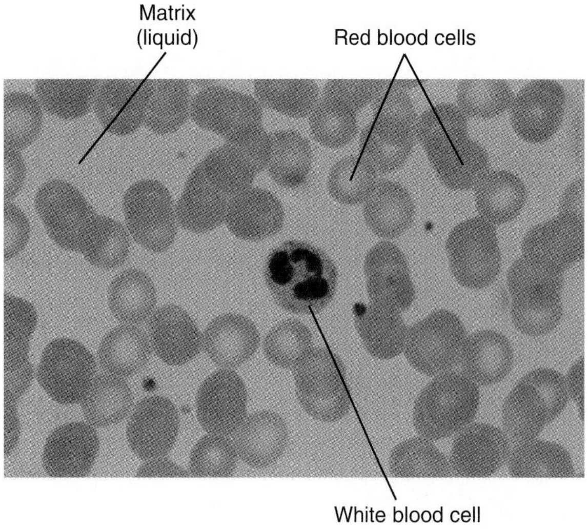

FIGURE 3-19

Skeletal muscle. Photomicrograph showing the striations of the muscle cell fibers in longitudinal section.

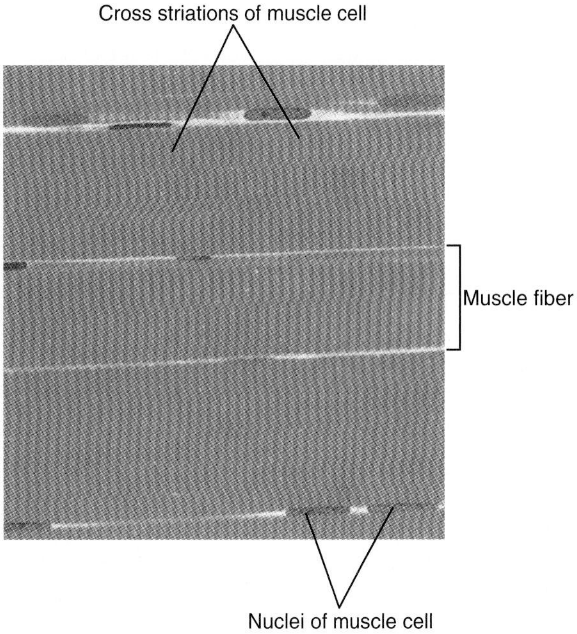

FIGURE 3-20

Cardiac muscle. Photomicrograph showing the branched, lightly striated fibers. The darker bands, called intercalated disks, which are characteristic of cardiac muscle, are easily identified in this tissue section.

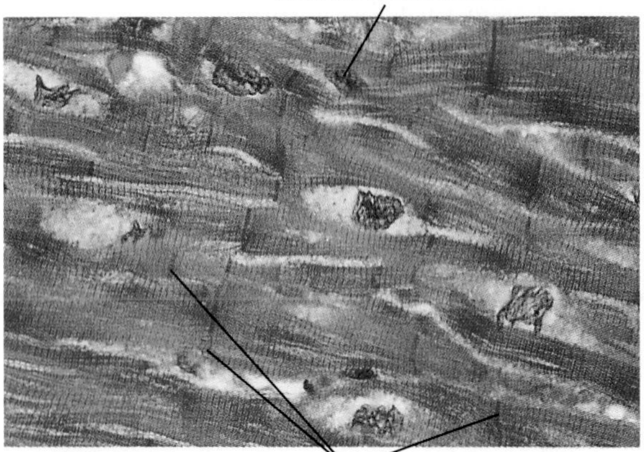

FIGURE 3-21

Smooth muscle. Photomicrograph, longitudinal section. Note the central placement of nuclei in the spindle-shaped smooth muscle fibers.

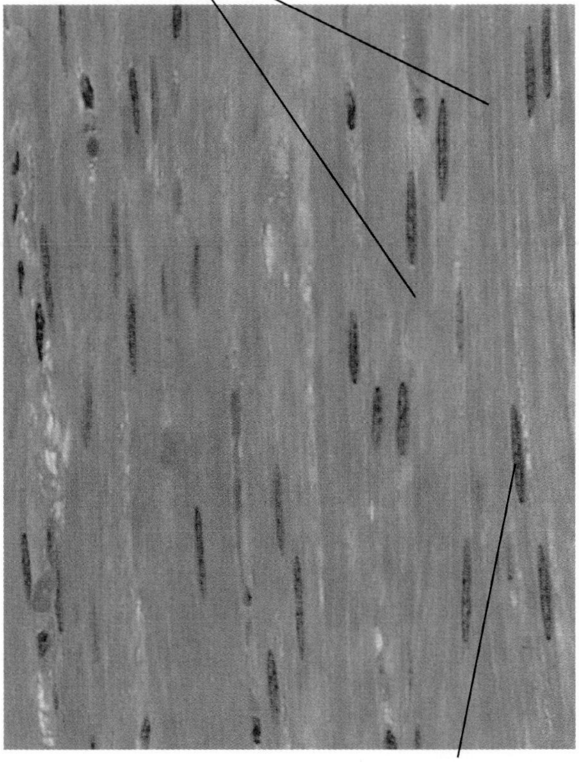

smooth muscle cells appear smooth (that is, without cross striations) and have only one nucleus per fiber. Smooth muscle helps form the walls of blood vessels and hollow organs such as the intestines and other tube-shaped structures in the body. Contractions of smooth (visceral) muscle propel food material through the digestive tract and help regulate the diameter of blood vessels. Contraction of smooth muscle in the tubes of the respiratory system, such as the bronchioles in the lungs, can impair breathing and result in asthma attacks and labored respiration.

Nervous Tissue

The function of **nervous tissue** is to provide rapid communication between body structures and control of body functions (Table 3-8). Nervous tissue consists of two kinds of cells: nerve cells, or **neurons** (NOO-rons), which are the conducting units of the system, and special connecting and supporting cells called **glia** (GLEE-ah) or neuroglia.

All neurons are characterized by a **cell body** and two types of processes: one **axon,** which transmits a nerve impulse away from the cell body, and one or more **dendrites** (DEN-drites), which carry impulses toward the cell body. Both neurons in Figure 3-22 have many dendrites extending from the cell body.

Quick Check

1. What is the difference between a simple and stratified epithelial tissue? Between squamous and cuboidal epithelial tissue?
2. Which main tissue type of the body is mostly matrix?
3. What are the three main types of muscle tissue?
4. What are the two main types of cell found in nervous tissue? Their functions?

FIGURE 3-22

Nervous tissue. Photomicrograph of neurons in a smear of the spinal cord. Both neurons in this slide show characteristic cell bodies and multiple cell processes.

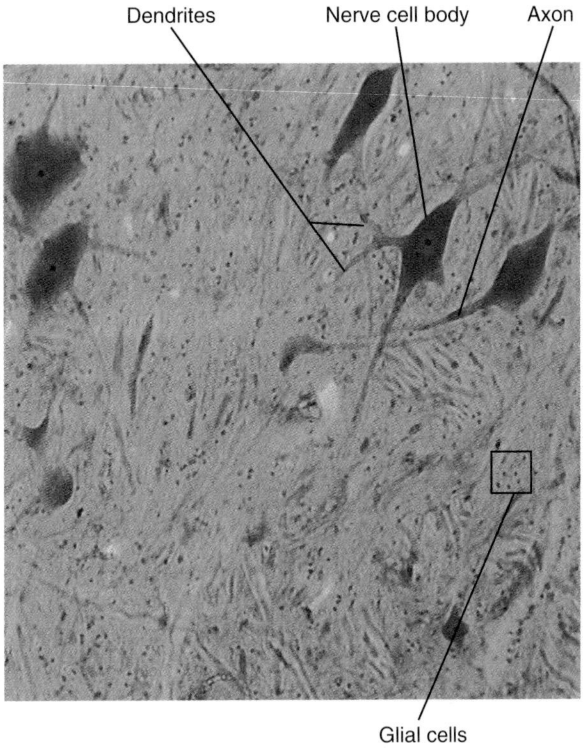

Health & Well-Being

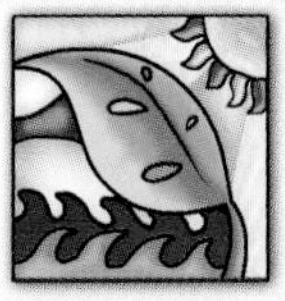

Tissues and Fitness

Achieving and maintaining an ideal body weight is a health-conscious goal. However, a better indicator of health and fitness is **body composition.** Exercise physiologists assess body composition to identify the percentage of the body made of lean tissue and the percentage made of fat. Body-fat percentage is often determined by using calipers to measure the thickness of skin folds at certain places on the body. A person with low body weight may still have a high ratio of fat to muscle, an unhealthy condition. In this case the individual is "underweight" but "overfat." In other words, fitness depends more on the percentage and ratio of specific tissue types than the overall amount of tissue present.

Therefore one goal of a good fitness program is a desirable body-fat percentage. For men, the ideal is 12% to 18%, and for women, the ideal is 18% to 24%. Because fat contains stored energy (measured in calories), a low fat percentage means a low energy reserve. High body-fat percentages are associated with several life-threatening conditions, including cardiovascular disease, diabetes, and cancer. A balanced diet and an exercise program ensure that the ratio of fat to muscle tissue stays at a level appropriate for maintaining homeostasis.

OUTLINE SUMMARY

CELLS

A. Size and shape
   1. Human cells vary considerably in size
   2. All are microscopic
   3. Cells differ notably in shape

B. Composition
   1. Cytoplasm containing specialized organelles surrounded by a plasma membrane
   2. Organization of cytoplasmic substances important for life

C. Structural parts
   1. Plasma membrane (Figure 3-1)
      a. Forms outer boundary of cell
      b. Thin, two-layered membrane of phospholipids containing proteins
      c. Is selectively permeable
   2. Cytoplasm (Figure 3-2)
      a. Organelles
         (1) Ribosomes
            (a) May attach to rough ER or lie free in cytoplasm
            (b) Manufacture proteins
            (c) Often called *protein factories*
         (2) Endoplasmic reticulum (ER)
            (a) Network of connecting sacs and canals
            (b) Carry substances through cytoplasm
            (c) Types are rough and smooth
            (d) Rough ER collects and transports proteins made by ribosomes
            (e) Smooth ER synthesizes chemicals; makes new membrane
         (3) Golgi apparatus
            (a) Group of flattened sacs near nucleus
            (b) Collect chemicals that move from the smooth ER in vesicles
            (c) Called the *chemical processing and packaging center*
         (4) Mitochondria
            (a) Composed of inner and outer membranes
            (b) Involved with energy-releasing chemical reactions
            (c) Often called *power plants* of the cell
            (d) Contains one DNA molecule
         (5) Lysosomes
            (a) Membranous-walled organelles
            (b) Contain digestive enzymes
            (c) Have protective function (eat microbes)
            (d) Formerly thought to be responsible for apoptosis (programmed cell death)
         (6) Centrioles
            (a) Paired organelles
            (b) Lie at right angles to each other near nucleus
            (c) Function in cell reproduction
         (7) Cilia
            (a) Fine, hairlike extensions found on free or exposed surfaces of some cells
            (b) Capable of moving in unison in a wavelike fashion
         (8) Flagella
            (a) Single projections extending from cell surfaces
            (b) Much larger than cilia
            (c) "Tails" of sperm cells only example of flagella in humans
   3. Nucleus
      a. Controls cell because it contains the genetic code—instructions for making proteins, which in turn determine cell structure and function
      b. Component structures include nuclear envelope, nucleoplasm, nucleolus, and chromatin granules
      c. 46 chromosomes contain DNA, which contains the genetic code

D. Relationship of cell structure and function
   1. Regulation of life processes

OUTLINE SUMMARY—*cont'd*

2. Survival of species through reproduction of the individual
3. Relationship of structure to function apparent in number and type of organelles seen in different cells
    - **a.** Heart muscle cells contain many mitochondria required to produce adequate energy needed for continued contractions
    - **b.** Flagellum of sperm cell gives motility, allowing movement of sperm through female reproductive tract, thus increasing chances for fertilization (Figure 3-3)

MOVEMENTS OF SUBSTANCES THROUGH CELL MEMBRANES

A. Passive transport processes do not require added energy and result in movement "down a concentration gradient"
1. Diffusion (Figure 3-4)
    - **a.** Substances scatter themselves evenly throughout an available space
    - **b.** It is unnecessary to add energy to the system
    - **c.** Movement is from high to low concentration
    - **d.** Osmosis and dialysis are specialized examples of diffusion across a selectively permeable membrane
    - **e.** Osmosis is diffusion of water (when some solutes cannot cross the membrane)
    - **f.** Dialysis is diffusion of solutes
2. Filtration
    - **a.** Movement of water and solutes caused by hydrostatic pressure on one side of membrane
    - **b.** Responsible for urine formation

B. Active transport processes occur only in living cells; movement of substances is "up the concentration gradient"; requires energy from ATP
1. Ion pumps (Figure 3-5)
    - **a.** An ion pump is protein complex in cell membrane
    - **b.** Ion pumps use energy from ATP to move substances across cell membranes against their concentration gradients
    - **c.** Examples: sodium-potassium pump, calcium pump
    - **d.** Some ion pumps work with other carriers so that glucose or amino acids are transported along with ions
2. Phagocytosis and pinocytosis
    - **a.** Both are active transport mechanisms because they require cell energy
    - **b.** Phagocytosis is a protective mechanism often used to destroy bacteria
    - **c.** Pinocytosis is used to incorporate fluids or dissolved substances into cells

CELL REPRODUCTION

A. DNA structure—large molecule shaped like a spiral staircase; sugar (deoxyribose), and phosphate units compose sides of the molecule; base pairs (adenine-thymine or guanine-cytosine) compose "steps"; base pairs always the same but sequence of base pairs differs in different DNA molecules; a gene is a specific sequence of base pairs within a DNA molecule; genes dictate formation of enzymes and other proteins by ribosomes, thereby indirectly determining a cell's structure and functions; in short, genes are heredity determinants (Figure 3-6)

B. Genetic code
1. Genetic information—stored in base-pair sequences on genes—expressed through protein synthesis
2. RNA molecules and protein synthesis
    - **a.** DNA—contained in cell nucleus
    - **b.** Protein synthesis—occurs in cytoplasm, thus genetic information must pass from the nucleus to the cytoplasm

Continued

OUTLINE SUMMARY—*cont'd*

   c. Process of transferring genetic information from nucleus to cytoplasm where proteins are produced requires completion of *transcription* and *translation* (Figure 3-6).
  3. Transcription
   a. Double-stranded DNA separates to form messenger RNA or mRNA
   b. Each strand of mRNA duplicates a particular gene (base-pair sequence) from a segment of DNA
   c. mRNA molecules pass from the nucleus to the cytoplasm where they direct protein synthesis in ribosomes and ER
  4. Translation
   a. Involves synthesis of proteins in cytoplasm by ribosomes
   b. Requires use of information contained in mRNA
 C. Cell division—reproduction of cell involving division of the nucleus (mitosis) and the cytoplasm; period when the cell is not actively dividing is called interphase
 D. DNA replication—process by which each half of a DNA molecule becomes a whole molecule identical to the original DNA molecule; precedes mitosis
 E. Mitosis—process in cell division that distributes identical chromosomes (DNA molecules) to each new cell formed when the original cell divides; enables cells to reproduce their own kind; makes heredity possible
 F. Stages of mitosis (Figure 3-7)
  1. Prophase—first stage
   a. Chromatin granules become organized
   b. Chromosomes (pairs of linked chromatids) appear
   c. Centrioles move away from nucleus
   d. Nuclear envelope disappears, freeing genetic material
   e. Spindle fibers appear
  2. Metaphase—second stage
   a. Chromosomes align across center of cell
   b. Spindle fibers attach themselves to each chromatid
  3. Anaphase—third stage
   a. Centromeres break apart
   b. Separated chromatids now called chromosomes
   c. Chromosomes are pulled to opposite ends of cell
   d. Cleavage furrow develops at end of anaphase
  4. Telophase—fourth stage
   a. Cell division is completed
   b. Nuclei appear in daughter cells
   c. Nuclear envelope and nucleoli appear
   d. Cytoplasm is divided (cytokinesis)
   e. Daughter cells become fully functional

TISSUES (Tables 3-5 through 3-7)
 A. Epithelial tissue
  1. Covers body and lines body cavities
  2. Cells packed closely together with little matrix
  3. Classified by shape of cells (Figure 3-8)
   a. Squamous
   b. Cuboidal
   c. Columnar
   d. Transitional
  4. Classified by arrangement of cells
   a. Simple
   b. Stratified
  5. Simple squamous epithelium (Figure 3-9)
   a. Single layer of scalelike cells
   b. Transport (e.g., absorption) is function

OUTLINE SUMMARY—*cont'd*

6. Stratified squamous epithelium (Figure 3-10)
   a. Several layers of closely packed cells
   b. Protection is primary function
7. Simple columnar epithelium (Figure 3-11)
   a. Columnar cells arranged in a single layer
   b. Line stomach and intestines
   c. Contain mucus-producing goblet cells
   d. Specialized for absorption
8. Stratified transitional epithelium (Figure 3-12)
   a. Found in body areas that stretch, such as urinary bladder
   b. Up to 10 layers of roughly cuboidal-shaped cells that distort to squamous shape when stretched
9. Pseudostratified epithelium
   a. Each cell touches basement membrane
   b. Lines the trachea
10. Simple cuboidal epithelium (Figure 3-13)
   a. Often specialized for secretory activity
   b. Cuboidal cells may be grouped into glands
   c. May secrete into ducts, directly into blood, and on body surface
   d. Examples of secretions include saliva, digestive juice, and hormones
   e. Cuboidal epithelium also forms the urine-producing tubules of the kidney

B. Connective tissue
1. Most abundant tissue in body
2. Most widely distributed tissue in body
3. Multiple types, appearances, and functions
4. Relatively few cells in intercellular matrix
5. Types
   a. Areolar—glue that holds organs together
   b. Adipose (fat)—lipid storage is primary function (Figure 3-14)
   c. Fibrous—strong fibers; example is tendon (Figure 3-15)
   d. Bone—matrix is calcified; function in support and protection (Figure 3-16)
   e. Cartilage—chondrocyte is cell type (Figure 3-17)
   f. Blood—matrix is fluid; function is transportation (Figure 3-18)

C. Muscle tissue (Figures 3-19 to 3-21)
1. Types
   a. Skeletal—attaches to bones; also called striated or *voluntary;* control is voluntary; striations apparent when viewed under a microscope (Figure 3-19)
   b. Cardiac—also called *striated involuntary;* composes heart wall; ordinarily cannot control contractions (Figure 3-20)
   c. Smooth—also called *nonstriated (visceral)* or *involuntary;* no cross striations; found in blood vessels and other tube-shaped organs (Figure 3-21)

D. Nervous tissue (Figure 3-22)
1. Cell types
   a. Neurons—conducting cells
   b. Glia (neuroglia)—supportive and connecting cells
2. Neurons
   a. Cell components
      (1) Cell body
      (2) Axon (one) carries nerve impulse away from cell body
      (3) Dendrites (one or more) carry nerve impulse toward the cell body
3. Function—rapid communication between body structures and control of body functions

NEW WORDS

adenosine
  triphosphate (ATP)
adipose
areolar
axon
centriole
centromere
chondrocyte
chromatid
chromatin
collagen
columnar
crenation
cuboidal
cytoplasm
dendrite
deoxyribonucleic acid
  (DNA)
glia
goblet cell
hemopoietic
hypertonic
hypotonic
interphase
lyse
matrix
mitosis
  prophase
  metaphase
  anaphase
  telophase
neuron
nucleoplasm
organelle
  cilia
  endoplasmic
    reticulum (ER)
  flagellum
  Golgi apparatus
  lysosome
  mitochondria
  nucleolus
  nucleus
  plasma membrane
  ribosome
osteon
ribonucleic acid
  (RNA)
spindle fiber
squamous
transcription
translation
transport
  dialysis
  diffusion
  filtration
  osmosis
  phagocytosis
  pinocytosis

REVIEW QUESTIONS

1. Describe the structure of the plasma membrane.
2. List three functions of the plasma membrane.
3. Give the function of the following organelles: *ribosome, Golgi apparatus, mitochondria, lysosomes,* and *centrioles.*
4. Give the function of the *nucleus* and *nucleolus.*
5. Explain the difference between *chromatin* and *chromosomes.*
6. Describe the processes of *diffusion* and *filtration.*
7. Describe the functioning of the *ion pump* and explain the process of *phagocytosis.*
8. Define *gene* and *genome.*
9. Describe the process of transcription.
10. Describe the process of translation.
11. List the four stages in active cell division (mitosis) and briefly describe what occurs in each stage.
12. What important event in mitosis occurs during interphase?
13. Name and describe three epithelial tissues.
14. Name and describe three connective tissues.
15. Name and describe two muscle tissues.
16. Name the two types of nervous tissue. Which is the functional nerve tissue and which is support tissue?

CRITICAL THINKING

17. Explain what is meant by tissue typing. Why has this become so important in recent years?
18. Explain what would happen if a cell containing 97% water were placed in a 10% salt solution.
19. If one side of a DNA molecule had a base sequence of adenine-adenine-guanine-cytosine-thymine-cytosine-thymine, what would the sequence of bases on the opposite side of the molecule be?
20. If a molecule of mRNA were made from the base sequence in Question 19, what would be the sequence of bases in the RNA?

100%

CHAPTER TEST

1. Phospholipids and Cholesterol are two fat-based molecules that make up part of the structure of the plasma membrane.
2. Organelles is a term that refers to small structures inside the cell; it means "little organs."
3. Active Transport is the movement of substances across a cell membrane using cell energy, while Passive Transport is the movement of substances across the cell membrane without using cell energy.
4. Pinocytosis refers to the movement of fluids or dissolved molecules into the cell by trapping them in the plasma membrane.
5. DNA and RNA are the two nucleic acids that are involved in transcription.
6. Transcription is the process in protein synthesis that uses the information in mRNA to build a protein molecule.
7. Translation is the process in protein synthesis that forms the mRNA molecule.
8. Gene is a segment of base pairs in a chromosome.
9. DNA is the total genetic information package in a cell.
10. Epithelium, Connective, Nerve, and Muscle are the four main types of tissues in the body.
11. Which of the following is not a specialized form of diffusion?
    - **a.** filtration
    - **b.** dialysis
    - **c.** osmosis
    - **d.** all of these are specialized forms of diffusion
12. During this stage of mitosis the chromosomes move away from the center of the cell:
    - **a.** interphase
    - **b.** metaphase
    - **c.** anaphase
    - **d.** telophase
13. During this stage the DNA replicates:
    - **a.** interphase
    - **b.** metaphase
    - **c.** prophase
    - **d.** telophase
14. During this stage of mitosis, the chromosomes align in the center of the cell:
    - **a.** interphase
    - **b.** metaphase
    - **c.** prophase
    - **d.** telophase
15. During this stage of mitosis the chromatin condenses into chromosomes:
    - **a.** interphase
    - **b.** metaphase
    - **c.** prophase
    - **d.** telophase
16. During this stage of mitosis the nuclear envelope and nuclei reappear:
    - **a.** interphase
    - **b.** prophase
    - **c.** anaphase
    - **d.** telophase

Continued

CHAPTER TEST—*cont'd*

Match the function in Column B with the proper cell structure in Column A.

COLUMN A

17. __G__ Ribosome
18. __C__ Endoplasmic reticulum
19. __E__ Golgi apparatus
20. __I__ Mitochondria
21. __B__ Lysosomes
22. __A__ Flagella
23. __D__ Cilia
24. __F__ Nucleus
25. __H__ Nucleoli

COLUMN B

a. A long cell projection used to propel sperm cells
b. Bags of digestive enzymes in the cell
c. Tubelike passages that carry substances through the cytoplasm
d. Short hairlike structures on the free surface of some cells
e. Chemically process and package substances from the endoplasmic reticulum
f. Directs protein synthesis; the brain of the cell
g. "Protein factories" in the cell, made of RNA
h. Small structure in the nucleus; helps in the formation of ribosomes
i. "Powerhouse" of the cell; most of the cell's ATP is formed here

STUDY TIPS

Chapter Three should be a review of your general biology course; most of what is in this chapter should sound familiar.

The section on cell structures begins with the plasma membrane. It is made up mostly of phospholipids, but the most important part of the membrane structure to remember is the proteins embedded in the phospholipids. They play important roles in a number of systems in the body such as the nervous or endocrine systems. The organelles may seem to have strange-sounding names, but many of the names can give you a clue about what they do. For example, *–some* means "body" or "structure" and *lysis* means "to digest" or "destroy," so the name *lysosome* tells you what it does. Ribosomes are made of ribonucleic acid. *Endo-* means "inside of," *plasmic* means "liquid," and *reticulum* means "net-like," so *endoplasmic reticulum* is self-explaining. Flash cards are probably helpful in learning this material. The transport processes of osmosis and dialysis are special cases of diffusion, osmosis with water and dialysis with solutes. Filtration uses a pressure rather than a concentration difference to move substances. *Phago* means "eat," *pino* means "drink," *cyto* means "cell," and *–asis* means "condition." *Phagocytosis* and *pinocytosis* are descriptions of what is going on in the cell. When studying protein synthesis, keep the goal of the process in mind. The cell wants a protein made. The DNA has the plans, but the ribosome is the factory. The DNA needs to tell the ribosome what to build (transcription), and the factory needs to have the pieces in the correct order (translation). Use flash cards to study the phases of mitosis; remember that the phases in mitosis are based on what is happening to the chromosomes. Tissue types are also a flash card topic. It may help to remember that epithelial tissues are covering or protective tissues and that the important thing about connective tissues is the matrix surrounding the cells.

In your study groups, go over the flash cards for the organelles, mitosis, and tissues. Be sure to discuss the steps of protein synthesis and the cell transport processes. Go over the questions in the back of the chapter and discuss possible test questions.

4 Organ Systems of the Body

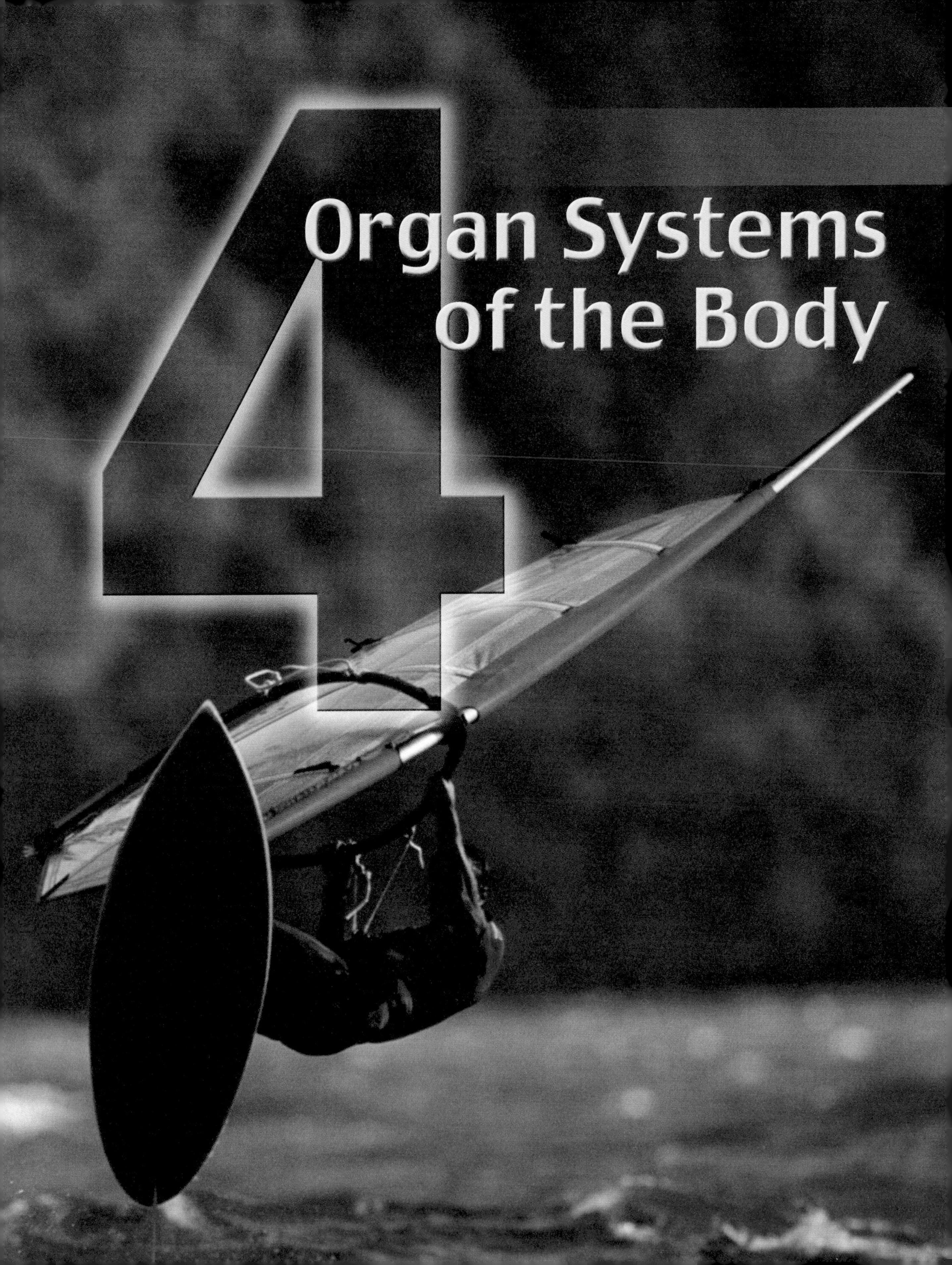

Outline

Objectives

AFTER YOU HAVE COMPLETED THIS CHAPTER, YOU SHOULD BE ABLE TO:

1. Define and contrast the terms *organ* and *organ system*.
2. List the 11 major organ systems of the body.
3. Identify and locate the major organs of each major organ system.
4. Briefly describe the major functions of each major organ system.
5. Identify and discuss the major subdivisions of the reproductive system.

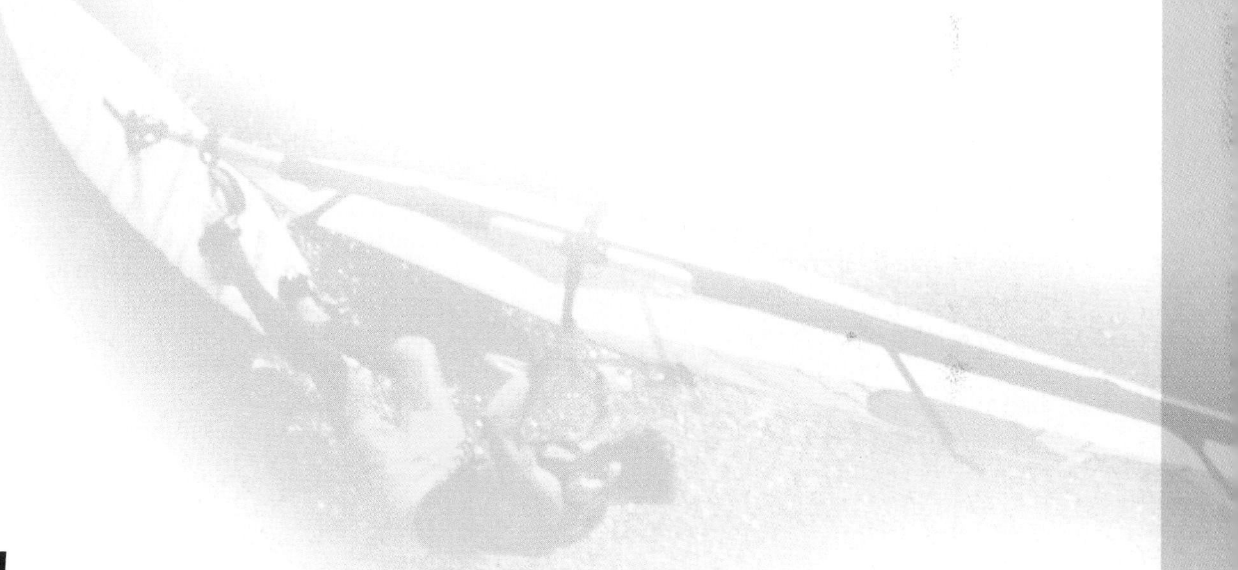

The words *organ* and *system* were discussed in Chapter 1 as having special meanings when applied to the body. An **organ** is a structure made up of two or more kinds of tissues organized in such a way that the tissues can together perform a more complex function than can any tissue alone. A **system** is a group of organs arranged in such a way that they can together perform a more complex function than can any organ alone. This chapter gives an overview of the 11 major organ systems of the body.

In the chapters that follow, the presentation of information on individual organs and an explanation of how they work together to accomplish complex body functions will form the basis for the discussion of each organ system. For example, a detailed description of the skin as the primary organ of the integumentary system will be covered in Chapter 5, and information on the bones of the body as organs of the skeletal system will be presented in Chapter 6. Knowledge of individual organs and how they are organized into groups makes much more meaningful the understanding of how a particular organ system functions as a unit in the body.

Recent discoveries that have allowed scientists to culture embryonic "stem cells" in the laboratory and then control the differentiation of these primitive cells into specific cell and tissue types, such as muscle or nerve, are exciting and complex advances in biology that will have a profound impact on human health. Although many scientific and ethical questions remain unanswered, the potential now exists for cell, tissue, and organ "engineering" that may well permit repair or total replacement of diseased or damaged organs in a functioning organ system.

When you have completed your study of the major organ systems in the chapters that follow, it will be possible to view the body not as an assembly of individual parts but as an integrated and functioning whole. This chapter names the systems of the body and the major organs that compose them, and it briefly describes the functions of each system. It is intended to provide a basic "road map" to help you anticipate and prepare for the more detailed information that follows in the remainder of the text.

ORGAN SYSTEMS OF THE BODY

In contrast to cells, which are the smallest structural units of the body, organ systems are its largest and most complex structural units. The 11 major organ systems that compose the human body are listed here.

1. Integumentary
2. Skeletal
3. Muscular
4. Nervous
5. Endocrine
6. Cardiovascular (circulatory)
7. Lymphatic
8. Respiratory
9. Digestive
10. Urinary
11. Reproductive
    a. Male subdivision
    b. Female subdivision

Examine Figure 4-1 to find a diagrammatic listing of the body systems and the major organs in each. In addition to the information contained in Figure 4-1, each system is presented in visual form in Figures 4-2 through 4-13. Visual presentation of material is often useful in understanding the interrelationships that are so important in anatomy and physiology.

Integumentary System

Note in Figure 4-2 that the skin is the largest and most important organ in the **integumentary** (integ-yoo-MEN-tar-ee) **system.** Its weight in most adults is 20 pounds or more, accounting for about 16% of total body weight and making it the body's heaviest organ. The integumentary system includes the skin and its **appendages,** which include the hair, nails, and specialized sweat- and oil-producing glands. In addition, a number of microscopic and highly specialized sense organs are embedded in the skin. They permit the body to respond to various stimuli such as pain, pressure, touch, and changes in temperature.

The integumentary system is crucial to survival. Its primary function is *protection.* The skin protects underlying tissue against invasion by harmful bacteria, bars entry of most chemicals, and minimizes the chances of mechanical injury to underlying structures. In addition, the skin regulates body temperature by sweating, synthesizes important chemicals, and functions as a sophisticated sense organ.

Skeletal System

The sternum or breastbone, the humerus, and the femur shown in Figure 4-3 are examples of the 206 individual organs (bones) found in the **skeletal system.** The system includes not only bones but also related tissues such as cartilage and ligaments that together provide the body with a rigid framework for support and protection. In addition, the skeletal system, through the existence of **joints** between bones, makes possible the movements of body parts. Without joints, we could make no movements; our bodies would be rigid, immobile hulks. Bones also serve

FIGURE 4-1

Body systems and their organs.

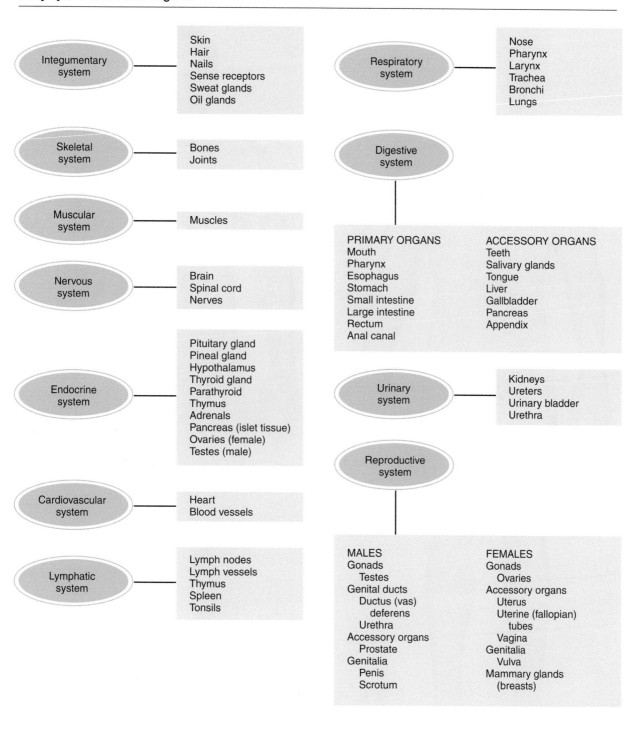

Integumentary system	Skin Hair Nails Sense receptors Sweat glands Oil glands
Skeletal system	Bones Joints
Muscular system	Muscles
Nervous system	Brain Spinal cord Nerves
Endocrine system	Pituitary gland Pineal gland Hypothalamus Thyroid gland Parathyroid Thymus Adrenals Pancreas (islet tissue) Ovaries (female) Testes (male)
Cardiovascular system	Heart Blood vessels
Lymphatic system	Lymph nodes Lymph vessels Thymus Spleen Tonsils
Respiratory system	Nose Pharynx Larynx Trachea Bronchi Lungs
Digestive system	PRIMARY ORGANS Mouth Pharynx Esophagus Stomach Small intestine Large intestine Rectum Anal canal ACCESSORY ORGANS Teeth Salivary glands Tongue Liver Gallbladder Pancreas Appendix
Urinary system	Kidneys Ureters Urinary bladder Urethra

Reproductive system	MALES
	Gonads
	  Testes
	Genital ducts
	  Ductus (vas) deferens
	  Urethra
	Accessory organs
	  Prostate
	Genitalia
	  Penis
	  Scrotum
	
	FEMALES
	Gonads
	  Ovaries
	Accessory organs
	  Uterus
	  Uterine (fallopian) tubes
	  Vagina
	Genitalia
	  Vulva
	Mammary glands (breasts)

FIGURE 4-2

Integumentary system.

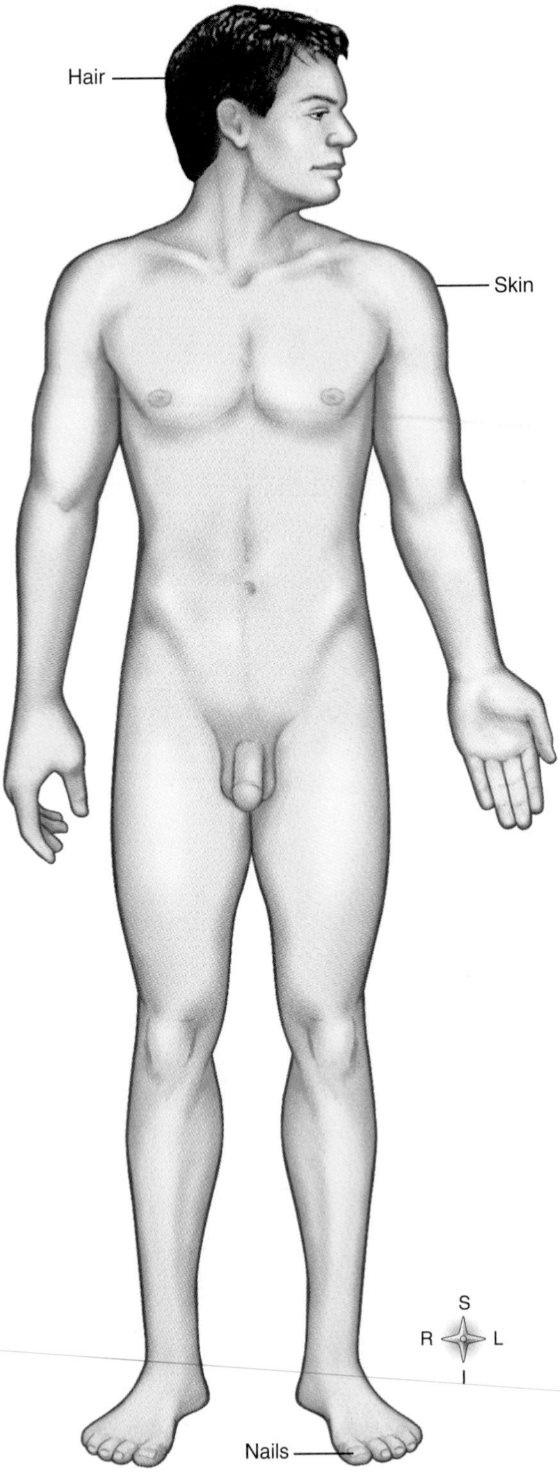

FIGURE 4-3

Skeletal system.

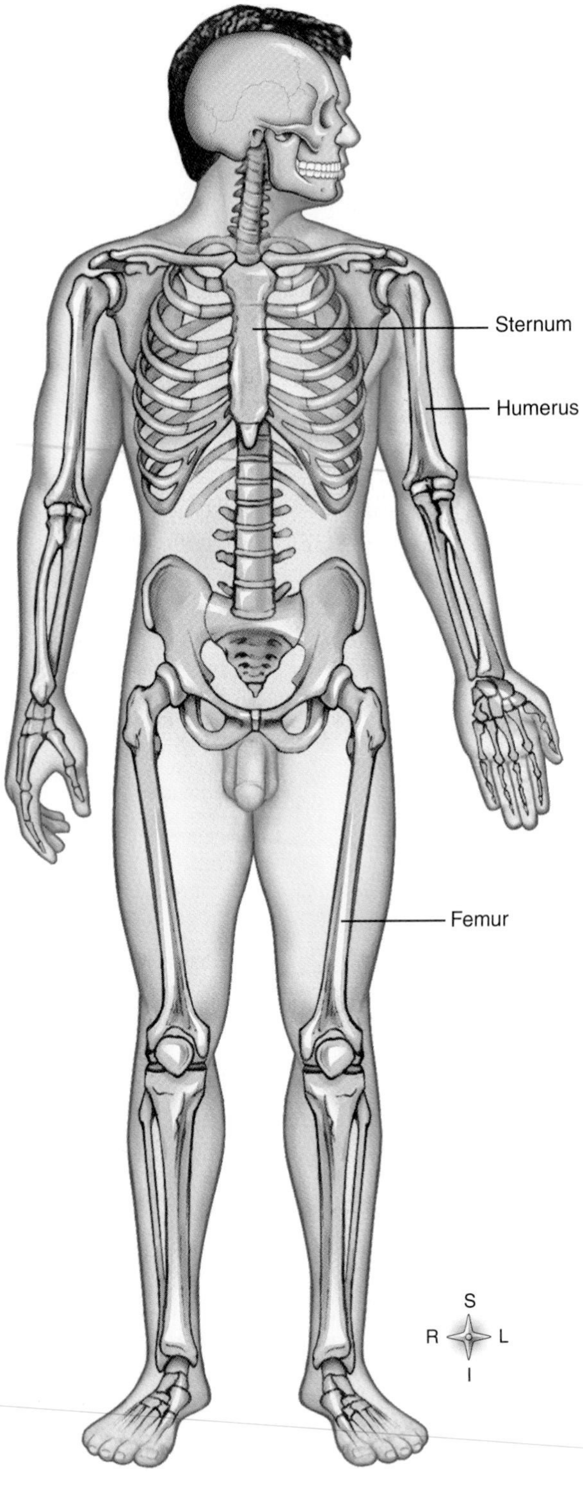

as storage areas for important minerals such as calcium and phosphorus. The formation of blood cells in the red marrow of certain bones is another crucial function of the skeletal system.

Muscular System

Individual skeletal muscles are the organs of the muscular system. Muscles not only produce movement and maintain body posture but also generate the heat required for maintaining a constant core body temperature. The skeletal muscles are called **voluntary muscles** because their contractions are under conscious control. In addition to the skeletal or voluntary muscles that constitute the muscular system, two other important types of muscle tissue are found in the body. **Involuntary** or **smooth muscle** tissue is found in blood vessel walls, other tubular structures, and in the lining of hollow organs such as the stomach and small intestine. **Cardiac muscle** is the specialized muscle tissue of the heart.

The tendon labeled in Figure 4-4 represents how tendons attach muscles to bones. When stimulated by a nervous impulse, muscle tissue shortens or contracts. Voluntary movement occurs when skeletal muscles contract because of the way muscles are attached to bones and the way bones articulate or join together with one another in joints.

Nervous System

The brain, spinal cord, and nerves are the organs of the **nervous system.** As you can see in Figure 4-5, nerves extend from the brain and spinal cord to every area of the body. The extensive networking of the components of the nervous system makes it possible for this complex system to perform its primary functions. These include the following:

1. Communication between body functions
2. Integration of body functions
3. Control of body functions
4. Recognition of sensory stimuli

These functions are accomplished by specialized signals called **nerve impulses.** In general, the functions of the nervous system result in rapid

FIGURE 4-4

Muscular system.

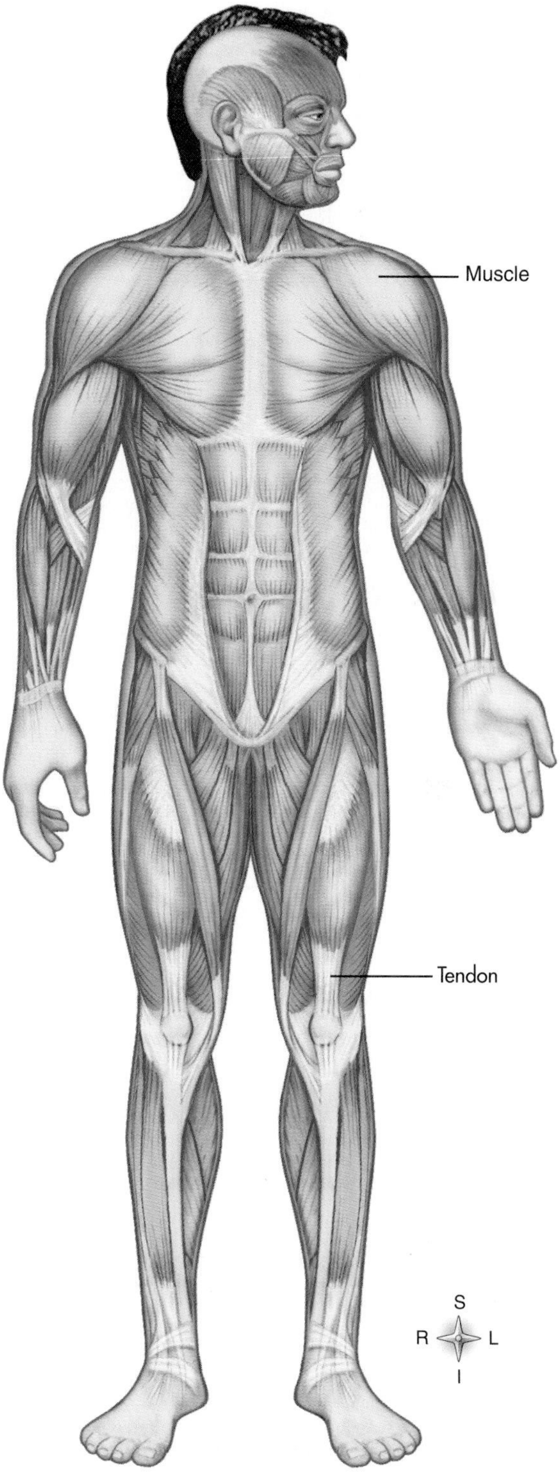

FIGURE 4-5

Nervous system.

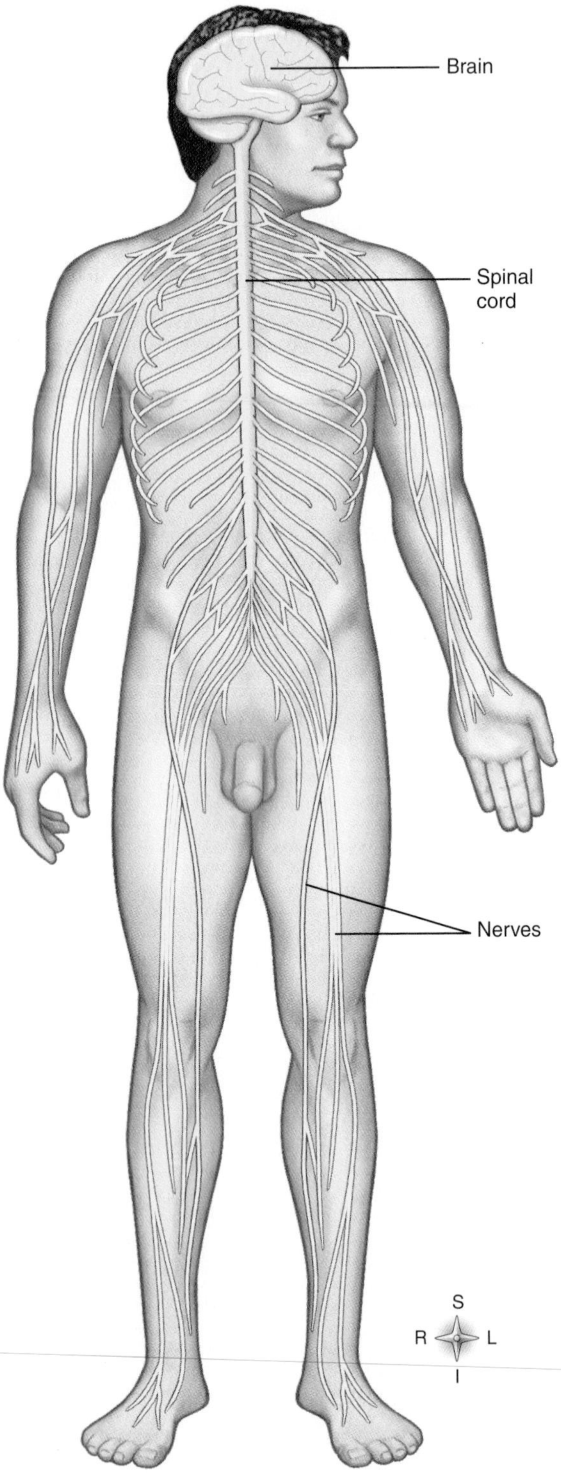

activity that lasts usually for a short duration. For example, we can chew our food normally, walk, and perform coordinated muscular movements only if our nervous system functions properly. The nerve impulse permits the rapid and precise control of diverse body functions. Other types of nerve impulses cause glands to secrete fluids. In addition, elements of the nervous system can recognize certain **stimuli** (STIM-yoo-lye), such as heat, light, pressure, or temperature, that affect the body. When stimulated, these specialized components of the nervous system, called **sense organs** (discussed in Chapter 9), generate nervous impulses that travel to the brain or spinal cord where analysis or relay occurs and, if needed, appropriate action is initiated.

Endocrine System

The **endocrine system** is composed of specialized glands that secrete chemicals known as **hormones** directly into the blood. Sometimes called *ductless glands*, the organs of the endocrine system perform the same general functions as the nervous system: communication, integration, and control. The nervous system provides rapid, brief control by fast-traveling nerve impulses. The endocrine system provides slower but longer-lasting control by hormone secretion; for example, secretion of growth hormone controls the rate of development over long periods of gradual growth.

In addition to controlling growth, hormones are the main regulators of metabolism, reproduction, and other body activities. They play important roles in fluid and electrolyte balance, acid-base balance, and energy metabolism.

As you can see in Figure 4-6, the endocrine glands are widely distributed throughout the body. The **pituitary** (pi-TOO-i-TAIR-ee) **gland, pineal** (PIN-e-al) **gland,** and **hypothalamus** (hi-po-THAL-ah-mus) are located in the skull. The **thyroid** (THY-roid) and **parathyroid** (PAIR-ah-THY-roid) **glands** are in the neck, and the **thymus** (THY-mus) **gland** is in the thoracic cavity, specifically in the mediastinum (see Figure 1-4, p. 8). The **adrenal** (ah-DRE-nal) **glands** and **pancreas** (PAN-kree-as) are found in the abdominal cavity. Note in Figure 4-6 that the ovaries in the female and

FIGURE 4-6

Endocrine system.

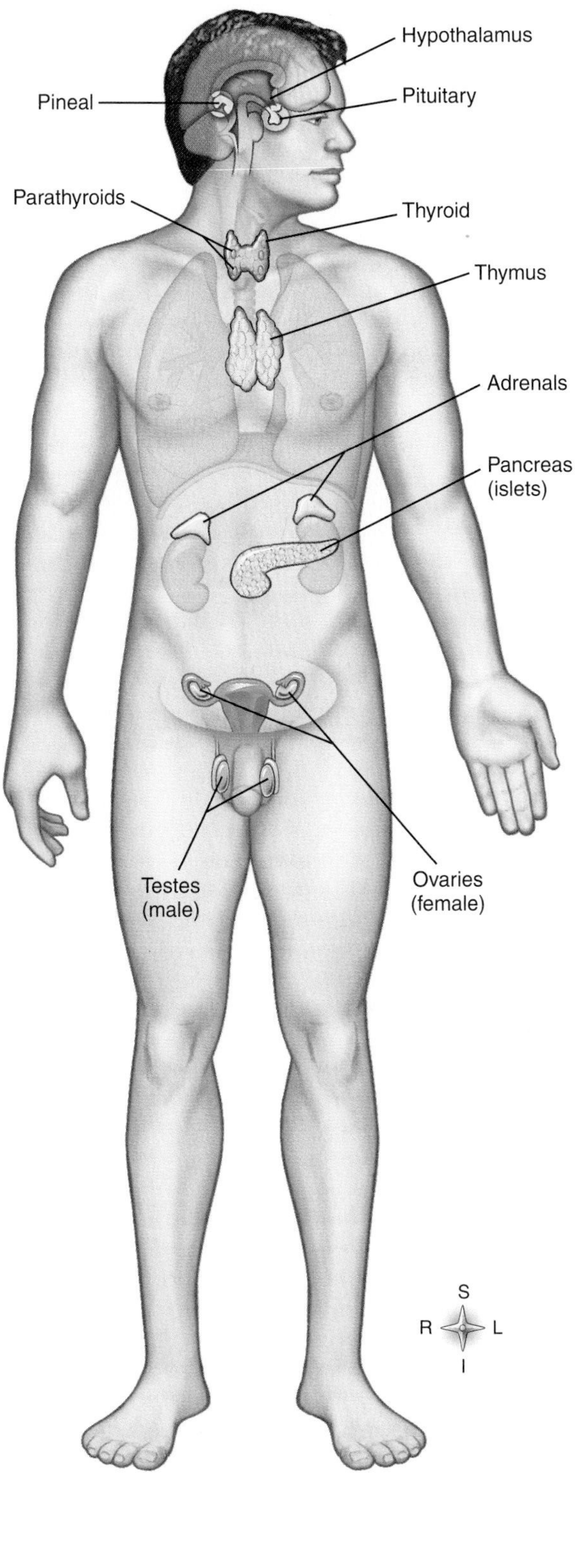

the testes in the male also function as endocrine glands.

Cardiovascular (Circulatory) System

The **cardiovascular** or **circulatory system** consists of the heart, which is a muscular pumping device as shown in Figure 4-7, and a closed system of vessels made up of **arteries, veins,** and **capillaries.** As the name implies, blood contained in this system is pumped by the heart around a closed circle or circuit of vessels as it passes through the body.

The primary function of the circulatory system is *transportation.* The need for an efficient transportation system in the body is critical. Transportation needs include continuous movement of oxygen and carbon dioxide, nutrients, hormones, and other important substances. Wastes produced by the cells are released into the bloodstream on an ongoing basis and are transported by the blood to the excretory organs. The circulatory system also helps regulate body temperature by distributing heat throughout the body and by assisting in retaining or releasing heat from the body by regulating blood flow near the body surface. Certain cells of the circulatory system can also become involved in the defense of the body or immunity.

Quick

1. What is the *integument*?
2. Give examples of organs of the skeletal system.
3. What are the major functions of the nervous system?
4. What organs make up the cardiovascular system?

Lymphatic System

The **lymphatic system** is composed of **lymph nodes, lymphatic vessels,** and specialized lymphatic organs such as the **tonsils, thymus,** and **spleen.** Note that the thymus in Figure 4-8 functions as an endocrine and as a lymphatic gland. Instead of containing blood, the lymphatic vessels are filled with lymph, a whitish, watery fluid that contains lymphocytes, proteins, and some fatty molecules. No red blood cells are pres-

FIGURE 4-7

Cardiovascular (circulatory) system.

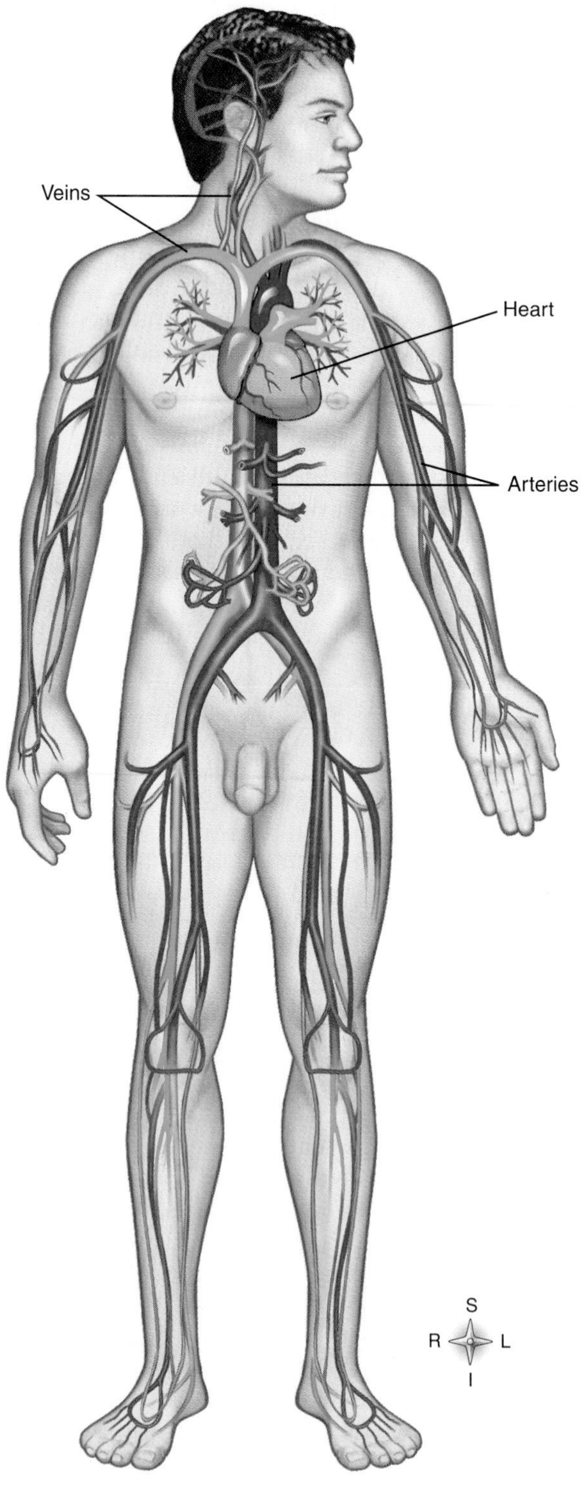

FIGURE 4-8

Lymphatic system.

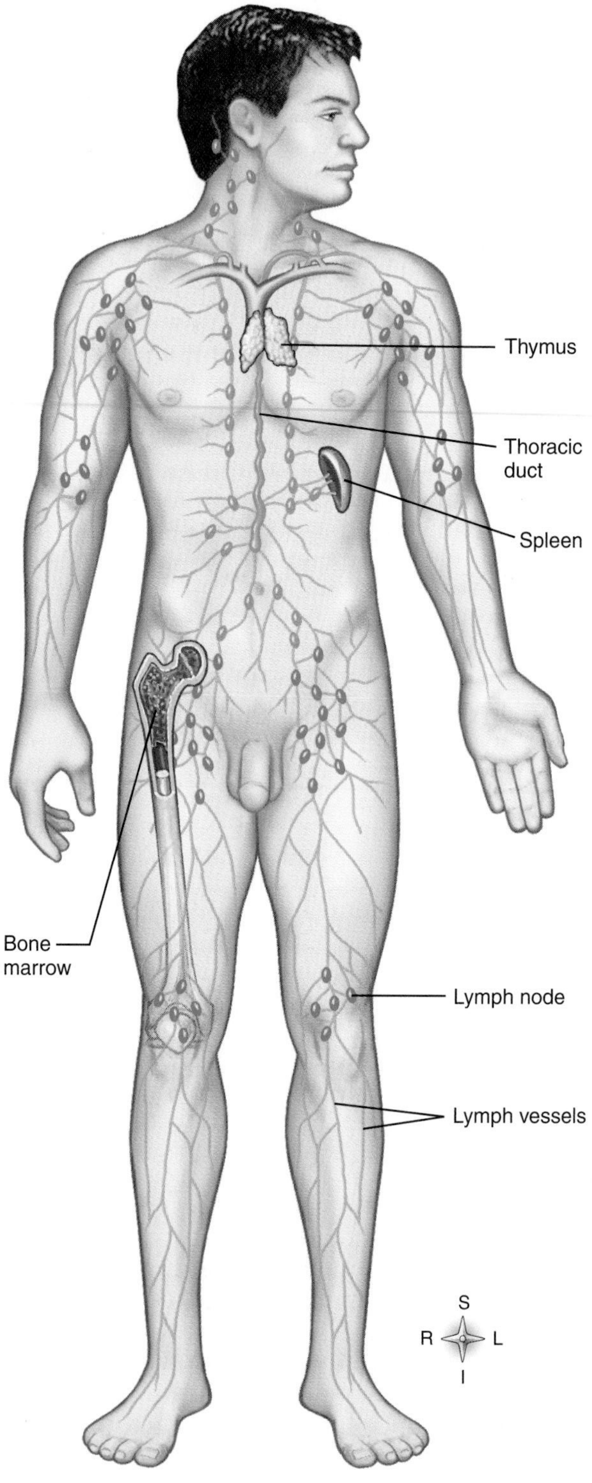

ent. The lymph is formed from the fluid around the body cells and diffuses into the lymph vessels. However, unlike blood, lymph does not circulate repeatedly through a closed circuit or loop of vessels. Instead, lymph flowing through lymphatic vessels eventually enters the circulatory system by passing through large ducts, including the **thoracic duct** shown in Figure 4-8, which in turn connect with veins in the upper area of the thoracic cavity. Collections of lymph nodes can be seen in the axillary (armpit) and in the inguinal (groin) areas of the body in Figure 4-8. The formation and movement of lymph are discussed in Chapter 13.

The functions of the lymphatic system include movement of fluids and certain large molecules from the tissue spaces around the cells and movement of fat-related nutrients from the digestive tract back to the blood. The lymphatic system is also involved in the functioning of the immune system, which plays a critical role in the defense mechanism of the body against disease.

Respiratory System

The organs of the **respiratory system** include the **nose**, **pharynx** (FAIR-inks), **larynx** (LAR-inks), **trachea** (TRAY-kee-ah), **bronchi** (BRON-ki), and **lungs** (Figure 4-9). Together these organs permit the movement of air into the tiny, thin-walled sacs of the lungs called **alveoli** (al-VE-o-li). In the alveoli, oxygen from the air is exchanged for the waste product carbon dioxide, which is carried to the lungs by the blood so that it can be eliminated from the body. The organs of the respiratory system perform a number of functions in addition to permitting movement of air into the alveoli. For example, if you live in a cold or dry environment, incoming air can be warmed and humidified as it passes over the lining of the respiratory air passages. In addition, inhaled irritants such as pollen or dust passing through the respiratory tubes can be trapped in the sticky mucus that covers the lining of many respiratory passages and then eliminated from the body. The respiratory system is also involved in regulating the acid-base balance of the body—a function that will be discussed in Chapter 19.

FIGURE 4-9

Respiratory system.

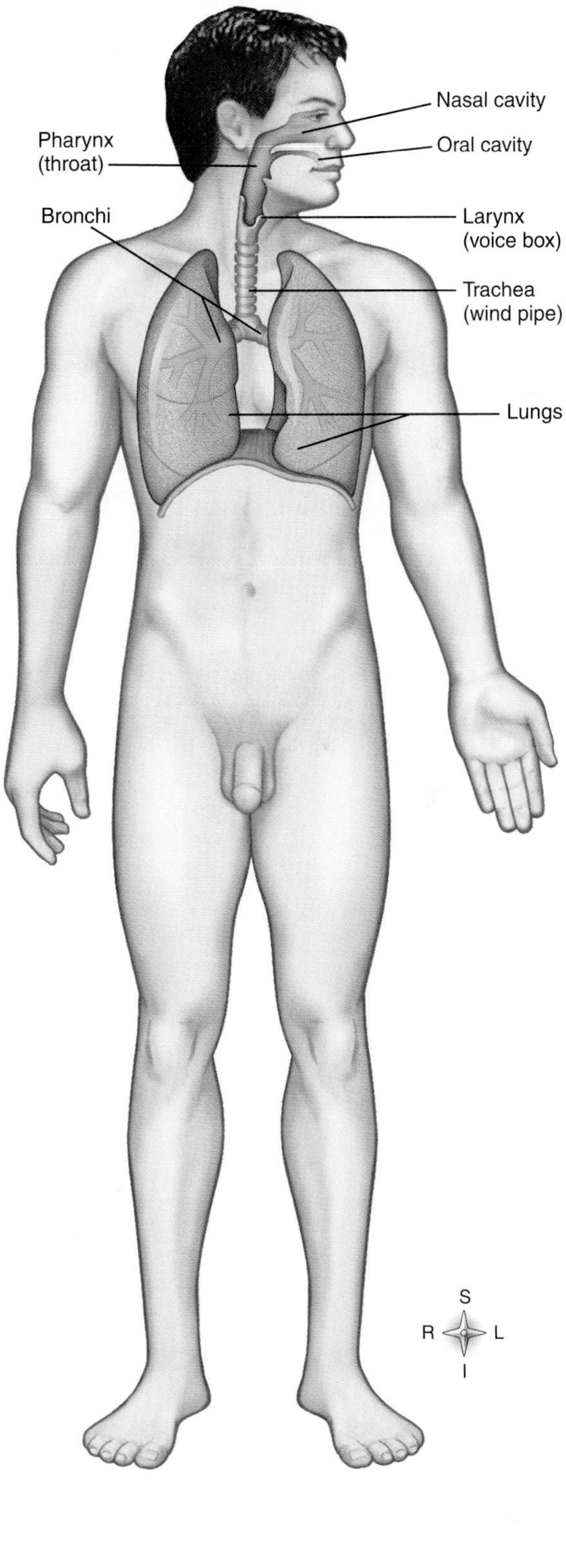

FIGURE 4-10

Digestive system.

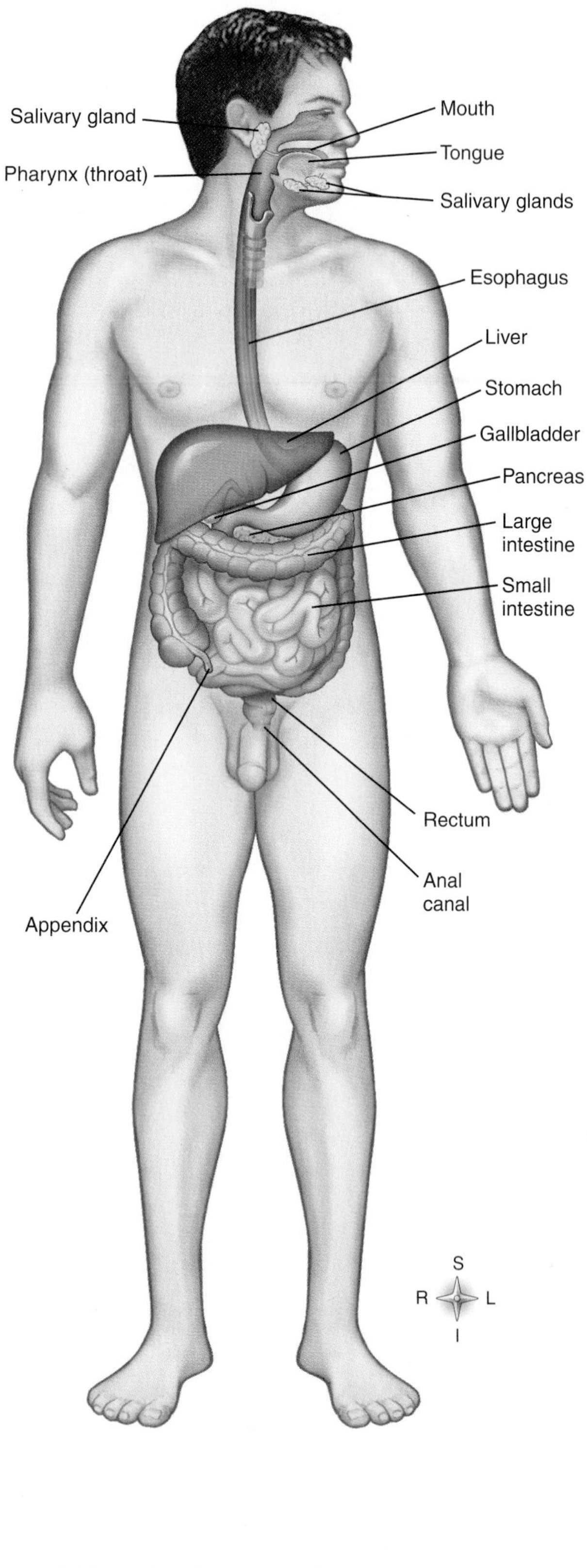

Digestive System

The organs of the **digestive system** (Figure 4-10) are often separated into two groups: the *primary organs* and the *secondary* or *accessory organs* (see Figure 4-1). They work together to ensure proper digestion and absorption of nutrients. The primary organs include the mouth, pharynx, esophagus, stomach, small intestine, large intestine, rectum, and anal canal. The accessory organs of digestion include the teeth, salivary glands, tongue, liver, gallbladder, pancreas, and appendix.

The primary organs of the digestive system form a tube, open at both ends, called the **gastrointestinal** (GAS-tro-in-TES-ti-nal) or **GI tract.** Food that enters the tract is digested, its nutrients are absorbed, and the undigested residue is eliminated from the body as waste material called feces (FEE-seez). The accessory organs assist in the mechanical or chemical breakdown of ingested food. The appendix, although classified as an accessory organ of digestion and physically attached to the digestive tube, is not functionally important in the digestive process. However, inflammation of the appendix, called **appendicitis** (ah-PEN-di-SYE-tis) is a very serious clinical condition and frequently requires surgery.

Urinary System

The organs of the **urinary system** include the **kidneys, ureters** (u-REE-ters), **bladder,** and **urethra** (yoo-RE-thrah).

The kidneys (Figure 4-11) "clear" or clean the blood of the waste products continually produced by the metabolism of nutrients in the body cells. The kidneys also play an important role in maintaining the electrolyte, water, and acid-base balances in the body.

The waste product produced by the kidneys is called **urine** (YOOR-in). After it is produced by the kidneys, it flows out of the kidneys through the ureters into the urinary bladder, where it is stored. Urine passes from the bladder to the outside of the body through the urethra. In the male the urethra passes through the penis, which has a double function: it transports urine and semen or seminal fluid. Therefore it has urinary and reproductive

Science Applications

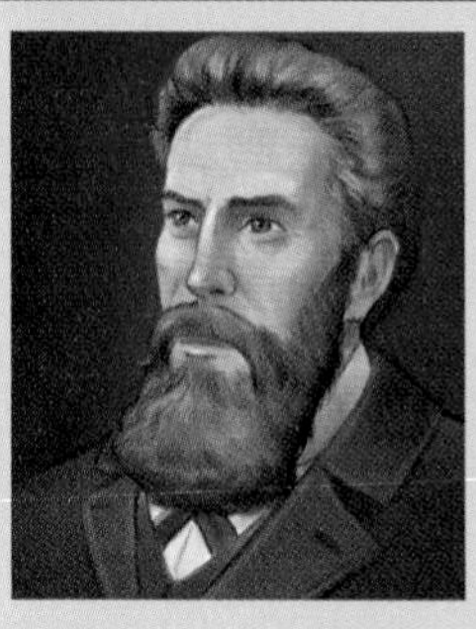

Radiography

Wilhelm Röntgen (1845–1923).

In 1895, the German physicist Wilhelm Röntgen (RENT-gen) made one of the most important medical discoveries of the modern age—radiographic imaging of the body. **Radiography,** or x-ray photography, is the oldest and still the most widely used method of noninvasive imaging of internal body structures and earned Röntgen a Nobel prize. While studying the effects of electricity passing through gas under low pressures, Röntgen accidentally discovered x-rays when they caused a plate coated with special chemicals to glow. Not long after that, he showed that they could produce shadows of internal organs such as bones on photographic film. His first, and most famous, radiograph was of his wife Bertha's hand. Although a little fuzzy, it clearly showed Bertha's finger bones and the outline of her ring. When this radiograph was published by a Vienna newspaper, the entire world became instantly aware of his breakthrough discovery.

The figure at right shows how radiography works. A source of waves in the x band of the radiation spectrum beams the x-rays through a body and to a piece of photographic film or phosphorescent screen. The resulting image shows the outlines of bones and other dense structures that absorb the x-rays. As the figure shows, one way to make soft, hollow structures such as digestive organs more visible is to use radiopaque contrast material. For example, barium sulfate (which absorbs x-rays) can be injected into the colon to make it more visible in a radiograph.

Today, many variations of Röntgen's invention are used to study internal organs without having to cut into the body. For example, computed tomography (CT) scanning is a modern, computerized type of x-ray photography. Radiographic technicians are health professionals whose chief responsibility is to make radiographs and radiologists are responsible for interpreting these images. Many medical, veterinary, and dental professionals rely on these images and interpretations in their diagnosis, assessment, and treatment of patients. In addition, radiography is used in many industrial and investigative settings—and even by archaeologists studying mummies.

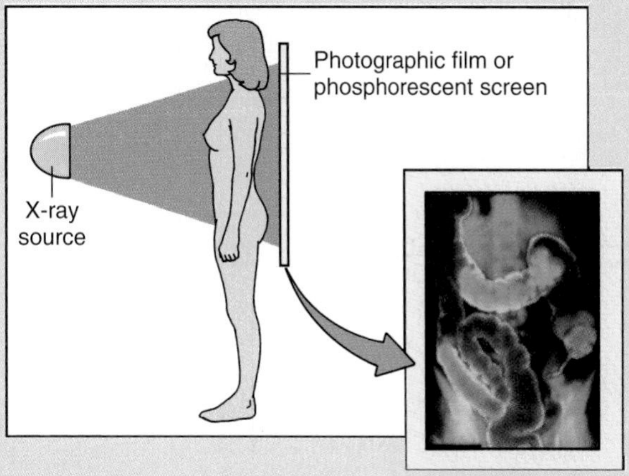

Radiography

purposes. In the female the urinary and reproductive passages are completely separate, so the urethra performs only a urinary function.

In addition to the organs of the urinary system, other organs are also involved in the elimination of body wastes. Undigested food residues and metabolic wastes are eliminated from the intestinal tract as feces, and the lungs rid the body of carbon dioxide. The skin also serves an excretory function by eliminating water and some salts in sweat.

Reproductive System

The normal function of the **reproductive system** is different from the normal function of other organ systems of the body. The proper functioning of the reproductive systems ensures survival, not of the individual but of the species—the human race. In addition, production of the hormones that permit the development of sexual characteristics occurs as a result of normal reproductive system activity.

FIGURE 4-11

Urinary system.

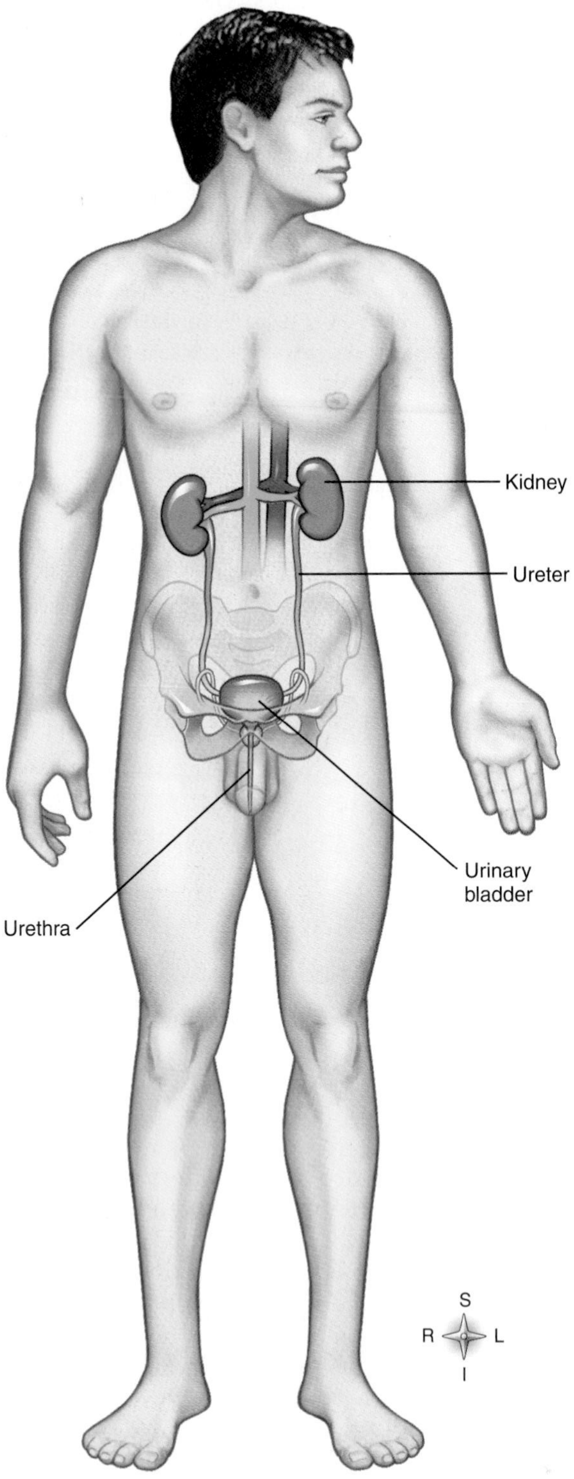

FIGURE 4-12

Male reproductive system.

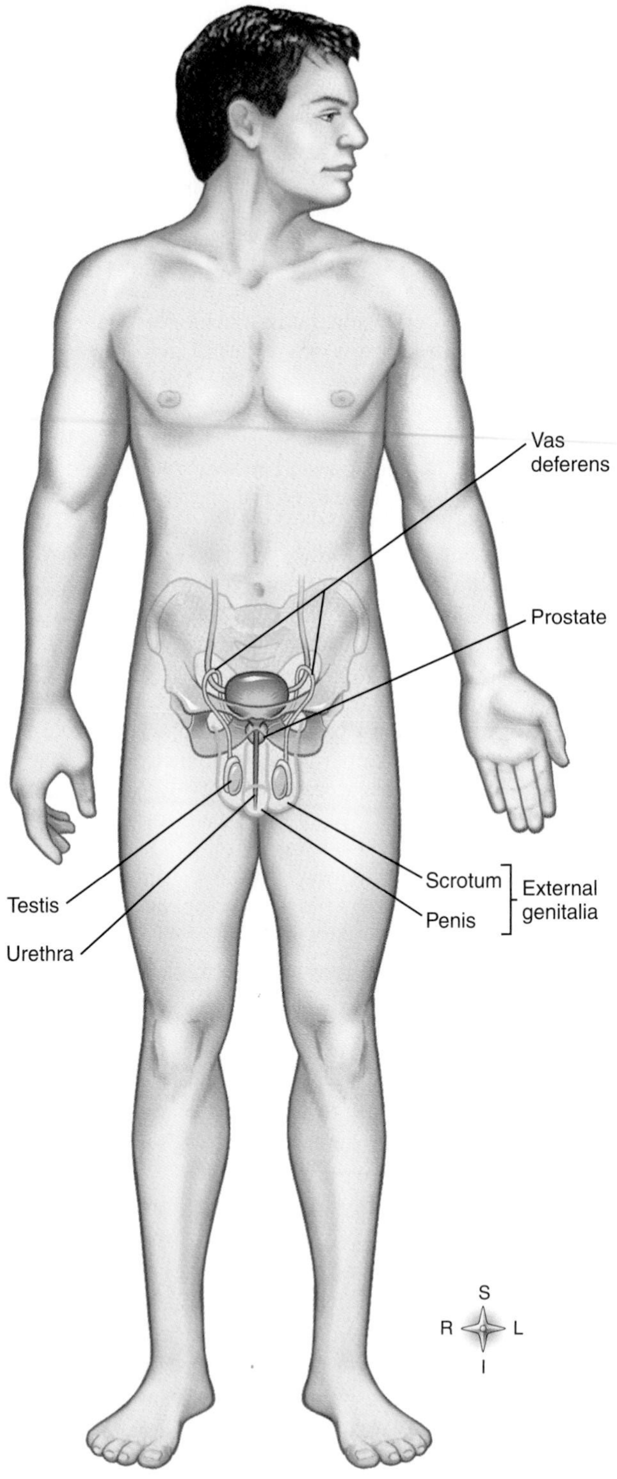

FIGURE 4-13

Female reproductive system.

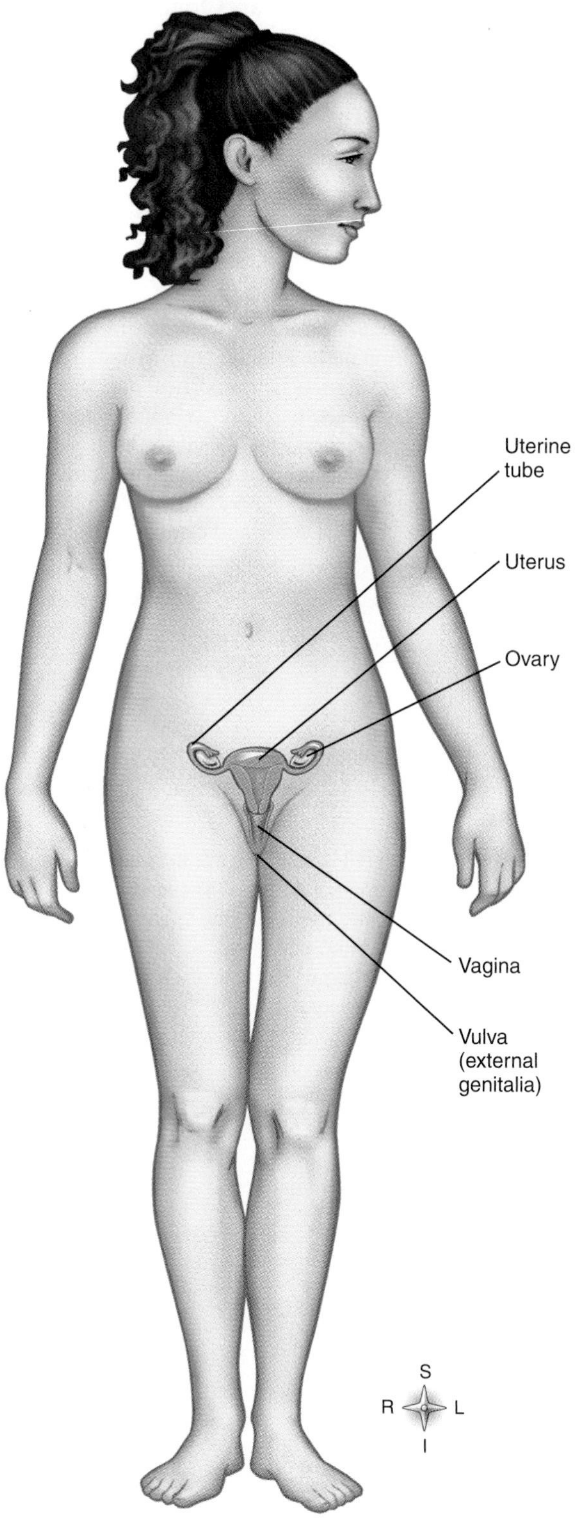

The male reproductive structures shown in Figure 4-12 include the **gonads** (GO-nads), called **testes** (TES-teez), which produce the sex cells or **sperm;** one of the important *genital ducts,* called the **vas deferens** (vas DEF-er-enz); and the **prostate** (PROSS-tate), which is classified as an **accessory organ** in the male. The **penis** (PEE-nis) and **scrotum** (SKRO-tum) are supporting structures and together are known as the **genitalia** (jen-i-tail-yah). The urethra, which is identified in Figure 4-11 as part of the urinary system, passes through the penis. It serves as a genital duct that carries sperm to the exterior and as a passageway for the elimination of urine. Functioning together, these structures produce, transfer, and ultimately introduce sperm into the female reproductive tract, where fertilization can occur. Sperm produced by the testes travel through a number of genital ducts, including the vas deferens, to exit the body. The prostate and other accessory organs, which add fluid and nutrients to the sex cells as they pass through the ducts and the supporting structures (especially the penis), permit transfer of sex cells into the female reproductive tract.

Female Reproductive System

The female **gonads** are the **ovaries.** The **accessory organs** shown in Figure 4-13 include the **uterus** (YOO-ter-us), **uterine** (YOO-ter-in) or **fallopian tubes,** and the **vagina** (vah-JYE-nah). In the female the term ***vulva*** (VUL-vah) is used to describe the external genitalia. The breasts or **mammary glands** are also classified as external accessory sex organs in the female.

The reproductive organs in the female produce the sex cells or **ova**; receive the male sex cells (sperm); transfer the sex cells to the uterus; permit fertilization; and allow for the development, birth, and nourishment of offspring.

Quick Check

1. What are the functions of the lymphatic system?
2. What functions besides gas exchange are performed by the respiratory system?
3. What are some of the accessory organs of the digestive system?
4. What organ in males is shared by both the urinary system and the reproductive system?

THE BODY AS A WHOLE

As you study the more detailed structure and function of the organ systems in the chapters that follow, always relate the system and its component organs to the body as a whole. No one body system functions entirely independently of other systems. Instead, you will find that they are structurally and functionally interrelated and interdependent.

Health & Well-Being

Cancer Screening Tests

A knowledge of the structure and function of the body organ systems is a critically important "first step" in understanding and using information that empowers us to become more sophisticated guardians of our own health and well-being. For example, a better understanding of the reproductive system helps individuals participate in a more direct and personal way in cancer prevention screening techniques.

Breast and testicular self-examinations to detect cancer are two important ways that women and men can participate directly in protecting their own health. Instruction in these techniques is an important part of many home health care educational outreach services. Although specific instructions for these self-tests lie beyond the scope of a textbook of normal anatomy and physiology, it is important to note that this information is readily available from the American Cancer Society and from most hospitals, clinics, and health care providers.

Health & Well-Being

Paired Organs

Have you ever wondered what advantage there might be in having two kidneys, two lungs, two eyes, and two of many other organs? Although the body could function well with only one of each, most of us are born with a pair of these organs. For paired organs that are vital to survival, such as the kidneys, this arrangement allows for the accidental loss of one organ without immediate threat to the survival of the individual. Athletes who have lost one vital organ through injury or disease are often counseled against participating in contact sports that carry the risk of damaging the remaining organ. If the second organ is damaged, total loss of a vital function, such as sight, or even death may result.

OUTLINE SUMMARY

DEFINITIONS AND CONCEPTS

A. Organ—a structure made up of two or more kinds of tissues organized in such a way that they can together perform a more complex function than can any tissue alone

B. Organ system—a group of organs arranged in such a way that they can together perform a more complex function than can any organ alone

C. Knowledge of individual organs and how they are organized into groups makes the understanding of how a particular organ system functions as a whole more meaningful

ORGAN SYSTEMS

A. Integumentary system (Figure 4-2)
- **1.** Structure—organs
  - **a.** Skin
  - **b.** Hair
  - **c.** Nails
  - **d.** Sense receptors
  - **e.** Sweat glands
  - **f.** Oil glands
- **2.** Functions
  - **a.** Protection
  - **b.** Regulation of body temperature
  - **c.** Synthesis of chemicals
  - **d.** Sense organ

B. Skeletal system (Figure 4-3)
- **1.** Structure
  - **a.** Bones
  - **b.** Joints
- **2.** Functions
  - **a.** Support
  - **b.** Movement (with joints and muscles)
  - **c.** Storage of minerals
  - **d.** Blood cell formation

C. Muscular system (Figure 4-4)
- **1.** Structure
  - **a.** Muscles
    - **(1)** Voluntary or striated
    - **(2)** Involuntary or smooth
    - **(3)** Cardiac
- **2.** Functions
  - **a.** Movement
  - **b.** Maintenance of body posture
  - **c.** Production of heat

D. Nervous system (Figure 4-5)
- **1.** Structure
  - **a.** Brain
  - **b.** Spinal cord
  - **c.** Nerves
  - **d.** Sense organs
- **2.** Functions
  - **a.** Communication
  - **b.** Integration
  - **c.** Control
  - **d.** Recognition of sensory stimuli
- **3.** System functions by production of nerve impulses caused by stimuli of various types
- **4.** Control is fast-acting and of short duration

E. Endocrine system (Figure 4-6)
- **1.** Structure
  - **a.** Pituitary gland
  - **b.** Pineal gland
  - **c.** Hypothalamus
  - **d.** Thyroid gland
  - **e.** Parathyroid glands
  - **f.** Thymus gland
  - **g.** Adrenal glands
  - **h.** Pancreas
  - **i.** Ovaries (female)
  - **j.** Testes (male)

Continued

OUTLINE SUMMARY—*cont'd*

2. Functions
   a. Secretion of special substances called hormones directly into the blood
   b. Same as nervous system—communication, integration, control
   c. Control is slow and of long duration
   d. Examples of hormone regulation:
      (1) Growth
      (2) Metabolism
      (3) Reproduction
      (4) Fluid and electrolyte balance

F. Cardiovascular (circulatory) system (Figure 4-7)
1. Structure
   a. Heart
   b. Blood vessels
2. Functions
   a. Transportation
   b. Regulation of body temperature
   c. Immunity (body defense)

G. Lymphatic system (Figure 4-8)
1. Structure
   a. Lymph nodes
   b. Lymphatic vessels
   c. Thymus
   d. Spleen
2. Functions
   a. Transportation
   b. Immunity (body defense)

H. Respiratory system (Figure 4-9)
1. Structure
   a. Nose
   b. Pharynx
   c. Larynx
   d. Trachea
   e. Bronchi
   f. Lungs
2. Functions
   a. Exchange of waste gas (carbon dioxide) for oxygen in the lungs
   b. Area of gas exchange in the lungs called alveoli
   c. Filtration of irritants from inspired air
   d. Regulation of acid-base balance

I. Digestive system (Figure 4-10)
1. Structure
   a. Primary organs
      (1) Mouth
      (2) Pharynx
      (3) Esophagus
      (4) Stomach
      (5) Small intestine
      (6) Large intestine
      (7) Rectum
      (8) Anal canal
   b. Accessory organs
      (1) Teeth
      (2) Salivary glands
      (3) Tongue
      (4) Liver
      (5) Gallbladder
      (6) Pancreas
      (7) Appendix
2. Functions
   a. Mechanical and chemical breakdown (digestion) of food
   b. Absorption of nutrients
   c. Undigested waste product that is eliminated is called *feces*
   d. Appendix is a structural but not a functional part of digestive system
   e. Inflammation of appendix is called *appendicitis*

OUTLINE SUMMARY—*cont'd*

J. Urinary system (Figure 4-11)
  1. Structure
    a. Kidneys
    b. Ureters
    c. Urinary bladder
    d. Urethra
  2. Functions
    a. "Clearing" or cleaning blood of waste products—waste product excreted from body is called *urine*
    b. Electrolyte balance
    c. Water balance
    d. Acid-base balance
    e. In males, urethra has urinary and reproductive functions

K. Reproductive system (Figures 4-12 and 4-13)
  1. Structure
    a. Male
      (1) Gonads—testes
      (2) Genital ducts—vas deferens, urethra
      (3) Accessory gland—prostate
      (4) Supporting structures—genitalia (penis and scrotum)
    b. Female
      (1) Gonads—ovaries
      (2) Accessory organs—uterus, uterine (fallopian) tubes, vagina
      (3) Supporting structures—genitalia (vulva), mammary glands (breasts)
  2. Functions
    a. Survival of genes
    b. Production of sex cells (male: sperm; female: ova)
    c. Transfer and fertilization of sex cells
    d. Development and birth of offspring
    e. Nourishment of offspring
    f. Production of sex hormones

NEW WORDS

appendix	gastrointestinal (GI) tract	integumentary	urine
cardiovascular	genitalia	lymphatic	
endocrine	hormone	nerve impulse	
feces		stimuli	

REVIEW QUESTIONS

Review the names of organ systems and individual organs in Figures 4-1 through 4-13.

1. Define *organ* and *organ system*.
2. Give examples of the stimuli to which the skin organs can respond.
3. How is the skin able to assist in the body's ability to regulate temperature?
4. What is the function of tendons?
5. What are some of the differences between the lymphatic and cardiovascular systems?
6. Name the organs that help rid the body of waste. What type of waste does each organ remove?
7. Besides bone, what other types of tissues are included in the skeletal system
8. List the eleven organ systems discussed in this chapter.
9. Most of the organ systems have more than one function. List two functions for the following systems: integumentary system, skeletal system, muscular system, lymphatic system, respiratory system and urinary system.
10. What is unique about the reproductive system?

CRITICAL THINKING

11. Explain the differences between the nervous and endocrine systems. Include what types of functions are regulated and the "message carriers" for each system.
12. The term *balance* is used in this chapter. This is another term for *homeostasis*. Go through the functions of the systems and list the homeostatic functions they have.

CHAPTER TEST

1. The primary organs of the digestive system make a long tube called the ___________ .
2. ___________ is another term for voluntary muscle.
3. ___________ is another term for involuntary muscle.
4. The nervous system can generate special electrochemical signals called ___________ .
5. The ______________, ______________, ______________, and ______________ are called the appendages of the skin.
6. The ___________ is part of both the lymphatic and endocrine systems.
7. The ___________ is part of both the male reproductive and urinary systems.
8. The gonads for the male reproductive system are the ___________ ; for the female reproductive system the gonads are the ___________ .
9. The skeletal system is composed of bone tissue and these two related tissues: ___________ and ___________ .

CHAPTER TEST—*cont'd*

Match the function in Column B with the correct system in Column A.

COLUMN A		COLUMN B
10. ______	Integumentary	**a.** Provides movement, body posture, and heat
11. ______	Skeletal	**b.** Uses hormones to regulate body functions
12. ______	Muscular	**c.** Transports fatty nutrients from the digestive system to the blood
13. ______	Nervous	**d.** Physical and chemical change in nutrients and absorption of
14. ______	Endocrine nutrients	**e.** Cleans the blood of metabolic wastes and regulates electrolyte balance
15. ______	Cardiovascular	**f.** Protection of underlying structures, sensory reception, and regulation of body temperature
16. ______	Lymphatic	**g.** Transports substances from one part of the body to another
17. ______	Respiratory	**h.** Ensures the survival of the species rather than the individual
18. ______	Digestive	**i.** Uses electrochemical signals to integrate and control body functions
19. ______	Urinary	**j.** Exchanges oxygen and carbon dioxide and regulates acid-base balance
20. ______	Reproductive	**k.** Provides a rigid framework for the body and stores minerals

STUDY TIPS

Chapter Four is the perfect "big picture" chapter. It is a preview for most of the remaining chapters in the text. Put the name of the system on one side of a flash card and the function of that system and its organs on the other side. Notice how each organ contributes to the function of the system. Before you begin the chapter dealing with a particular system, it would be helpful to get an overview of that system by reviewing the synopsis of that system in this chapter.

In your study groups, go over the flash cards. Discuss how several systems need to be involved in accomplishing one function in the body such as getting food or oxygen to the cells. Go over the questions in the back of the chapter and discuss possible test questions.

The Integumentary System and Body Membranes

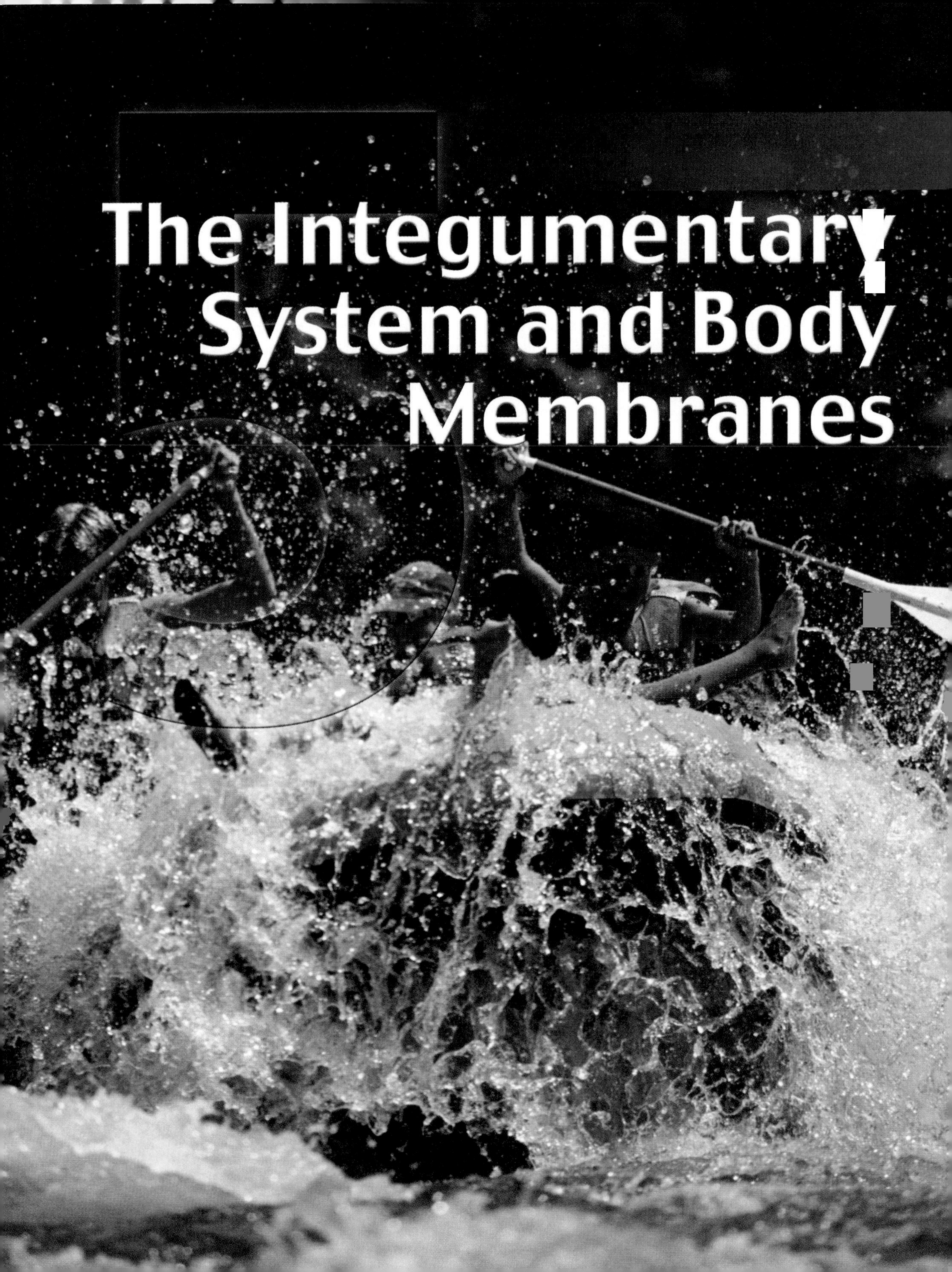

Outline

Objectives

AFTER YOU HAVE COMPLETED THIS CHAPTER, YOU SHOULD BE ABLE TO:

1. Classify, compare the structure of, and give examples of each type of body membrane.
2. Describe the structure and function of the epidermis and dermis.
3. List and briefly describe each accessory organ of the skin.
4. List and discuss the three primary functions of the integumentary system.
5. Classify burns and describe how to estimate the extent of a burn injury.

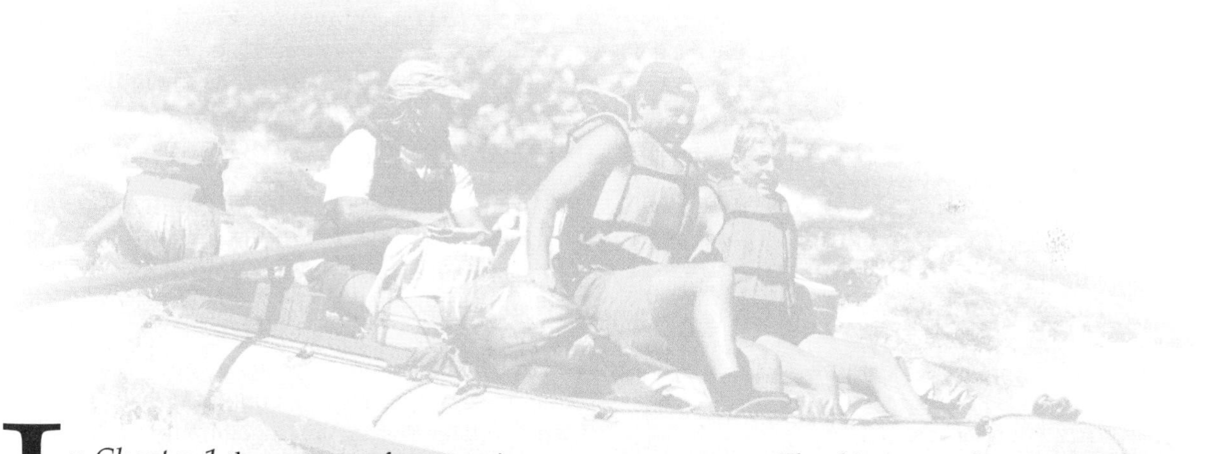

In Chapter 1 the concept of progressive organization of body structures from simple to complex was established. Complexity in body structure and function progresses from cells to tissues and then to organs and organ systems. This chapter discusses the skin and its **appendages**—the hair, the nails, and the skin glands—as an organ system. This system is called the **integumentary system. Integument** (in-TEG-yoo-ment) is another name for the skin, and the skin itself is the principal organ of the integumentary system. The skin is one of a group of anatomically simple but functionally important sheetlike structures called **membranes.** This chapter will begin with classification and discussion of the important body membranes. Study of the structure and function of the integument will follow. Ideally, you should study the skin and its appendages before proceeding to the more traditional organ systems in the chapters that follow to improve your understanding of how structure is related to function.

CLASSIFICATION OF BODY MEMBRANES

The term *membrane* refers to a thin, sheetlike structure that may have many important functions in the body. Membranes cover and protect the body surface, line body cavities, and cover the inner surfaces of the hollow organs such as the digestive, reproductive, and respiratory passageways. Some membranes anchor organs to each other or to bones, and others cover the internal organs. In certain areas of the body, membranes secrete lubricating fluids that reduce friction during organ movements such as the beating of the heart or lung expansion and contraction. Membrane lubricants also decrease friction between bones in joints. There are two major categories or types of body membranes:

1. **Epithelial membranes,** composed of epithelial tissue and an underlying layer of specialized connective tissue
2. **Connective tissue membranes,** composed exclusively of various types of connective tissue; no epithelial cells are present in this type of membrane

Epithelial Membranes

There are three types of epithelial tissue membranes in the body:

1. Cutaneous membrane
2. Serous membranes
3. Mucous membranes

Cutaneous Membrane

The **cutaneous** (kyoo-TAY-nee-us) **membrane** or **skin** is the primary organ of the integumentary system. It is one of the most important and certainly one of the largest and most visible organs. In most individuals the skin composes some 16% of the body weight. It fulfills the requirements necessary for an epithelial tissue membrane in that it has a superficial layer of epithelial cells and an underlying layer of supportive connective tissue. Its structure is uniquely suited to its many functions. The skin will be discussed in depth later in the chapter.

Serous Membranes

As with all epithelial membranes, a **serous** (SE-rus) **membrane** is composed of two distinct layers of tissue. The epithelial sheet is a thin layer of simple squamous epithelium. The connective tissue layer forms a very thin, gluelike **basement membrane** that holds and supports the epithelial cells.

The serous membrane that lines body cavities and covers the surfaces of organs in those cavities is in reality a single, continuous sheet of tissue covering two different surfaces. The name of the serous membrane is determined by its location. Using this criterion results in two types of serous membranes; the first type lines body cavities, and the second type covers the organs in those cavities. The serous membrane, which lines the walls of a body cavity much like wallpaper covers the walls of a room, is called the **parietal** (pah-RYE-i-tal) **portion.** The other type of serous membrane, which covers the surface of organs found in body cavities, is called the **visceral** (VIS-er-al) **portion.**

The serous membranes of the thoracic and abdominal cavities are identified in Figure 5-1. In the thoracic cavity the serous membranes are called **pleura** (PLOOR-ah); in the abdominal cavity, they are called **peritoneum** (pair-i-toe-NEE-um). Look again at Figure 5-1 to note the placement of the **parietal** and **visceral pleura** and the **parietal** and **visceral peritoneum.** In both cases the parietal layer forms the lining of the body cavity, and the visceral layer covers the organs found in that cavity.

Serous membranes secrete a thin, watery fluid that helps reduce friction and serves as a lubricant when organs rub against one another and against the walls of the cavities that contain them. **Pleurisy** (PLOOR-i-see) is a very painful pathological condition characterized by inflammation of the serous membranes (pleura) that line the chest cavity and cover the lungs. Pain is caused by irritation and friction as the lungs rub against the walls of the chest cavity. In severe cases the inflamed surfaces of the pleura fuse, and permanent damage may develop. The term *peritonitis* (pair-i-toe-NYE-tis) is used to describe inflammation of the serous membranes in the abdominal cavity. Peritonitis is sometimes a serious complication of an infected appendix.

FIGURE 5-1

Types of body membranes. A, Epithelial membranes, including cutaneous membrane (skin), serous membranes (parietal and visceral pleura and peritoneum), and mucous membranes. **B,** Connective tissue membranes, including synovial membranes. See text for explanation.

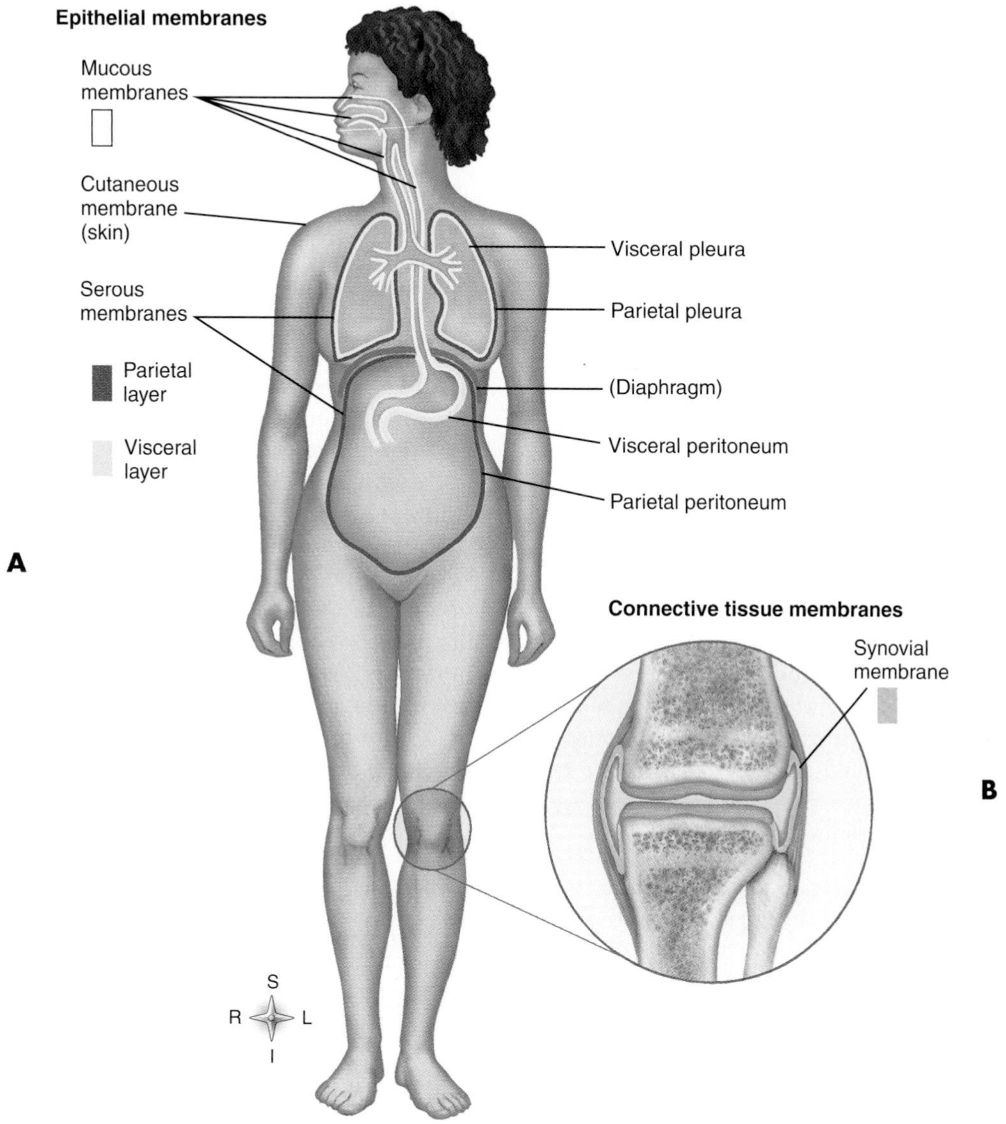

Mucous Membranes

Mucous (MYOO-kus) **membranes** are epithelial membranes that line body surfaces opening directly to the exterior. Examples of mucous membranes include those lining the respiratory, digestive, urinary, and reproductive tracts. The epithelial component of a mucous membrane varies, depending on its location and function. In the esophagus, for example, a tough, abrasion-resistant stratified squamous epithelium is found. A thin layer of simple columnar epithelium covers the walls of the lower segments of the digestive tract.

The epithelial cells of most mucous membranes secrete a thick, slimy material called **mucus** that keeps the membranes moist and soft.

The term **mucocutaneous** (myoo-ko-kyoo-TAY-nee-us) **junction** is used to describe the transitional area that serves as a point of "fusion" where skin and mucous membranes meet. Such junctions lack accessory organs such as hair or sweat glands that characterize skin. These transitional areas are generally moistened by mucous glands within the body orifices or openings where these junctions are located. The eyelids, nasal openings, vulva, and anus have mucocutaneous junctions that may become sites of infection or irritation.

Connective Tissue Membranes

Unlike cutaneous, serous, and mucous membranes, connective tissue membranes do not contain epithelial components. The **synovial** (si-NO-vee-al) **membranes** lining the spaces between bones and joints that move are classified as connective tissue membranes. These membranes are smooth and slick and secrete a thick, colorless lubricating fluid called **synovial fluid.** The membrane itself, with its specialized fluid, helps reduce friction between the opposing surfaces of bones in movable joints. Synovial membranes also line the small, cushionlike sacs called **bursae** (BER-see) found between moving body parts.

Quick Check

1. What are the four main types of membranes in the body?
2. Which of the body's membranes are types of epithelial membranes?
3. What fluid(s) is/are produced by each of the four main membrane types? What is the function of each fluid?

THE SKIN

The brief description of the skin in Chapter 4 (see p. 80) identified it not only as the primary organ of the integumentary system but also as the largest and one of the most important organs of the body. Architecturally the skin is a marvel. Consider the incredible number of structures fitting into 1 square inch of skin: 500 sweat glands; more than 1,000 nerve endings; yards of tiny blood vessels; nearly 100 oil or **sebaceous** (se-BAY-shus) **glands;** 150 sensors for pressure, 75 for heat, and 10 for cold; along with millions of cells.

Structure of the Skin

The skin or cutaneous membrane is a sheetlike organ composed of the following layers of distinct tissue (Figure 5-2):

1. The **epidermis** is the outermost layer of the skin. It is a relatively thin sheet of stratified squamous epithelium.
2. The **dermis** is the deeper of the two layers. It is thicker than the epidermis and is made up largely of connective tissue.

As you can see in Figure 5-2, the layers of the skin are supported by a thick layer of loose connective tissue and fat called **subcutaneous** (sub-kyoo-TAY-nee-us) **tissue** or the **hypodermis** (hy-poh-DER-mis). Fat in the subcutaneous layer insulates the body from extremes of heat and cold. It also serves as a stored source of energy for the body and can be used as a food source if required. In addition, the subcutaneous tissue acts as a shock-absorbing pad and helps protect underlying tissues from injury caused by bumps and blows to the body surface.

Epidermis

The tightly packed epithelial cells of the epidermis are arranged in many distinct layers. The cells of the innermost layer, called the **stratum germinativum,** undergo mitosis and reproduce themselves (see Figure 5-2). As they move toward the surface of the skin, these new cells "specialize" in ways that increase their ability to provide protection for the body tissues that lie below them. This ability is of critical clinical significance. It enables the skin to repair itself if it is injured. The self-repairing characteristic of normal skin makes it possible for the body to maintain an effective barrier against infection, even when it is subjected to injury and normal wear and tear. As new cells are produced

FIGURE 5-2

Microscopic view of the skin. The epidermis, shown in longitudinal section, is raised at one corner to reveal the ridges in the dermis.

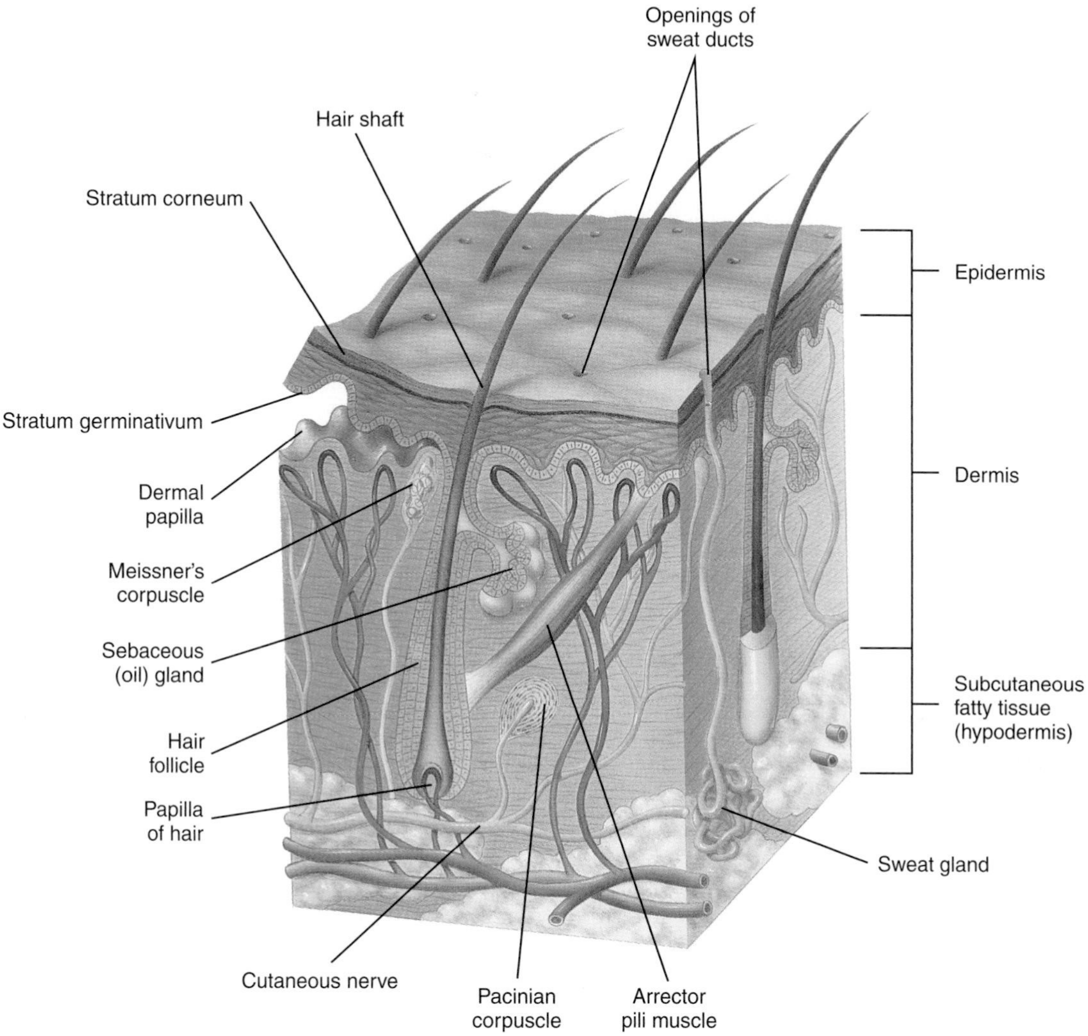

in the deep layer of the epidermis, they move upward through additional layers, or "strata" of cells. As they approach the surface, the cytoplasm is replaced by one of nature's most unique proteins, a substance called **keratin** (KARE-ah-tin). Keratin is a tough, waterproof material that provides cells in the outer layer of the skin with a horny, abrasion-resistant, and protective quality. The tough outer layer of the epidermis is called the **stratum corneum** (KOR-nee-um). Cells filled with keratin are continually pushed to the surface of the epidermis. In the photomicrograph of the skin shown in Figure 5-3, many of the outermost cells of the stratum corneum have been dislodged. These dry, dead cells filled with keratin "flake off" by the thousands onto our clothes, our bath water,

FIGURE 5-3

Photomicrograph of the skin. Many dead cells of the stratum corneum have flaked off from the surface of the epidermis. Note that the epidermis is very cellular. The dermis has fewer cells and more connective tissue.

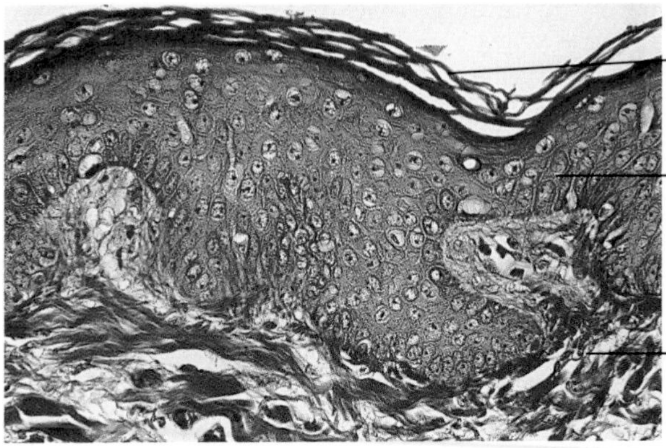

and things we handle. Millions of epithelial cells reproduce daily to replace the millions shed—just one example of the work our bodies do without our knowledge, even when we seem to be resting.

The deepest cell layer of the epidermis identified in Figure 5-2 is responsible for the production of a specialized **pigment** substance that gives color to the skin. The term *pigment* comes from a Latin word meaning "paint." It is this epidermal layer that gives color to the skin. The brown pigment **melanin** (MEL-ah-nin) is produced by specialized cells in this layer. These cells are called **melanocytes** (MEL-ah-no-sites). The higher the concentration of melanin, the deeper is the color of skin. The primary function of melanin is to absorb harmful ultraviolet (UV) radiation from sunlight before it reaches tissues below the outer layers of the skin. The amount of melanin in your skin depends first on the skin color genes you have inherited. That is, heredity determines how dark or light your basic skin color is. However, other factors such as sunlight can modify this hereditary effect. Prolonged exposure to sunlight in light-skinned people darkens the exposed area because it leads to increased melanin deposits in the epidermis—a protective mechanism that keeps deeper tissues safe from UV radiation. If the skin contains little melanin, as under the nails where there is no melanin at all, a change in color can occur if the volume of blood in the skin changes significantly or if the amount of oxygen in the blood is increased or decreased. In these individuals increased blood flow to the skin or increased blood oxygen levels can cause a pink flush to appear. However, if blood oxygen levels decrease or if actual blood flow is reduced dramatically, the skin turns a bluish gray color—a condition called **cyanosis** (SYE-ah-NO-sis). In general, the less abundant the melanin deposits in the skin, the more visible the changes in color caused by the change in skin blood volume or oxygen level. Conversely, the richer the skin's pigmentation, the less noticeable such changes will be.

The cells of the epidermis are packed tightly together. They are held firmly to one another and to the dermis below by specialized junctions between the membranes of adjacent cells. If these links, sometimes described as "spot welds," are weakened or destroyed, the skin falls apart. When this occurs because of burns, friction injuries, or exposure to irritants, **blisters** may result.

The junction that exists between the thin epidermal layer of the skin above and the dermal layer below is called the **dermal-epidermal junction.** The area of contact between dermis and epidermis "glues" them together and provides support for the epidermis, which is attached to its upper surface. Blister formation also occurs if this junction is damaged or destroyed. The junction is

Science Applications

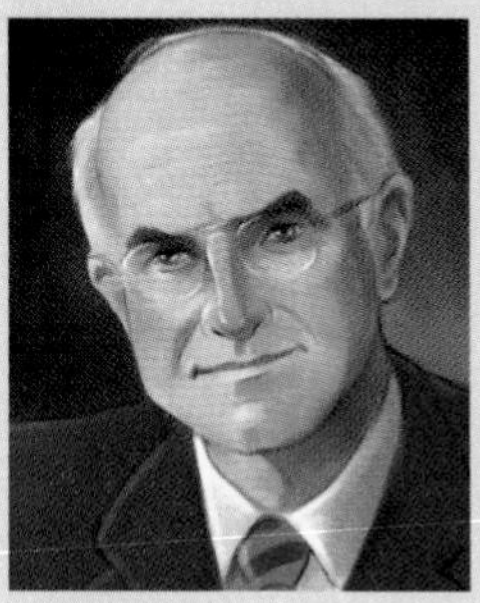

Secrets of the Skin

Dr. Joseph E. Murray (b. 1919).

The skin is our most visible organ, so it is no wonder that observing the structure and function of skin has generated sparks that have lit the fires of scientific discovery through the ages. The ancient Romans outlined the process of inflammation in detail after observing it first in the skin. In the twentieth century, Joseph Murray (see figure) noticed that skin he grafted onto burned soldiers he treated during World War II would eventually be rejected by the body. After the war, Murray tried to understand the body's immune reactions to transplanted tissues; his work led to the first successful kidney transplants. His breakthroughs in transplanting kidneys not only earned him a Nobel Prize in 1990, it also paved the way for all the different types of tissue and organ transplantation that we see today.

Many scientists continue to study the secrets of the skin and many physicians and other health care professionals also pioneer new methods of skin care and treatment in the fields of dermatology, allergy, burn medicine, and reconstructive and cosmetic surgery. Additional practical applications of some of this skin science are practiced by people working with cosmetics and other skin treatments, nail treatments, and hair treatments. For example, industrial researchers, product developers, cosmeticians, spa specialists, and hair stylists all require some knowledge of current skin science to do their jobs effectively.

visible in Figure 5-2, which shows the epidermis lifted up on one corner to reveal the underlying dermis more clearly.

Dermis

The dermis is the deeper of the two primary skin layers and is much thicker than the epidermis. It is composed largely of connective tissue. Instead of cells being crowded close together like the epithelial cells of the epidermis, they are scattered far apart, with many fibers in between. Some of the fibers are tough and strong (collagen or white fibers), and others are stretchable and elastic (elastic or yellow fibers).

The upper region of the dermis is characterized by parallel rows of tiny bumps called **dermal papillae** (pah-PIL-ee), which are visible in Figure 5-2. These upward projections are interesting and useful features. They form an important part of the dermal-epidermal junction that helps bind the skin layers together. In addition, they form the ridges and grooves that make up your fingerprints and footprints.

You can observe these ridges on the tips of the fingers and on the skin covering the palms of your hands. Observe in Figure 5-2 how the epidermis follows the contours of the dermal papillae. These ridges develop sometime before birth. Not only is their pattern unique in each individual, but also the pattern never changes except to grow larger—two facts that explain why our fingerprints or footprints can provide positive identification of who we are. The biological function of skin ridges is to improve our grip when making or using tools, for example, or walking bare-footed on smooth surfaces.

The deeper area of the dermis is filled with a dense network of interlacing fibers. Most of the fibers in this area are collagen that gives toughness to the skin. However, elastic fibers are also present. These make the skin stretchable and elastic (able to rebound). As we age, the number of elastic fibers in the dermis decreases, and the amount of fat stored in the subcutaneous tissue is reduced. Wrinkles develop as the skin loses elasticity, sags, and becomes less soft and pliant.

In addition to connective tissue elements, the dermis contains a specialized network of nerves and nerve endings to process sensory information such as pain, pressure, touch, and temperature. At various levels of the dermis, there are muscle fibers, hair follicles, sweat and sebaceous glands, and many blood vessels.

Clinical Application

Subcutaneous Injection

Although the subcutaneous layer is not part of the skin, it carries the major blood vessels and nerves to the skin above it. The rich blood supply and loose, spongy texture of the subcutaneous layer make it an ideal site for the rapid and relatively pain-free absorption of injected material. Liquid medicines such as insulin and pelleted implant materials are often administered by **subcutaneous injection** into the spongy and porous layer beneath the skin. Because the subcutaneous layer is also called the hypodermis, it is not surprising that subcutaneous injections are given with a *hypodermic needle*.

Appendages of the Skin

Hair

The human body is covered with millions of hairs. Indeed, at the time of birth most of the specialized structures called **follicles** (FOL-li-kuls) that are required for hair growth are already present. They develop early in fetal life and by birth are present in most parts of the skin. The hair of a newborn infant is extremely fine and soft; it is called **lanugo** (lah-NOO-go) from the Latin word meaning "down." In premature infants, lanugo may be noticeable over most of the body, but soon after birth the lanugo is lost and replaced by new hair that is stronger and more pigmented. Although only a few areas of the skin are hairless—notably the lips, the palms of the hands, and the soles of the feet—most body hair remains almost invisible. Hair is most visible on the scalp, eyelids, and eyebrows. The coarse hair that first appears in the pubic and axillary regions at the time of puberty develops in response to the secretion of hormones.

Hair growth begins when cells of the epidermal layer of the skin grow down into the dermis, forming a small tube called the hair follicle. The relationship of a hair follicle and its related structures to the epidermal and dermal layers of the skin is shown in Figure 5-4. Hair growth begins from a small, cap-shaped cluster of cells called the **hair papilla** (pah-PIL-ah), which is located at the base of the follicle. The papilla is nourished by a dermal blood vessel. Note in Figure 5-4 that part of the hair, namely the **root**, lies hidden in the follicle. The visible part of a hair is called the **shaft.** Figure 5-5 shows shafts of hair extending from their follicles.

As long as cells in the papilla of the hair follicle remain alive, new hair will replace any that is cut or plucked. Contrary to popular belief, frequent cutting or shaving does not make hair grow faster or become coarser. Why? Because neither process affects the epithelial cells that form the hairs, because they are embedded in the dermis.

A tiny, smooth (involuntary) muscle can be seen in Figure 5-4. It is called an **arrector pili** (ah-REK-tor PYE-lie) muscle. It is attached to the base of a dermal papilla above and to the side of a hair follicle below. Generally, these muscles contract only when we are frightened or cold. When contraction occurs, each muscle simultaneously pulls on its two points of attachment (that is, up on a hair follicle but down on a part of the skin). This produces little raised places, called *goose bumps*, between the depressed points of the skin and at the same time pulls the hairs up until they are more or less straight. The name *arrector pili* describes the function of these muscles; it is Latin for "erectors of the hair." We unconsciously recognize these facts in expressions such as "I was so frightened my hair stood on end."

Receptors

Receptors in the skin make it possible for the body surface to act as a sense organ, relaying messages to the brain concerning sensations such as touch, pain, temperature, and pressure. Receptors differ in structure from the highly complex to the very simple. Figure 5-6 shows enlarged views of a **Meissner's** (MIZE-ners) **corpuscle** and a **Pacinian** (pah-SIN-ee-an) **corpuscle.** Look again at Figure 5-2 and find these receptors. The Pacinian corpuscle is deep in the dermis. It is capable of detecting *pressure* on the skin surface. The Meissner's corpuscle is generally located close to the skin surface. It is capable of detecting sensations of *light touch.* Both specialized receptors are widely distributed in skin. Additional receptors in the skin respond to other types of stimuli. For example, **free nerve endings** respond to pain and temperature, and receptors called **Krause's end**

FIGURE 5-4

Hair follicle. Relationship of a hair follicle and related structures to the epidermal and dermal layers of the skin.

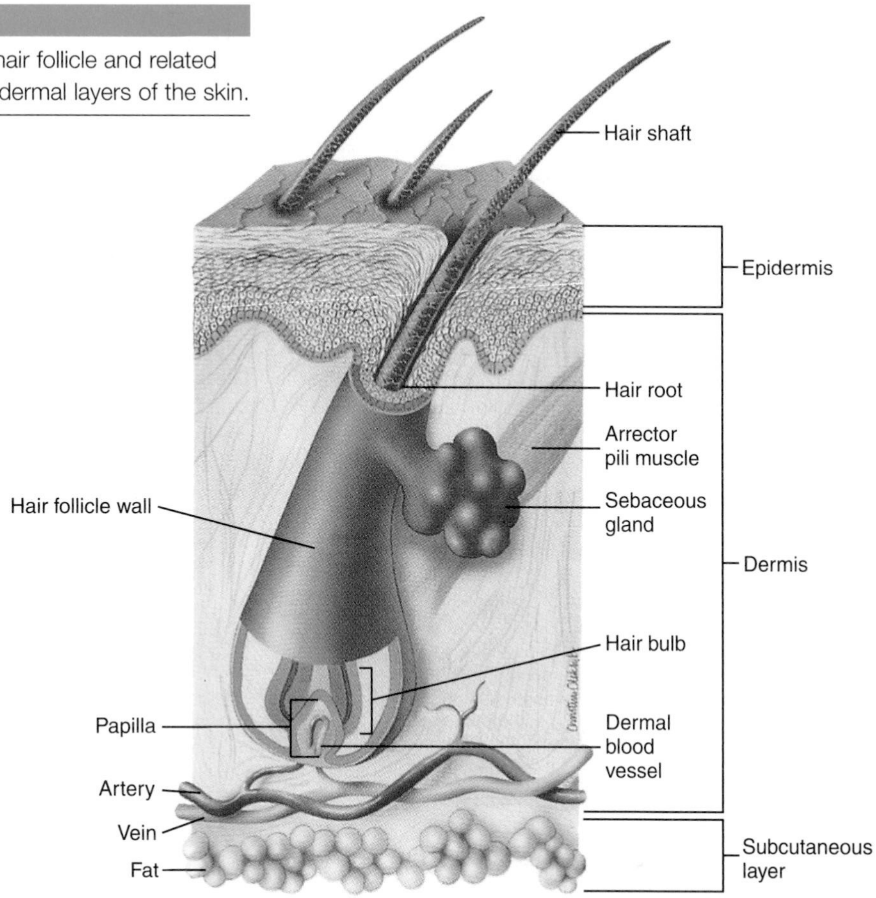

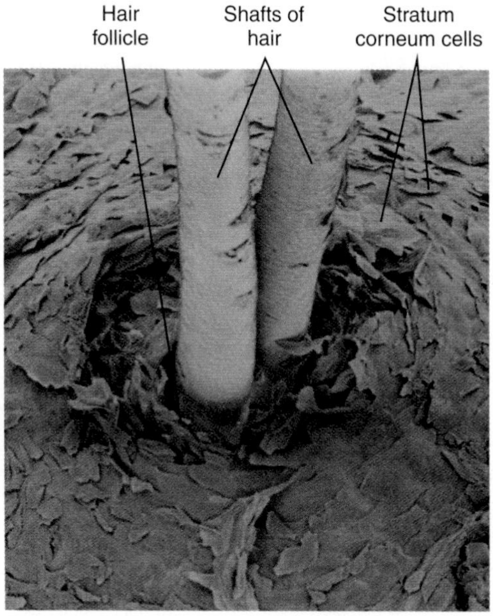

FIGURE 5-5

Hair shaft and follicle. Scanning electron micrograph showing shafts of hair extending from their follicles.

Health & Well-Being

Healthy Skin

Skin, as with any organ, is blemish-free in its ideal, healthy condition. But because it faces our external environment, it is subject to all kinds of injuries and insults. For example, viruses called *papillomaviruses* often cause benign neoplasms (bumps) called **warts.** Various fungi can cause itchy rashes on the skin, especially where the skin is wet and in the dark. For example, in **tinea pedis** (TIN-ee-ah PED-is) or **athlete's foot,** the wet, dark conditions inside an athletic sneaker can produce a mild fungal infection. Minor bacterial infections (such as **acne**) or more serious *Staphylococcus* or **staph** infections can cause skin damage or even body-wide infections. Perhaps the most serious problem in skin is skin cancer. The most serious type of skin cancer is **malignant melanoma** (mel-ah-NO-mah), which is a malignant neoplasm involving the melanin-producing cells of the skin. Melanoma (*A*) is triggered by the long-term effects of childhood exposure to the ultraviolet radiation of the sun and has reached epidemic proportions recently as the first generation of serious sunbathers has reached later adulthood. Another type of skin cancer is **Kaposi sarcoma (KS)** (KAP-oh-see sar-KO-mah), which produces a purplish tumor on the skin (*B*). Historically, KS only rarely affected older men of Mediterranean heritage, but now it often affects people of all ages who have lost their immune function because of acquired immunodeficiency syndrome (AIDS).

Malignant melanoma

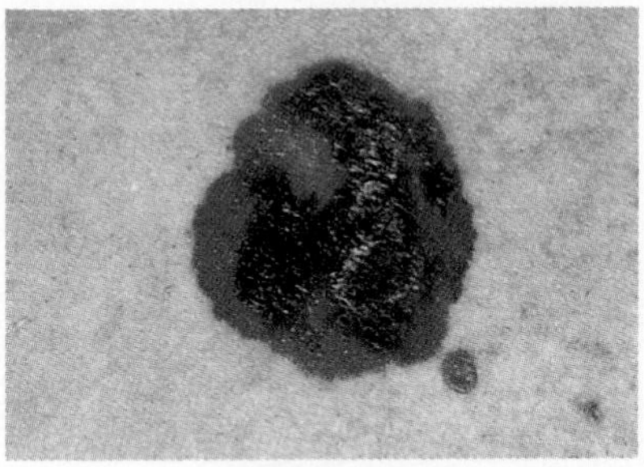

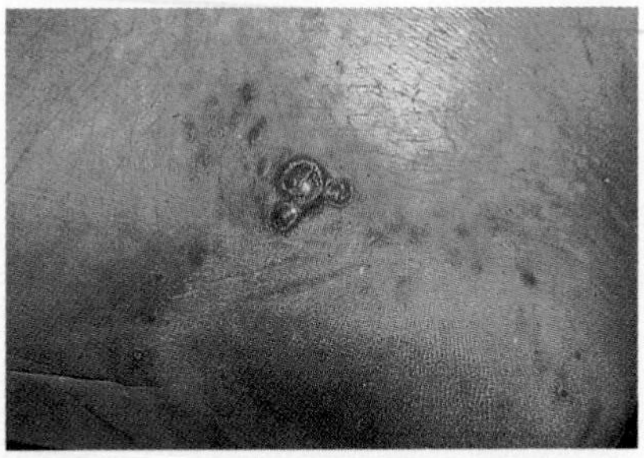

Kaposi sarcoma

FIGURE 5-6

Skin receptors. Receptors are specialized nerve endings that make it possible for the skin to act as a sense organ. **A,** Meissner's corpuscle. **B,** Pacinian corpuscle. (See also Figure 5-2.)

A

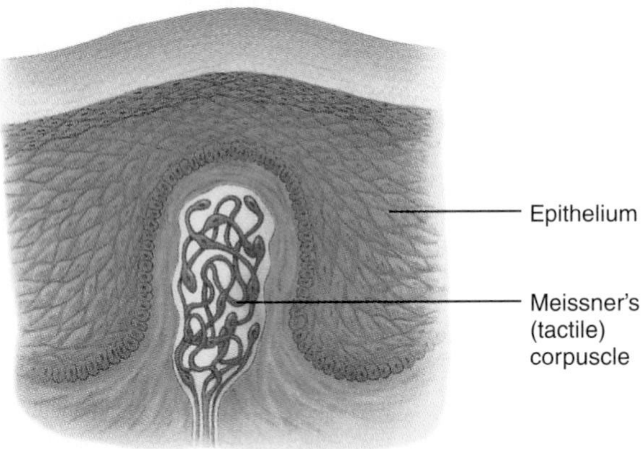

B

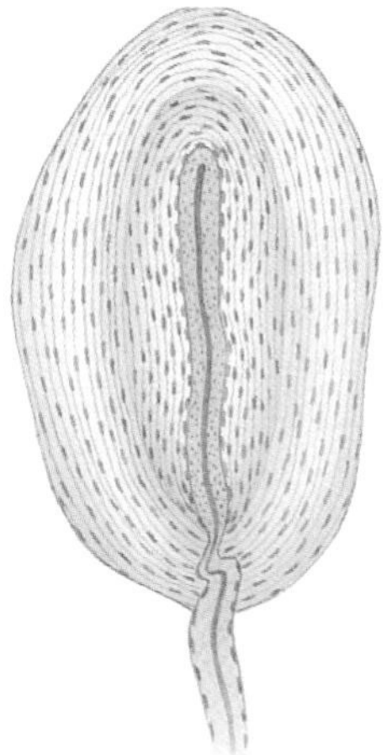

bulbs detect low-frequency vibration. Other receptors mediate sensations such as crude touch, and vibration.

Nails

Nails are classified as accessory organs of the skin and are produced by cells in the epidermis. They form when epidermal cells over the terminal ends of the fingers and toes fill with keratin and become hard and platelike. The components of a typical fingernail and its associated structures are shown in Figure 5-7. In this illustration the fingernail of the index finger is viewed from above and in sagittal section. (Recall that a sagittal section divides a body part into right and left portions.) Look first at the nail as seen from above. The visible part of the nail is called the **nail body.** The rest of the nail, namely, the **root,** lies in a groove and is hidden by a fold of skin called the **cuticle** (KYOO-ti-kul). In the sagittal section you can see the nail root from the side and note its relationship to the cuticle, which is folded back over its upper surface. The nail body nearest the root has a crescent-shaped white area known as the **lunula** (LOO-nyoo-lah), or "little moon." You should be able to identify this area easily on your own nails; it is most noticeable on the thumbnail. Under the nail lies a layer of epithelium called the **nail bed,** which is labeled on the sagittal section in Figure 5-7. Because it contains abundant blood vessels, it appears pink in color through the translucent nail bodies. If blood oxygen levels drop and cyanosis develops, the nail bed will turn blue.

Skin Glands

The skin glands include the two varieties of **sweat** or **sudoriferous** (soo-doe-RIF-er-us) **glands** and the microscopic **sebaceous glands.**

Sweat (sudoriferous) glands. Sweat glands are the most numerous of the skin glands. They can be classified into two groups—**eccrine** (EK-rin) and **apocrine** (AP-o-krin)—based on type of secretion and location. **Eccrine sweat glands** are by far the more numerous, important, and widespread sweat glands in the body. They are quite small and, with few exceptions, are distributed over the total body surface. Throughout life they produce a transparent, watery liquid called **perspiration,** or **sweat.** Sweat assists in the elimination of waste products such as ammonia and uric acid. In addition to elimination of waste, sweat plays a critical role in helping the body maintain a constant temperature. Anatomists estimate that a single square inch of skin on the palms of the hands contains about 3,000 eccrine sweat glands. With a magnifying glass you can locate the pinpoint-size openings on the skin that you probably call **pores.** The pores are outlets of small ducts from the eccrine sweat glands.

Apocrine sweat glands are found primarily in the skin in the armpit (axilla) and in the pigmented skin areas around the genitals. They are larger than

FIGURE 5-7

Structure of nails. A, Fingernail viewed from above. **B,** Sagittal section of fingernail and associated structures.

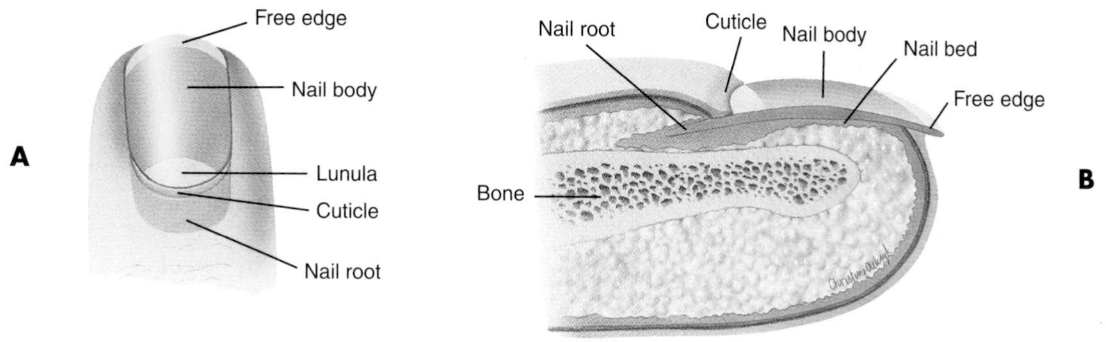

Health & Well-Being

Exercise and the Skin

Excess heat produced by the skeletal muscles during exercise increases the core body temperature far beyond the normal range. Because blood in vessels near the skin's surface dissipates heat well, the body's control centers adjust blood flow so that more warm blood from the body's core is sent to the skin for cooling. During exercise, blood flow in the skin can be so high that the skin takes on a redder coloration.

To help dissipate even more heat, sweat production increases to as high as 3 liters per hour during exercise. Although each sweat gland produces very little of this total, more than 3 million individual sweat glands are found throughout the skin. Sweat evaporation is essential to keeping body temperature in balance, but excessive sweating can lead to a dangerous loss of fluid. Because normal amounts of drinking may not replace the water lost through sweating, it is important to increase fluid consumption during and after any type of exercise to avoid **dehydration.**

the eccrine glands, and instead of watery sweat, they secrete a thicker secretion. The odor associated with apocrine gland secretion is not caused by the secretion itself. Instead, it is caused by the contamination and decomposition of the secretion by skin bacteria. Apocrine glands enlarge and begin to function at puberty.

Sebaceous glands. Sebaceous glands secrete oil for the hair and skin. Oil or sebaceous glands grow where hairs grow. Their tiny ducts open into hair follicles (see Figure 5-4) so that their secretion, called **sebum** (SEE-bum), lubricates the hair and skin. Someone aptly described sebum as "nature's skin cream" because it prevents drying and cracking of the skin. Sebum secretion increases during adolescence, stimulated by the increased blood levels of the sex hormones. Frequently sebum accumulates in and enlarges some of the ducts of the sebaceous glands, forming white pimples. This sebum often darkens, forming a **blackhead.** Sebum secretion decreases in late adulthood, contributing to increased wrinkling and cracking of the skin.

Quick Check

1. What are the two major layers of the skin?
2. Where in the skin would you find layers of dead, keratinized cells?
3. How is hair formed?
4. Where in the skin would you find sensory nerve receptors?

Functions of the Skin

The skin or cutaneous membrane serves three important functions that contribute to survival. The most important functions are:

1. Protection
2. Temperature regulation
3. Sense organ activity

Protection

The skin as a whole is often described as our "first line of defense" against a multitude of hazards. It protects us against the daily invasion of deadly microbes. The tough, keratin-filled cells of the stratum corneum also resist the entry of harmful chemicals and protect against physical tears and cuts. Because it is waterproof, **keratin** also protects the body from excessive fluid loss. Melanin in the pigment layer of the skin prevents the sun's harmful ultraviolet rays from penetrating the interior of the body.

Temperature Regulation

The skin plays a key role in regulating the body's temperature. Incredible as it seems, on a hot and humid day the skin can serve as a means for releasing almost 3,000 calories of body heat—enough heat energy to boil more than 20 liters of water! It accomplishes this feat by regulating sweat secretion and by regulating the flow of blood close to the body surface. When sweat evaporates from the body surface, heat is also lost. The principle of heat loss through evaporation is basic to many cooling systems. When increased quantities of blood are allowed to fill the vessels close to the skin, heat is also lost by radiation. Blood supply to the skin far exceeds the amount needed by the skin. Such an abundant blood supply primarily enables the regulation of body temperature.

Sense Organ Activity

The skin functions as an enormous sense organ. Its millions of nerve endings serve as antennas or receivers for the body, keeping it informed of changes in its environment. The specialized receptors shown in Figures 5-2 and 5-6 make it possible for the body to detect sensations of light touch (Meissner's corpuscles) and pressures (Pacinian corpuscles). Other receptors make it possible for us to respond to the sensations of pain, heat, and cold.

Clinical Application

Decubitus Ulcers

Family members, nurses, or other professionals who provide home health care services for bedridden or otherwise immobilized individuals need to be aware of the causes and nature of **decubitus** (de-KU-bi-tus) **ulcers** or pressure sores. Decubitus means "lying down," a name that hints at a common cause of pressure sores: lying in one position for long periods. Also called *bedsores*, these lesions appear after blood flow to a local area of skin slows because of pressure on skin covering a bony prominence such as the heel (see illustration). Ulcers form and infections develop as lack of blood flow causes tissue damage. Frequent changes in body position and soft support cushions help prevent decubitus ulcers.

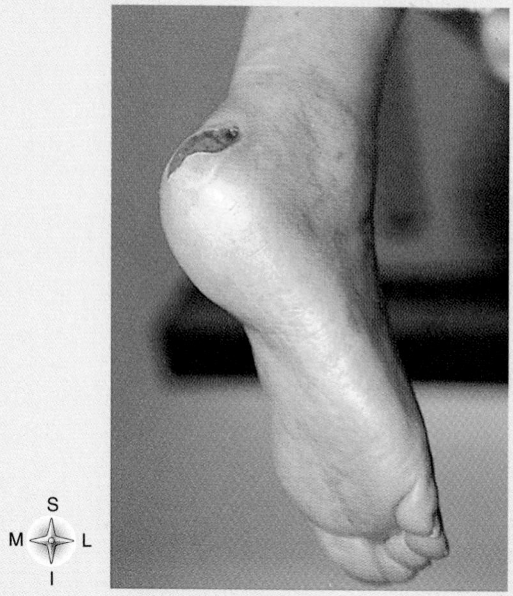

Burns

Burns constitute one of the most serious and frequent problems that affect the skin. Typically, we think of a burn as an injury caused by fire or by contact of the skin with a hot surface. However, overexposure to ultraviolet light (sunburn) or contact of the skin with an electric current or a harmful chemical such as an acid can also cause burns.

Estimating Body Surface Area

When burns involve large areas of the skin, treatment and the possibility for recovery depend in large part on the **total area involved** and the **severity of the burn.** The severity of a burn is determined by the depth of the injury, as well as by the amount of body surface area affected.

The **"rule of nines"** is one of the most frequently used methods of determining the extent of a burn injury. With this technique (Figure 5-8) the body is divided into 11 areas of 9% each, with the area around the genitals representing the additional 1% of body surface area. As you can see in Figure 5-8, in the adult 9% of the skin covers the head and each upper extremity, including front and back surfaces. Twice as much, or 18%, of the total skin area covers the front and back of the trunk and each lower extremity, including front and back surfaces.

FIGURE 5-8

The "rule of nines." Dividing the body into 11 areas of 9% each helps to estimate the amount of skin surface burned in an adult.

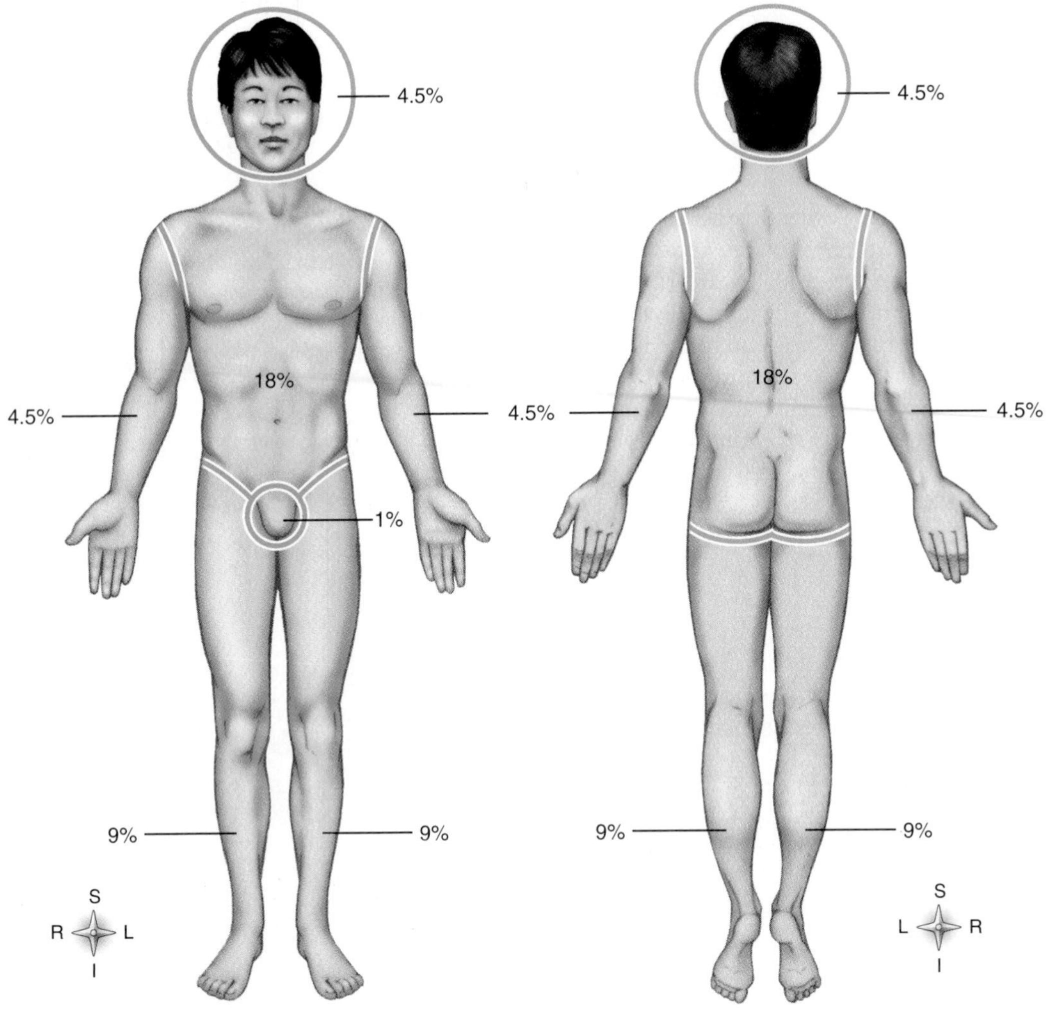

Classification of Burns

The classification system used to describe the severity of burns is based on the number of tissue layers involved. The most severe burns destroy not only layers of the skin and subcutaneous tissue but underlying tissues, as well.

First-degree burns. A **first-degree burn** (for example, a typical sunburn) causes minor discomfort and some reddening of the skin. Although the surface layers of the epidermis may peel in 1 to 3 days, no blistering occurs, and actual tissue destruction is minimal.

Second-degree burns. A **second-degree burn** involves the deep epidermal layers and always causes injury to the upper layers of the dermis. Although deep second-degree burns damage sweat

FIGURE 5-9

Classification of burns. Thickness of the damaged skin is one way to classify burns. **A,** First-degree or partial-thickness burn. **B,** Second-degree or partial-thickness burn. **C,** Third-degree or full-thickness burn.

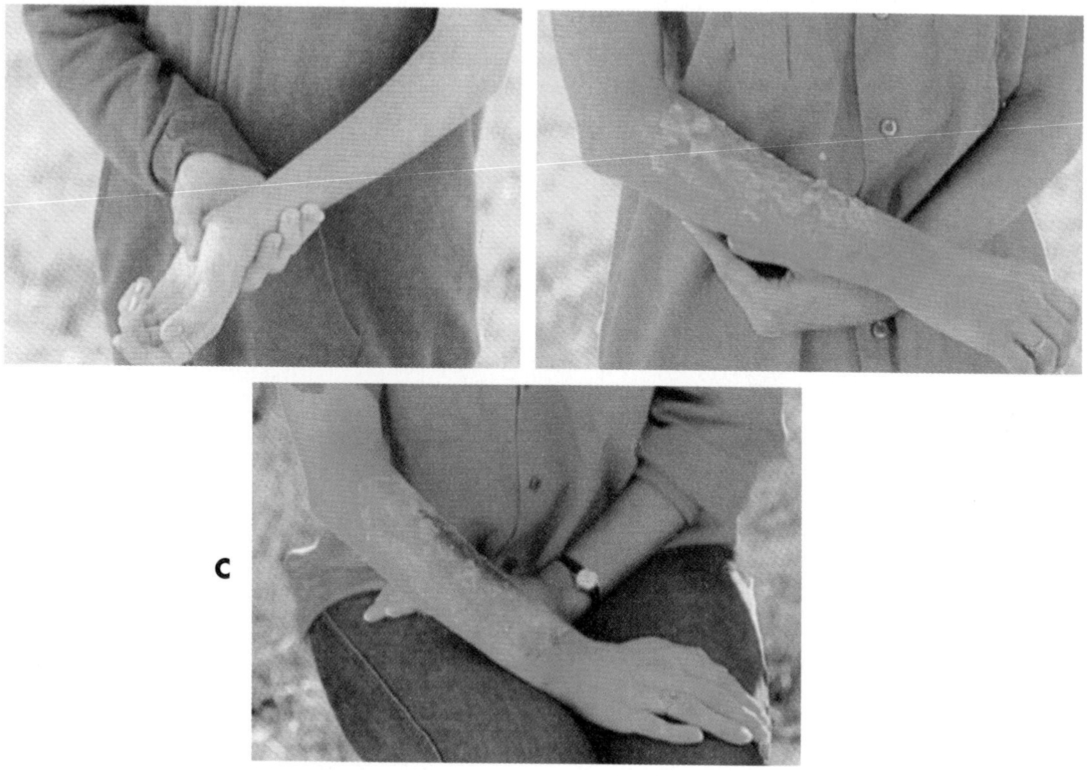

glands, hair follicles, and sebaceous glands, complete destruction of the dermis does not occur. Blisters, severe pain, generalized swelling, and fluid loss characterize this type of burn. Scarring is common. First- and second-degree burns are called **partial-thickness burns.**

Third-degree burns. A **third-degree,** or **full-thickness burn,** is characterized by complete destruction of the epidermis and dermis. In addition, tissue death extends below the primary skin layers into the subcutaneous tissue. Third-degree burns often involve underlying muscles and even bone. One distinction between second- and third-degree burns is that third-degree lesions are insensitive to pain immediately after injury because of the destruction of nerve endings. The fluid loss that results from third-degree burns is a very serious problem. Another serious problem with third-degree burns is the great risk of infection.

Quick Check

1. What are the three most important functions of the skin?
2. Can you list some of the sensory stimuli that can be detected by the skin?
3. How can the amount of skin surface area covered by a burn be estimated?

OUTLINE SUMMARY

CLASSIFICATION OF BODY MEMBRANES

A. Classification of body membranes (Figure 5-1)
   1. Epithelial membranes—composed of epithelial tissue and an underlying layer of connective tissue
   2. Connective tissue membranes—composed largely of various types of connective tissue

B. Epithelial membranes
   1. Cutaneous membrane—the skin
   2. Serous membranes—simple squamous epithelium on a connective tissue basement membrane
      a. Types
         (1) Parietal—line walls of body cavities
         (2) Visceral—cover organs found in body cavities
      b. Examples
         (1) Pleura—parietal and visceral layers line walls of thoracic cavity and cover the lungs
         (2) Peritoneum—parietal and visceral layers line walls of abdominal cavity and cover the organs in that cavity
      c. Diseases
         (1) Pleurisy—inflammation of the serous membranes that line the chest cavity and cover the lungs
         (2) Peritonitis—inflammation of the serous membranes in the abdominal cavity that line the walls and cover the abdominal organs
   3. Mucous membranes
      a. Line body surfaces that open directly to the exterior
      b. Produce mucus, a thick secretion that keeps the membranes soft and moist

C. Connective tissue membranes
   1. Do not contain epithelial components
   2. Produce a lubricant called *synovial fluid*
   3. Examples are the synovial membranes in the spaces between joints and in the lining of bursal sacs

THE SKIN

A. Structure (Figure 5-2)—two primary layers called *epidermis* and *dermis*
   1. Epidermis
      a. Outermost and thinnest primary layer of skin
      b. Composed of several layers of stratified squamous epithelium
      c. Stratum germinativum—innermost layer of cells that continually reproduce, and new cells move toward the surface
      d. As cells approach the surface, they are filled with a tough, waterproof protein called *keratin* and eventually flake off
      e. Stratum corneum—outermost layer of keratin-filled cells
      f. Pigment-containing layer—epidermal layer that contains pigment cells called *melanocytes*, which produce the brown pigment melanin
      g. Blisters—caused by breakdown of union between cells or primary layers of skin
      h. Dermal-epidermal junction—specialized area between two primary skin layers
   2. Dermis
      a. Deeper and thicker of the two primary skin layers and composed largely of connective tissue
      b. Upper area of dermis characterized by parallel rows of peglike dermal papillae
      c. Ridges and grooves in dermis form pattern unique to each individual
         (1) Basis of fingerprinting
         (2) Improves grip for tool use and walking
      d. Deeper areas of dermis filled with network of tough collagenous and stretchable elastic fibers
      e. Number of elastic fibers decreases with age and contributes to wrinkle formation
      f. Dermis also contains nerve endings, muscle fibers, hair follicles, sweat and sebaceous glands, and many blood vessels

OUTLINE SUMMARY—*cont'd*

B. Appendages of the skin
- **1.** Hair (Figures 5-4 and 5-5)
  - **a.** Soft hair of fetus and newborn is called *lanugo*
  - **b.** Hair growth requires epidermal tubelike structure called *hair follicle*
  - **c.** Hair growth begins from hair papilla
  - **d.** Hair root lies hidden in follicle and visible part of hair called *shaft*
  - **e.** Arrector pili—specialized smooth muscle that produces "goose bumps" and causes hair to stand up straight
- **2.** Receptors (Figure 5-6)
  - **a.** Specialized nerve endings—make it possible for skin to act as a sense organ
  - **b.** Meissner's corpuscle—capable of detecting light touch
  - **c.** Pacinian corpuscle—capable of detecting pressure
- **3.** Nails (Figure 5-7)
  - **a.** Produced by epidermal cells over terminal ends of fingers and toes
  - **b.** Visible part is called *nail body*
  - **c.** Root lies in a groove and is hidden by cuticle
  - **d.** Crescent-shaped area nearest root is called *lunula*
  - **e.** Nail bed may change color with change in blood flow
- **4.** Skin glands
  - **a.** Types
    - **(1)** Sweat or sudoriferous
    - **(2)** Sebaceous
  - **b.** Sweat or sudoriferous glands
    - **(1)** Types
      - **(a)** Eccrine sweat glands
        - Most numerous, important, and wide-spread of the sweat glands
        - Produce perspiration or sweat, which flows out through pores on skin surface
        - Function throughout life and assist in body heat regulation
      - **(b)** Apocrine sweat glands
        - Found primarily in axilla and around genitalia
        - Secrete a thicker secretion quite different from eccrine perspiration
        - Breakdown of secretion by skin bacteria produces odor
  - **c.** Sebaceous glands
    - **(1)** Secrete oil or sebum for hair and skin
    - **(2)** Level of secretion increases during adolescence
    - **(3)** Amount of secretion is regulated by sex hormones
    - **(4)** Sebum in sebaceous gland ducts may darken to form a blackhead

C. Functions of the skin
- **1.** Protection—first line of defense
  - **a.** Against infection by microbes
  - **b.** Against ultraviolet rays from sun
  - **c.** Against harmful chemicals
  - **d.** Against cuts and tears
- **2.** Temperature regulation
  - **a.** Skin can release almost 3,000 calories of body heat per day
    - **(1)** Mechanisms of temperature regulation
      - **(a)** Regulation of sweat secretion
      - **(b)** Regulation of flow of blood close to the body surface
- **3.** Sense organ activity
  - **a.** Skin functions as an enormous sense organ
  - **b.** Receptors serve as receivers for the body, keeping it informed of changes in its environment

D. Burns
- **1.** Treatment and recovery or survival depend on total area involved and severity or depth of the burn
- **2.** Body surface area is estimated using the "rule of nines" (Figure 5-8) in adults
  - **a.** Body is divided into 11 areas of 9% each

Continued

OUTLINE SUMMARY—*cont'd*

b. Additional 1% of body surface area is around genitals
3. Classification of burns
   a. First-degree (partial-thickness) burns—only the surface layers of epidermis involved
   b. Second-degree (partial-thickness) burns—involve the deep epidermal layers and always cause injury to the upper layers of the dermis
   c. Third-degree (full-thickness) burns—characterized by complete destruction of the epidermis and dermis
      (1) May involve underlying muscle and bone
      (2) Lesion is insensitive to pain because of destruction of nerve endings immediately after injury—intense pain is soon experienced
      (3) Risk of infection is increased

NEW WORDS

apocrine sweat gland
arrector pili
blister
bursa
cutaneous
cuticle
cyanosis
dehydration
dermis
eccrine sweat gland
epidermis
follicle
hypodermis
Kaposi sarcoma (KS)
keratin
Krause's end bulb
lanugo
lunula
malignant melanoma
Meissner's corpuscle
melanin
melanocyte
mucocutaneous junction
mucous membrane
mucus
Pacinian corpuscle
papilla
parietal
peritoneum
peritonitis
pleura
pleurisy
sebaceous gland
serous membrane
stratum corneum
subcutaneous
sudoriferous gland
synovial membrane
tinea pedis
visceral portion

REVIEW QUESTIONS

1. Define *membrane.*
2. Explain the structure of a serous membrane. Include the difference between the parietal and visceral membranes.
3. Explain the structure of a mucous membrane. Include an explanation of the mucocutaneous junction.
4. Explain the structure of a synovial membrane. What is the function of synovial fluid?
5. Name and briefly describe the layers of the epidermis.
6. Explain the structure of the dermis.
7. Differentiate between the *hair papilla,* the *hair root,* and the *hair shaft.*
8. Explain what occurs when the arrector pili contract.
9. Name the four receptors of the skin. To what type of stimuli does each respond?
10. Give the location of the eccrine glands and their function, and describe the type of fluid they produce.
11. Give the location of the apocrine glands and their function, and describe the type of fluid they produce.
12. Give the location of the sebaceous glands and their function, and describe the type of fluid they produce.
13. Explain the difference between a second-degree and third-degree burn. Which is considered a "full-thickness" burn?

CRITICAL THINKING

14. Explain the protective function of melanin.
15. Explain fully the role of the skin in temperature regulation.
16. If a person burned all of his back, the back of his right arm, and the back of his right thigh, approximately what percent of his body surface area was involved? How did you determine this?

CHAPTER TEST

20/20

1. The mucous, serous, and cutaneous are the three types of epithelial membranes.
2. Epithelial membranes are usually composed of two distinct layers: the epithelial layer and a supportive connective tissue layer called the basement membrane
3. The membrane lining the interior of the chest wall is called the parietal pleura
4. The membrane covering the organs of the abdomen is called the visceral. peritoneum
5. The connective tissue membrane that lines the space between the bone and joints is called the synovial. membrane
6. The two main layers of the epidermis of the skin are the stratum corneum and the stratum germinativum
7. As new skin cells approach the surface of the skin, their cytoplasm is replaced by a unique waterproof protein called keratin.
8. The upper region of the dermis forms projections called Dermal papillae that form unique fingerprints.
9. The eccrine are sweat glands that can be found all over the body and produce a transparent watery liquid.
10. The apocrine are sweat glands that can be found in the armpits and produce a thicker secretion.
11. The sebaceous glands secrete an oil called sebum.
12. protection, sensation, and Temperature regulation are the three functions of the skin.
13. The receptors in the skin that respond to pain are the:
    a. Meissner's corpuscle
    b. Pacinian corpuscle
    c. free nerve endings (circled)
    d. Krause's end bulbs
14. The receptors in the skin that respond to touch and cold are the:
    a. Meissner's corpuscle
    b. Pacinian corpuscle
    c. free nerve endings
    d. Krause's end bulbs (circled)
15. The receptors in the skin that respond to light touch are the:
    a. Meissner's corpuscle (circled)
    b. Pacinian corpuscle
    c. free nerve endings
    d. Krause's end bulbs
16. The receptors in the skin that respond to deep pressure are the:
    a. Meissner's corpuscle
    b. Pacinian corpuscle (circled)
    c. free nerve endings
    d. Krause's end bulbs

CHAPTER TEST—*cont'd*

Match the description of the part of the hair in Column B with the name of the structure in Column A.

COLUMN A	COLUMN B
17. _B_ Hair follicle	**a.** The part of the hair hidden in the follicle
18. _D_ Hair papilla	**b.** The growth of the epidermal cells into the dermis forming a small tube
19. _A_ Hair root	**c.** The part of the hair that is visible extending from the follicle
20. _C_ Hair shaft	**d.** A cuplike cluster of cells where hair growth begins

STUDY TIPS

Before starting your study of Chapter 5, go back to Chapter 4 and review the synopsis of the integumentary system. The body membranes are either epithelial or connective. The epithelial membranes cover or protect; this is the general function of epithelial tissue (Chapter 3). The difference between mucous and serous membranes is where they are; if the membrane is exposed to the environment in any way, it is mucous membrane. Connective membranes cover joints. The skin is divided into two parts. *Epi* means "on," so the epidermis is *on* the dermis. Its job is protective. The dermis contains most of the skin structures; nails, sense receptors, hair, glands, blood vessels, and muscles. The functions of the skin—protection, sensation, and heat regulation—are related to its location. Burns are classified by how much damage has been done to the skin and how deeply the damage occurred.

In your study groups, have a photocopy of the figures on the membranes, the microscopic view of the skin, the hair, and the nails. Blacken out the labels and quiz each other on the location and function of various structures. Go over the questions in the back of the chapter and discuss possible test questions.

The Skeletal System

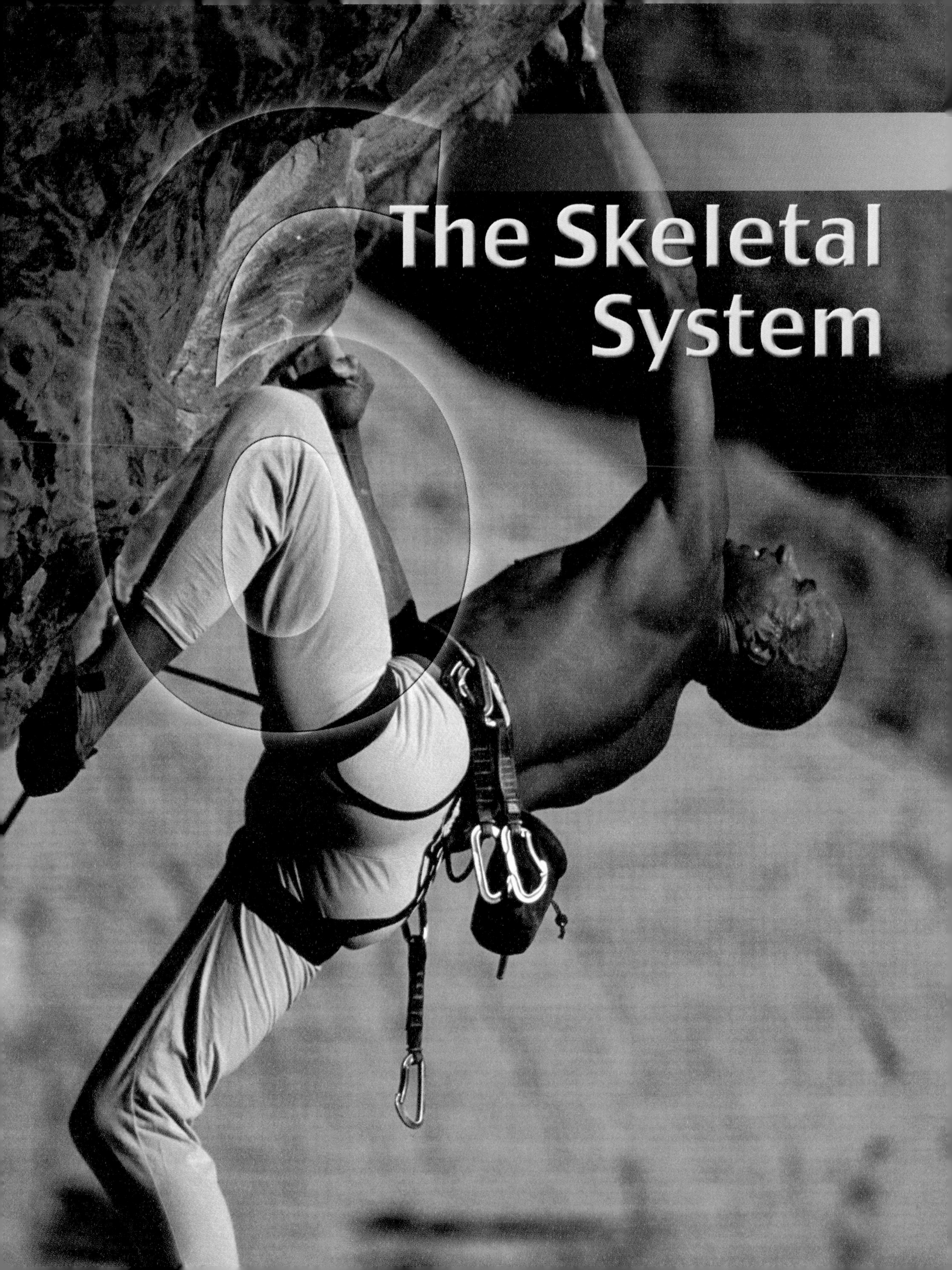

Outline

Objectives

AFTER YOU HAVE COMPLETED THIS CHAPTER, YOU SHOULD BE ABLE TO:

1. List and discuss the generalized functions of the skeletal system.
2. Identify the major anatomical structures found in a typical long bone.
3. Discuss the microscopic structure of bone and cartilage, including the identification of specific cell types and structural features.
4. Explain how bones are formed, how they grow, and how they are remodeled.
5. Identify the two major subdivisions of the skeleton and list the bones found in each area.
6. List and compare the major types of joints in the body and give an example of each.

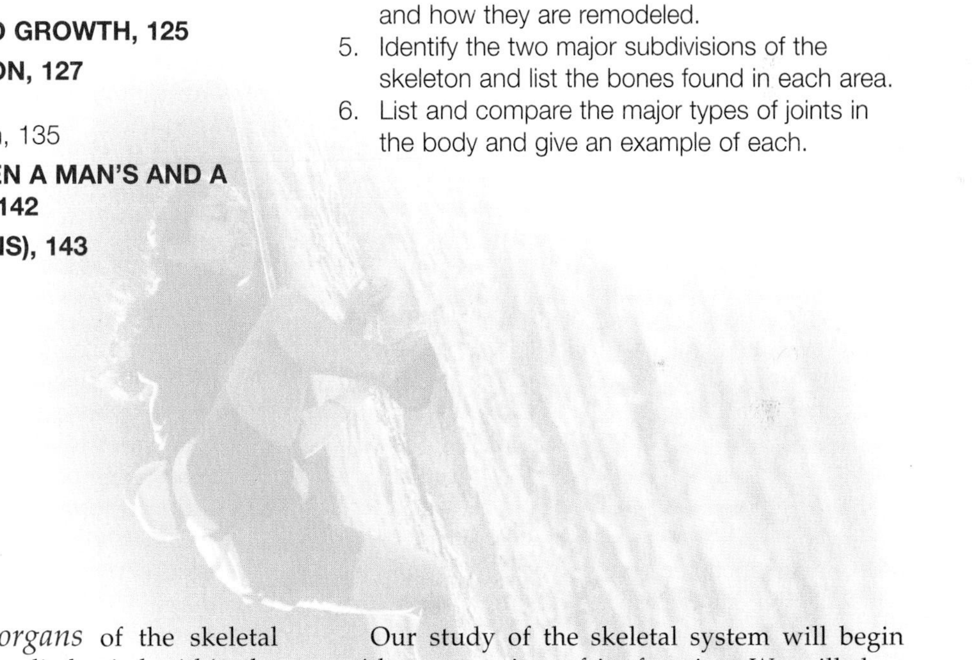

T*he primary organs* of the skeletal system—bones—lie buried within the muscles and other soft tissues, providing a rigid framework and support structure for the whole body. In this respect the skeletal system functions like steel girders in a building; however, unlike steel girders, bones can be moved. Bones are also living organs. They can remodel themselves and help the body respond to a changing environment. This ability of bones to change allows our bodies to grow and adapt to new situations.

Our study of the skeletal system will begin with an overview of its function. We will then classify bones by their structure and describe the characteristics of a typical bone. After discussing the microscopic structure of skeletal tissues, we will briefly outline bone growth and formation. With this information, the study of specific bones and the way they are assembled in the skeleton will be more meaningful. The chapter will end with a discussion of skeletal functions and an overview of joints or **articulations** (ar-tick-yoo-LAY-shuns).

An understanding of how bones articulate with one another in joints and how they relate to other body structures provides a basis for understanding the functions of many other organ systems. Coordinated movement, for example, is possible only because of the way bones are joined to one another and because of the way muscles are attached to those bones. In addition, knowing where specific bones are in the body will assist you in locating other body structures that will be discussed later.

FUNCTIONS OF THE SKELETAL SYSTEM

Support

Bones form the body's supporting framework. All the softer tissues of the body literally hang from the skeletal framework.

Protection

Hard, bony "boxes" protect delicate structures enclosed within them. For example, the skull protects the brain. The breastbone and ribs protect vital organs (heart and lungs) and also a vital tissue (red bone marrow, the blood cell–forming tissue).

Movement

Muscles are anchored firmly to bones. As muscles contract and shorten, they pull on bones and thereby move them.

Storage

Bones play an important part in maintaining homeostasis of blood calcium, a vital substance required for normal nerve and muscle function. They serve as a safety-deposit box for calcium. When the amount of calcium in blood increases above normal, calcium moves out of the blood and into the bones for storage. Conversely, when blood calcium decreases below normal, calcium moves in the opposite direction. It comes out of storage in bones and enters the blood.

Hemopoiesis

The term ***hemopoiesis*** (hee-mo-poy-EE-sis) is used to describe the process of blood cell formation. It is a combination of two Greek words: *hemo* (HEE-mo) meaning "blood" and *poiesis* (poy-EE-sis) meaning "to make." Blood cell formation is a vital process carried on in **red bone marrow.** Red bone marrow is soft connective tissue inside the hard walls of some bones.

TYPES OF BONES

There are four types of bones. Their names suggest their shapes: *long* (for example, humerus or upper arm bone), *short* (for example, carpals or wrist bones), *flat* (for example, frontal or skull bone), and *irregular* (for example, vertebrae or spinal bones). Many important bones in the skeleton are classified as long bones, and all have several common characteristics. By studying a typical long bone, you can become familiar with the structural features of the entire group.

STRUCTURE OF LONG BONES

Figure 6-1 will help you learn the names of the main parts of a long bone. Identify each of the following:

1. **Diaphysis** (dye-AF-i-sis) or shaft—a hollow tube made of hard, compact bone, hence a rigid and strong structure light enough in weight to permit easy movement
2. **Medullary cavity**—the hollow area inside the diaphysis of a bone; contains soft **yellow bone marrow,** an inactive, fatty form of marrow found in the adult skeleton
3. **Epiphyses** (e-PIF-i-sees) or the ends of the bone—red bone marrow fills in small spaces in the spongy bone composing the epiphyses
4. **Articular cartilage**—a thin layer of cartilage covering each epiphysis; functions like a small rubber cushion would if it were placed over the ends of bones where they form a joint
5. **Periosteum**—a strong fibrous membrane covering a long bone except at joint surfaces, where it is covered by articular cartilage
6. **Endosteum**—a fibrous membrane that lines the medullary cavity

FIGURE 6-1

Longitudinal section of a long bone.

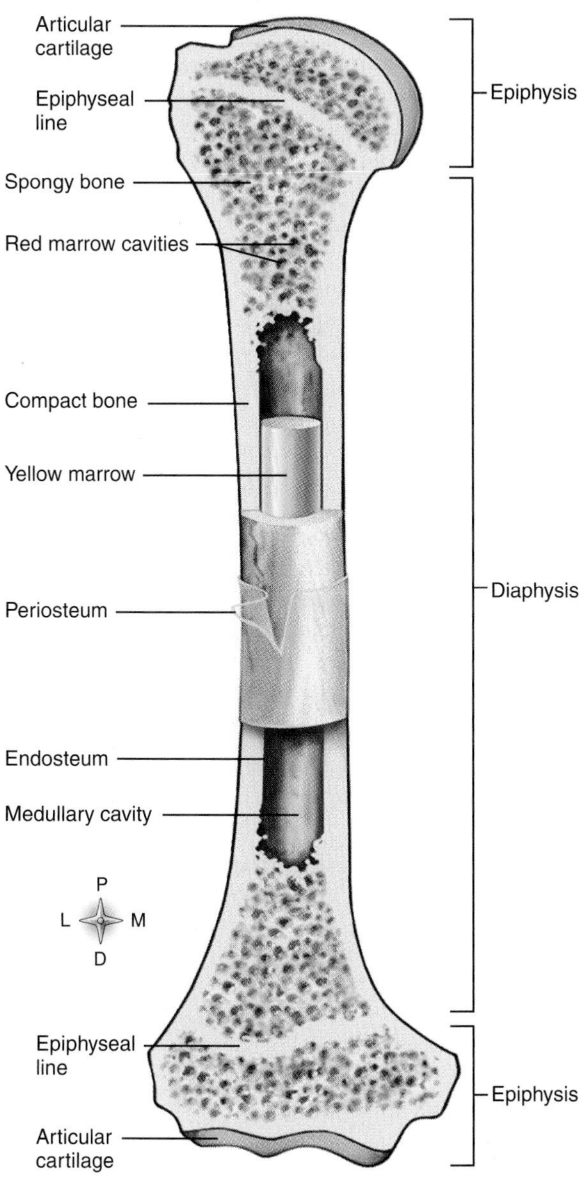

Quick
1. Can you name some of the organs of the skeletal system?
2. What are the five major functions of the skeletal system?
3. What are the four categories of bones in the skeleton?
4. Can you describe the major features of a long bone?

MICROSCOPIC STRUCTURE OF BONE AND CARTILAGE

The skeletal system contains two major types of connective tissue: **bone** and **cartilage.** Bone has different appearances and textures, depending on its location. In Figure 6-2, *A,* the outer layer of bone is hard and dense. Bone of this type is called **dense** or **compact bone.** The porous bone in the end of the long bone is called *spongy bone.* As the name implies, spongy bone contains many spaces that may be filled with marrow. Compact or dense bone appears solid to the naked eye. Figure 6-2, *B,* shows the microscopic appearance of spongy and compact bone. The needlelike threads of spongy bone that surround a network of spaces are called **trabeculae** (trah-BEK-yoo-lee).

As you can see in Figures 6-2 and 6-3, compact or dense bone does not contain a network of open spaces. Instead, the matrix is organized into numerous structural units called **osteons** or *Haversian systems.* Each circular and tubelike osteon is composed of calcified matrix arranged in multiple layers resembling the rings of an onion. Each ring is called a **concentric lamella** (lah-MEL-ah). The circular rings or lamellae surround the **central canal,** which contains a blood vessel.

Bones are not lifeless structures. Within their hard, seemingly lifeless matrix are many living bone cells called **osteocytes** (OS-tee-o-sites). Osteocytes lie between the hard layers of the lamellae in little spaces called **lacunae** (lah-KOO-nee). In Figures 6-2, *B,* and 6-3, note that tiny passageways or canals called **canaliculi** (kan-ah-LIK-yoo-lye) connect the lacunae with one other and with the central canal in each Haversian system. Nutrients pass from the blood vessel in the Haversian canal through the canaliculi to the osteocytes. Note also in Figure 6-2, *B,* that numerous blood vessels from the outer **periosteum** (pair-ee-OS-tee-um) enter the bone and eventually pass through the Haversian canals.

Cartilage both resembles and differs from bone. As with bone, it consists more of intercellular substance than of cells. Innumerable collagenous fibers reinforce the matrix of both tissues. However, in cartilage the fibers are embedded in a firm gel instead of in a calcified cement sub-

FIGURE 6-2

Microscopic structure of bone. A, Longitudinal section of a long bone shows the location of the microscopic section illustrated in **B,** Note that the compact bone forming the hard shell of the bone is constructed of cylindrical units called *osteons*. Spongy bone is constructed of bony projections called *trabeculae*.

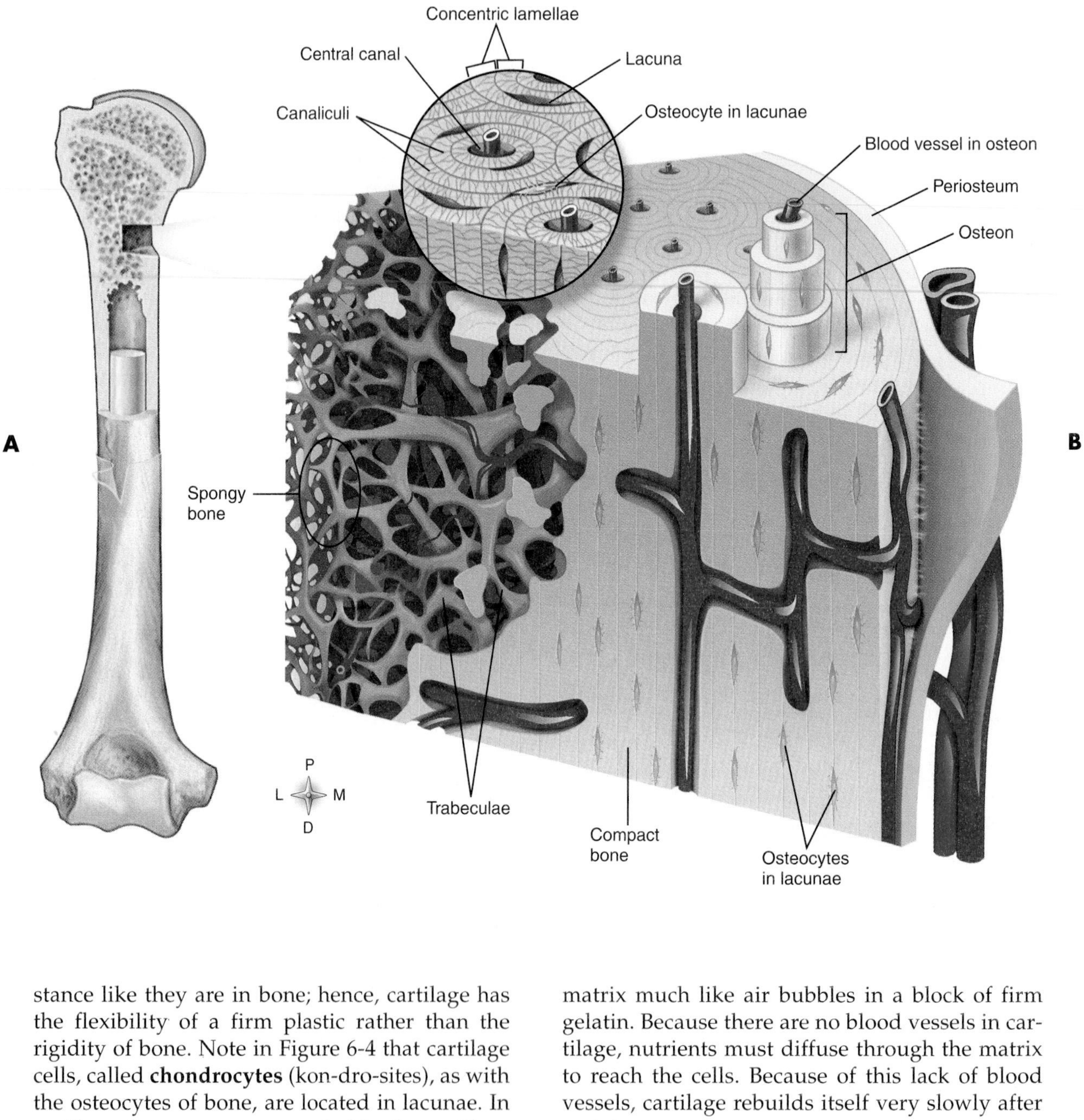

stance like they are in bone; hence, cartilage has the flexibility of a firm plastic rather than the rigidity of bone. Note in Figure 6-4 that cartilage cells, called **chondrocytes** (kon-dro-sites), as with the osteocytes of bone, are located in lacunae. In cartilage, lacunae are suspended in the cartilage matrix much like air bubbles in a block of firm gelatin. Because there are no blood vessels in cartilage, nutrients must diffuse through the matrix to reach the cells. Because of this lack of blood vessels, cartilage rebuilds itself very slowly after an injury.

FIGURE 6-3

Compact bone. Photomicrograph shows osteon system of organization. (The letter C shows the central canal.)

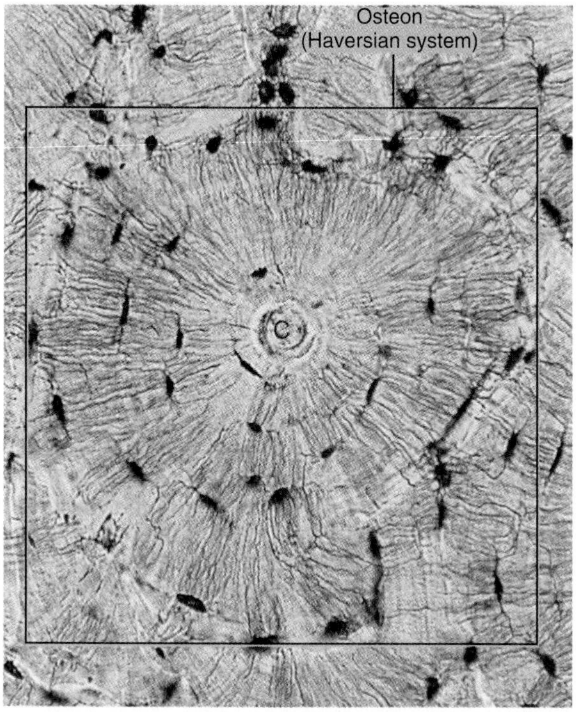

FIGURE 6-4

Cartilage tissue. Photomicrograph shows chondrocytes scattered around the tissue matrix in spaces called lacunae.

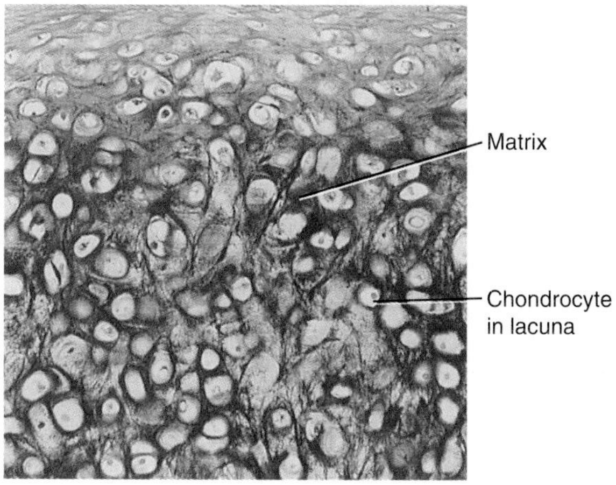

BONE FORMATION AND GROWTH

When the skeleton begins to form in a baby before its birth, it consists not of bones but of cartilage and fibrous structures shaped like bones. Gradually these cartilage "models" become transformed into real bones when the cartilage is replaced with calcified bone matrix. This process of constantly "remodeling" a growing bone as it changes from a small cartilage model to the characteristic shape and proportion of the adult bone requires continuous activity by bone-forming cells called **osteoblasts** (OS-tee-o-blasts) and bone-resorbing cells called **osteoclasts** (OS-tee-o-clasts). The laying down of calcium salts in the gel-like matrix of the forming bones is an ongoing process. This calcification process is what makes bones as "hard as bone." The combined action of the osteoblasts and osteoclasts sculpts bones into their adult shapes (Figure 6-5). The process of "sculpting" by the bone-forming and bone-resorbing cells allows bones to respond to stress or injury by changing size, shape, and density. The stresses placed on certain bones during exercise increase the rate of bone deposition. For this reason, athletes or dancers may have denser, stronger bones than less active people.

Most bones of the body are formed from cartilage models, as illustrated in Figures 6-5 and 6-6. This process is called **endochondral** (en-doe-KON-dral) **ossification** (os-i-fi-KAY-shun), meaning "formed in cartilage." A few flat bones, such as the skull bones illustrated in Figure 6-6, are formed by another process in connective tissue membranes.

As you can see in Figure 6-5, a long bone grows and ultimately becomes "ossified" from small centers located in both ends of the bone, called **epiphyses,** and from a larger center located in the shaft or the **diaphysis** of the bone. As long as any cartilage, called an **epiphyseal plate,** remains between the epiphyses and the diaphysis, growth continues. Growth ceases when all epiphyseal cartilage is transformed into bone. All that remains is an *epiphyseal line* that marks the location where the two centers of ossification have fused together. Physicians sometimes use this knowledge to determine whether a child is going to grow any more. They have an x-ray study performed on the

FIGURE 6-5

Endochondral ossification. A, Bone formation begins with a cartilage model. **B** and **C,** Invasion of the diaphysis (shaft) by blood vessels and the combined action of osteoblast and osteoclast cells result in cavity formation, calcification, and the appearance of bone tissue. **D** and **E,** centers of ossification also appear in the epiphyses (ends) of the bone. **F,** Note the epiphyseal plate, indications that this bone is not yet mature and that additional growth is possible. **G,** In a mature bone, only a faint epiphyseal line marks where the cartilage has disappeared and the centers of ossification have fused together.

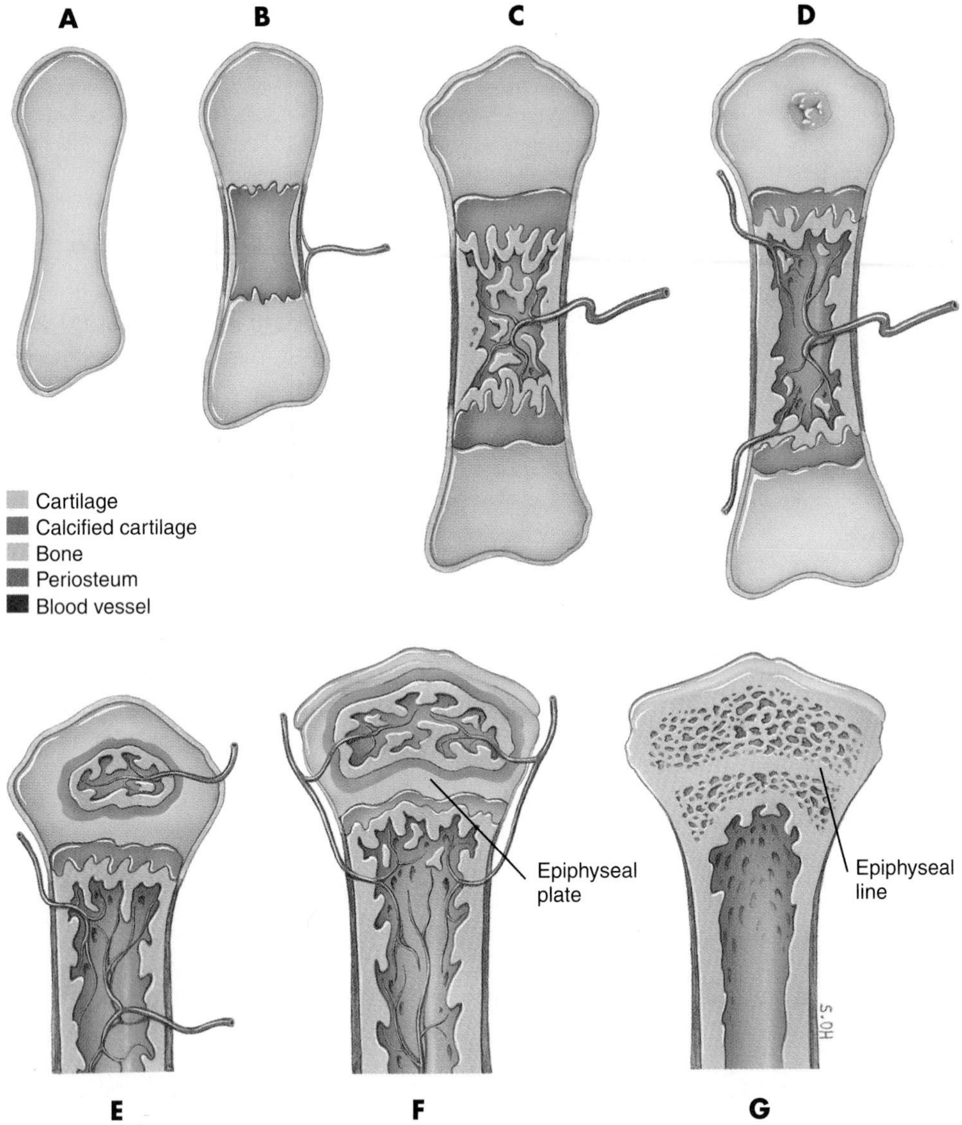

FIGURE 6-6

Bone development in a newborn. An infant's skeleton has many bones that are not yet completely ossified.

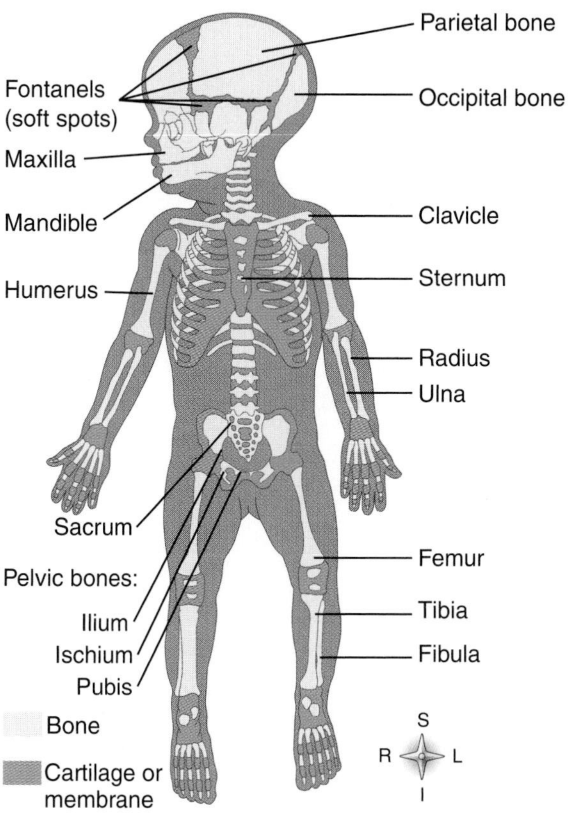

child's wrist; if it shows a layer of epiphyseal cartilage, they know that additional growth will occur. However, if it shows no epiphyseal cartilage, they know that growth has stopped and that the individual has attained adult height.

Quick

1. What is the basic structural unit of compact bone tissue called?
2. What are osteocytes? Where would you find them in bone tissue?
3. How does cartilage differ from bone?
4. What is ossification? What is the role of the osteoblast?

DIVISIONS OF SKELETON

The human skeleton has two divisions: the **axial skeleton** and the **appendicular skeleton.** Bones of the center or axis of the body make up the axial skeleton. The bones of the skull, spine, and chest and the hyoid bone in the neck are all in the axial skeleton. The bones of the upper and lower extremities or appendages make up the appendicular skeleton. The appendicular skeleton consists of the bones of the upper extremities (shoulder, pectoral girdles, arms, wrists, and hands) and the lower extremities (hip, pelvic girdles, legs, ankles, and feet) (Table 6-1). Locate the various parts of the axial skeleton and the appendicular skeleton in Figure 6-7.

Health & Well-Being

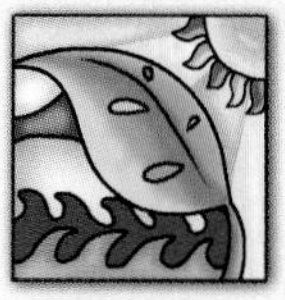

Osteoporosis

Osteoporosis (os-tee-o-po-RO-sis) is one of the most common and serious of all bone diseases. It is characterized by excessive loss of calcified matrix and collagenous fibers from bone. Osteoporosis occurs most frequently in elderly white females. Although white and black males are also susceptible, black women are seldom affected by it.

Because sex hormones play important roles in stimulating osteoblast activity after puberty, decreasing levels of these hormones in the blood of elderly persons reduces new bone growth and the maintenance of existing bone mass. Therefore some resorption of bone and subsequent loss of bone mass is an accepted consequence of advancing years. However, bone loss in osteoporosis goes far beyond the modest decrease normally seen in old age. The result is a dangerous pathological condition resulting in bone degeneration, increased susceptibility to "spontaneous fractures," and pathological curvature of the spine. Treatment may include drug therapy and dietary supplements of calcium and vitamin D to replace deficiencies or to offset intestinal malabsorption.

FIGURE 6-7

Human skeleton. The axial skeleton is distinguished by its bluer tint. **A,** Anterior view.

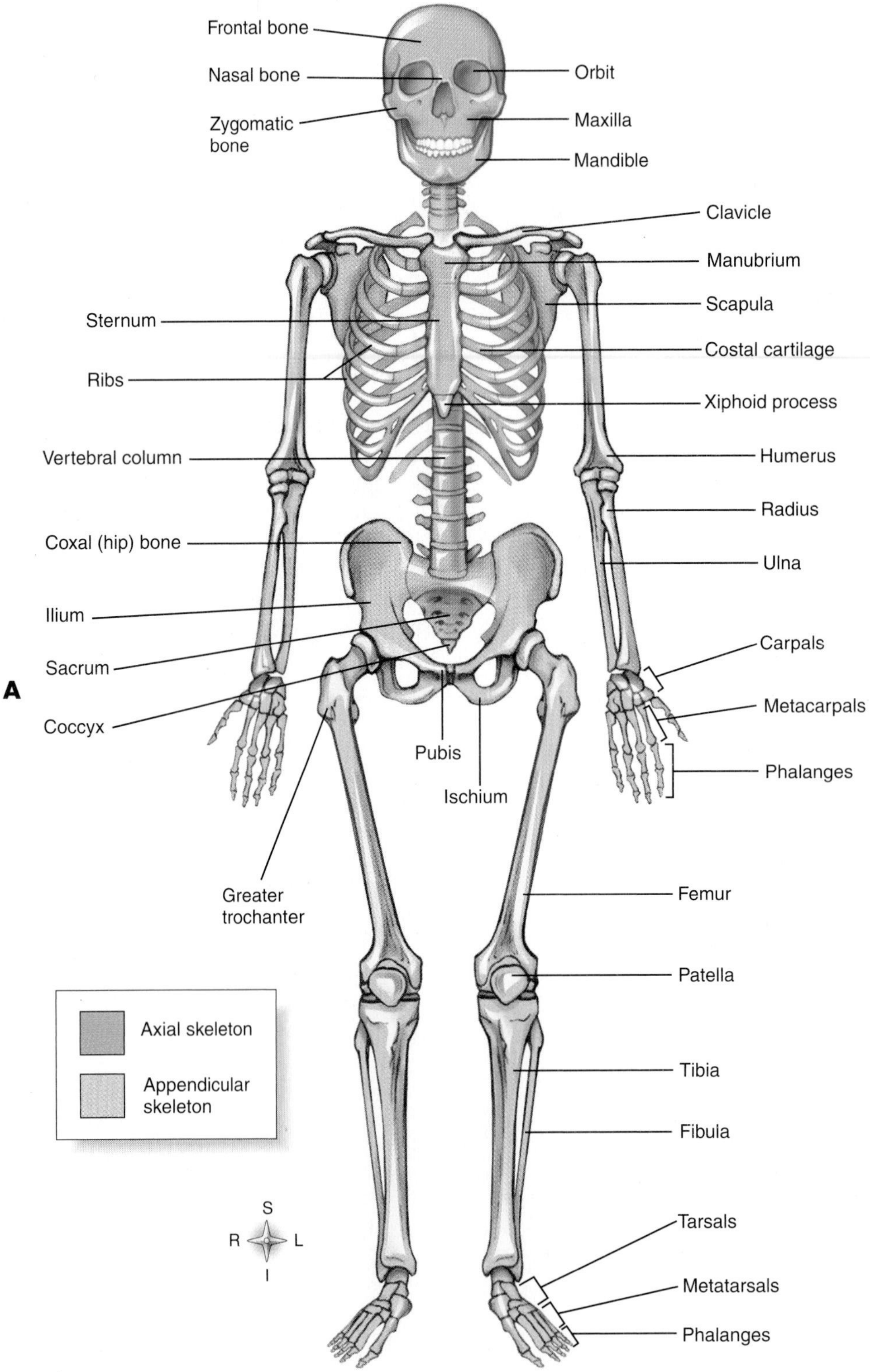

FIGURE 6-7—*cont'd*

B, Posterior view.

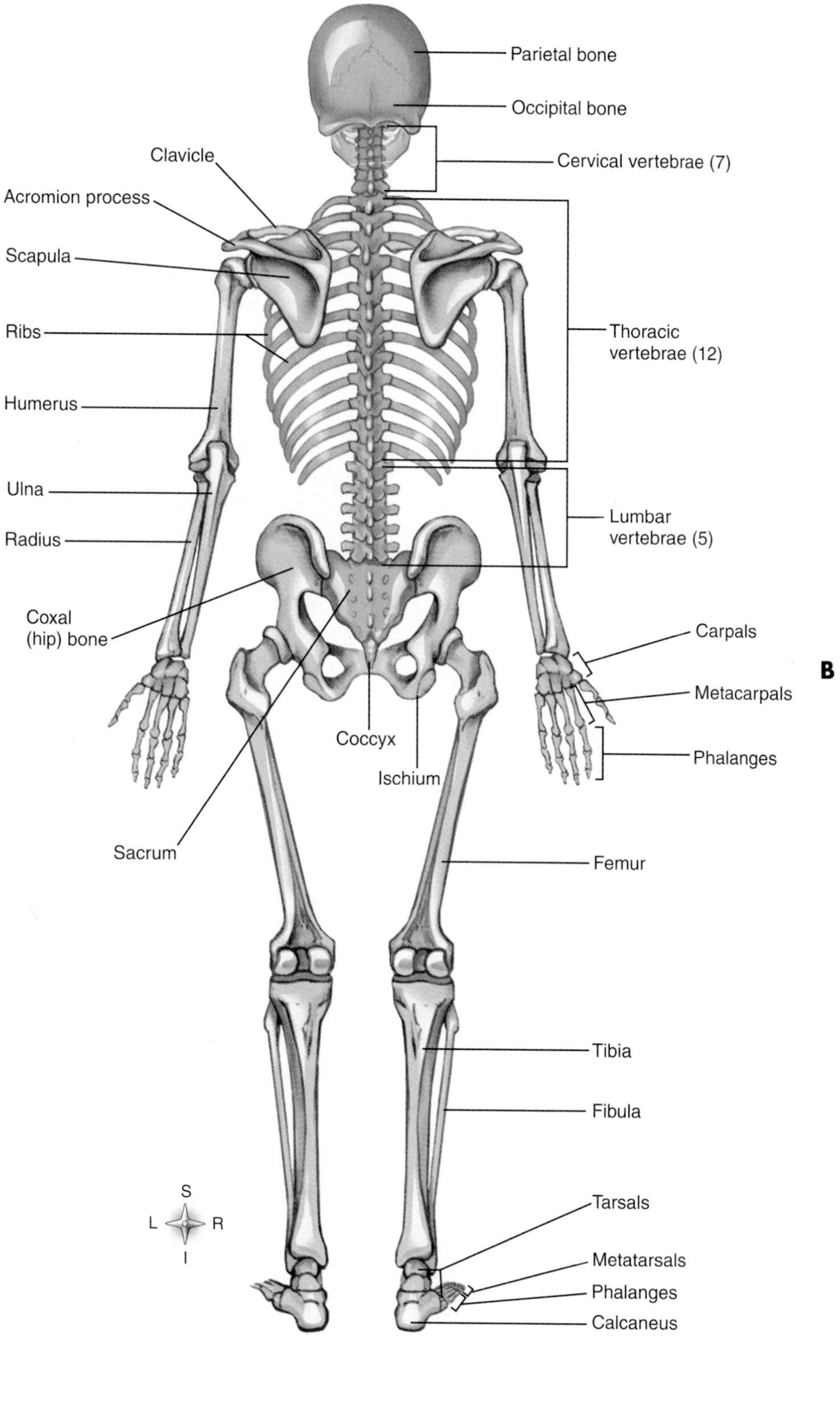

TABLE 6-1

Main Parts of the Skeleton*

AXIAL SKELETON†	APPENDICULAR SKELETON‡
Skull	Upper Extremities
Cranium	Shoulder (pectoral) girdle
Ear bones	Arm
Face	Wrists
Spine	Hands
Vertebrae	Lower Extremities
Thorax	Hip (pelvic) girdle
Ribs	Legs
Sternum	Ankles
Hyoid bone	Feet

*Total bones = 206.
†Total = 80 bones.
‡Total = 126 bones.

Clinical Application

Epiphyseal Fracture

The point of articulation between the epiphysis and diaphysis of a growing long bone is susceptible to injury if overstressed, especially in the young child or preadolescent athlete. In these individuals the epiphyseal plate can be separated from the diaphysis or epiphysis, causing an epiphyseal fracture. This x-ray study shows such a fracture in a young boy. Without successful treatment, an epiphyseal fracture may inhibit normal growth. Stunted bone growth in turn may cause the affected limb to be shorter than the normal limb.

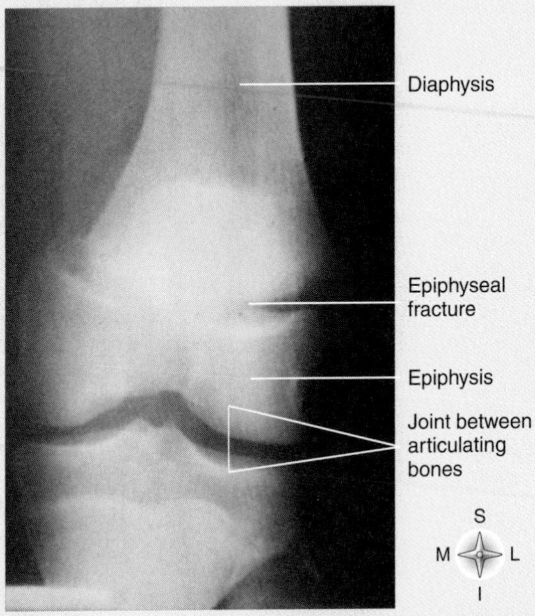

Axial Skeleton

Skull

The skull consists of 8 bones that form the **cranium,** 14 bones that form the **face,** and 6 tiny bones in the **middle ear.** You will probably want to learn the names and locations of these bones; they are given in Table 6-2. Find as many of them as you can on Figure 6-8. Feel their outlines in your own body where possible. Examine them on a skeleton if you have access to one.

"My sinuses give me so much trouble." Have you ever heard this complaint or perhaps uttered it yourself? **Sinuses** are spaces or cavities inside some of the cranial bones. Four pairs of them (those in the frontal, maxillary, sphenoid, and ethmoid bones) have openings into the nose and thus are referred to as **paranasal sinuses.** Sinuses give trouble when the mucous membrane that lines them becomes inflamed, swollen, and painful. For example, inflammation in the frontal sinus (*frontal sinusitis*) often starts from a common cold. The suffix *-itis* added to a word means "inflammation of." Turn to p. 365 in Chapter 14 for a figure showing the size and location of the paranasal sinuses.

Note in Figure 6-8 that the two parietal bones, which give shape to the bulging topside of the skull, form immovable joints called **sutures** with several bones: the *lambdoidal suture* with the occipital bone, the *squamous suture* with the temporal bone and part of the sphenoid, and the *coronal suture* with the frontal bone.

You may be familiar with the "soft spots" on a baby's skull. These are six **fontanels,** or areas where ossification is incomplete at birth. You can

TABLE 6-2
Bones of the Skull

NAME	NUMBER	DESCRIPTION
CRANIAL BONES		
Frontal	1	Forehead bone; also forms front part of floor of cranium and most of upper part of eye sockets; cavity inside bone above upper margins of eye sockets (orbits) called *frontal sinus*; lined with mucous membrane
Parietal	2	Form bulging topsides of cranium
Temporal	2	Form lower sides of cranium; contain *middle* and *inner ear structures*; *mastoid sinuses* are mucosa-lined spaces in *mastoid process*, the protuberance behind ear; *external auditory canal* is tube leading into temporal bone; muscles attach to *styloid process*
Occipital	1	Forms back of skull; spinal cord enters cranium through large hole *(foramen magnum)* in occipital bone
Sphenoid	1	Forms central part of floor of cranium; pituitary gland located in small depression in sphenoid called *sella turcica* (*Turkish saddle*); muscles attach to *pterygoid process*
Ethmoid	1	Uniquely shaped bone that helps form floor of cranium; side walls, roof of nose, and part of its middle partition (nasal septum—made up of the *vomer* and the *perpendicular plate*); and part of orbit. Contains honeycomblike spaces, the *ethmoid sinuses*; *superior* and *middle conchae* are projections of ethmoid bone; form "ledges" along side wall of each nasal cavity
FACE BONES		
Nasal	2	Small bones that form upper part of bridge of nose
Maxilla	2	Upper jawbones; also help form roof of mouth, floor, and side walls of nose and floor of orbit; large cavity in maxillary bone is *maxillary sinus*
Zygomatic	2	Cheek bones; also help form orbit
Mandible	1	Lower jawbone articulates with temporal bone at *condyloid process;* small anterior hole for passage of nerves and vessels is the *mental foramen*
Lacrimal	2	Small bones; help form medial wall of eye socket and side wall of nasal cavity
Palatine	2	Form back part of roof of mouth and floor and side walls of nose and part of floor of orbit
Inferior concha	2	Form curved "ledge" along inside of side wall of nose, below middle concha
Vomer	1	Forms lower, back part of nasal septum
EAR BONES		
Malleus	2	Malleus, incus, and stapes are tiny bones in middle ear cavity in temporal bone; *malleus* means "hammer"—shape of bone
Incus	2	*Incus* means "anvil"—shape of bone
Stapes	2	*Stapes* means "stirrup"—shape of bone

FIGURE 6-8

The skull. A, Right side. **B,** Front.

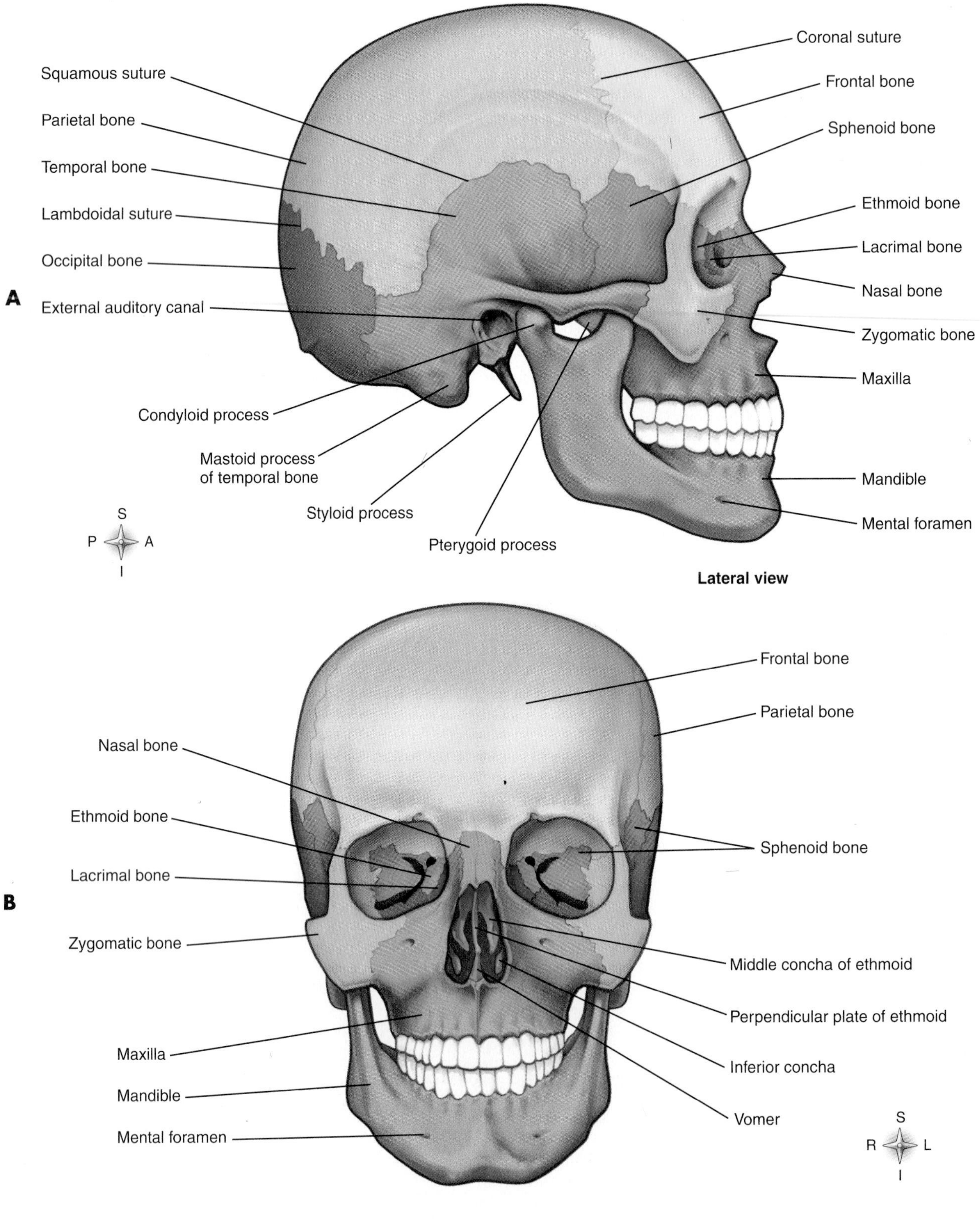
A
Squamous suture
Parietal bone
Temporal bone
Lambdoidal suture
Occipital bone
External auditory canal
Condyloid process
Mastoid process of temporal bone
Styloid process
Pterygoid process
Coronal suture
Frontal bone
Sphenoid bone
Ethmoid bone
Lacrimal bone
Nasal bone
Zygomatic bone
Maxilla
Mandible
Mental foramen
S
P
A
I
Lateral view
B
Nasal bone
Ethmoid bone
Lacrimal bone
Zygomatic bone
Maxilla
Mandible
Mental foramen
Frontal bone
Parietal bone
Sphenoid bone
Middle concha of ethmoid
Perpendicular plate of ethmoid
Inferior concha
Vomer
S
R
L
I

FIGURE 6-9

The spinal column. View shows the 4 spinal curves, 7 cervical vertebrae, 12 thoracic vertebrae, 5 lumbar vertebrae, sacrum, and coccyx. **A,** Lateral view. **B,** Anterior view. **C,** Posterior view.

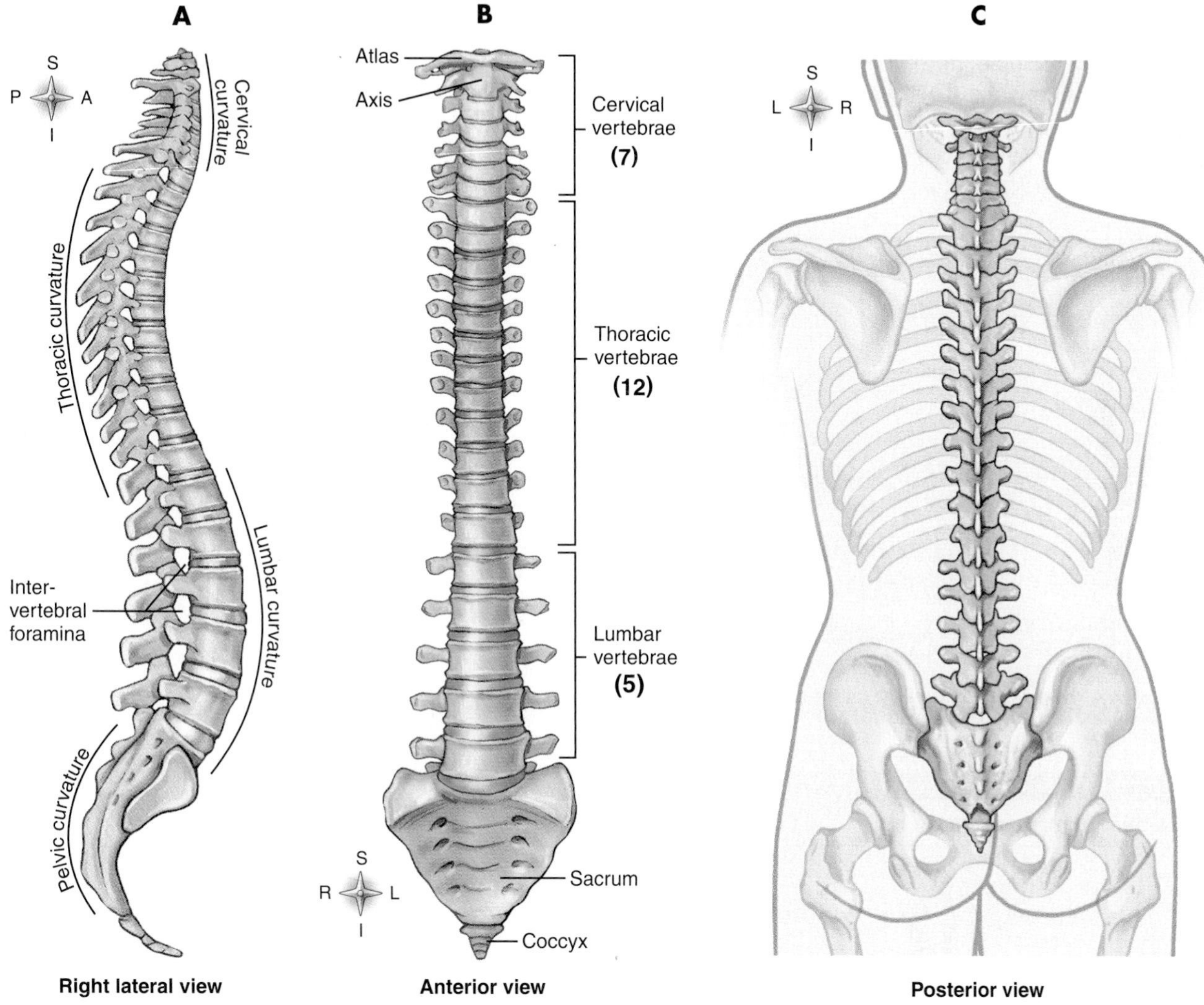

see them in Figure 6-6. Fontanels allow some compression of the skull during birth without much risk of breaking the skull bones. They may also be important in determining the position of the baby's head before delivery. The fontanels fuse to form sutures before a baby is 2 years old.

Spine (Vertebral Column)

The term *vertebral column* may conjure up a mental picture of the spine as a single long bone shaped like a column in a building, but this is far from true. The vertebral column consists of a series of separate bones or **vertebrae** connected in such a way that they form a flexible curved rod (Figure 6-9). Different sections of the spine have different names: cervical region, thoracic region, lumbar region, sacrum, and coccyx. They are illustrated in Figure 6-9 and described in Table 6-3.

Although individual vertebrae are small bones that are irregular in shape, they have several well-defined parts. Note, for example, in Figure 6-10, the body of the lumbar vertebra shown there, its spinous process (or spine), its two transverse processes, and the hole in its center, called the *vertebral foramen*.

The superior and inferior articular processes permit limited and controlled movement between adjacent vertebrae. To feel the tip of the spinous process of one of your vertebrae, simply bend your head forward and run your fingers down the back of your neck until you feel a projection of bone at shoulder level. This is the tip of the seventh cervical vertebra's long spinous process. The seven cervical vertebrae form the supporting framework of the neck.

Have you ever noticed the four curves in your spine? Your neck and the small of your back curve slightly inward or forward, whereas the chest region of the spine and the lowermost portion curve in the opposite direction (Figure 6-9). The cervical and lumbar curves of the spine are called *concave curves*, and the thoracic and sacral curves are called *convex curves*. This is not true, however, of a newborn baby's spine. It forms a continuous convex curve from top to bottom (Figure 6-11). Gradually, as the baby learns to hold up his or her head, a reverse or concave curve develops in the neck, (cervical region). Later, as the baby learns to stand, the

TABLE 6-3

Bones of the Vertebral Column

NAME	NUMBER	DESCRIPTION
Cervical	7	Upper seven vertebrae, in neck region; first cervical vertebra called *atlas*; second, *axis*
Thoracic vertebrae	12	Next 12 vertebrae; ribs attach to these
Lumbar vertebrae	5	Next five vertebrae; are in small of back
Sacrum	1	In child, five separate vertebrae; in adult, fused into one
Coccyx	1	In child, three to five separate vertebrae; in adult, fused into one

FIGURE 6-10

The third lumbar vertebra. A, From above. **B,** From the side.

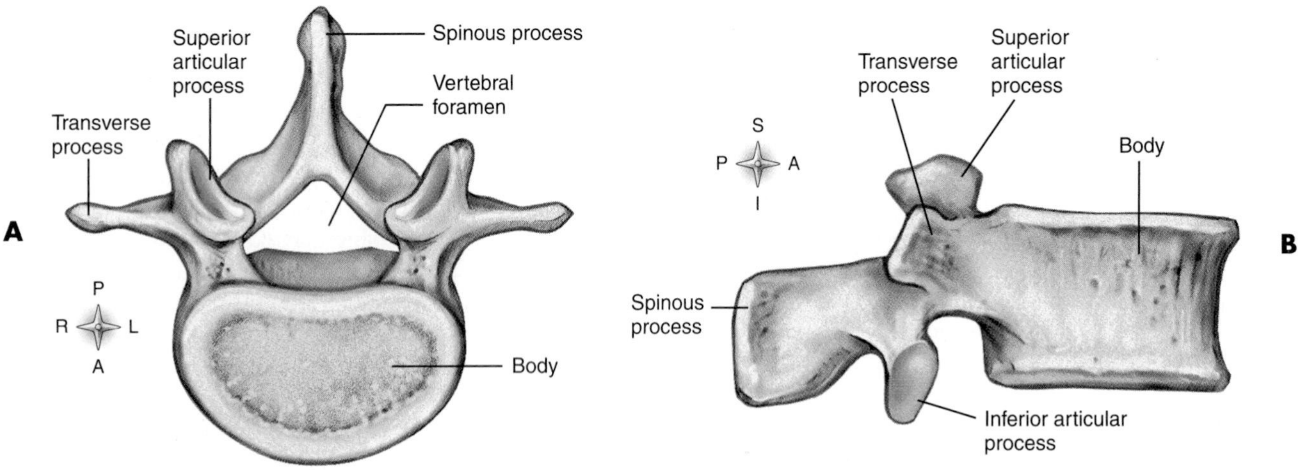

lumbar region of his or her spine also becomes concave.

The normal curves of the spine have important functions. They give it enough strength to support the weight of the rest of the body. They also provide the balance necessary for us to stand and walk on two feet instead of having to crawl on all fours. A curved structure has more strength than a straight one of the same size and materials. (The next time you pass a bridge, look to see whether or not its supports form a curve.) Clearly the spine needs to be a strong structure. It supports the head that is balanced on top of it, the ribs and internal organs that are suspended from it in front, and the hips and legs that are attached to it below.

Thorax

Twelve pairs of ribs, the sternum (breastbone), and the thoracic vertebrae form the bony cage known as the **thorax** or **chest.** Each of the 12 pairs of ribs is attached posteriorly to a vertebra. Also, all the ribs except the lower two pairs are attached to the sternum and so have anterior and posterior anchors. Look closely at Figure 6-12 and you can see that the first seven pairs of ribs (sometimes referred to as the *true ribs*) are attached to the sternum by costal cartilage. The eighth, ninth, and tenth pairs of ribs are attached to the cartilage of the seventh ribs and are sometimes called *false ribs*. The last two pairs of ribs, in contrast, are not attached to any costal cartilage but seem to float free in front, hence their descriptive name, *floating ribs* (Table 6-4).

FIGURE 6-11

Spinal curvature of an infant. The spine of the newborn baby forms a continuous convex curve.

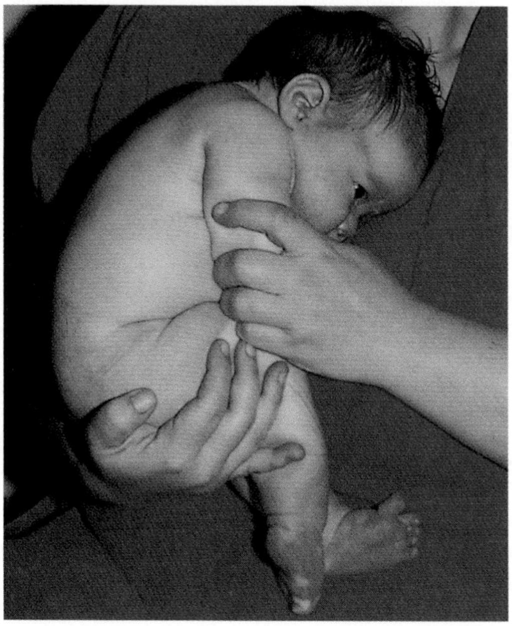

Quick

1. What is the difference between the axial skeleton and the appendicular skeleton?
2. What is a suture? A fontanel? A sinus?
3. What are the three major categories of vertebrae? How many bones in each?
4. How is a false rib different from a true rib?

Appendicular Skeleton

Of the 206 bones that form the skeleton as a whole, 126 are contained in the appendicular subdivision. Look again at Figure 6-7 to identify the appendicular components of the skeleton. Note that the bones in the shoulder or pectoral girdle connect the bones of the arm, forearm, wrist, and hands to the axial skeleton of the thorax, and the hip or pelvic girdle connects the bones of the thigh, leg, ankle, and foot to the axial skeleton of the pelvis.

Upper Extremity

The **scapula** (SKAP-yoo-lah) or shoulder blade and the **clavicle** (KLAV-ik-kul) or collarbone compose the *shoulder* or *pectoral girdle*. This connects the upper extremity to the axial skeleton. The only direct point of attachment between bones occurs at the **sternoclavicular** (ster-no-klah-VIK-yoo-lar) **joint** between the clavicle and the sternum or breastbone. As you can see in Figures 6-7 and 6-12, this joint is very small. Because the upper extremity is capable of a wide range of motion, great pressures can occur at or near the joint. As a result, fractures of the clavicle are very common.

The **humerus** (HYOO-mer-us) is the long bone of the arm and the second longest bone in the

FIGURE 6-12

Bones of the thorax. Rib pairs 1 through 7, the true ribs, are attached by cartilage to the sternum. Rib pairs 8 through 10, the false ribs, are attached to the cartilage of the seventh pair. Rib pairs 11 and 12 are called floating ribs because they have no anterior cartilage attachments.

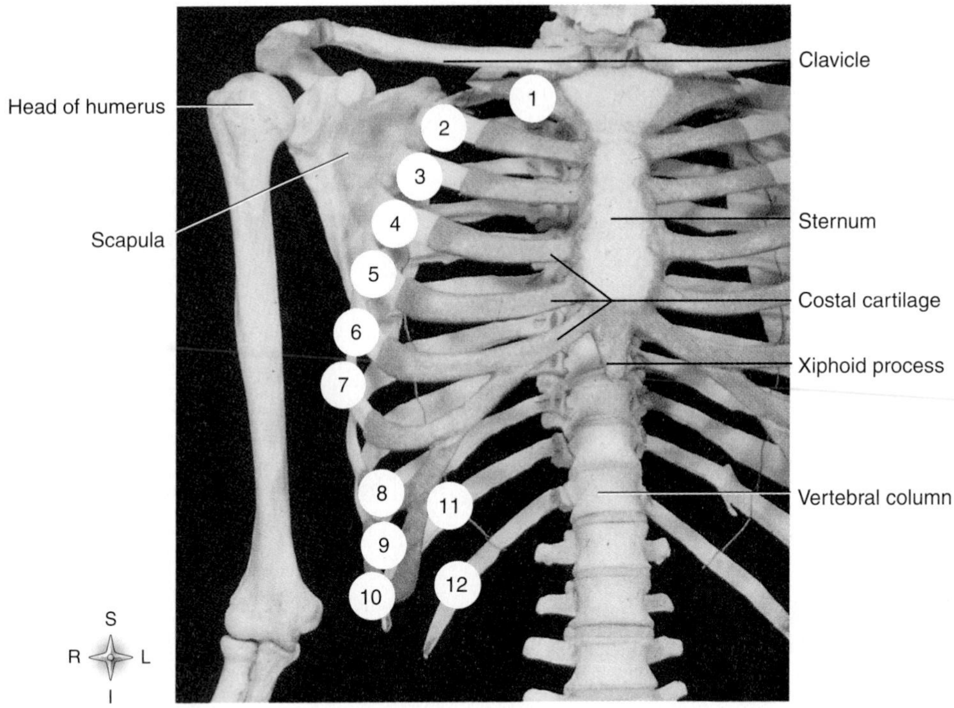

TABLE 6-4

Bones of the Thorax

NAME	NUMBER	DESCRIPTION
True ribs	14	Upper seven pairs; attached to sternum by *costal cartilages*
False ribs	10	Lower five pairs; lowest two pairs do not attach to sternum, therefore, called *floating ribs*; next three pairs attached to sternum by costal cartilage of seventh ribs
Sternum	1	Breastbone; shaped like a dagger; piece of cartilage at lower end of bone called *xiphoid process*; superior portion called the *manubrium*

body. It is attached to the scapula at its proximal end and articulates with the two bones of the forearm at the elbow joint. The bones of the forearm are the **radius** and the **ulna.** The anatomy of the elbow is a good example of how structure is related to function. Note in Figure 6-13 that the large bony process of the ulna, called the **olecranon** (o-LEK-rah-non) **process,** fits nicely into a

FIGURE 6-13

Bones of the arm, elbow joint, and forearm. Posterior aspect of **A,** right humerus; **B,** right radius and ulna; and **C,** right elbow.

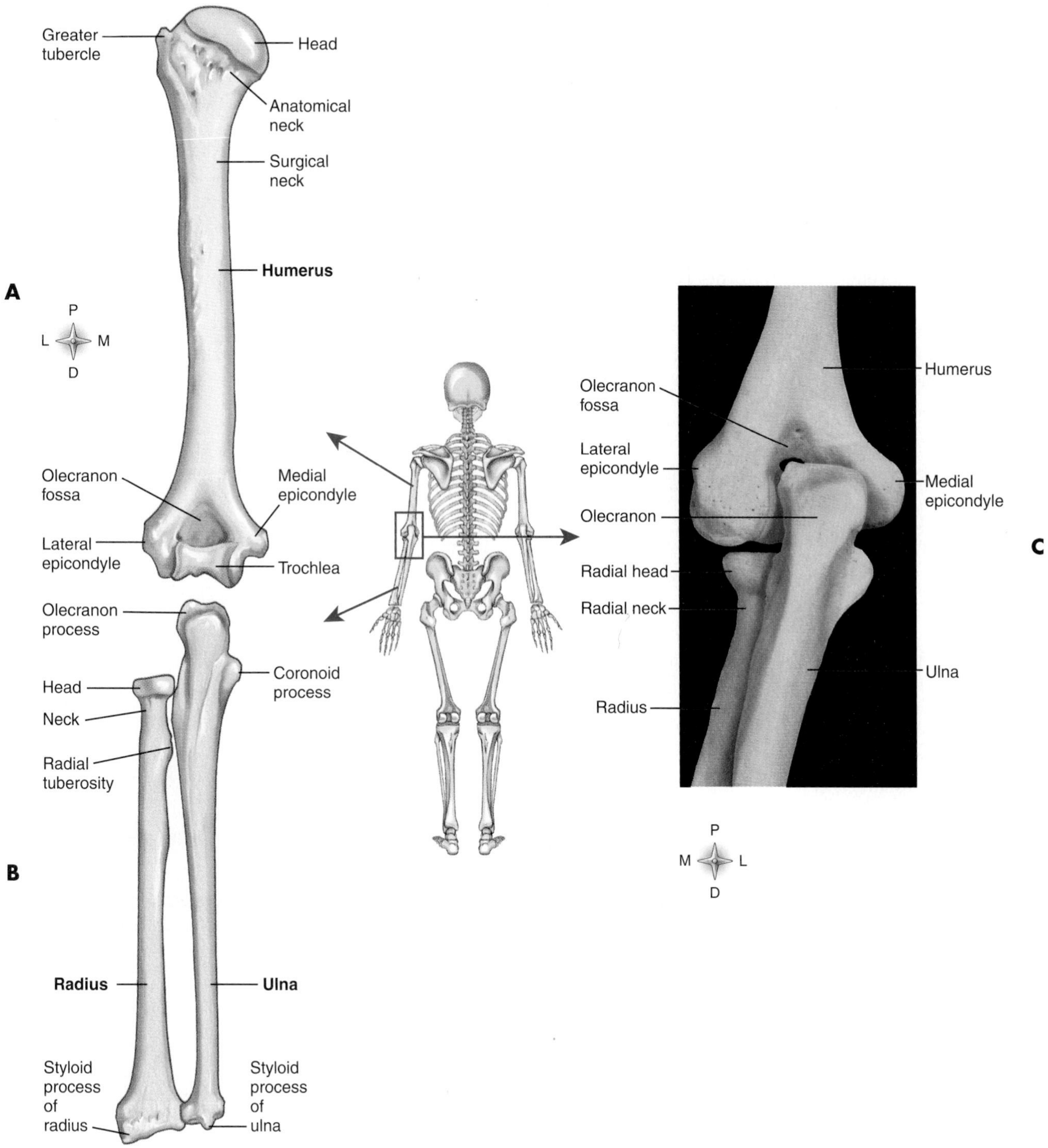

large depression on the posterior surface of the humerus, called the **olecranon fossa.** This structural relationship makes possible movement at the joint.

The radius and the ulna of the forearm articulate with each other and with the distal end of the humerus at the elbow joint. In addition, they also touch each another distally where they articulate with the bones of the wrist. In the anatomical position, with the arm at the side and the palm facing forward, the radius runs along the lateral side of the forearm, and the ulna is located along the medial border.

The wrist and the hand have more bones in them for their size than any other part of the body—8 **carpal** (KAR-pal) or wrist bones, 5 **metacarpal** (met-ah-KAR-pal) bones that form the support structure for the palm of the hand, and 14 **phalanges** (fah-LAN-jeez) or finger bones—27 bones in all (Table 6-5). This composition is very important structurally. The presence of many small bones in the hand and wrist and the many movable joints between them makes the human hand highly maneuverable. Some anatomists refer to the hand and wrist as the functional "reason" for the upper extremity. Figure 6-14 shows the relationships between the bones of the wrist and hand.

Lower Extremity

The *hip* or *pelvic girdle* connects the legs to the trunk. The hip girdle as a whole consists of two large **coxal** or pelvic bones, one located on each side of the pelvis. These two bones, with the sacrum and coccyx behind, provide a strong base of support for the torso and connect the lower extremities to the axial skeleton. In an infant's body each coxal bone consists of three separate bones—the **ilium** (ILL-ee-um), the **ischium** (IS-kee-um), and the **pubis** (PYOO-bis) (Figure 6-6). These

TABLE 6-5

Bones of the Upper Extremities

NAME	NUMBER	DESCRIPTION
Clavicle	2	Collarbones; only joints between shoulder girdle and axial skeleton are those between each clavicle and sternum (*sternoclavicular joints*)
Scapula	2	Shoulder blades; scapula plus clavicle forms *shoulder girdle*; *acromion process*—tip of shoulder that forms joint with clavicle; *glenoid cavity*—arm socket
Humerus	2	Upper arm bone (Muscles are attached to the *greater tubercle* and to the *medial* and *lateral epicondyles*; the *trochlea* articulates with the ulna; the *surgical neck* is a common fracture site.)
Radius	2	Bone on thumb (lateral) side of lower arm (Muscles are attached to the *radial tuberosity* and to the *styloid process*.)
Ulna	2	Bone on little finger (medial) side of lower arm; *olecranon process*— projection of ulna known as elbow or "funny bone" (Muscles are attached to the *coronoid process* and to the *styloid process*.)
Carpal bones	16	Short bones at upper end of hand; anatomical wrist
Metacarpals	10	Form framework of palm of hand
Phalanges	28	Finger bones; three in each finger, two in each thumb

bones grow together to become one bone in an adult (Figures 6-7 and 6-18).

Just as the humerus is the only bone in the arm, the **femur** (FEE-mur) is the only bone in the thigh (Figure 6-15). It is the longest bone in the body and articulates proximally (toward the hip) with the coxal bone in a deep, cup-shaped socket called the **acetabulum** (as-e-TAB-yoo-lum). The articulation of the head of the femur in the acetabulum is more stable than the articulation of the head of the humerus with the scapula in the upper extremity. As a result, dislocation of the hip occurs less often than does disarticulation of the shoulder. Distally, the femur articulates with the knee cap or **patella** (pah-TEL-ah) and the **tibia** or "shinbone." The tibia forms a rather sharp edge or crest along the front of your lower leg. A slender, non–weight-bearing, and rather fragile bone named the **fibula** lies along the outer or lateral border of the lower leg.

Toe bones have the same name as finger bones—**phalanges.** There is the same number of toe bones as finger bones, a fact that might surprise you because toes are shorter than fingers. Foot bones comparable to the metacarpals and carpals of the hand have slightly different names. They are called **metatarsals** and **tarsals** in the foot (Figure 6-16). Just as each hand contains five metacarpal bones, each foot contains five metatarsal bones. However, the foot has only seven tarsal bones, in contrast to the hand's eight carpals. The largest tarsal bone is the **calcaneus** or heel bone. The bones of the lower extremities are summarized in Table 6-6.

FIGURE 6-14

Bones of the right hand and wrist. There are 14 phalanges in each hand. Each of these bones is called a phalanx.

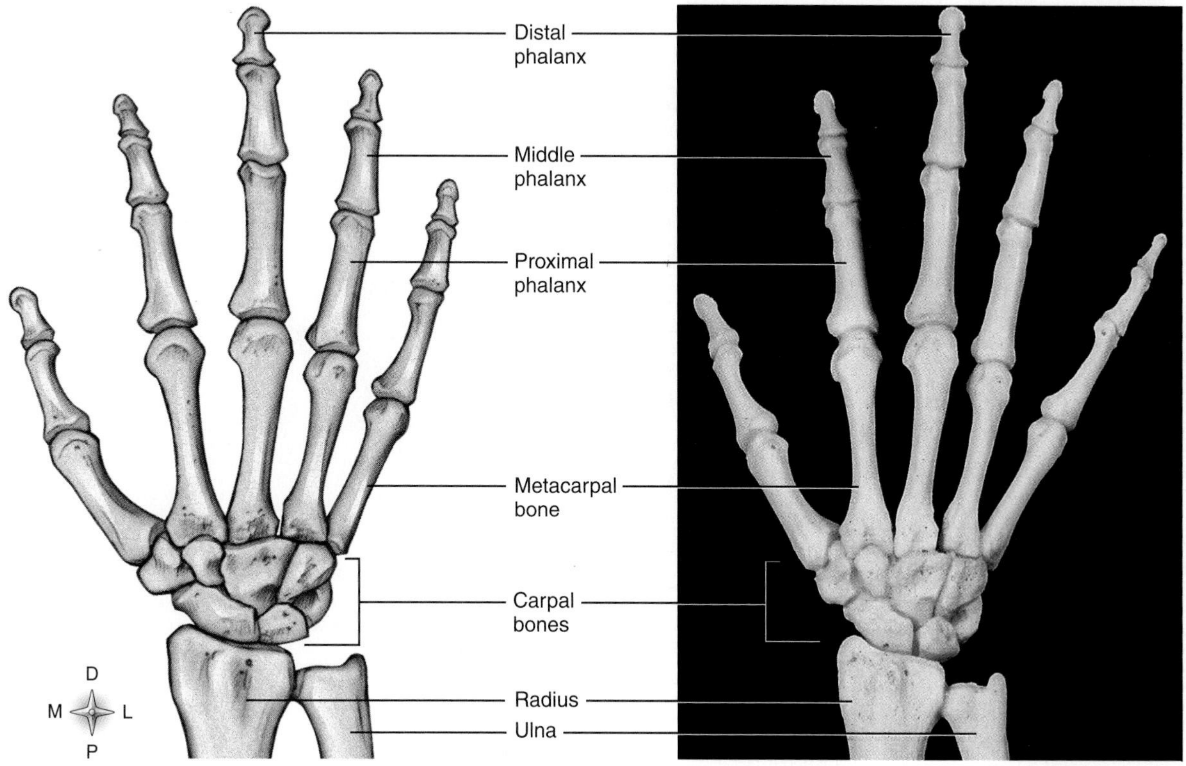

FIGURE 6-15

Bones of the thigh, knee joint, and leg. A, Anterior aspect of right femur; **B,** anterior aspect of the knee; **C,** right tibia and fibula; **D,** posterior aspect of the right knee.

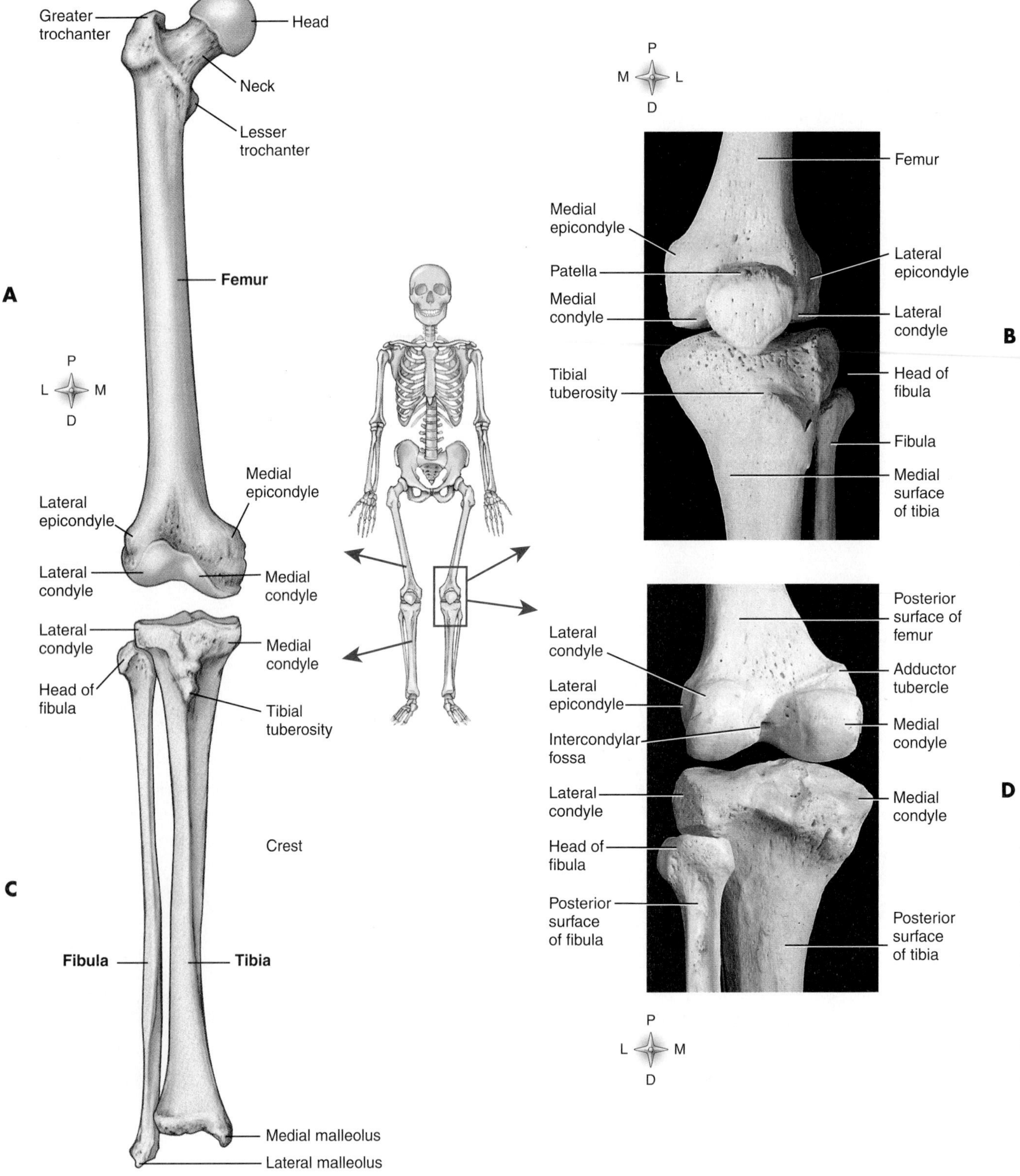

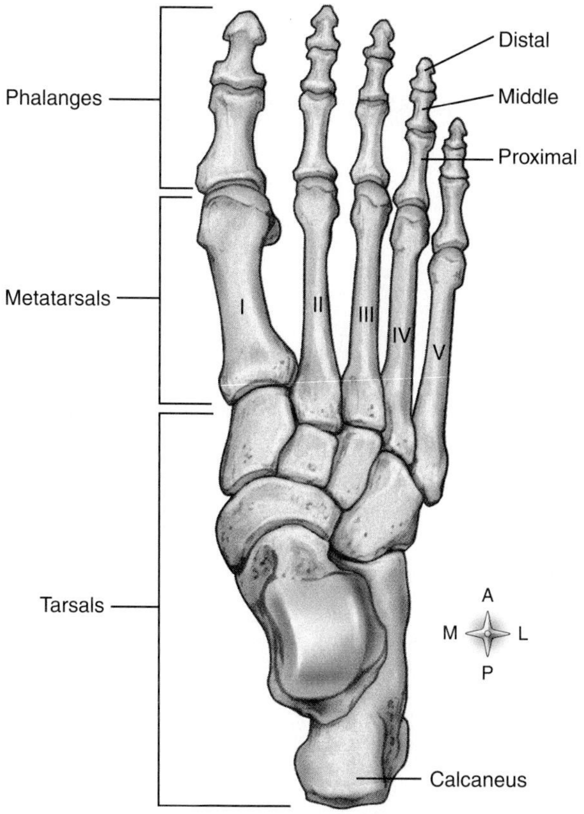

FIGURE 6-16

Bones of the right foot. Compare the names and numbers of foot bones (viewed here from above) with those of the hand bones shown in Figure 16-14.

TABLE 6-6

Bones of the Lower Extremities

NAME	NUMBER	DESCRIPTION
Coxal bone	2	Hipbones; *ilium*—upper flaring part of pelvic bone; *ischium*—lower back part; *pubic bone*—lower front part; *acetabulum*—hip socket; *symphysis pubis*—joint in midline between two pubic bones; *pelvic inlet*—opening into *true pelvis* or pelvic cavity; if pelvic inlet is misshapen or too small, infant skull cannot enter true pelvis for natural birth
Femur	2	Thigh or upper leg bones; *head of femur*—ball-shaped upper end of bone; fits into acetabulum (Muscles are attached to the *greater* and *lesser trochanters* and to the *lateral* and *medial epicondyles*; the *lateral* and *medial condyles* form articulations at the knee.)
Patella	2	Kneecap
Tibia	2	Shinbone; *medial malleolus*—rounded projection at lower end of tibia commonly called *inner anklebone*; muscles are attached to the *tibial tuberosity*
Fibula	2	Long slender bone of lateral side of lower leg; *lateral malleolus*—rounded projection at lower end of fibula commonly called *outer anklebone*
Tarsal bones	14	Form heel and back part of foot; anatomical ankle; largest is the *calcaneus*
Metatarsals	10	Form part of foot to which toes are attached; tarsal and metatarsal bones arranged so that they form three arches in foot; *inner longitudinal arch* and *outer longitudinal arch*, which extend from front to back of foot, and transverse or *metatarsal arch*, which extends across foot
Phalanges	28	Toe bones; three in each toe, two in each great toe

FIGURE 6-17

Arches of the foot. A, Medial and lateral longitudinal arches. **B,** "Flatfoot" occurs when tendons and ligaments weaken and the arches fall. **C,** Transverse arch. (Arrows show direction of force.)

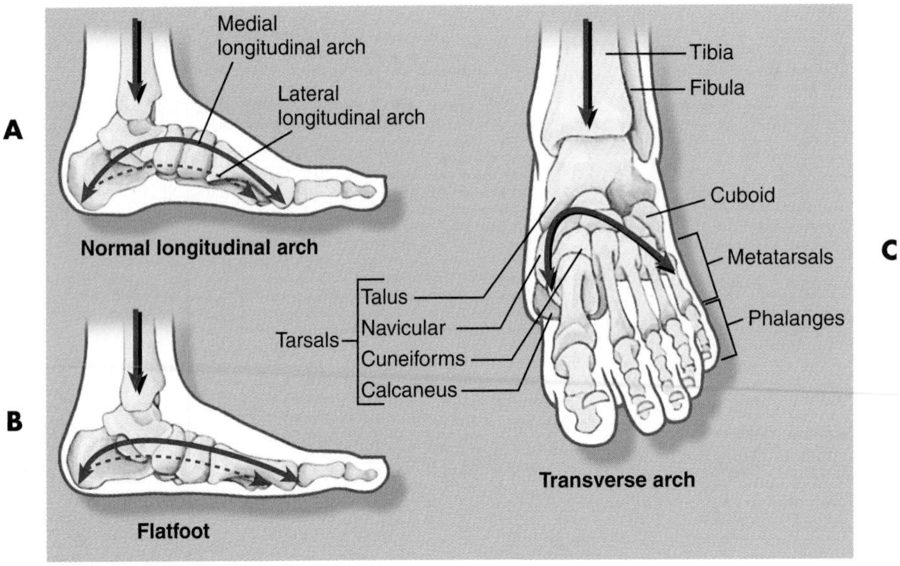

You stand on your feet, so certain features of their structure make them able to support the body's weight. The great toe, for example, is considerably more solid and less mobile than the thumb. The foot bones are held together in such a way as to form springy lengthwise and crosswise arches. These provide great supporting strength and a highly stable base. Strong ligaments and leg muscle tendons normally hold the foot bones firmly in their arched positions. Frequently, however, the foot ligaments and tendons weaken. The arches then flatten, a condition appropriately called *fallen arches* or *flatfeet*.

Two arches extend in a lengthwise direction in the foot (Figure 6-17, *A*). One lies on the inside part of the foot and is called the **medial longitudinal arch.** The other lies along the outer edge of the foot and is named the **lateral longitudinal arch.** Another arch extends across the ball of the foot; this arch is called the **transverse** or **metatarsal arch** (Figure 6-17, *B*).

DIFFERENCES BETWEEN A MAN'S AND A WOMAN'S SKELETON

A man's skeleton and a woman's skeleton differ in several ways. If you were to examine a male skeleton and a female skeleton placed side by side, you would probably first notice the difference in their sizes. Most male skeletons are larger than most female skeletons, a structural difference that seems to have no great functional importance. Structural differences between the male and female hipbones, however, do have functional importance. The female pelvis is made so that the body of a baby can be cradled in it before birth and can pass through it during birth. Although the individual male hipbones (coxal bones) are generally larger than the individual female hipbones, together the male hipbones form a narrower structure than do the female hipbones. A man's pelvis is shaped something like a funnel, but a woman's pelvis has a broader, shal-

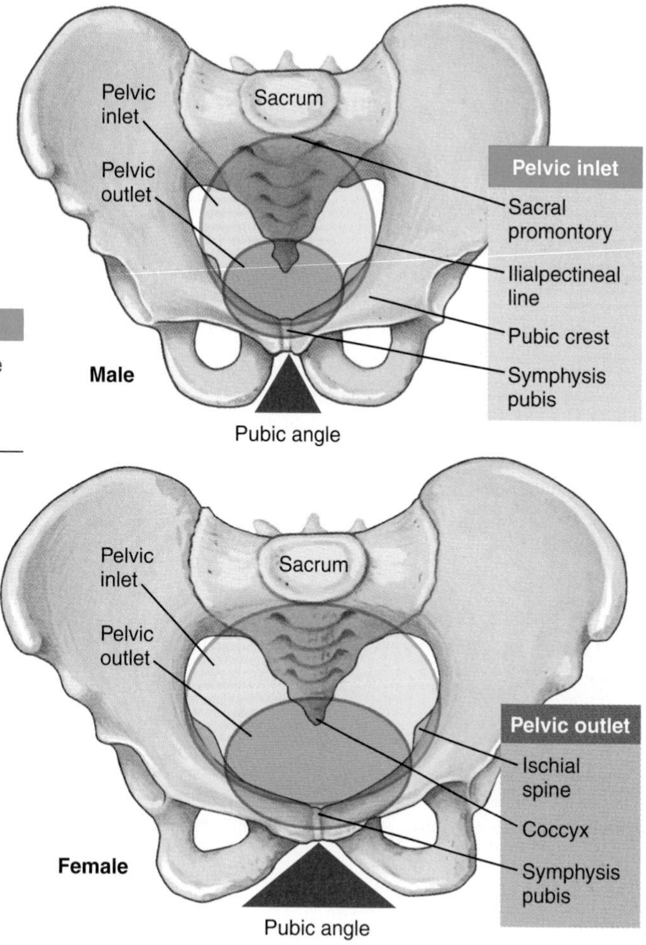

FIGURE 6-18

Comparison of the male and female pelvis. Notice the narrower width of the male pelvis, giving it a more funnel-like shape than the female pelvis.

lower shape, more like a basin. (Incidentally, the word *pelvis* means "basin.") Another difference is that the pelvic inlet and pelvic outlet are both normally much wider in the female than in the male. Figure 6-18 shows this difference clearly. The angle at the front of the female pelvis where the two pubic bones join is wider than it is in the male.

Quick Check

1. Can you name some of the bones of the upper extremity? The lower extremity?
2. What are the phalanges? Why are there two different sets of phalanges?
3. What are metacarpal bones? How do they differ from metatarsal bones?
4. How does the female pelvis differ from the male pelvis?

JOINTS (ARTICULATIONS)

Every bone in the body, except one, connects to at least one other bone. In other words, every bone but one forms a joint with some other bone. (The exception is the hyoid bone in the neck, to which the tongue anchors.) Most of us probably never think much about our joints unless something goes wrong with them and they do not function properly. Then their tremendous importance becomes painfully clear. Joints hold our bones together securely and at the same time make it possible for movement to occur between the bones—between most of them, that is. Without joints we could not move our arms, legs, or many other of our body parts. Our bodies would, in short, be rigid, immobile hulks. Try, for example, to move your arm at your shoulder joint in as many directions as you can. Try to do the same thing at your elbow joint. Now examine the shape of the bones at each of these joints on a skeleton or in Figure 6-7. Do you see why you cannot move your arm at your elbow in nearly as many directions as you can at your shoulder?

Kinds of Joints

One method classifies joints into three types according to the degree of movement they allow:

1. Synarthroses (no movement)
2. Amphiarthroses (slight movement)
3. Diarthroses (free movement)

Differences in joint structure account for differences in the degree of movement that is possible.

Synarthroses

A synarthrosis is a joint in which fibrous connective tissue grows between the articulating (joining) bones holding them close together. The joints between cranial bones are synarthroses, commonly called *sutures* (Figure 6-19, *A*).

Amphiarthroses

An amphiarthrosis is a joint in which cartilage connects the articulating bones. The symphysis pubis, the joint between the two pubic bones, is an amphiarthrosis (Figure 6-19, *B*).

Joints between the bodies of the vertebrae are also amphiarthroses. These joints make it possible to flex the trunk forward or sideways and even to circumduct and rotate it. Strong ligaments connect the bodies of the vertebrae, and fibrous disks lie between them. The central core of these intervertebral disks consists of a pulpy, elastic substance that loses some of its resiliency with age.

Diarthroses

Fortunately most of our joints by far are diarthroses. Such joints allow considerable movement, sometimes in many directions and sometimes in only one or two directions.

FIGURE 6-19

Joints of the skeleton. A, Synarthrotic joint. **B,** Amphiarthrotic joint.

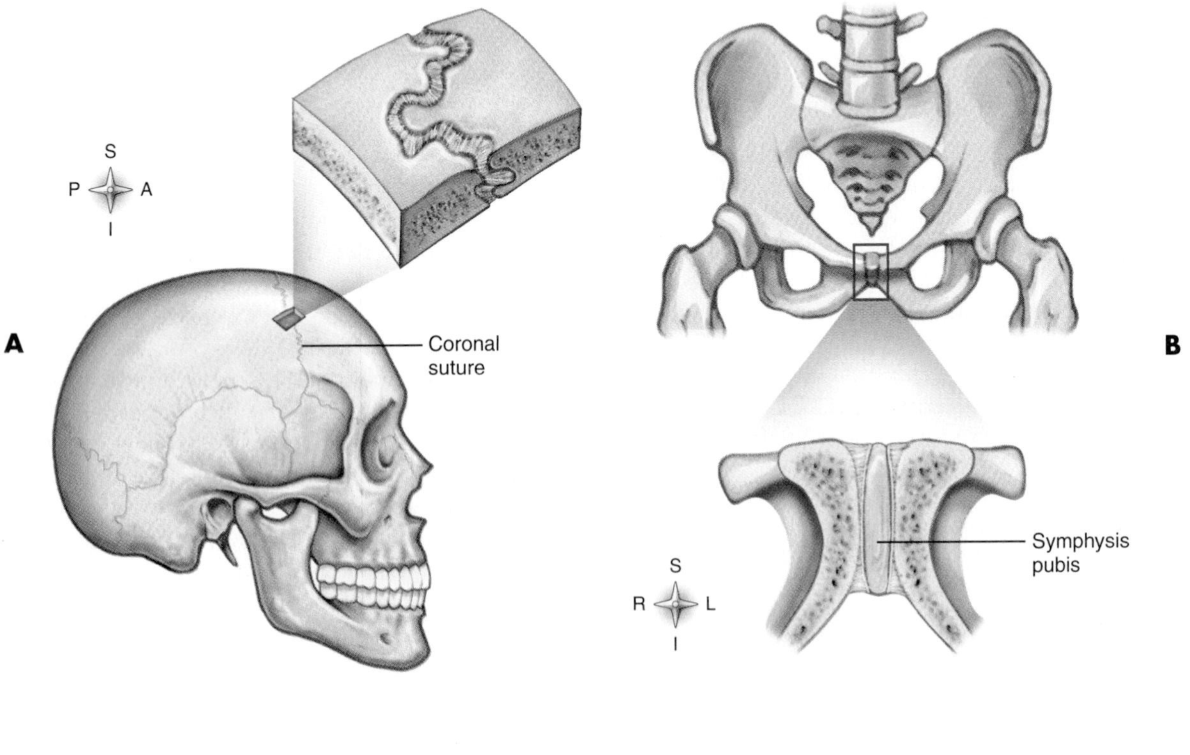

Clinical Application

Palpable Bony Landmarks

Health professionals often identify externally palpable bony landmarks when dealing with the sick and injured. **Palpable** bony landmarks are bones that can be touched and identified through the skin. They serve as reference points in identifying other body structures.

There are externally palpable bony landmarks throughout the body. Many skull bones such as the zygomatic bone can be palpated. The medial and lateral epicondyles of the humerus, the olecranon process of the ulna, and the styloid process of the ulna and the radius at the wrist can be palpated on the upper extremity. The highest corner of the shoulder is the acromion process of the scapula.

When you put your hands on your hips, you can feel the superior edge of the ilium called the *iliac crest*. The anterior end of the crest, called the *anterior superior iliac spine*, is a prominent landmark used often as a clinical reference. The medial malleolus of the tibia and the lateral malleolus of the fibula are prominent at the ankle. The calcaneus or heel bone is easily palpated on the posterior aspect of the foot. On the anterior aspect of the lower extremity, examples of palpable bony landmarks include the patella or knee cap, the anterior border of the tibia or shin bone, and the metatarsals and phalanges of the toes. Try to identify as many of the externally palpable bones of the skeleton as possible on your own body. Using these as points of reference will make it easier for you to visualize the placement of other bones that cannot be touched or palpated through the skin.

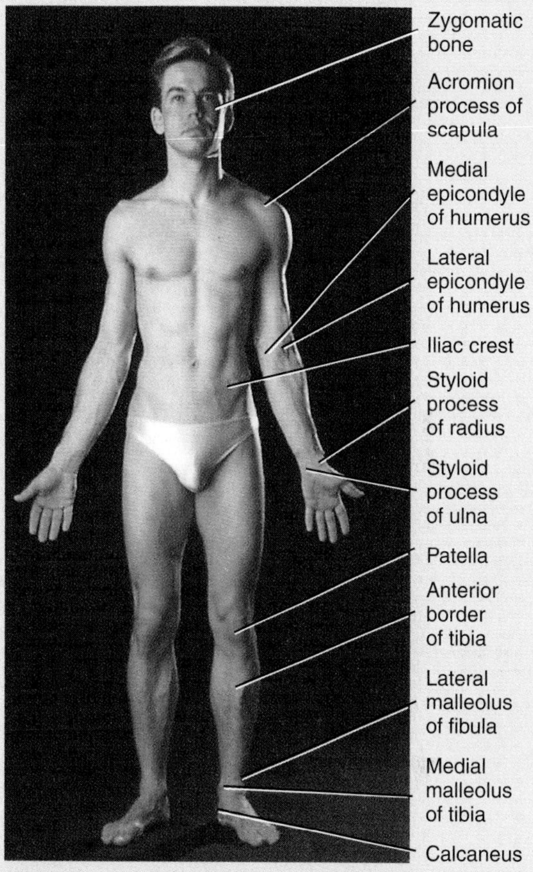

Structure. Diarthroses (freely movable joints) are made alike in certain ways. All have a joint capsule, a joint cavity, and a layer of cartilage over the ends of two joining bones (Figure 6-20). The **joint capsule** is made of the body's strongest and toughest material—fibrous connective tissue—and is lined with a smooth, slippery synovial membrane. The capsule fits over the ends of the two bones somewhat like a sleeve. Because it attaches firmly to the shaft of each bone to form its covering (called the *periosteum; peri* means "around," and *osteum* means "bone"), the joint capsule holds the bones securely together but at the same time permits movement at the joint. The structure of the joint capsule, in other words, helps make possible the joint's function.

Ligaments (cords or bands made of the same strong fibrous connective tissue as the joint capsule) also grow out of the periosteum and lash the two bones together even more firmly.

The layer of **articular cartilage** over the joint ends of bones acts like a rubber heel on a shoe—it absorbs jolts. The articular cartilage also provides a smooth surface so the bones of the joint can

FIGURE 6-20

Structure of a diarthrotic joint. Each diarthrosis has a joint capsule, a joint cavity, and a layer of cartilage over the ends of the joined bones.

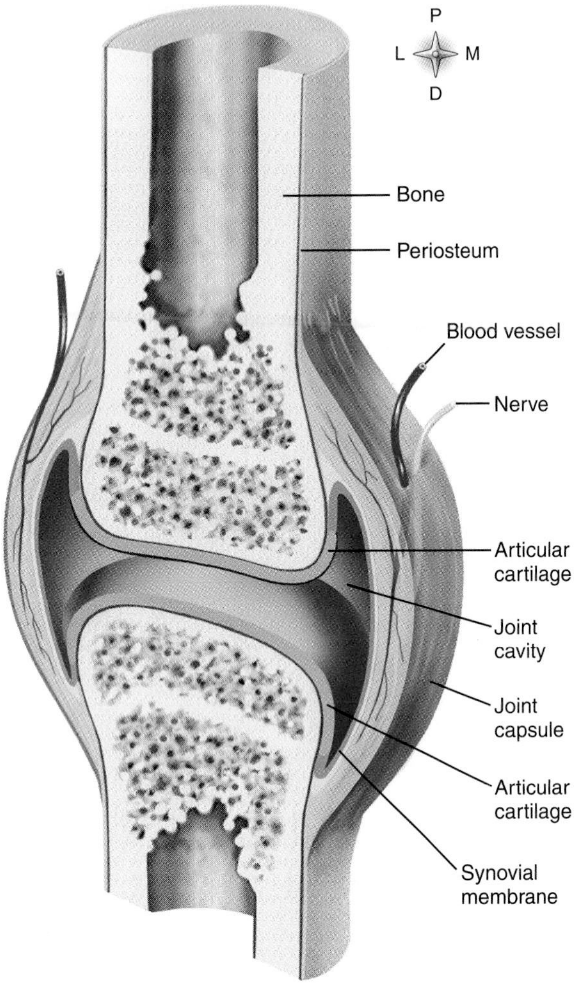

move with little friction. The **synovial membrane** secretes a lubricating fluid (synovial fluid) that allows easier movement with less friction.

There are several types of diarthroses: ball-and-socket, hinge, pivot, saddle, gliding, and condyloid (Figure 6-21). Because they differ in structure, they differ also in their possible range of movement. In a ball-and-socket joint, a ball-shaped head of one bone fits into a concave socket of another bone. Shoulder and hip joints, for example, are ball-and-socket joints. Of all the joints in our bodies, these permit the widest range of movements. Think for a moment about how many ways you can move your upper arms. You can move them forward, you can move them backward, you can move them away from the sides of your body, and you can move them back down to your sides. You can also move them around so as to describe a circle with your hands.

Hinge joints, like the hinges on a door, allow movements in only two directions, namely, **flexion** and **extension.** Flexion is bending a joint; extension is straightening it out (Table 6-7). Elbow

Clinical Application

Total Hip Replacement

Because total hip replacement (THR) is the most common orthopedic operation performed on older persons (more than 200,000 procedures per year in the United States), home health care professionals often work with patients recovering from THR surgery.

The THR procedure involves replacement of the femoral head by a metal prosthesis and the acetabular socket by a polyethylene cup. The prostheses are usually coated with a porous material that allows natural growth of bone to mesh with the artificial material. Such meshing of tissue and prostheses ensures stability of the parts without the loosening that the use of glues in the past often allowed. First introduced in 1953, THR technique has advanced to the state that the procedure has a success rate of about 85%.

Patients at home after THR surgery should progress through proper surgical healing and recovery, including stabilization of the prostheses as new tissue grows into their porous surfaces. THR patients should also expect some improvement in regained use of the affected hip, including weight-bearing and walking movements.

FIGURE 6-21

Types of diarthrotic joints. Notice that the structure of each type dictates its function (movement).

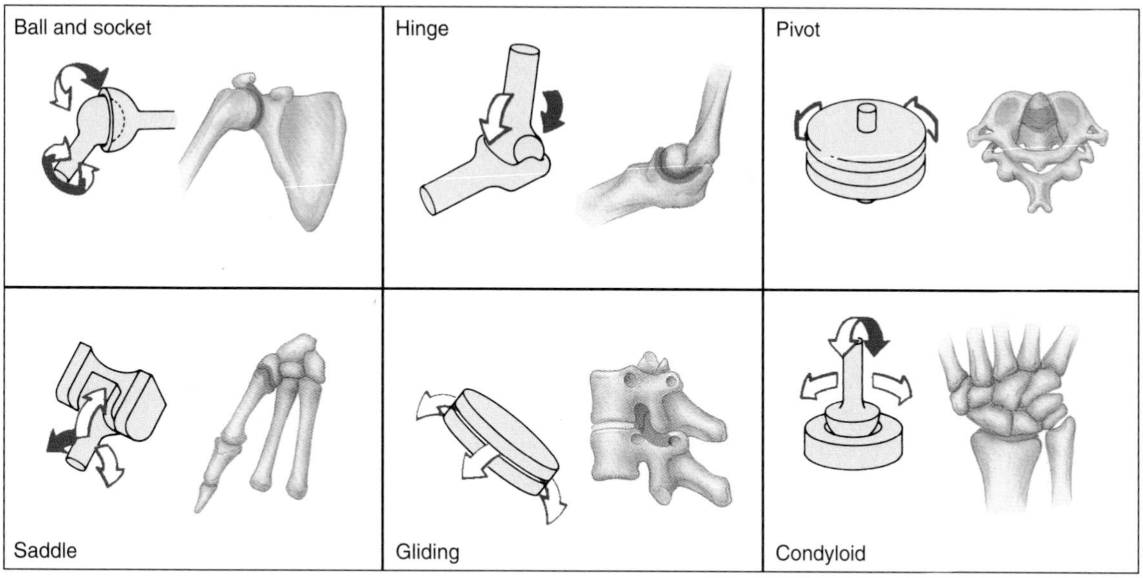

and knee joints and the joints in the fingers are hinge joints.

Pivot joints are those in which a small projection of one bone pivots in an arch of another bone. For example, a projection of the axis, the second vertebra in the neck, pivots in an arch of the atlas, the first vertebra in the neck. This **rotates** the head, which rests on the atlas.

Only one pair of saddle joints exists in the body—between the metacarpal bone of each thumb and a carpal bone of the wrist (the name of this carpal bone is the *trapezium*). Because the articulating surfaces of these bones are saddle-shaped, they make possible the human thumb's great mobility, a mobility no animal's thumb possesses. We can **flex, extend, abduct, adduct,** and **circumduct** our thumbs, and most important of all, we can move our thumbs to touch the tip of any one of our fingers. (This movement is called *opposing the thumb to the fingers.*) Without the saddle joints at the base of each of our thumbs, we could not do such a simple act as picking up a pin or grasping a pencil between thumb and forefinger.

Gliding joints are the least movable diarthrotic joints. Their flat articulating surfaces allow limited gliding movements, such as that at the superior and inferior articulating processes between successive vertebrae.

Condyloid joints are those in which a condyle (an oval projection) fits into an elliptical socket. An example is the fit of the distal end of the radius into depressions in the carpal bones.

Quick Check

1. What are the three major types of joints in the skeleton? Give an example of each.
2. What membrane in a diarthrotic joint provides lubrication for movement?
3. What is a ligament?
4. What is meant by "flexing" the elbow? Extending the elbow?

TABLE 6-7

Types of Joint Movements

MOVEMENT	EXAMPLE	DESCRIPTION
Flexion (to flex a joint)	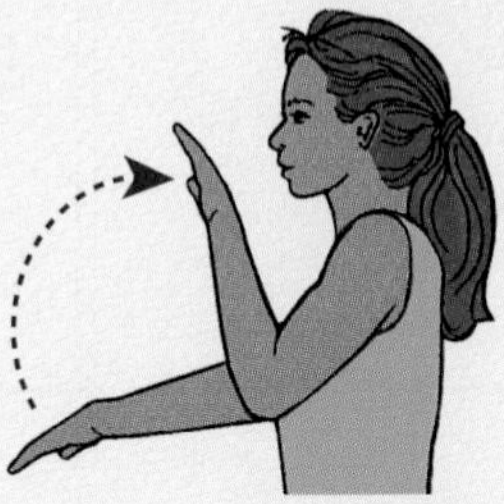	Reduces the angle of the joint, as in bending the elbow
Extension (to extend a joint)	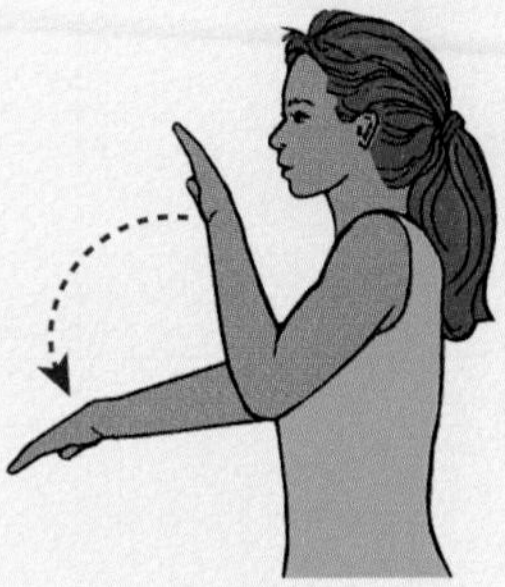	Increases the angle of a joint, as in straightening a bent elbow
Rotation (to rotate a joint)	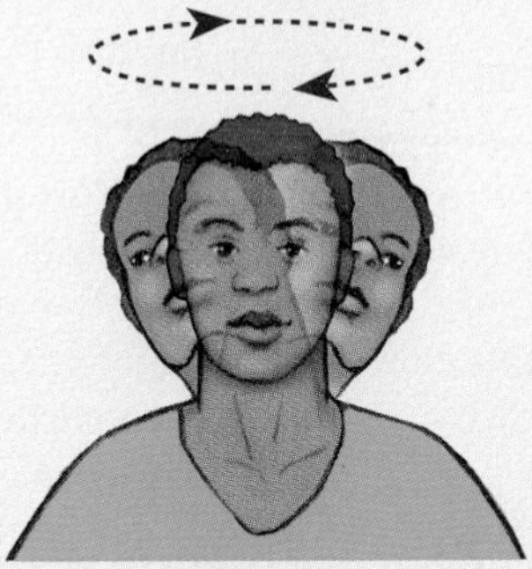	Spins one bone relative to another, as in rotating the head at the neck joint

TABLE 6-7—*cont'd*

Types of Joint Movements

MOVEMENT	EXAMPLE	DESCRIPTION
Circumduction (to circumduct a joint)	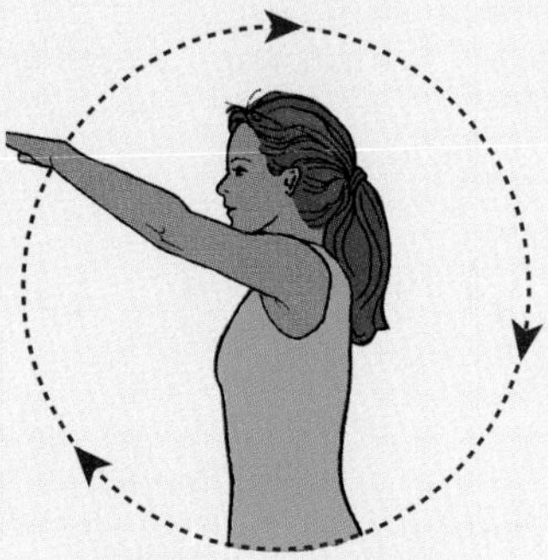	Moves the distal end of a bone in a circle, while keeping the proximal end relatively stable, as in moving the arm in a circle and thus circumducting the shoulder joint
Abduction (to abduct a joint)	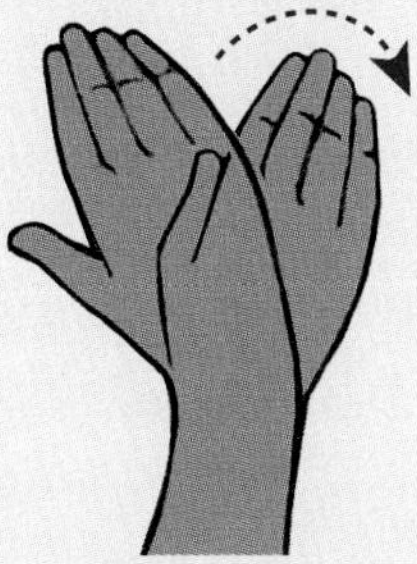	Increases the angle of a joint to move a part away from the midline, as in moving the hand to the side and away from the body
Adduction (to adduct a joint)	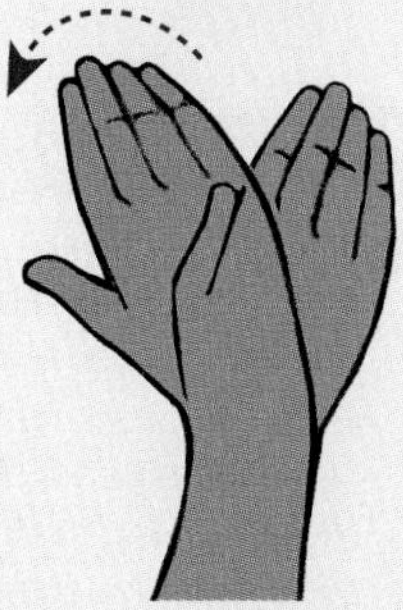	Decreases the angle of a joint to move a part toward the midline, as in moving the hand in and down from the side

Your study of these movements continues in Chapter 7, beginning on p. 173.

Health & Well-Being

The Knee Joint

The knee is the largest and most vulnerable joint. Because the knee is often subjected to sudden, strong forces during athletic activity, knee injuries are among the most common type of athletic injury. Sometimes, the articular cartilages on the tibia become torn when the knee twists while bearing weight. The ligaments holding the tibia and femur together can also be injured in this way. Knee injuries may also occur when a weight-bearing knee is hit by another person.

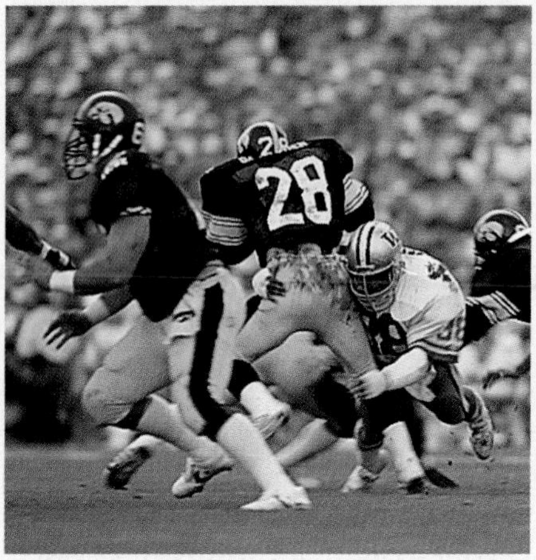

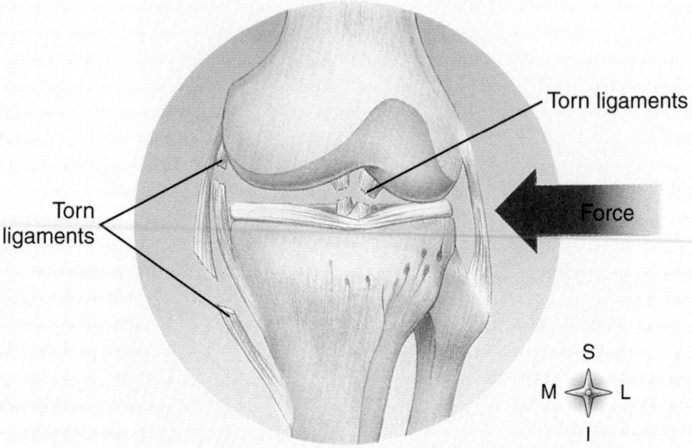

Science Applications

Bones and Joints

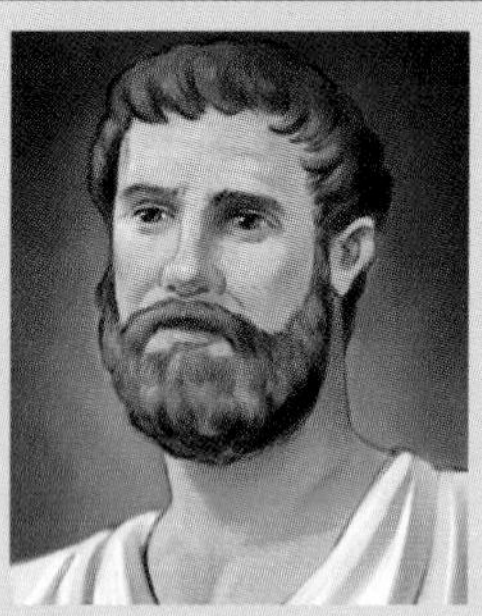

Hippocrates (ca. 460-377 BC).

Ever since 400 BCE, when Hippocrates (the Greek physician often regarded as a founder of the medical profession) first described treatments of human bone and joint disorders and injuries, many approaches to treating the human skeleton have been taken. For example, physical and occupational therapists help patients regain movement in joints through physical exercises and orthopedic surgeons help their patients by means of surgical operations. Because the skeleton, with its many bones and joints, is the framework of the entire body, it is not surprising to learn that many different health professionals deal directly with the skeleton. For example, podiatrists work with the bones and joints of the foot and ankle, sports trainers and physicians work with many parts of the skeleton, and chiropractic physicians often work closely with the alignment of the vertebral column. Of course, radiographic technicians and radiologists are often called upon to make medical images of the bones and joints and interpret the meaning of the images.

OUTLINE SUMMARY

FUNCTIONS OF BONE
A. Supports and gives shape to the body
B. Protects internal organs
C. Helps make movements possible
D. Stores calcium
E. Hemopoiesis or blood cell formation

TYPES OF BONES
A. Long—Example: humerus (upper arm)
B. Short—Example: carpals (wrist)
C. Flat—Example: frontal (skull)
D. Irregular—Example: vertebrae (spinal cord)

STRUCTURE OF LONG BONES
A. Structural components (Figure 6-1)
  1. Diaphysis or shaft
  2. Medullary cavity containing yellow marrow
  3. Epiphyses or ends of the bone; spongy bone contains red bone marrow
  4. Articular cartilage—covers epiphyses as a cushion
  5. Periosteum—strong membrane covering bone except at joint surfaces
  6. Endosteum—lines medullary cavity

MICROSCOPIC STRUCTURE OF BONE AND CARTILAGE
A. Bone types (Figure 6-2)
  1. Spongy
    a. Texture results from needlelike threads of bone called *trabeculae* surrounded by a network of open spaces
    b. Found in epiphyses of bones
    c. Spaces contain red bone marrow
  2. Compact
    a. Structural unit is Haversian system—composed of concentric lamella, lacunae containing osteocytes, and canaliculi, all covered by periosteum
B. Cartilage (Figure 6-4)
  1. Cell type called *chondrocyte*
  2. Matrix is gel-like and lacks blood vessels

BONE FORMATION AND GROWTH
(Figures 6-5 and 6-6)
A. Sequence of development early—cartilage models replaced by calcified bone matrix
B. Osteoblasts form new bone, and osteoclasts resorb bone

DIVISIONS OF SKELETON
Skeleton composed of the following divisions and their subdivisions:
A. Axial skeleton
  1. Skull
  2. Spine
  3. Thorax
  4. Hyoid bone
B. Appendicular skeleton
  1. Upper extremities, including shoulder girdle
  2. Lower extremities, including hip girdle
C. Location and description of bones—see Figures 6-7 to 6-17 and Tables 6-2 to 6-6

DIFFERENCES BETWEEN A MAN'S AND A WOMAN'S SKELETON
A. Size—male skeleton generally larger
B. Shape of pelvis—male pelvis deep and narrow, female pelvis broad and shallow
C. Size of pelvic inlet—female pelvic inlet generally wider, normally large enough for baby's head to pass through it (Figure 6-18)
D. Pubic angle—angle between pubic bones of female generally wider

JOINT (ARTICULATIONS)
A. Kinds of joints (Figures 6-19 to 6-21)
  1. Synarthroses (no movement)—fibrous connective tissue grows between articulating bones; for example, sutures of skull
  2. Amphiarthroses (slight movement)—cartilage connects articulating bones; for example, symphysis pubis

Continued

OUTLINE SUMMARY—*cont'd*

3. Diarthroses (free movement)—most joints belong to this class
   a. Structures of freely movable joints—joint capsule and ligaments hold adjoining bones together but permit movement at joint
   b. Articular cartilage—covers joint ends of bones and absorbs joints
   c. Synovial membrane—lines joint capsule and secretes lubricating fluid
   d. Joint cavity—space between joint ends of bones

B. Types of freely movable joints—ball-and-socket, hinge, pivot, saddle, gliding, and condyloid

NEW WORDS

amphiarthroses	diaphysis	osteoblasts	sinus
appendicular skeleton	diarthroses	osteoclasts	skull
articular cartilage	epiphyses	osteocytes	spine
articulation	fontanels	osteon	synarthroses
axial skeleton	hemopoiesis	pectoral girdle	synovial membrane
canaliculi	lacunae	pelvic girdle	thorax
chondrocytes	lamella	periosteum	trabeculae
compact bone	medullary cavity	red bone marrow	yellow bone marrow

REVIEW QUESTIONS

1. List and briefly explain the five functions of the skeletal system.
2. Describe the structure of the osteon.
3. Describe the structure of cartilage.
4. Explain briefly the process on endochondral ossification. Include the function of the osteoblast and osteoclasts.
5. Explain the importance of the epiphyseal plate.
6. In general, what bones are included in the axial skeleton and the appendicular skeleton?
7. The vertebral column is divided into five sections based on location; name the sections and give the number of vertebrae in each section.
8. Distinguish between true, false, and floating ribs. How many of each are there?
9. Describe and give an example of a synarthrotic joint.
10. Describe and give an example of an amphiarthrotic joint.
11. Describe and give an example of two types of diarthrotic joints.
12. Briefly describe a joint capsule.

CRITICAL THINKING

13. When a patient receives a bone marrow transplant, what vital process is being restored?
14. Explain how the canaliculi allow bone to heal more efficiently than cartilage.
15. What effect does the task of childbearing have on the differences between the male and female skeleton?

Trisha Minium

CHAPTER TEST

1. The thin layer of cartilage on the end of bones where they form joints is called the articular cartilage.
2. The hollow area in the shaft of long bones where marrow is located is called the medullary cavity.
3. The needlelike threads of spongy bone are called __________.
4. The structural units of compact bone are called either osteons or __________.
5. Osteocytes and chondrocytes live in small spaces in the matrix called __________.
6. Bone-resorbing cells are called __________.
7. Bone-forming cells are called __________.
8. The process of forming bone from cartilage is called __________.
9. If an epiphyseal plate remains between the epiphysis and diaphysis, bone growth can continue.
10. The two major divisions of the human skeleton are the axial skeleton and the appendicular skeleton.
11. The three types of joints named based on the amount of movement they allow are synarthrodial, amphiarthodial and diarthrodial.
12. The ligaments are cords or bands made of strong connective tissue that holds two bones together.
13. Which of the following is not a function of the skeletal system?
    a. mineral storage
    b. blood formation
    (c.) heat regulation
    d. protection
14. The strong fibrous membrane covering a long bone except for the joint is called the:
    a. endosteum
    (b.) periosteum
    c. diaphysis
    d. epiphysis
15. The fibrous inner lining of the hollow tube in a long bone is called the:
    a. endosteum
    (b.) periosteum
    c. diaphysis
    d. epiphysis
16. The end of a long bone is called the:
    a. endosteum
    b. periosteum
    c. diaphysis
    (d.) epiphysis
17. The shaft of a long bone is called the:
    a. endosteum
    b. periosteum
    (c.) diaphysis
    d. epiphysis

Match the bones in Column A with their locations in Column B.

COLUMN A	COLUMN B
18. B ulna	a. skull
19. A mandible	b. upper extremity (arm, forearm, wrist, and hand)
20. B humerus	c. trunk
21. D metatarsals	d. lower extremity (thigh, leg, ankle, and foot)
22. D tibia	
23. C rib	
24. D fibula	
25. C sternum	
26. B scapula	
27. D femur	
28. B metacarpals	
29. A frontal bone	
30. B patella	
31. A zygomatic bone	
32. B clavicle	
33. A occipital bone	
34. B carpals	
35. A maxilla	

STUDY TIPS

Before starting your study of Chapter 6, go back to Chapter 4 and review the synopsis of the skeletal system. There are several terms in this chapter that use prefixes or suffixes that help explain their meaning. The prefixes *epi-* and *endo-* were discussed earlier. *Peri-* means "around," *osteo-* or *os-* refers to bone, and *chondro-* refers to cartilage. *-Cyte* means "cell," *-blast* means "young cell," and *-clast* means "to destroy." Using these prefixes or suffixes makes some of the terms self-explanatory. When studying the microscopic structures of bone, remember that bone tissue heals fairly easily, whereas cartilage doesn't. This is because there are living cells throughout the bone. These cells must have food and oxygen and a way to get rid of waste products. The structure of the osteon allows this to occur. Most of the names of the bones should be somewhat familiar to you. The figures of the full skeletons and the figure of the skull may be the best way to learn them. The joints are named based on the amount of movement they allow (*arthro-* means joint). The joint capsule is an example of a synovial membrane discussed in Chapter 4.

In your study groups you can use flash cards to study the terms in the bone structure and joints. Discuss bone formation and the structure of the osteon. A photocopy of the skeleton figures with the names blacked out will help with learning the bones. There is no real shortcut to learning the names and locations of the bones, but quizzing each other will help. Go over the questions at the end of the chapter and discuss possible test questions.

7 The Muscular System

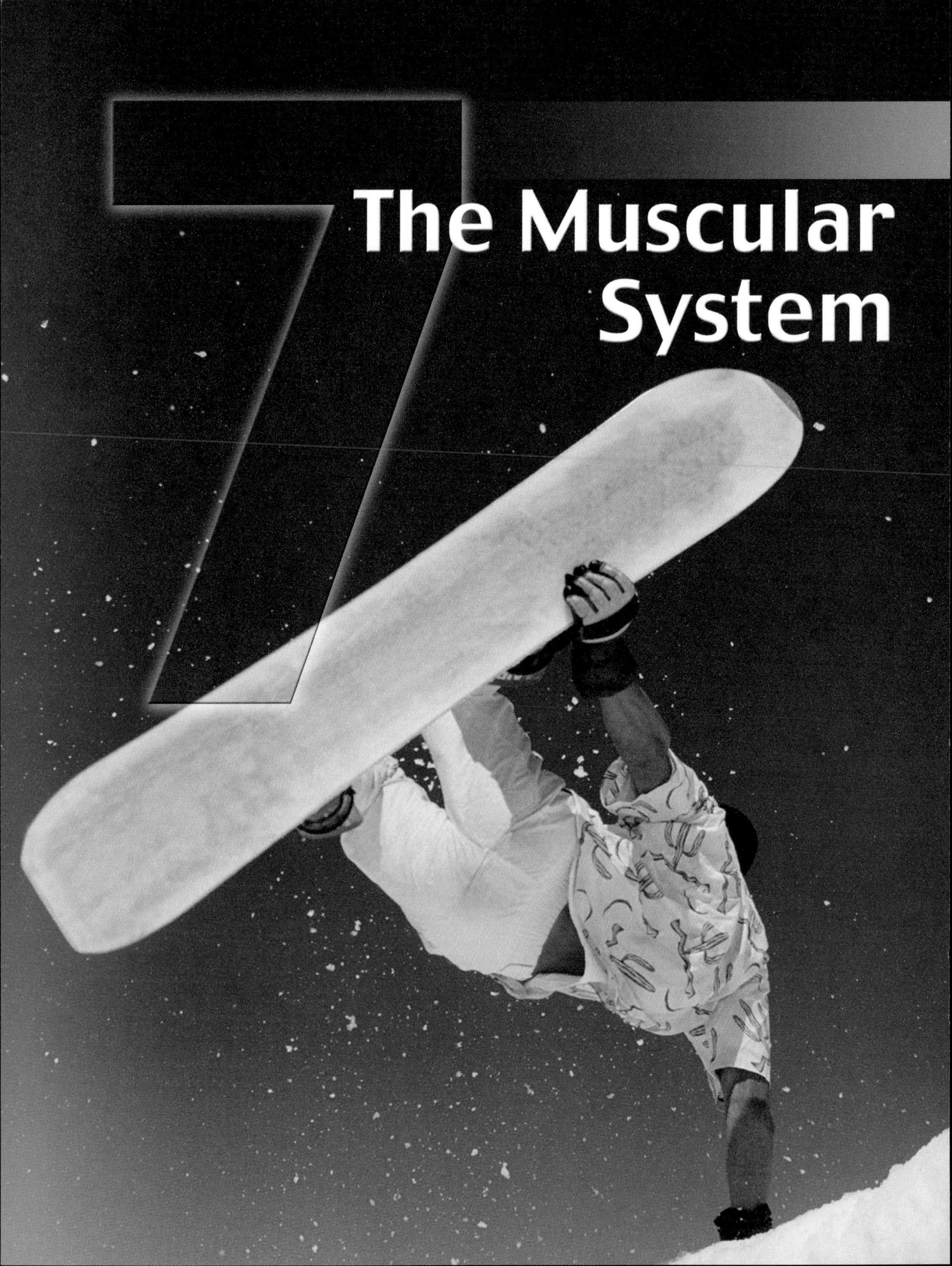

Outline

Objectives

AFTER YOU HAVE COMPLETED THIS CHAPTER, YOU SHOULD BE ABLE TO:

1. List, locate in the body, and compare the structure and function of the three major types of muscle tissue.
2. Discuss the microscopic structure of a skeletal muscle sarcomere and motor unit.
3. Discuss how a muscle is stimulated and compare the major types of skeletal muscle contractions.
4. Name, identify on a model or diagram, and give the function of the major muscles of the body discussed in this chapter.
5. List and explain the most common types of movement produced by skeletal muscles.

A*lthough we will* initially review the three types of muscle tissue introduced earlier (see Chapter 4), the plan for this chapter is to focus on skeletal or voluntary muscle—those muscle masses that attach to bones and actually move them about when contraction or shortening of muscle cells, or muscle fibers, occurs. If you weigh 120 pounds, about 50 pounds of your weight comes from your skeletal muscles, the "red meat" of the body that is attached to your bones.

Movements caused by skeletal muscle contraction vary in complexity from blinking an eye to the coordinated and fluid movements of a gifted athlete. Not many of our body structures can claim as great an importance for happy, useful living as can our voluntary muscles, and only a few can boast of greater importance for life itself. Our ability to survive often depends on our ability to adjust to the changing conditions of our environment. Movements frequently constitute a major part of this adjustment.

MUSCLE TISSUE

Under the microscope, threadlike and cylindrical skeletal muscle cells appear in bundles. They are characterized by many crosswise stripes and multiple nuclei (Figure 7-1, *A*). Each fine thread is a muscle cell or, as it is usually called, a *muscle fiber*. This type of muscle tissue has three names: *skeletal muscle*, because it attaches to bone; *striated muscle*, because of its cross stripes or striations; and *voluntary muscle*, because its contractions can be controlled voluntarily.

In addition to **skeletal muscle**, the body also contains two other kinds of muscle tissue: cardiac muscle and nonstriated, smooth, or involuntary muscle. **Cardiac muscle** composes the bulk of the heart. Cells in this type of muscle tissue are also cylindrical, branch frequently (Figure 7-1, *B*), and then recombine into a continuous mass of interconnected tissue. As with skeletal muscle cells, these cells have cross striations. They also have unique dark bands called *intercalated disks* where the plasma membranes of adjacent cardiac fibers come in contact with each other. Cardiac muscle tissue demonstrates the principle that "form follows function." The interconnected nature of cardiac muscle fibers helps the tissue to contract as a unit and increases the efficiency of the heart muscle in pumping blood.

Nonstriated or **smooth muscle** cells are tapered at each end, have a single nucleus, and lack the cross stripes or striations of skeletal muscle cells (Figure 7-1, *C*). They have a smooth, even appearance when viewed through a microscope. They are called *involuntary* because we normally do not have control over their contractions. Smooth or involuntary muscle forms an important part of blood vessel walls and of many hollow internal organs (viscera) such as the gut, urethra, and ureters. Because of its location in many visceral structures, it is sometimes called *visceral muscle*. Although we cannot willfully control the action of smooth mus-

FIGURE 7-1

Muscle tissue. A, Skeletal muscle. **B,** Cardiac muscle. **C,** Smooth muscle.

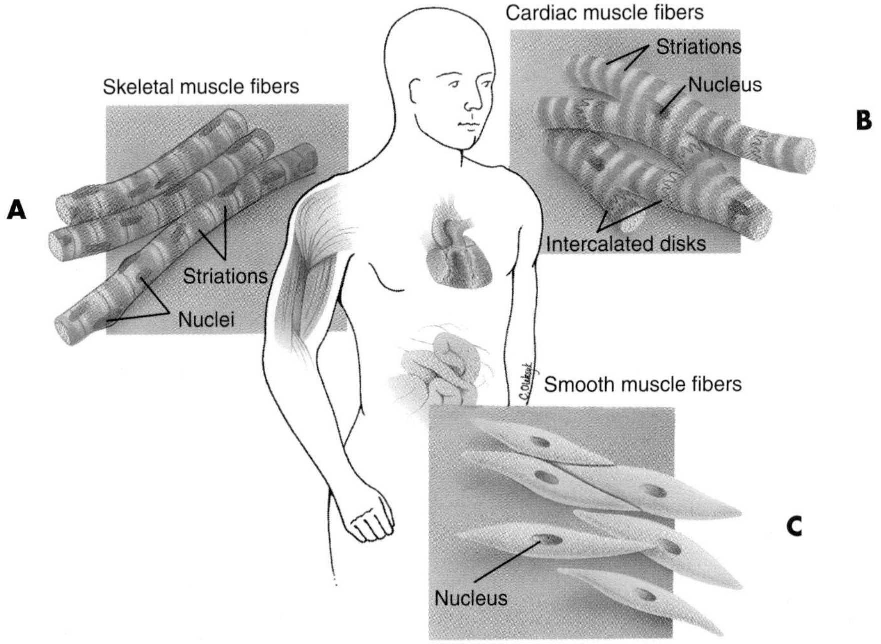

cle, its contractions are highly regulated so that, for example, food is passed through the digestive tract or urine is pushed through the ureters into the bladder.

Muscle cells specialize in contraction, or shortening. Every movement we make is produced by contractions of skeletal muscle cells. Contractions of cardiac muscle cells keep the blood circulating, and smooth muscle contractions do many things; for instance, they move food into and through the stomach and intestines and make a major contribution to the maintenance of normal blood pressure.

STRUCTURE OF SKELETAL MUSCLE

A skeletal muscle is an organ composed mainly of striated muscle cells and connective tissue. Most skeletal muscles attach to two bones that have a movable joint between them. In other words, most muscles extend from one bone across a joint to another bone. Also, one of the two bones is usually more stationary in a given movement than the other. The muscle's attachment to this more stationary bone is called its **origin.** Its attachment to the more movable bone is called the muscle's **insertion.** The rest of the muscle (all of it except its two ends) is called the *body* of the muscle (Figure 7-2).

Tendons anchor muscles firmly to bones. Made of dense fibrous connective tissue in the shape of heavy cords, tendons have great strength. They do not tear or pull away from bone easily. Yet any emergency room nurse or physician sees many tendon injuries—severed tendons and tendons torn loose from bones.

Small fluid-filled sacs called **bursae** lie between some tendons and the bones beneath them. These small sacs are made of connective tissue and are lined with **synovial membrane.** The synovial membrane secretes a slippery lubricating fluid (synovial fluid) that fills the bursa. Like a small, flexible cushion, a bursa makes it easier for a tendon to slide over a bone when the tendon's muscle shortens. **Tendon sheaths** enclose some tendons. Because these tube-shaped structures are also lined with synovial membrane and are moistened with synovial fluid, they, like the bursae, facilitate body movement.

Microscopic Structure

Muscle tissue consists of specialized contractile cells or **muscle fibers** that are grouped together and arranged in a highly organized way. Each skeletal muscle fiber is itself filled with two kinds of very fine and threadlike structures called **thick** and **thin myofilaments** (my-o-FIL-a-ments). The thick myofilaments are formed from a protein called **myosin**, and the thin myofilaments are composed mostly of the protein **actin.** Find the label **sarcomere** (SAR-ko-meer) in Figure 7-3. Think of the sarcomere as the basic functional or *contractile unit* of skeletal muscle. Recall that the osteon (Haversian system) serves as the basic building block of compact bone; the sarcomere serves that function in skeletal muscle. The submicroscopic structure of a sarcomere consists of numerous actin and myosin myofilaments arranged so that, when viewed under a microscope, dark and light stripes or cross striations are seen. The repeating

FIGURE 7-2

Attachments of a skeletal muscle. A muscle originates at a relatively stable part of the skeleton (origin) and inserts at the skeletal part that is moved when the muscle contracts (insertion).

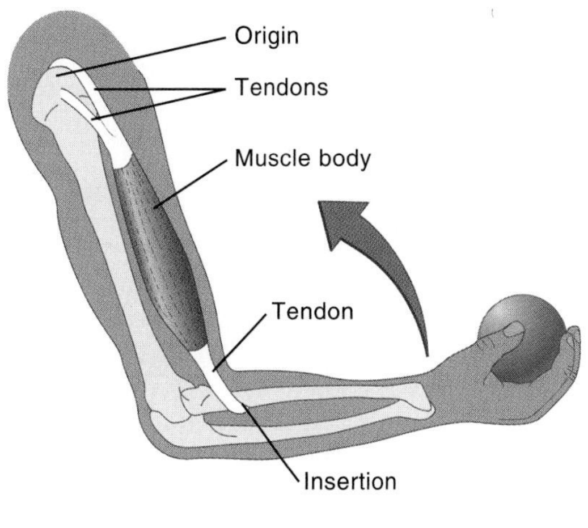

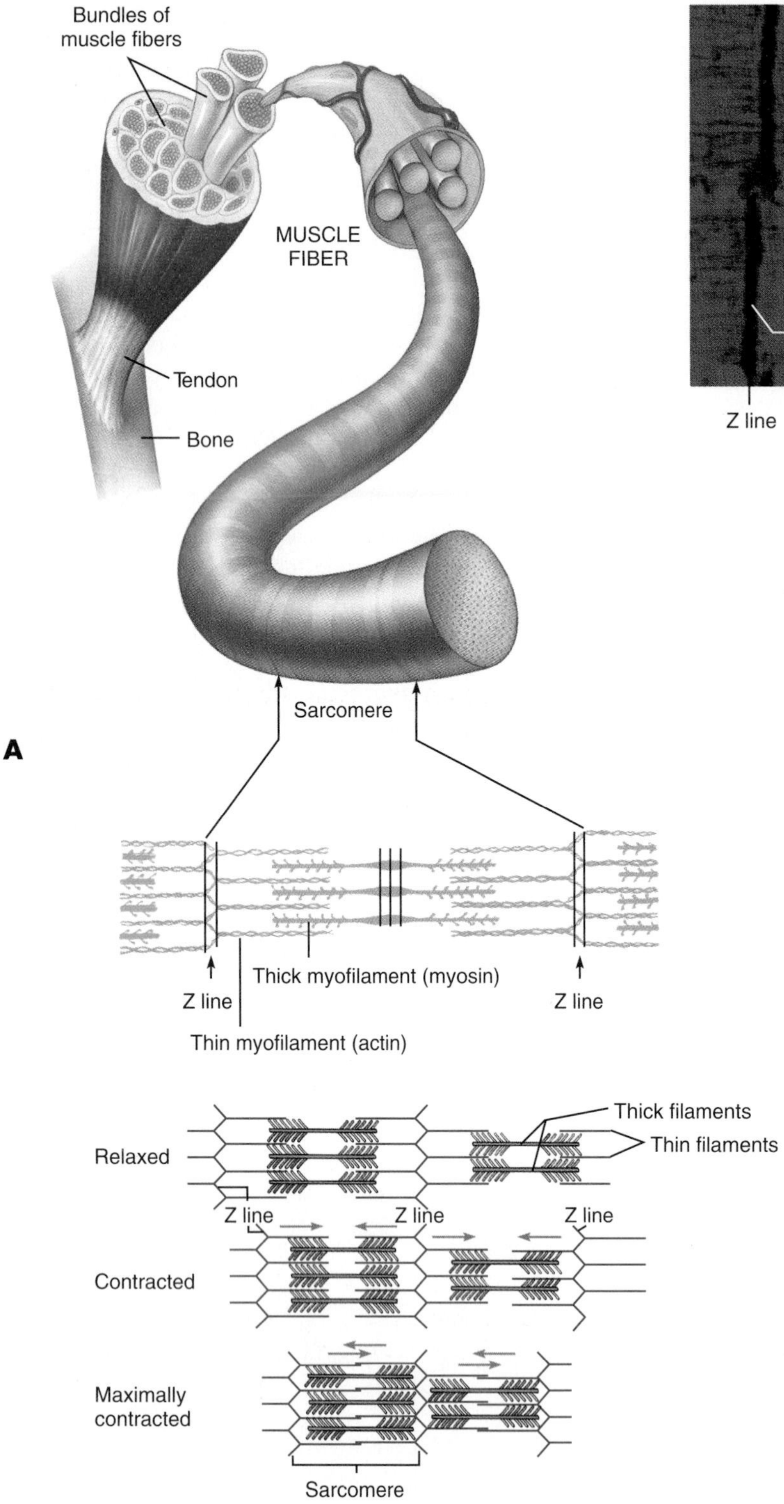

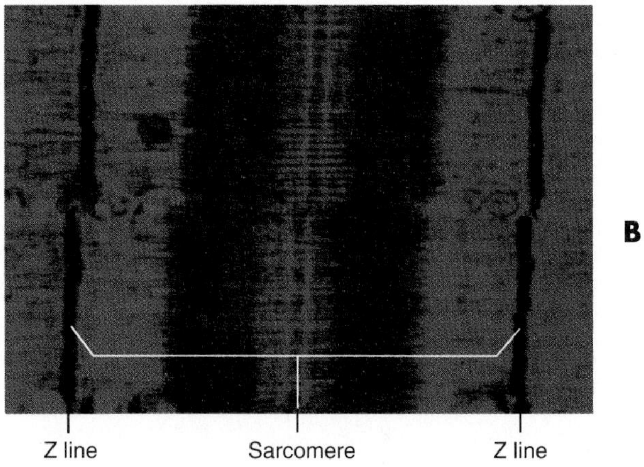

FIGURE 7-3

Structure of skeletal muscle. A, Each muscle organ has many muscle fibers, each containing many bundles of thick and thin filaments. The diagrams show the overlapping thick and thin filaments arranged to form adjacent segments called *sarcomeres*. During contraction, the thin filaments are pulled toward the center of each sarcomere, shortening the whole muscle. **B,** This electron micrograph shows that the overlapping thick and thin filaments within each sarcomere create a pattern of dark striations in the muscle. The extreme magnification allowed by electron microscopy has revolutionized our concept of the structure and function of skeletal muscle and other tissues.

units or sarcomeres are separated from each other by dark bands called *Z lines.*

Although the sarcomeres in the upper portion (Figure 7-3, *A*) and in the electron photomicrograph (EM) of Figure 7-3, *B*, are in a relaxed state, the thick and thin myofilaments, which are lying parallel to each other, still overlap. Now look at the diagrams in the lower portion of Figure 7-3, *A*. Note that contraction of the muscle causes the two types of myofilaments to slide toward each other and shorten the sarcomere and thus the entire muscle. When the muscle relaxes, the sarcomeres can return to resting length, and the filaments resume their resting positions.

An explanation of how a skeletal muscle contracts is provided by the **sliding filament model.** According to this model, during contraction, the thick and thin myofilaments in a muscle fiber first attach to one another by forming "bridges" that then act as levers to ratchet or pull the myofilaments past each other. The connecting bridges between the myofilaments form properly only if calcium is present. During the relaxed state, calcium is within the endoplasmic reticulum (see Chapter 3) in the muscle cell. It is released into the cytoplasm when the muscle is stimulated by a nerve to contract. The shortening of a muscle cell also requires energy. This is supplied by the breakdown of adenosine triphosphate (ATP) molecules, the energy storage molecules of the cell.

Quick

1. What are the three main types of muscle tissue? How do they differ?
2. What is a muscle's origin? Its insertion?
3. How do a muscle's myofilaments provide the mechanism for movement?

FUNCTIONS OF SKELETAL MUSCLE

The three primary functions of the muscular system are:

1. Movement
2. Posture or muscle tone
3. Heat production

Movement

Muscles move bones by pulling on them. Because the length of a skeletal muscle becomes shorter as its fibers contract, the bones to which the muscle attaches move closer together. As a rule, only the insertion bone moves. Look again at Figure 7-2. As the ball is lifted, the shortening of the muscle body pulls the insertion bone toward the origin bone. The origin bone stays put, holding firm, while the insertion bone moves toward it. One tremendously important function of skeletal muscle contractions therefore is to produce body movements. Remember this simple rule: a muscle's insertion bone moves toward its origin bone. It can help you understand muscle actions.

Voluntary muscular movement is normally smooth and free of jerks and tremors because skeletal muscles generally work in coordinated teams, not singly. Several muscles contract while others relax to produce almost any movement that you can imagine. Of all the muscles contracting simultaneously, the one that is mainly responsible for producing a particular movement is called the **prime mover** for that movement. The other muscles that help in producing the movement are called **synergists** (SIN-er-jists). As prime movers and synergist muscles at a joint contract, other muscles, called **antagonists** (an-TAG-o-nists), relax. When antagonist muscles contract, they produce a movement opposite to that of the prime movers and their synergist muscles.

Locate the biceps brachii, brachialis, and triceps brachii muscles in Figure 7-6. All of these muscles are involved in bending and straightening the forearm at the elbow joint. The biceps brachii is the prime mover during bending, and the brachialis is its helper or synergist muscle. When the biceps brachii and brachialis muscles bend the forearm, the triceps brachii relaxes. Therefore while the forearm bends, the triceps brachii is the antagonistic muscle. While the forearm straightens, these three muscles continue to work as a team. However, during straightening, the triceps brachii becomes the prime mover and the biceps brachii and brachialis become the antagonistic muscles. This combined and coordinated activity is what makes our muscular movements smooth and graceful.

Posture

We are able to maintain our body position because of a specialized type of skeletal muscle contraction called **tonic contraction.** Because relatively few of a muscle's fibers shorten at one time in a tonic contraction, the muscle as a whole does not shorten, and no movement occurs. Consequently, tonic contractions do not move any body parts. They do hold muscles in position, however. In other words, muscle tone maintains **posture.** Good posture means that body parts are held in the positions that favor best function. These positions balance the distribution of weight and therefore put the least strain on muscles, tendons, ligaments, and bones.

Skeletal muscle tone maintains posture by counteracting the pull of gravity. Gravity tends to pull the head and trunk down and forward, but the tone in certain back and neck muscles pulls just hard enough in the opposite direction to overcome the force of gravity and hold the head and trunk erect.

Heat Production

Healthy survival depends on our ability to maintain a constant body temperature. A fever or elevation in body temperature of only a degree or two above 37° C (98.6° F) is almost always a sign of illness. Just as serious is a fall in body temperature. Any decrease below normal, a condition called **hypothermia** (hy-po-THER-mee-ah), drastically affects cellular activity and normal body function. The contraction of muscle fibers produces most of the heat required to maintain body temperature. Energy required to produce a muscle contraction is obtained from ATP. Most of the energy released during the breakdown of ATP during a muscular contraction is used to shorten the muscle fibers; however, some of the energy is lost as heat during the reaction. This heat helps us to maintain our body temperature at a constant level.

FATIGUE

If muscle cells are stimulated repeatedly without adequate periods of rest, the strength of the muscle contraction decreases, resulting in **fatigue.** If repeated stimulation occurs, the strength of the contraction continues to decrease, and eventually the muscle loses its ability to contract.

During exercise, the stored ATP required for muscle contraction becomes depleted. Formation of more ATP results in a rapid consumption of oxygen and nutrients, often outstripping the ability of the muscle's blood supply to replenish them. When oxygen supplies run low, the muscle cells switch to a type of energy conversion that does not require oxygen. This process produces lactic acid that may result in muscle soreness after exercise. The term ***oxygen debt*** describes the continued increased metabolism that must occur in a cell to remove excess lactic acid that accumulates during prolonged exercise. Thus the depleted energy reserves are replaced. Labored breathing after the cessation of exercise is required to "pay the debt" of oxygen required for the metabolic effort. This mechanism is a good example of homeostasis at work. The body returns the cells' energy and oxygen reserves to normal, resting levels.

ROLE OF OTHER BODY SYSTEMS IN MOVEMENT

Remember that muscles do not function alone. Other structures such as bones and joints must function with them. Most skeletal muscles cause movements by pulling on bones across movable joints.

The respiratory, circulatory, nervous, muscular, and skeletal systems play essential roles in producing normal movements. This fact has great practical importance. For example, a person might have perfectly normal muscles and still not be able to move normally. He or she might have a nervous system disorder that shuts off impulses to certain skeletal muscles and thereby results in **paralysis.** Multiple sclerosis acts in this way, but so do some other conditions such as a brain hemorrhage, a brain tumor, or a spinal cord injury. Skeletal system disorders, especially arthritis, have disabling effects on body movement. Muscle functioning, then, depends on the functioning of many other parts of the body. This fact illustrates a principle that is repeated often in this book. It can be simply stated: Each part of the body is one of many components in a large, interactive system. The normal function of one part depends on the normal function of the other parts.

Quick

1. What are the three primary functions of the muscular system?
2. When a prime mover muscle contracts, what does its antagonist do?
3. How would you define the term *posture*?
4. How does muscle function affect body temperature?
5. What is *oxygen debt*?

MOTOR UNIT

Before a skeletal muscle can contract and pull on a bone to move it, the muscle must first be stimulated by nerve impulses. Muscle cells are stimulated by a nerve fiber called a **motor neuron** (Figure 7-4). The point of contact between the nerve ending and the muscle fiber is called a **neuromuscular junction.** Specialized chemicals are released by the motor neuron in response to a nervous impulse. These chemicals then generate events within the muscle cell that result in contraction or shortening of the muscle cell. A single motor neuron, with the muscle cells it innervates, is called a **motor unit** (Figure 7-4).

MUSCLE STIMULUS

In a laboratory setting a single muscle fiber can be isolated and subjected to stimuli of varying intensities so that it can be studied. Such experiments show that a muscle fiber does not contract until an applied stimulus reaches a certain level of intensity. The minimal level of stimulation required to cause a fiber to contract is called the **threshold stimulus.**

FIGURE 7-4

Motor neuron. A motor unit consists of one motor neuron and the muscle fibers supplied by its branches.

A

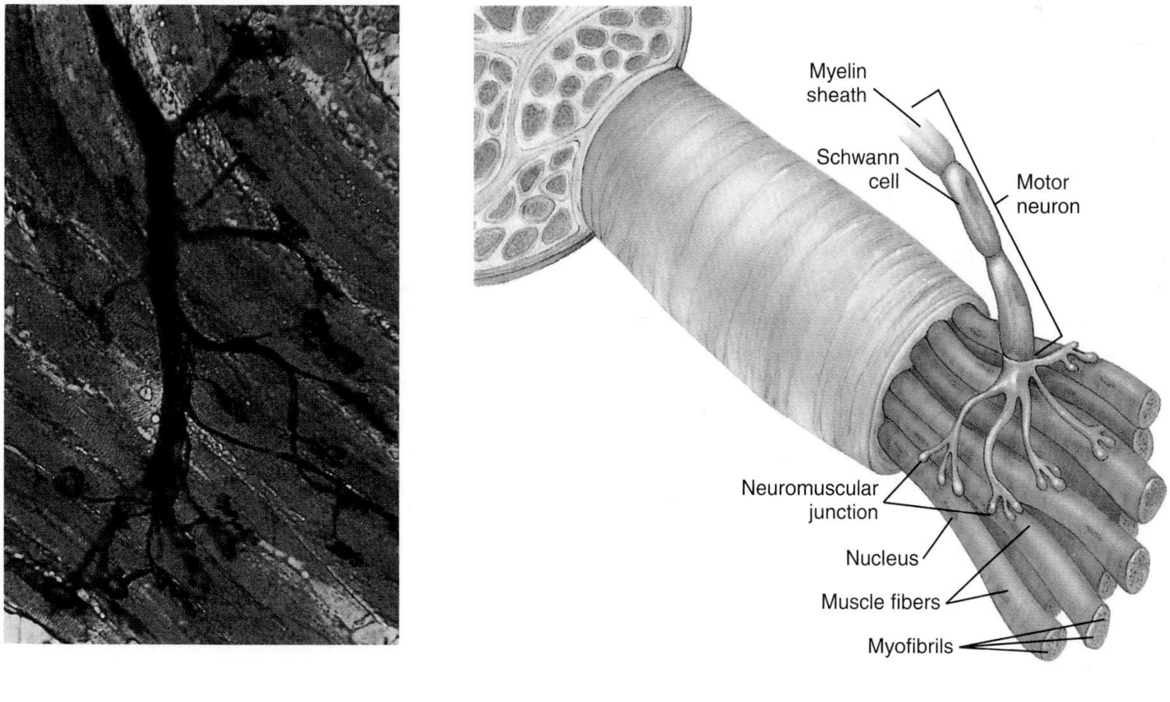

B

When a muscle fiber is subjected to a threshold stimulus, it contracts completely. Because of this, muscle cells are said to respond **"all or none."** However, a muscle is composed of many muscle cells that are controlled by different motor units and that have different threshold-stimulus levels. Although each fiber in a muscle such as the biceps brachii responds all or none when subjected to a threshold stimulus, the muscle as a whole does not. This fact has tremendous importance in everyday life. It allows you to pick up a 2-liter bottle of soda or a 20 kg weight because different numbers of motor units can be activated for different loads. Once activated, however, each fiber always responds all or none.

TYPES OF SKELETAL MUSCLE CONTRACTION

In addition to the specialized tonic contraction of muscle that maintains muscle tone and posture, other types of contraction also occur. Additional types of muscle contraction include the following:

1. Twitch contraction
2. Tetanic contraction
3. Isotonic contraction
4. Isometric contraction

Twitch and Tetanic Contractions

A **twitch** is a quick, jerky response to a stimulus. Twitch contractions can be seen in isolated muscles during research, but they play a minimal role in normal muscle activity. To accomplish the coordinated and fluid muscular movements needed for most daily tasks, muscles must contract not in a jerky but in a smooth and sustained way.

A **tetanic contraction** is a more sustained and steady response than a twitch. It is produced by a series of stimuli bombarding the muscle in rapid succession. Contractions "melt" together to produce a sustained contraction or *tetanus*. About 30 stimuli per second, for example, evoke a tetanic contraction in certain types of skeletal muscle. Tetanic contraction is not necessarily a maximal contraction in which each muscle fiber responds at the same time. In most cases, only a few groups of muscle fibers undergo contractions at any time.

Isotonic Contraction

In most cases, isotonic contraction of muscle produces movement at a joint. With this type of contraction the muscle changes length, and the insertion end moves relative to the point of origin (Figure 7-5, *A*). Walking, running, breathing, lifting, and twisting are examples of isotonic contraction.

Isometric Contraction

Contraction of a skeletal muscle does not always produce movement. Sometimes, it increases the tension within a muscle but does not shorten the muscle. When the muscle does not shorten and no movement results, it is called an *isometric contraction*. The word *isometric* comes from Greek words that mean "equal measure." In other words, a muscle's length during an isometric contraction and during relaxation is about equal. Although muscles do not shorten (and thus produce no movement) during isometric contractions, tension within them increases (Figure 7-5, *B*). Because of this, repeated isometric contractions make muscles grow larger and stronger. Pushing against a wall or other immovable object is a good example of isometric exercise. Although no movement occurs and the muscle does not shorten, its internal tension increases dramatically.

EFFECTS OF EXERCISE ON SKELETAL MUSCLES

We know that exercise is good for us. Some of the benefits of regular, properly practiced exercise are greatly improved muscle tone, better posture, more efficient heart and lung function, less fatigue, and looking and feeling better.

Skeletal muscles undergo changes that correspond to the amount of work that they normally do. During prolonged inactivity, muscles usually shrink in mass, a condition called **disuse atrophy.**

FIGURE 7-5

Types of muscle contraction. A, In isotonic contraction the muscle changes length, producing movement. **B,** In isometric contraction the muscle pulls forcefully against a load but does not shorten.

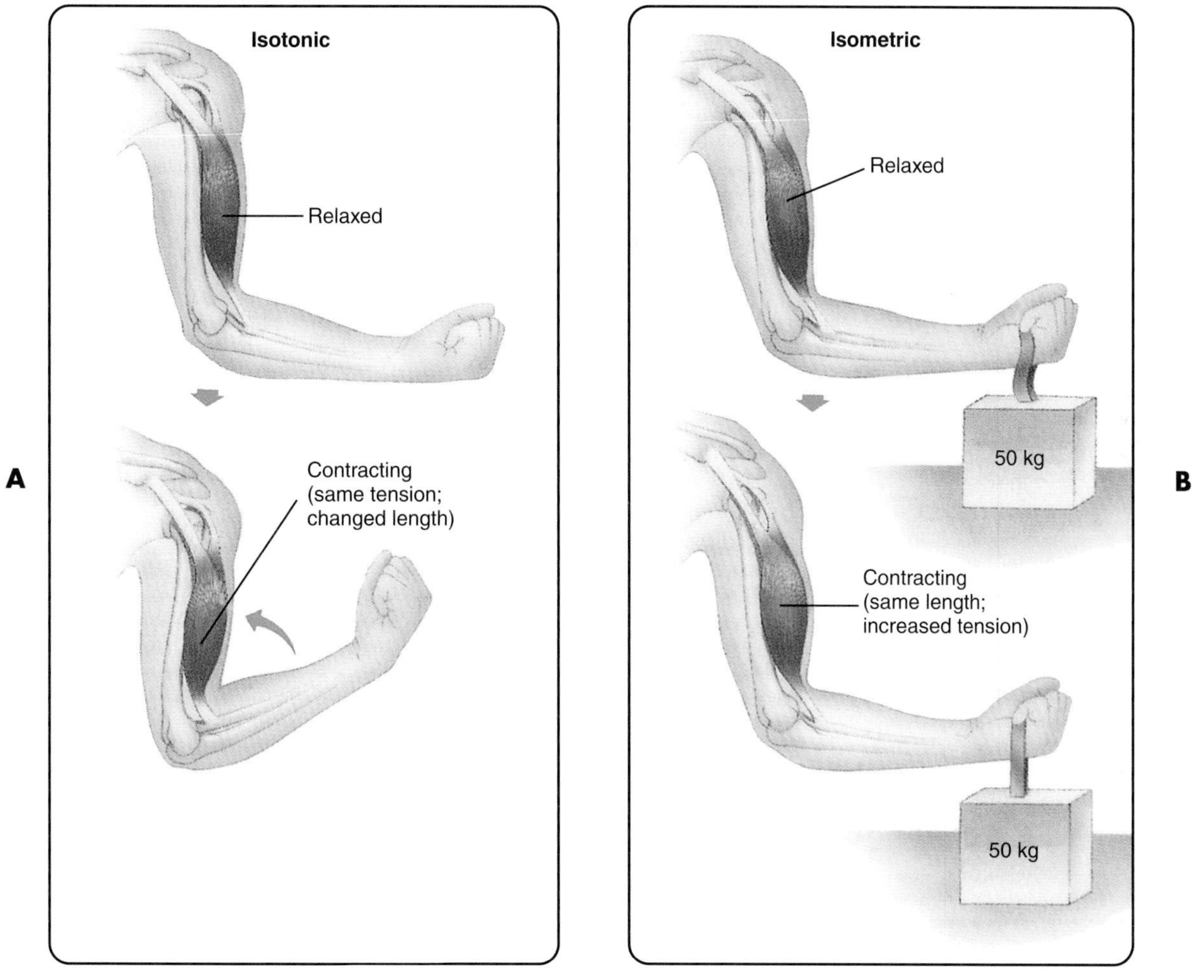

Exercise, on the other hand, may cause an increase in muscle size called **hypertrophy.**

Muscle hypertrophy can be enhanced by **strength training,** which involves contracting muscles against heavy resistance. Isometric exercises and weight lifting are common strength-training activities. This type of training results in increased numbers of myofilaments in each muscle fiber. Although the number of muscle fibers stays the same, the increased number of myofilaments greatly increases the mass of the muscle.

Endurance training, often called **aerobic training,** does not usually result in muscle hypertrophy. Instead, this type of exercise program increases a muscle's ability to sustain moderate exercise over a long period. Aerobic activities such as running, bicycling, or other primarily isotonic movements increase the number of blood vessels in a muscle without significantly increasing its size. The increased blood flow allows a more efficient delivery of oxygen and glucose to muscle fibers during exercise. Aerobic training also causes an increase in

Clinical Application

Carpal Tunnel Syndrome

Some physicians specialize in the field of occupational health, the study of health matters related to work or the workplace. Many problems seen by occupational health experts are caused by repetitive motions of the wrists or other joints. Word processors (typists) and meat cutters, for example, are at risk of developing conditions caused by repetitive motion injuries.

One common problem often caused by such repetitive motion is **tenosynovitis** (ten-o-sin-o-VYE-tis)—inflammation of the tendon sheath. Tenosynovitis can be painful, and the swelling characteristic of this condition can limit movement in affected parts of the body. For example, swelling of the tendon sheath around tendons in an area of the wrist known as the *carpal tunnel* can limit movement of the wrist, hand, and fingers. The figure shows the relative positions of the tendon sheath and medial nerve within the carpal tunnel. If this swelling, or any other lesion in the carpal tunnel, presses on the *median nerve*, a condition called **carpal tunnel syndrome** may result. Because the median nerve connects to the palm and radial side (thumb side) of the hand, carpal tunnel syndrome is characterized by weakness, pain, and tingling in this part of the hand. The pain and tingling may also radiate to the forearm and shoulder. Prolonged and severe cases of carpal tunnel syndrome may be relieved by injection of antiinflammatory agents. A permanent cure is sometimes accomplished by surgical cutting or removal of the swollen tissue pressing on the median nerve.

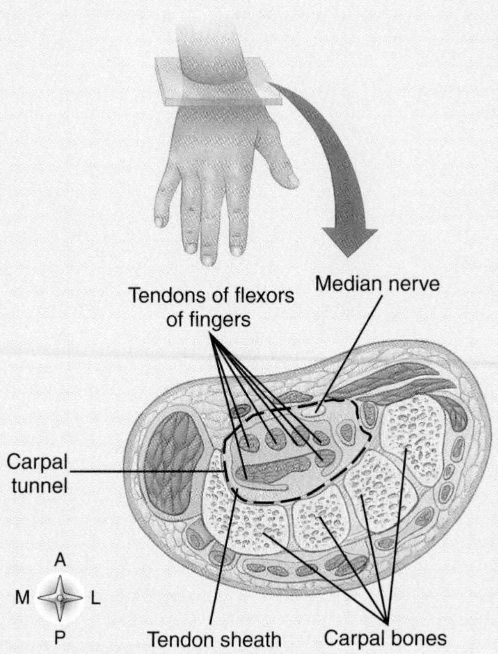

the number of mitochondria in muscle fibers. This allows production of more ATP as a rapid energy source.

Quick Check

1. What is a *motor unit?*
2. How does a muscle produce different levels of strength?
3. What is the difference between *isotonic* and *isometric* muscle contraction?
4. How does strength training affect a person's muscles?

SKELETAL MUSCLE GROUPS

In the paragraphs that follow, representative muscles from the most important skeletal muscle groups will be discussed. Refer to Figure 7-6 often so that you will be able to see a muscle as you read about its placement on the body and its function. Table 7-1 identifies and groups muscles according to function and provides information about muscle action and points of origin and insertion. Keep in mind that muscles move bones, and the bones that they move are their insertion bones.

Muscles of the Head and Neck

The **muscles of facial expression** (Figure 7-7) allow us to communicate many different emotions nonverbally. Contraction of the **frontal** muscle, for example, allows you to raise your eyebrows in surprise and furrow the skin of your forehead into a frown. The **orbicularis** (or-bik-yoo-LAIR-is) **oris** (OR-iss), called the *kissing muscle*, puckers the lips. The **zygomaticus** (zye-go-MAT-ik-us) elevates the corners of the mouth and lips and has been called the *smiling muscle*.

The **muscles of mastication** are responsible for closing the mouth and producing chewing move-

Text continued on p. 170

FIGURE 7-6

General overview of the body musculature. A, Anterior view.

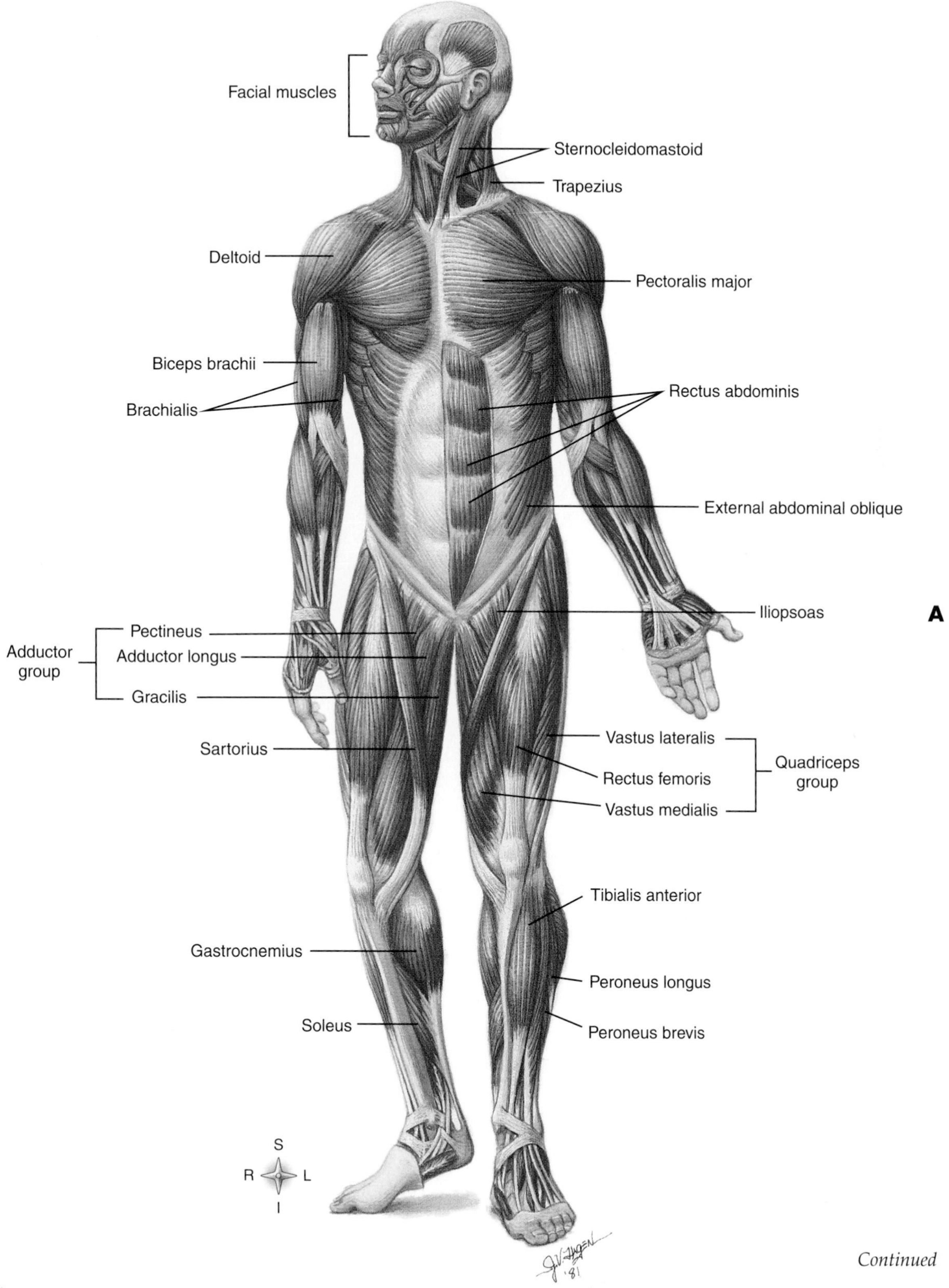

Continued

FIGURE 7-6—*cont'd*

General overview of the body musculature—*cont'd.* **B,** Posterior view.

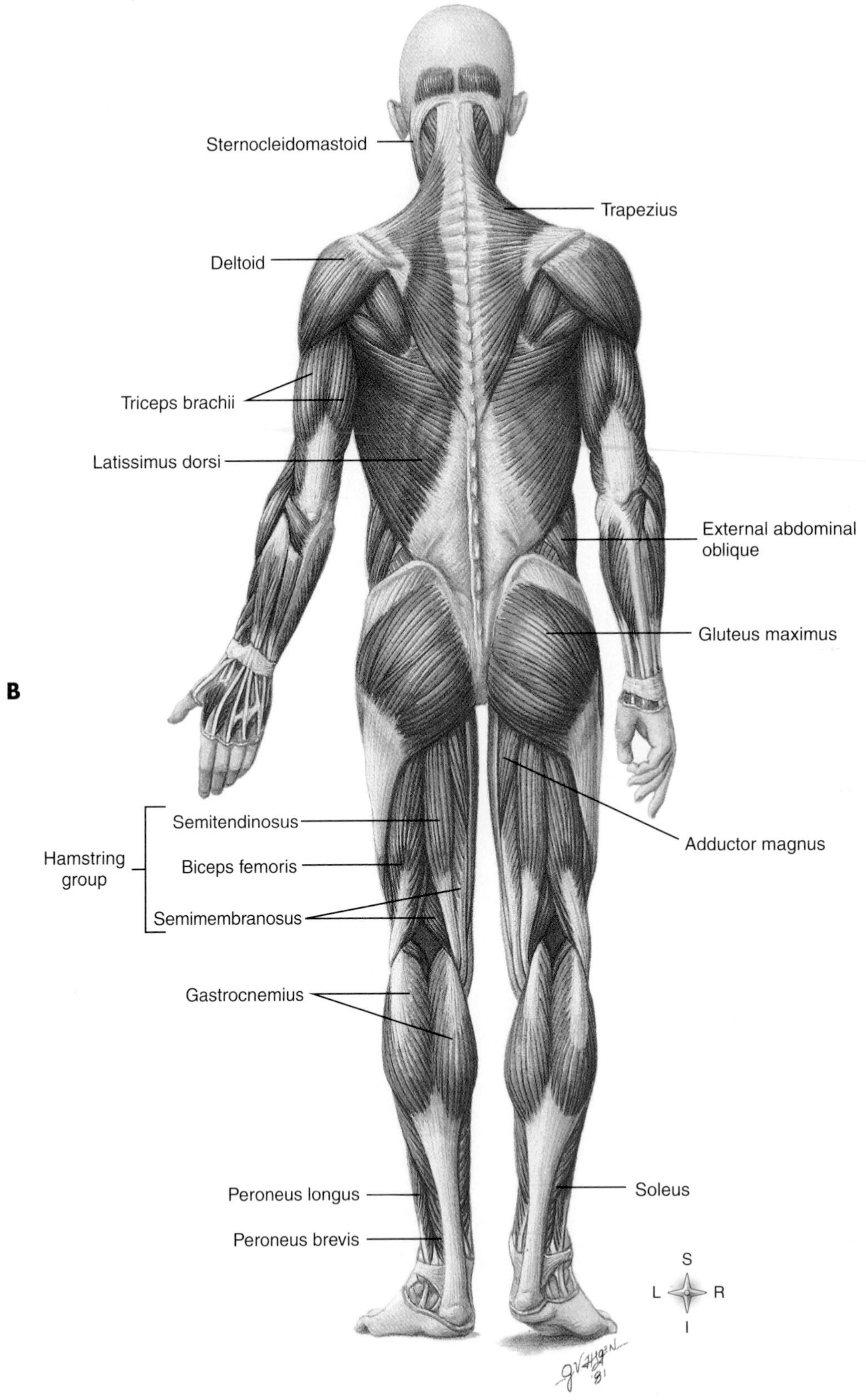

TABLE 7-1

Principal Muscles of the Body

MUSCLE	FUNCTION	INSERTION	ORIGIN
MUSCLES OF THE HEAD AND NECK			
Frontal	Raises eyebrow	Skin of eyebrow	Occipital bone
Orbicularis oculi	Closes eye	Maxilla and frontal bone	Maxilla and frontal bone (encircles eye)
Orbicularis oris	Draws lips together	Encircles lips	Encircles lips
Zygomaticus	Elevates corners of mouth and lips	Angle of mouth and upper lip	Zygomatic
Masseter	Closes jaw	Mandible	Zygomatic arch
Temporal	Closes jaw	Mandible	Temporal region of the skull
Sternocleidomastoid	Rotates and flexes head and neck	Mastoid process	Sternum and clavicle
Trapezius	Extends head and neck	Scapula	Skull and upper vertebrae
MUSCLES THAT MOVE THE UPPER EXTREMITIES			
Pectoralis major	Flexes and helps adduct upper arm	Humerus	Sternum, clavicle, and upper rib cartilages
Latissimus dorsi	Extends and helps adduct upper arm	Humerus	Vertebrae and ilium
Deltoid	Abducts upper arm	Humerus	Clavicle and scapula
Biceps brachii	Flexes elbow	Radius	Scapula
Triceps brachii	Extends elbow	Ulna	Scapula and humerus
MUSCLES OF THE TRUNK			
External oblique	Compresses abdomen	Midline of abdomen	Lower thoracic cage
Internal oblique	Compresses abdomen	Midline of abdomen	Pelvis
Transversus abdominis	Compresses abdomen	Midline of abdomen	Ribs, vertebrae, and pelvis
Rectus abdominis	Flexes trunk	Lower rib cage	Pubis
MUSCLES THAT MOVE THE LOWER EXTREMITIES			
Iliopsoas	Flexes thigh or trunk	Femur	Ilium and vertebrae
Sartorius	Flexes thigh and rotates lower leg	Tibia	Ilium
Gluteus maximus	Extends thigh	Femur	Ilium, sacrum, coccyx

Continued

TABLE 7-1—*cont'd*

Principal Muscles of the Body—*cont'd*

MUSCLE	FUNCTION	INSERTION	ORIGIN
MUSCLES THAT MOVE THE LOWER EXTREMITIES—*cont'd*			
Adductor Group			
Adductor longus	Adducts thigh	Femur	Pubis
Gracilis	Adducts thigh	Tibia	Pubis
Pectineus	Adducts thigh	Femur	Pubis
Hamstring Group			
Semimembranosus	Flexes knee	Tibia	Ischium
Semitendinosus	Flexes knee	Tibia	Ischium
Biceps femoris	Flexes knee	Fibula	Ischium and femur
Quadriceps Group			
Rectus femoris	Extends knee	Tibia	Ilium
Vastus lateralis, intermedius, and medialis	Extend knee	Tibia	Femur
TIBIALIS ANTERIOR	Dorsiflexes ankle	Metatarsals (foot)	Tibia
GASTROCNEMIUS	Plantar flexes ankle	Calcaneus (heel)	Femur
SOLEUS	Plantar flexes ankle	Calcaneus (heel)	Tibia and fibula
Peroneus Group			
Peroneus longus	Plantar flex ankle	Tarsal and metatarsals (ankle and foot)	Tibia and fibula and brevis

ments. As a group, they are among the strongest muscles in the body. The two largest muscles of the group, identified in Figure 7-7, are the **masseter** (mas-SEE-ter), which elevates the mandible, and the **temporal** (TEM-po-ral), which assists the masseter in closing the jaw.

The **sternocleidomastoid** (stern-o-kli-doe-MAS-toyd) and **trapezius** (tra-PEE-zee-us) muscles are easily identified in Figures 7-6 and 7-7. The two sternocleidomastoid muscles are located on the anterior surface of the neck. They originate on the sternum and then pass up and cross the neck to insert on the mastoid process of the skull. Working together, they flex the head on the chest. If only one contracts, the head is both flexed and tilted to the opposite side. The triangular-shaped trapezius muscles form the line from each shoulder to the neck on its posterior surface. They have a wide line of origin extending from the base of the skull down the spinal column to the last thoracic vertebra. When contracted, the trapezius muscles help elevate the shoulders and extend the head backwards.

FIGURE 7-7

Muscles of the head and neck. Muscles that produce most facial expressions surround the eyes, nose, and mouth. Large muscles of mastication stretch from the upper skull to the lower jaw. These powerful muscles produce chewing movements. The neck muscles connect the skull to the trunk of the body, rotating the head or bending the neck.

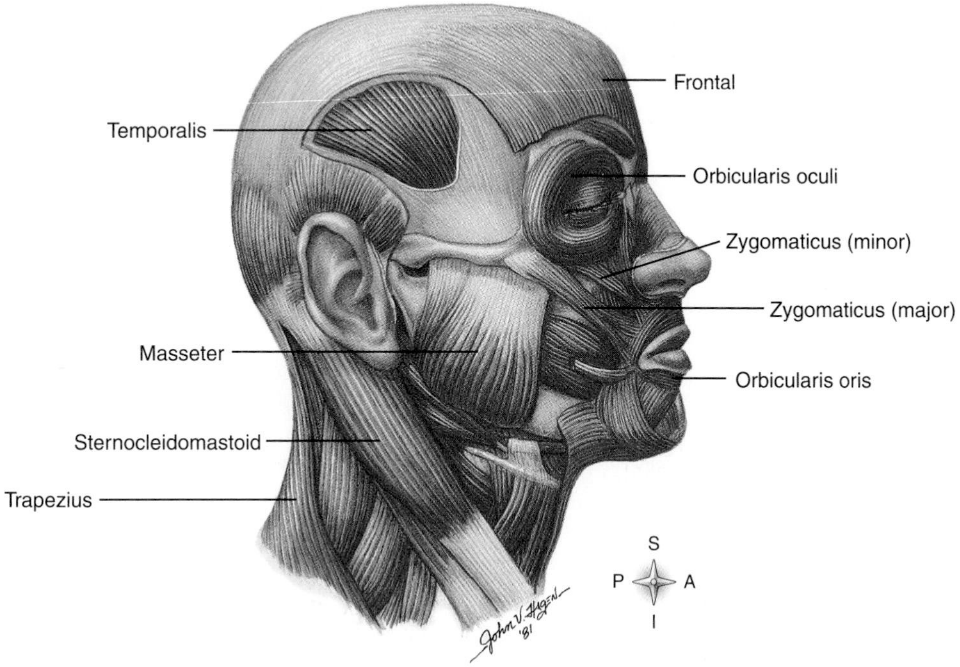

Muscles That Move the Upper Extremities

The upper extremity is attached to the thorax by the fan-shaped **pectoralis** (pek-tor-RAL-is) **major** muscle, which covers the upper chest, and by the **latissimus** (la-TIS-i-mus) **dorsi** muscle, which takes its origin from structures over the lower back (Figures 7-6 and 7-8). Both muscles insert on the humerus. The pectoralis major is a flexor, and the latissimus dorsi is an extensor of the upper arm.

The deltoid muscle forms the thick, rounded prominence over the shoulder and upper arm (see Figure 7-6). The muscle takes its origin from the scapula and clavicle and inserts on the humerus. It is a powerful abductor of the upper arm.

As the name implies, the biceps brachii (BRAY-kee-eye) is a two-headed muscle that serves as a primary flexor of the forearm (see Figure 7-6). It originates from the bones of the shoulder girdle and inserts on the radius in the forearm.

The **triceps brachii** is on the posterior or back surface of the upper arm. It has three heads of origin from the shoulder girdle and inserts into the olecranon process of the ulna. The triceps is an extensor of the elbow and thus performs a straightening function. Because this muscle is responsible for delivering blows during fights, it is often called the *boxer's muscle.*

Muscles of the Trunk

The muscles of the anterior or front side of the abdomen are arranged in three layers, with the fibers in each layer running in different directions much like the layers of wood in a sheet of plywood (see

FIGURE 7-8

Muscles of the trunk. A, Anterior view showing superficial muscles. **B,** Anterior view showing deeper muscles.

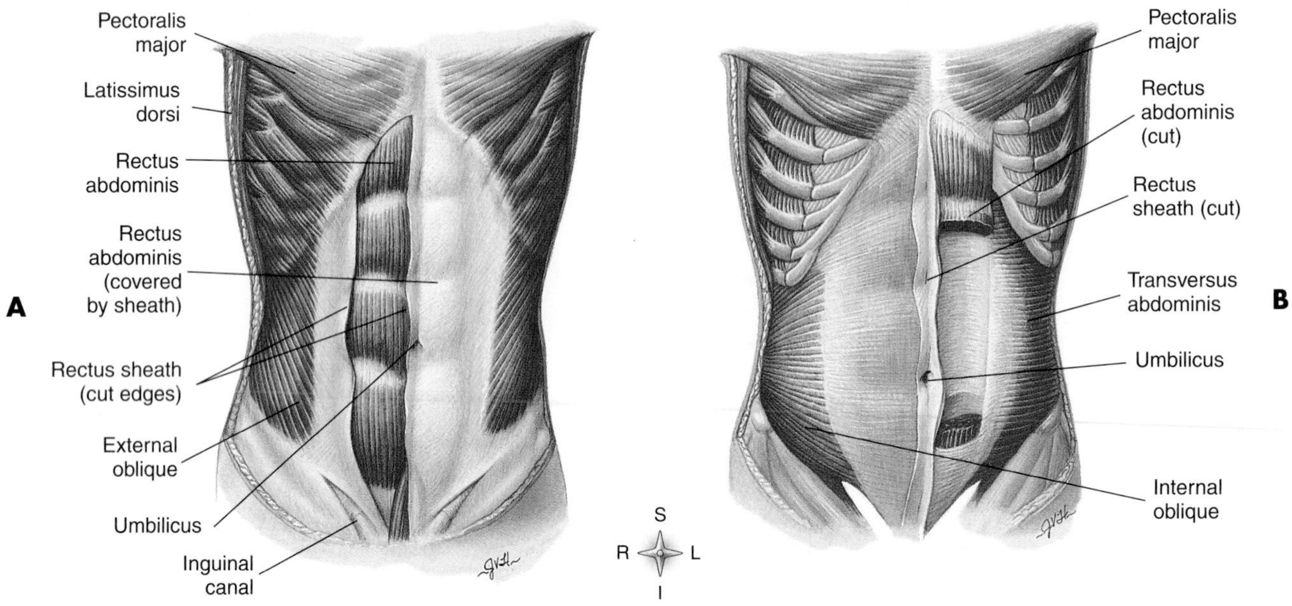

Figure 7-8). The result is a very strong "girdle" of muscle that covers and supports the abdominal cavity and its internal organs.

The three layers of muscle in the anterolateral (side) abdominal walls are arranged as follows: the outermost layer or **external oblique;** a middle layer or **internal oblique;** and the innermost layer or **transversus abdominis.** In addition to these sheetlike muscles, the band- or strap-shaped **rectus abdominis** muscle runs down the midline of the abdomen from the thorax to the pubis. The rectus abdominis and external oblique muscles can be seen in Figure 7-8. In addition to protecting the abdominal viscera, the rectus abdominis flexes the spinal column.

The *respiratory muscles* will be discussed in Chapter 14. **Intercostal muscles,** located between the ribs, and the sheetlike **diaphragm** separating the thoracic and abdominal cavities change the size and shape of the chest during breathing. As a result, air is moved into or out of the lungs.

Muscles That Move the Lower Extremities

The **iliopsoas** (il-ee-o-SO-us) originates from deep within the pelvis and the lower vertebrae to insert on the lesser trochanter of the femur and capsule of the hip joint. It is generally classified as a flexor of the thigh and an important postural muscle that stabilizes and keeps the trunk from falling over backward when you stand. However, if the thigh is fixed so that it cannot move, the iliopsoas flexes the *trunk*. An example would be doing sit-ups.

The **gluteus** (GLOO-tee-us) **maximus** (MAX-i-mus) forms the outer contour and much of the substance of the buttock. It is an important extensor of the thigh (see Figure 7-6) and supports the torso in the erect position.

The **adductor muscles** originate on the bony pelvis and insert on the femur. They are located on the inner or medial side of the thighs. These muscles adduct or press the thighs together.

Research, Issues & Trends

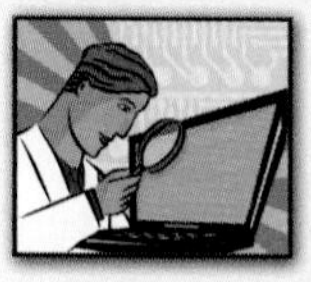

Enhancing Muscle Strength

The most obvious and effective way of increasing skeletal muscle strength is by strength training; that is, regularly pulling against heavy resistance. The maximal amount of muscular strength one can achieve is determined mainly by genetics. However, there are a number of chemical enhancements athletes have tried over the centuries to improve strength. An early fad among athletes in the twentieth century was the overuse of vitamin supplements. Although moderate vitamin supplementation will ensure adequate intake of vitamins necessary for good muscle function, overuse may lead to *hypervitaminosis* and possibly serious consequences.

Another type of chemical often abused by athletes is *anabolic steroids*. Anabolic steroids are usually synthetic derivatives of the male hormone *testosterone*. As with testosterone, they do in fact stimulate an increase in muscle size and strength, making them attractive to coaches and athletes wanting to win their events. However, prolonged use of these hormones can cause serious, even life-threatening, hormonal imbalances. For this reason, anabolic steroids are banned from most organized sports.

Sports physiologists are now investigating a whole variety of chemicals such as creatine phosphate and various coenzymes that are reported to enhance strength or endurance. Always carefully review the latest research findings on these substances with the help of a health or exercise professional before using them yourself, or you may suffer serious health consequences.

The three **hamstring muscles** are called the *semimembranosus*, *semitendinosus*, and *biceps femoris*. Acting together, they serve as powerful flexors of the lower leg (see Figure 7-6). They originate on the ischium and insert on the tibia or fibula.

The **quadriceps** (KWOD-re-seps) **femoris** muscle group covers the upper thigh. The four thigh muscles—the *rectus femoris* and three *vastus* muscles—extend the lower leg (see Figure 7-6 and Table 7-1). One component of the quadriceps group has its origin on the pelvis, and the remaining three originate on the femur; all four insert on the tibia. Only two of the vastus muscles are visible in Figure 7-6. The vastus intermedius is covered by the rectus femoris and is not visible.

The **tibialis** (tib-ee-AL-is) **anterior** muscle (see Figure 7-6) is located on the anterior or front surface of the leg. It dorsiflexes the foot. The **gastrocnemius** (gas-trok-NEE-mee-us) is the primary calf muscle. Note in Figure 7-6 that it has two fleshy components arising from both sides of the femur. It inserts through the Achilles tendon into the heel bone or calcaneus. The gastrocnemius is responsible for plantar flexion of the foot; because it is used to stand on tiptoe, it is sometimes called the toe dancer's muscle. A group of three muscles called the **peroneus** (pair-o-NEE-us) **group** (see Figure 7-6) is found along the sides of the lower leg. As a group, these muscles plantar flex the foot. A long tendon from one component of the group—the *peroneus longus* muscle tendon—forms a support arch for the foot (see Figure 6-17).

Quick Check

1. What do the *muscles of mastication* do for a person?
2. Why is the triceps brachii muscle sometimes called the "boxer's muscle?"
3. What action do the hamstring muscles perform?

MOVEMENTS PRODUCED BY SKELETAL MUSCLE CONTRACTIONS

The particular type of movement that at any joint depends on the muscle acting at that joint, on their origin and insertion points, on the shapes of the bones involved, and the joint type (see Chapter 6). Muscles acting on some joints produce movement in several directions, whereas only limited movement is possible at other joints. The terms most often used to describe body movements are as follows:

1. Flexion
2. Extension
3. Abduction
4. Adduction
5. Rotation
6. Supination and pronation
7. Dorsiflexion and plantar flexion

Clinical Application

Intramuscular Injections

Many drugs are administered by intramuscular injection. If the amount to be injected is 2 milliliters (ml) or less, the deltoid muscle is often selected as the site of injection. Note in Figure A that the needle is inserted into the muscle about two-fingers' breadth below the acromion process of the scapula and lateral to the tip of the acromion. If the amount of medication to be injected is 2 to 3 ml, the gluteal area shown in Figure B is often used. Injections are made into the gluteus medius muscle near the center of the upper outer quadrant, as shown in the illustration. Another technique of locating the proper injection site is to draw an imaginary diagonal line from a point of reference on the back of the bony pelvis (posterior superior iliac spine) to the greater trochanter of the femur. The injection is given about three-fingers' breadth above and one third of the way down the line. It is important that the sciatic nerve and the superior gluteal blood vessels be avoided during the injection. Proper technique requires knowledge of the underlying anatomy.

In addition to intramuscular injections, which are generally administered by a health care provider in an institutional setting, many individuals must self-administer injections of needed medications, such as insulin, on a regular basis in their homes. Educating these patients or their caregivers on how to correctly administer medication by injection is an important issue in the delivery of home health care services. Topics that must be covered include instruction on proper injection techniques, selection of needle length and gauge, identification of important anatomic landmarks in making injection site selections, and the preparation and rotation of selected injection sites.

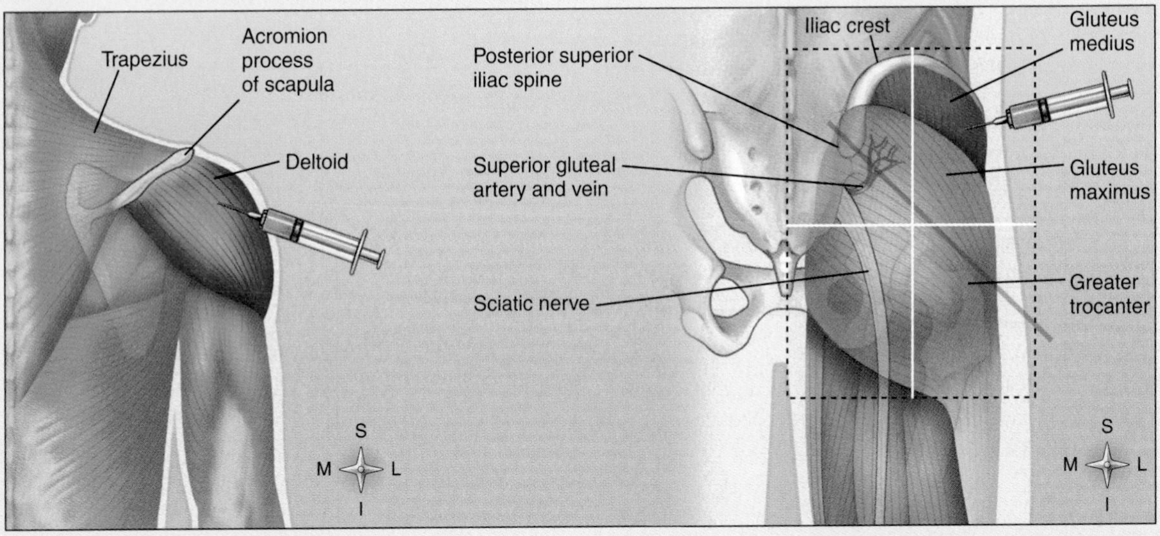

Flexion is a movement that makes the angle between two bones at their joint smaller than it was at the beginning of the movement. Most flexions are movements commonly described as bending. If you bend your elbow or your knee, you flex it. **Extension** movements are the opposite of flexions. They make the angle between two bones at their joint larger than it was at the beginning of the movement. Therefore, extensions are straightening or stretching movements rather than bending movements. Figures 7-9 and 7-10 illustrate flexion and extension of the elbow and knee.

Abduction means moving a part away from the midline of the body, such as moving your arm out to the side. **Adduction** means moving a part toward the midline, such as bringing your arms down to your sides from an elevated position. Figure 7-11, *A*, shows abduction and adduction.

FIGURE 7-9

Flexion and extension of the elbow. A and **B,** When the elbow is flexed, the biceps brachii contracts while its antagonist, the triceps brachii, relaxes. **B** and **C,** When the elbow is extended, the biceps brachii relaxes while the triceps brachii contracts.

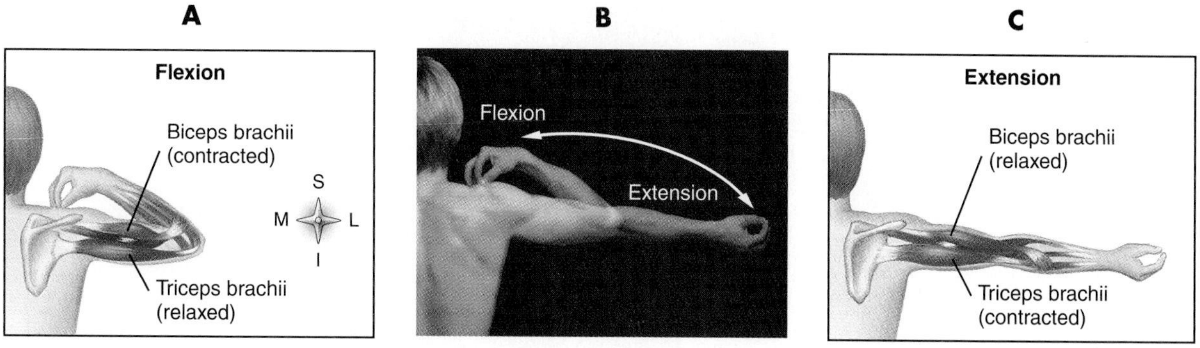

FIGURE 7-10

Flexion and extension of the knee. A and **B,** When the knee flexes, muscles of the hamstring group contract while their antagonists in the quadriceps femoris group relax. **B** and **C,** When the knee extends, the hamstring muscles relax while the quadriceps femoris muscle contracts.

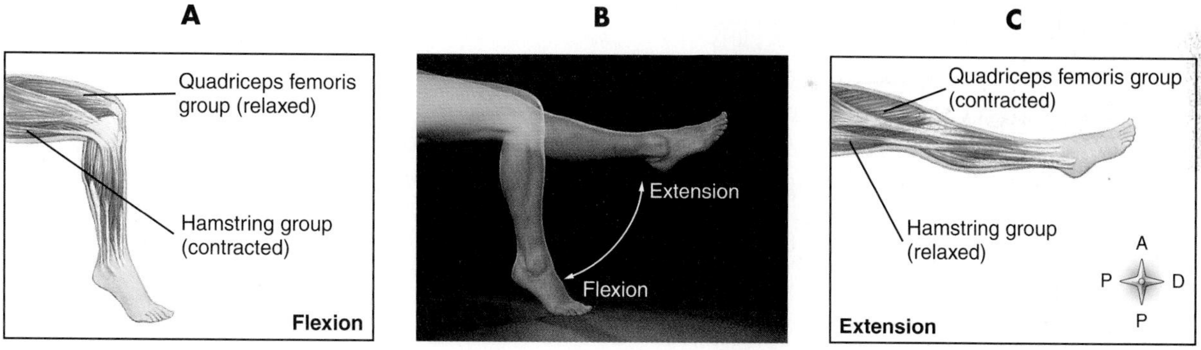

Rotation is movement around a longitudinal axis. You rotate your head and neck by moving your skull from side to side as in shaking your head "no" (Figure 7-11, *B*).

Supination and **pronation** refer to hand positions that result from rotation of the forearm. (The term *prone* refers to the body as a whole lying face down. *Supine* means lying face up.) Supination results in a hand position with the palm turned to the anterior position (as in the anatomical position), and pronation occurs when you turn the palm of your hand so that it faces posteriorly (Figure 7-11, *C*).

Dorsiflexion and **plantar flexion** refer to ankle movements. In dorsiflexion the dorsum or top of the foot is elevated with the toes pointing upward. In plantar flexion the bottom of the foot is directed downward so that you are in effect standing on your toes (Figure 7-11, *D*).

As you study the illustrations and learn to recognize the muscles discussed in this chapter, you

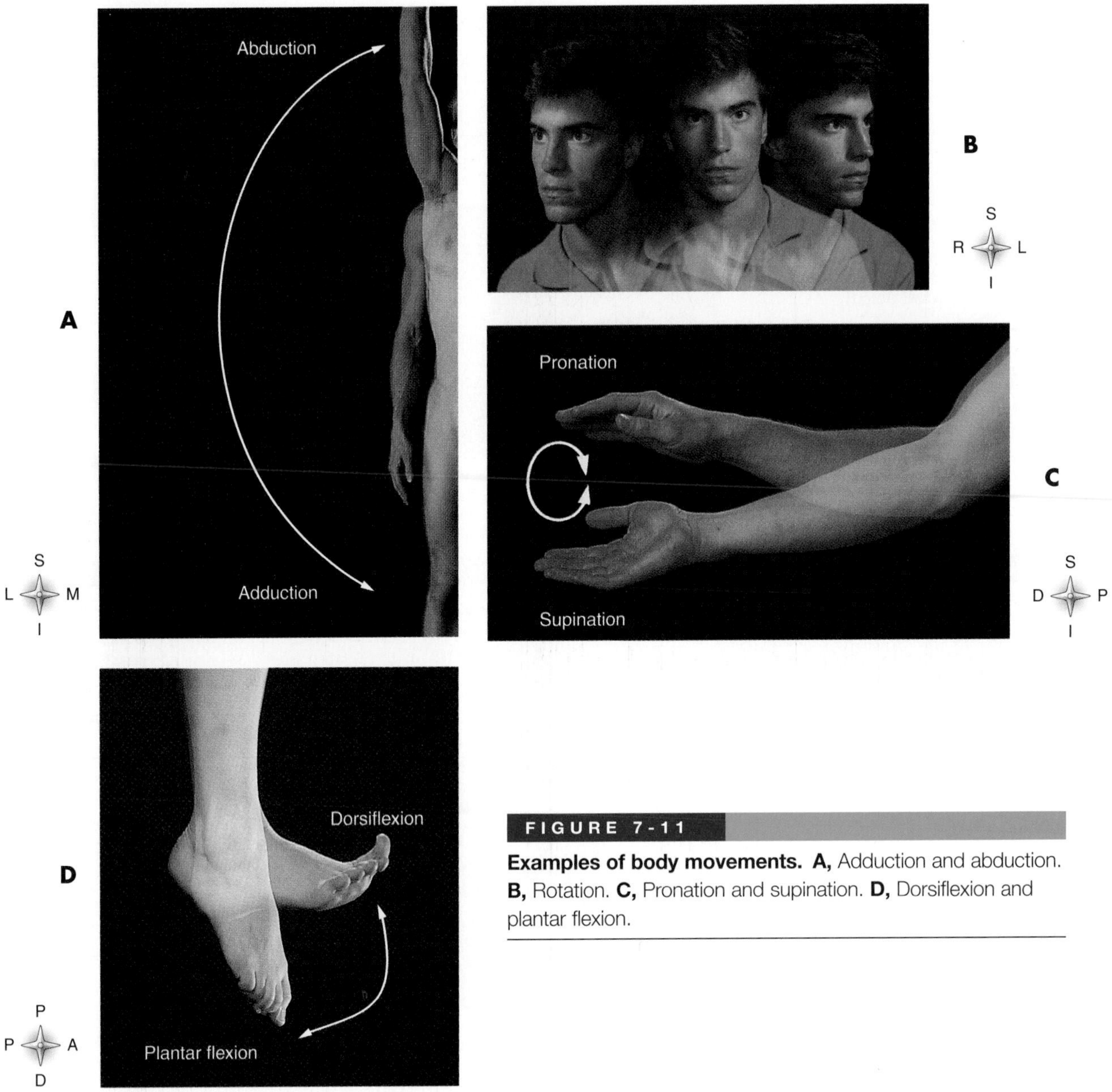

FIGURE 7-11

Examples of body movements. A, Adduction and abduction. **B,** Rotation. **C,** Pronation and supination. **D,** Dorsiflexion and plantar flexion.

should attempt to group them according to function, as in Table 7-2. You will note, for example, that flexors produce many of the movements used for walking, sitting, swimming, typing, and many other activities. Extensors also function in these activities but perhaps play their most important role in maintaining an upright posture.

Quick Check

1. When a person flexes the knee, what movement is this?
2. What happens when a person abducts his or her arm?
3. How is dorsiflexion of the foot performed?

TABLE 7-2

Muscles Grouped According to Function

PART MOVED	FLEXORS	EXTENSORS	ABDUCTORS	ADDUCTORS
Upper arm latissimus	Pectoralis major	Latissimus dorsi	Deltoid	Pectoralis major and dorsi contracting together
Lower arm	Biceps brachii	Triceps brachii	None	None
Thigh	Iliopsoas and sartorius	Gluteus maximus	Gluteus medius	Adductor group
Lower leg	Hamstrings	Quadriceps group	None	None
Foot	Tibialis anterior	Gastrocnemius and soleus	Peroneus longus	Tibialis anterior

Science Applications

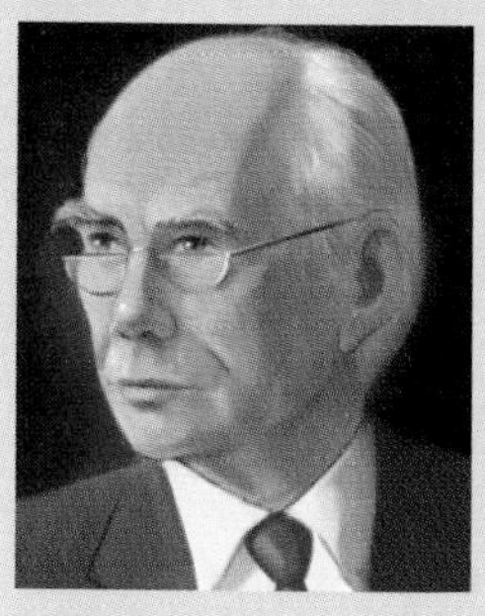

Muscle Function

Andrew F. Huxley
(b. 1917).

The British physiologist Andrew F. Huxley is largely responsible for explaining how muscle fibers contract. After making pioneering discoveries in how nerves conduct impulses, a feat for which he shared the 1963 Nobel Prize in Medicine or Physiology, Huxley turned his attention to muscle fibers. It was he who in the 1950s proposed the sliding filament model along with its mechanical explanation of muscle contraction.

Today, research physiologists continue to find out more about how muscle fibers work. These discoveries are being applied in many different professions. For example, nutritionists use this information in advising athletes and others what and when to eat to maximize muscular strength and endurance. Athletes themselves, along with their coaches and trainers, use current concepts of muscle science in helping them improve their performance. Of course, health professionals such as physicians, nurses, and physical therapists use information about muscular problems such a myasthenia gravis and muscular dystrophy to help treat patients. Many other professions, such as massage therapy, occupational therapy, ergonomics, physical education and fitness, dance, art, and biomechanical engineering also rely on up-to-date information on muscle structure and function.

OUTLINE SUMMARY

INTRODUCTION

A. Muscular tissue enables the body and its parts to move
   1. Movement caused by ability of muscle cells (called *fibers*) to shorten or contract
   2. Muscle cells shorten by converting chemical energy (obtained from food) into mechanical energy, which causes movement
   3. Three types of muscle tissue exist in body (see Chapter 3)

MUSCLE TISSUE

A. Types of muscle tissue (Figure 7-1)
   1. Skeletal muscle—also called *striated* or *voluntary muscle*
      a. Is 40% to 50% of body weight ("red meat" attached to bones)
      b. Microscope reveals crosswise stripes or striations
      c. Contractions can be voluntarily controlled
   2. Cardiac muscle—composes bulk of heart
      a. Cardiac muscle cells branch frequently
      b. Characterized by unique dark bands called *intercalated disks*
      c. Interconnected nature of cardiac muscle cells allows heart to contract efficiently as a unit
   3. Nonstriated muscle or involuntary muscle—also called *smooth* or *visceral muscle*
      a. Lacks cross stripes or striations when seen under a microscope; appears smooth
      b. Found in walls of hollow visceral structures such as digestive tract, blood vessels, and ureters
      c. Contractions not under voluntary control; movement caused by contraction is involuntary

B. Function—all muscle cells specialize in contraction (shortening)

STRUCTURE OF SKELETAL MUSCLE

A. Structure
   1. Each skeletal muscle is an organ composed mainly of skeletal muscle cells and connective tissue
   2. Most skeletal muscles extend from one bone across a joint to another bone
   3. Parts of a skeletal muscle
      a. Origin—attachment to the bone that remains relatively stationary or fixed when movement at the joint occurs
      b. Insertion—point of attachment to the bone that moves when a muscle contracts
      c. Body—main part of the muscle
   4. Muscles attach to bone by tendons—strong cords of fibrous connective tissue; some tendons enclosed in synovial-lined tubes and are lubricated by synovial fluid; tubes called *tendon sheaths*
   5. Bursae—small synovial-lined sacs containing a small amount of synovial fluid; located between some tendons and underlying bones

B. Microscopic structure (Figure 7-3)
   1. Contractile cells called *fibers*—grouped into bundles
   2. Fibers contain thick myofilaments (containing the protein myosin) and thin myofilaments (composed of actin)
   3. Basic functional (contractile) unit called *sarcomere*; sarcomeres separated from each other by dark bands called *Z lines*
      a. Sliding filament model explains mechanism of contraction
         (1) Thick and thin myofilaments slide past each other as a muscle contracts
         (2) Contraction requires calcium and energy-rich ATP molecules

FUNCTIONS OF SKELETAL MUSCLE

A. Movement
   1. Muscles produce movement; as a muscle contracts, it pulls the insertion bone closer to the origin bone; movement occurs at the joint between the origin and the insertion
      a. Groups of muscles usually contract to produce a single movement
         (1) Prime mover—muscle whose contraction is mainly responsible for producing a given movement

OUTLINE SUMMARY—*cont'd*

(2) Synergist—muscle whose contractions help the prime mover produce a given movement
(3) Antagonist—muscle whose actions oppose the action of a prime mover in any given movement

B. Posture
1. A specialized type of muscle contraction, called *tonic contraction*, enables us to maintain body position
   a. In tonic contraction, only a few of a muscle's fibers shorten at one time
   b. Tonic contractions produce no movement of body parts
   c. Tonic contractions maintain muscle tone called *posture*
      (1) Good posture reduces strain on muscles, tendons, ligaments, and bones
      (2) Poor posture causes fatigue and may lead to deformity

C. Heat production
1. Survival depends on the body's ability to maintain a constant body temperature
   a. Fever—an elevated body temperature—often a sign of illness
   b. Hypothermia—a reduced body temperature
2. Contraction of muscle fibers produces most of the heat required to maintain normal body temperature

FATIGUE
A. Reduced strength of muscle contraction
B. Caused by repeated muscle stimulation without adequate periods of rest
C. Repeated muscular contraction depletes cellular ATP stores and outstrips the ability of the blood supply to replenish oxygen and nutrients
D. Contraction in the absence of adequate oxygen produces lactic acid, which contributes to muscle soreness
E. *Oxygen debt*—term used to describe the metabolic effort required to burn excess lactic acid that may accumulate during prolonged periods of exercise; the body is attempting to return the cells' energy and oxygen reserves to pre-exercise levels

ROLE OF OTHER BODY SYSTEMS IN MOVEMENT
A. Muscle functioning depends on the functioning of many other parts of the body
1. Most muscles cause movements by pulling on bones across movable joints
2. Respiratory, circulatory, nervous, muscular, and skeletal systems play essential roles in producing normal movements
3. Multiple sclerosis, brain hemorrhage, and spinal cord injury are examples of how pathological conditions in other body organ systems can dramatically affect movement

MOTOR UNIT (Figure 7-4)
A. Stimulation of a muscle by a nerve impulse is required before a muscle can shorten and produce movement
B. A motor neuron is the specialized nerve that transmits an impulse to a muscle, causing contraction
C. A neuromuscular junction is the specialized point of contact between a nerve ending and the muscle fiber it innervates
D. A motor unit is the combination of a motor neuron with the muscle cell or cells it innervates

MUSCLE STIMULUS
A. A muscle will contract only if an applied stimulus reaches a certain level of intensity
1. A threshold stimulus is the minimal level of stimulation required to cause a muscle fiber to contract

B. Once stimulated by a threshold stimulus, a muscle fiber will contract completely, a response called *all or none*
C. Different muscle fibers in a muscle are controlled by different motor units having different threshold-stimulus levels
1. Although individual muscle fibers always respond all or none to a threshold stimulus, the muscle as a whole does not

Continued

OUTLINE SUMMARY—*cont'd*

2. Different motor units responding to different threshold stimuli permit a muscle as a whole to execute contractions of graded force

TYPES OF SKELETAL MUSCLE CONTRACTION

A. Twitch and tetanic contractions
   1. Twitch contractions are laboratory phenomena and do not play a significant role in normal muscular activity; they are a single contraction of muscle fibers caused by a single threshold stimulus
   2. Tetanic contractions are sustained and steady muscular contractions caused by a series of stimuli bombarding a muscle in rapid succession
B. Isotonic contractions
   1. Contraction of a muscle that produces movement at a joint
   2. During isotonic contractions, the muscle changes length, causing the insertion end of the muscle to move relative to the point of origin
   3. Most types of body movements such as walking and running are caused by isotonic contractions
C. Isometric contractions
   1. Isometric contractions are muscle contractions that do not produce movement; the muscle as a whole does not shorten
   2. Although no movement occurs during isometric contractions, tension within the muscle increases

EFFECTS OF EXERCISE ON SKELETAL MUSCLES

A. Exercise, if regular and properly practiced, improves muscle tone and posture, results in more efficient heart and lung functioning, and reduces fatigue
   1. Muscles undergo changes related to the amount of work they normally do
      a. Prolonged inactivity causes disuse atrophy
      b. Regular exercise increases muscle size, called *hypertrophy*
   2. Strength training is exercise involving contraction of muscles against heavy resistance
      a. Strength training increases the numbers of myofilaments in each muscle fiber, and as a result, the total mass of the muscle increases
      b. Strength training does not increase the number of muscle fibers
   3. Endurance training is exercise that increases a muscle's ability to sustain moderate exercise over a long period; it is sometimes called *aerobic training*
      a. Endurance training allows more efficient delivery of oxygen and nutrients to a muscle via increased blood flow
      b. Endurance training does not usually result in muscle hypertrophy

SKELETAL MUSCLE GROUPS (Table 7-1)

A. Muscles of the head and neck (Figure 7-7)
   1. Facial muscles
      a. Orbicularis oculi
      b. Orbicularis oris
      c. Zygomaticus
   2. Muscles of mastication
      a. Masseter
      b. Temporal
   3. Sternocleidomastoid—flexes head
   4. Trapezius—elevates shoulders and extends head
B. Muscles that move the upper extremities
   1. Pectoralis major—flexes upper arm
   2. Latissimus dorsi—extends upper arm
   3. Deltoid—abducts upper arm
   4. Biceps brachii—flexes forearm
   5. Triceps brachii—extends forearm
C. Muscles of the trunk (Figure 7-8)
   1. Abdominal muscles
      a. Rectus abdominis
      b. External oblique
      c. Internal oblique
      d. Transversus abdominis
   2. Respiratory muscles
      a. Intercostal muscles
      b. Diaphragm

OUTLINE SUMMARY—*cont'd*

D. Muscles that move the lower extremities
  1. Iliopsoas—flexes thigh
  2. Gluteus maximus—extends thigh
  3. Adductor muscles—adduct thighs
  4. Hamstring muscles—flex lower leg
     a. Semimembranosus
     b. Semitendinosus
     c. Biceps femoris
  5. Quadriceps femoris group—extend lower leg
     a. Rectus femoris
     b. Vastus muscles
  6. Tibialis anterior—dorsiflexes foot
  7. Gastrocnemius—plantar flexes foot
  8. Peroneus group—flex foot

TYPES OF MOVEMENTS PRODUCED BY SKELETAL MUSCLE CONTRACTIONS

(Figures 7-9 through 7-11)

A. Flexion—movement that decreases the angle between two bones at their joint: bending

B. Extension—movement that increases the angle between two bones at their joint: straightening

C. Abduction—movement of a part away from the midline of the body

D. Adduction—movement of a part toward the midline of the body

E. Rotation—movement around a longitudinal axis

F. Supination and pronation—hand positions that result from rotation of the forearm; supination results in a hand position with the palm turned to the anterior position; pronation occurs when the palm faces posteriorly

G. Dorsiflexion and plantar flexion—foot movements; dorsiflexion results in elevation of the dorsum or top of the foot; during plantar flexion, the bottom of the foot is directed downward

NEW WORDS

abduction	flexion	neuromuscular junction	sarcomere
actin	hypertrophy	origin	sliding filament theory
adduction	hypothermia	oxygen debt	stimulus
all or none	insertion	paralysis	supination
antagonist	isometric	plantar flexion	synergist
atrophy	isotonic	posture	tendon
bursa	motor neuron	prime mover	tenosynovitis
dorsiflexion	motor unit	pronation	tetanic contraction
extension	myofilaments	rotation	tonic contraction
fatigue	myosin		

REVIEW QUESTIONS

1. Briefly describe the structure of cardiac muscle.
2. Briefly describe the structure of smooth muscle.
3. Briefly describe the structure and give the function of tendons, bursae, and synovial membranes.
4. Explain how tonic contractions help maintain posture.
5. Give an example of how two other body systems contribute to the movement of the body.
6. Explain twitch and tetanic contractions.

Continued

REVIEW QUESTIONS—*cont'd*

7. Explain isotonic contractions.
8. Explain isometric contractions.
9. What is strength training and what are its results?
10. What is endurance training and what are its results?
11. Name two muscles of the head or neck and give their origin, insertion, and function.
12. Name two muscles that move the upper extremity and give their origin, insertion, and function.
13. Name two muscles of the trunk and give their origin, insertion, and function.
14. Name three muscles that move the lower extremity and give their origin, insertion, and function.
15. Describe the following movements: flexion, extension, abduction, adduction, and rotation.

CRITICAL THINKING

16. Draw and label a relaxed sarcomere; include actin, myosin, and Z lines. Explain the process that causes the sarcomere to contract.
17. Explain the interaction of the prime mover, the synergist, and the antagonist in efficient movement.
18. Describe the conditions that cause a muscle to develop an "oxygen debt." How is the oxygen debt "paid off"?

CHAPTER TEST

1. Muscle fiber is another name for muscle cell.
2. Cardiac muscle makes up the bulk of the tissue of the heart.
3. The muscle attachment to the more movable bone is called the insertion
4. The muscle attachment to the more stationary bone is called the origin.
5. actin is the protein that makes up the thin myofilaments.
6. Myosin is the protein that makes up the thick myofilaments.
7. The sarcomere is the basic functional unit of contraction in a skeletal muscle.
8. The three functions of the skeletal system are protection, support, and movement
9. The molecule ATP supplies energy for muscle contraction.
10. Lactic acid is the waste product produced when the muscle must switch to an energy supplying process that does not require oxygen.
11. A single motor neuron with all the muscle cells it innervates is called a motor unit
12. threshold stimulus is the minimal level of stimulation required to cause a muscle fiber to contract.
13. isotonic is a type of muscle contraction that produces movement in a joint and allows the muscle to shorten.
14. Isometric is a type of muscle contraction that does not produce movement and does not allow the muscle to shorten but increases muscle tension.
15. Abduction is a term describing movement of a body part away from the midline of the body.
16. Extension is a term used to describe the movement that is the opposite of flexion.
17. Supination describes the hand position when the body is in anatomical position.
18. Skeletal muscles can also be called:
    - **a.** visceral muscles
    - **b.** voluntary muscles
    - **c.** cardiac muscles
    - **d.** all of the above
19. Smooth muscles can also be called:
    - **a.** visceral muscles
    - **b.** involuntary muscles
    - **c.** nonstriated muscles
    - **d.** all of the above

CHAPTER TEST—*cont'd*

Match the muscles in Column A with the locations in Column B.

COLUMN A

20. _A_ temporal muscle
21. _B_ biceps brachii
22. _D_ sartorius
23. _D_ gastrocnemius
24. _A_ masseter
25. _B_ pectoralis major
26. _C_ external oblique
27. _C_ gluteus maximus
28. _A._ sternocleidomastoid
29. _C_ rectus abdominis
30. _C_ rectus femoris
31. _B_ triceps brachii

COLUMN B

a. muscles of the head or neck
b. muscles that move the upper extremity
c. muscles of the trunk
d. muscles that move the lower extremity

STUDY TIPS

Before starting Chapter 7, go back to Chapter 4 and review the synopsis of the muscular system. The three types of muscle tissue were covered in Chapter 3.

There are two prefixes that refer to muscle: *myo-* and *sarco-*. Several terms in the chapter have one of these prefixes. Make sure you understand the terms *origin* and *insertion*; they will come up frequently later in the chapter. Movement is one of the functions of the muscle system. In order to create movement, muscle cells must get shorter. The sarcomere is the structure in the muscle that actually shortens. The sliding filament model explains how this shortening occurs. The shortening of the sarcomere requires energy. ATP supplies this energy. ATP is most efficiently formed when oxygen is supplied to the muscle. When you can't supply the muscle with enough oxygen, your muscle "borrows" energy, using a process that creates lactic acid and develops an "oxygen debt." The names of the muscles are probably less familiar to you than the names of the bones. But muscle names can give you some information about the muscles. Muscles are named for their shape: *deltoid, trapezius*. They are named for a bone they are near: rectus *femoris, tibialis* anterior. They are named for their number of origins: *triceps* brachii; their points of attachments: *sternocleidomastoid*; their size: gluteus *maximus*; and the direction of the muscle fibers: *rectus* abdominus (*rectus* means having fibers running parallel to the midline of the body). When you are learning the muscles, try to look for meaning in the muscle names. Most of the terms for muscle movement are fairly straightforward. One way to remember the difference between supination and pronation is that when your hand is supinated, you can hold a bowl of soup. And in *add*uction, you *add* to your body; you pull the appendage into the trunk (silly, but effective).

In your study group you should go over flash cards for the terms in the chapter. Discuss the processes of contraction and fatigue, and be sure you understand the movement terms. If you are asked to learn just the names and locations of the muscles, a photocopy of the muscle figures with the labels blackened out can be used to quiz each other. If you are asked to learn the functions, origins, and insertions, you need to add flash cards along with the figures. Go over the questions at the end of the chapter and discuss possible test questions.

8 The Nervous System

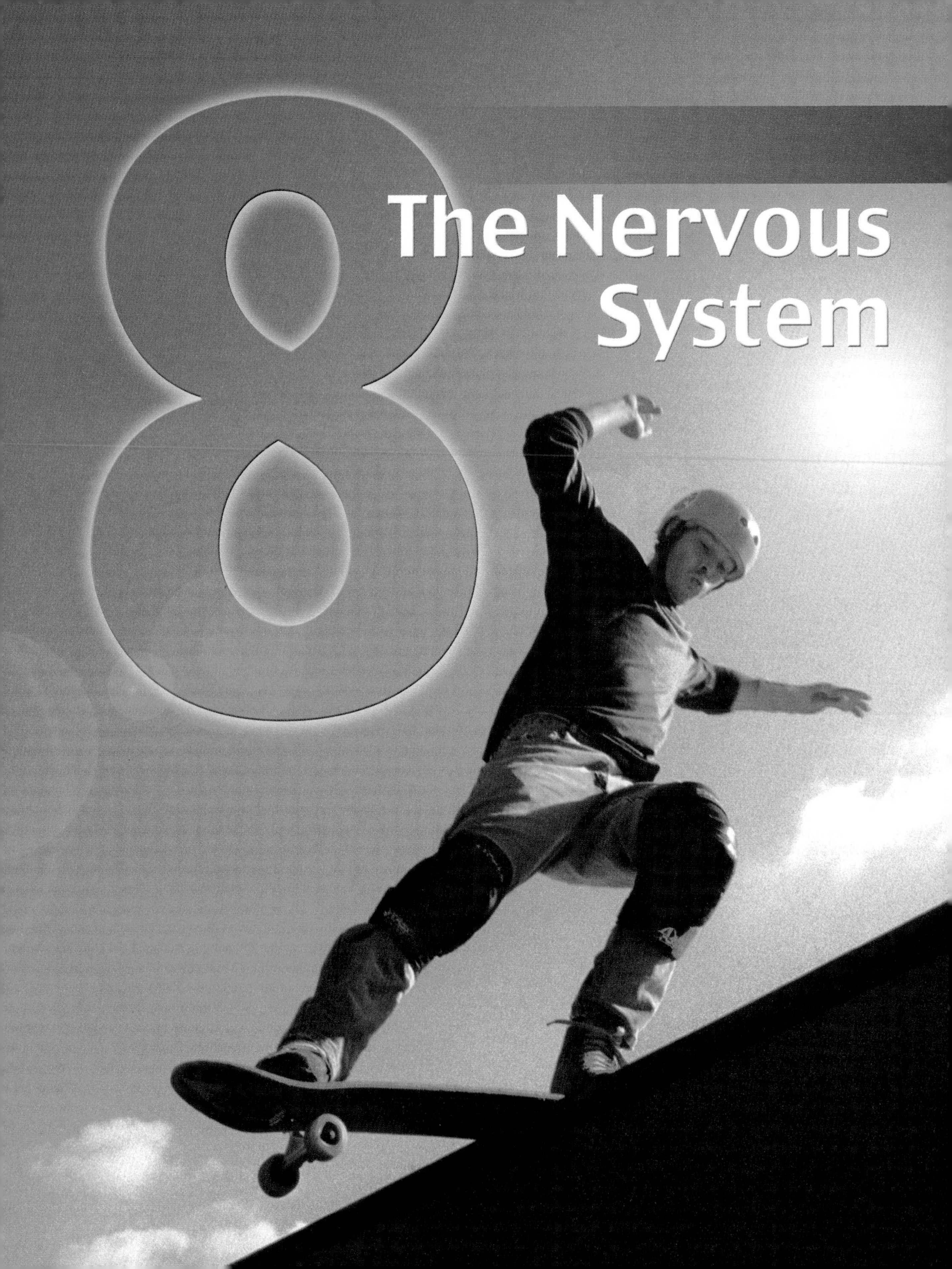

Outline

Objectives

AFTER YOU HAVE COMPLETED THIS CHAPTER, YOU SHOULD BE ABLE TO:

1. List the organs and divisions of the nervous system and describe the generalized functions of the system as a whole.
2. Identify the major types of cells in the nervous system and discuss the function of each.
3. Identify the anatomical and functional components of a three-neuron reflex arc. Compare and contrast the propagation of a nerve impulse along a nerve fiber and across a synaptic cleft.
4. Identify the major anatomical components of the brain and spinal cord and briefly comment on the function of each.
5. Compare and contrast spinal and cranial nerves.
6. Discuss the anatomical and functional characteristics of the two divisions of the autonomic nervous system.

T*he normal body* must accomplish a gigantic and enormously complex job—keeping itself alive and healthy. Each one of its billions of cells performs some activity that is a part of this function. Control of the body's billions of cells is accomplished mainly by two communication systems: the nervous system and the endocrine system. Both systems transmit information from one part of the body to another, but they do it in different ways. The nervous system transmits information very rapidly by nerve impulses conducted from one body area to another. The endocrine system transmits information more slowly by chemicals secreted by ductless glands into the bloodstream and circulated from the glands to other parts of the body. Nerve impulses and hormones communicate information to body structures, increasing or decreasing their activities as needed for healthy survival. In other words, the communication systems of the body are also its control and integrating systems. They weld the body's hundreds of functions into its one overall function of keeping itself alive and healthy.

Recall that homeostasis is the balanced and controlled internal environment of the body that is basic to life itself. Homeostasis is possible only if our physiological control and integration systems function properly. Our plan for this chapter is to name the cells, organs, and divisions of the nervous system; discuss the generation of nervous impulses; and then discover how these impulses move between one area of the body and another. We will study not only the major components of the nervous system, such as the brain, spinal cord, and nerves, but also learn about how they function to maintain and regulate homeostasis. In Chapter 9, we will consider the special senses.

ORGANS AND DIVISIONS OF THE NERVOUS SYSTEM

The organs of the nervous system as a whole include the brain and spinal cord, the numerous nerves of the body, the specialized sense organs such as the eyes and ears, and the microscopic sense organs such as those found in the skin. The system as a whole consists of two principal divisions called the central nervous system and the peripheral nervous system (Figure 8-1). Because the brain and spinal cord occupy a midline or central

FIGURE 8-1

Divisions of the nervous system.

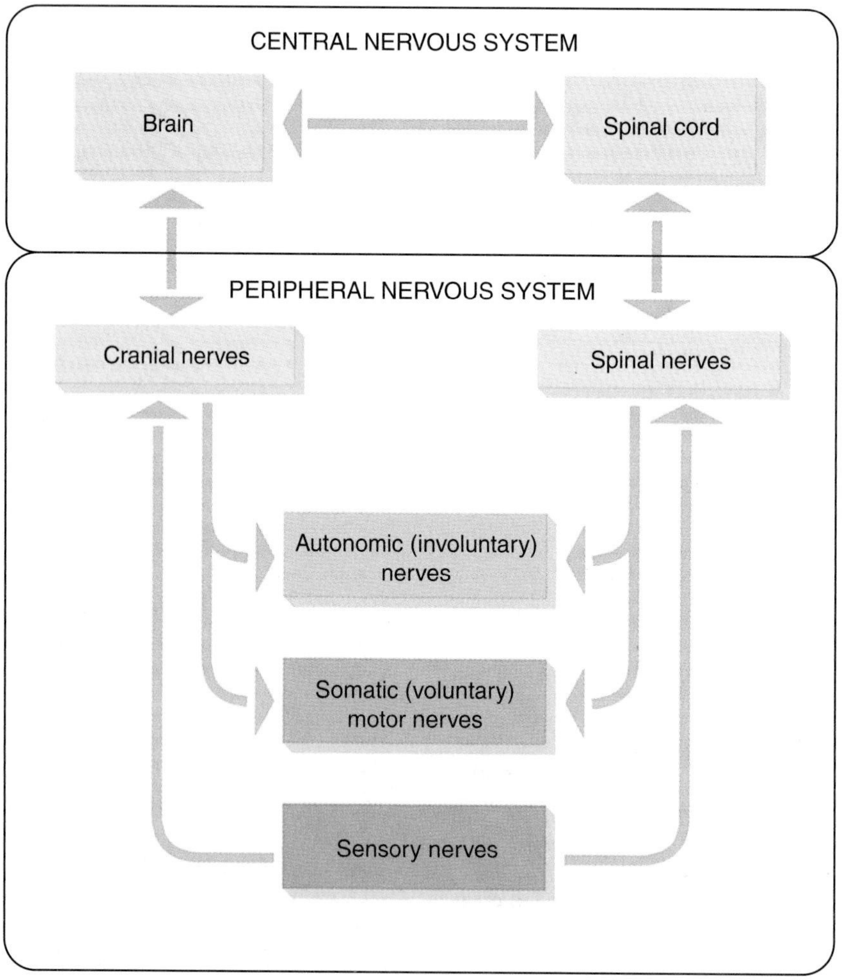

location in the body, they are together called the **central nervous system** or **CNS.** Similarly, the usual designation for the nerves of the body is the **peripheral nervous system** or **PNS.** Use of the term *peripheral* is appropriate because nerves extend to outlying or peripheral parts of the body. A subdivision of the peripheral nervous system, called the **autonomic nervous system** or **ANS,** consists of structures that regulate the body's automatic or involuntary functions (for example, the heart rate, the contractions of the stomach and intestines, and the secretion of chemical compounds by glands).

CELLS OF THE NERVOUS SYSTEM

The two types of cells found in the nervous system are called **neurons** (NOO-rons) or nerve cells and **glia** (GLEE-ah), which are specialized connective tissue cells. Neurons conduct impulses, whereas glia support neurons.

Neurons

Each neuron consists of three parts: a main part called the neuron **cell body,** one or more branching projections called **dendrites** (DEN-drites), and one elongated projection known as an **axon**. Identify each part on the neuron shown in Figure 8-2. Dendrites are the processes or projections that transmit impulses to the neuron cell bodies, and axons are the processes that transmit impulses away from the neuron cell bodies.

The three types of neurons are classified according to the direction in which they transmit impulses: **sensory neurons, motor neurons,** and **interneurons.** Sensory neurons transmit impulses to the spinal cord and brain from all parts of the body. Motor neurons transmit impulses in the opposite direction—away from the brain and spinal cord. They do not conduct impulses to all parts of the body but only to two kinds of tissue—muscle and glandular epithelial tissue. Interneurons conduct impulses from sensory neurons to motor neurons. Sensory neurons are also called *afferent* neurons; motor neurons are called *efferent* neurons, and interneurons are called *central* or *connecting* neurons.

The axon shown in Figure 8-2, *B*, is surrounded by a segmented wrapping of a material called **myelin** (MY-e-lin). Myelin is a white, fatty substance formed by **Schwann cells** that wrap around some axons outside the central nervous system. Such fibers are called **myelinated fibers.** In Figure 8-2, *B*, one such axon has been enlarged to show additional detail. **Nodes of Ranvier** (rahn-vee-AY) are indentations between adjacent Schwann cells.

The outer cell membrane of a Schwann cell is called the **neurilemma** (noo-ri-LEM-mah). That axons in the brain and cord have no neurilemma is clinically significant because it plays an essential part in the regeneration of cut and injured axons. Therefore the potential for regeneration in the brain and spinal cord is far less than it is in the peripheral nervous system.

Glia

Glia—or *neuroglia* (noo-ROG-lee-ah)—do not specialize in transmitting impulses. Instead, they are special types of supporting cells. Their name is appropriate because it is derived from the Greek word *glia* meaning "glue." One function of glia cells is to hold the functioning neurons together and protect them. An important reason for discussing glia is that one of the most common types of brain tumor—called **glioma** (glee-O-mah)—develops from them. We now know that glia perform many different functions, including the regulation of neuron function. Therefore, they are not just "glue" in the physical sense but also the cells that help bring the functions of nervous tissue together into a coordinated whole.

Glia vary in size and shape (Figure 8-3). Some are relatively large cells that look somewhat like stars because of the threadlike extensions that jut out from their surfaces. These glia cells are called astrocytes (AS-tro-sites), a word that means "star cells" (see Figure 8-3). Their threadlike branches attach to neurons and to small blood vessels, holding these structures close to each other. Along with the walls of the blood vessels, astrocyte branches form a two-layer structure called the

FIGURE 8-2

Neuron. A, Diagram of a typical neuron showing dendrites, a cell body, and an axon. **C,** Segment of a myelinated axon cut to show detail of the concentric layers of the Schwann cell filled with myelin. **B,** Photomicrograph of a neuron.

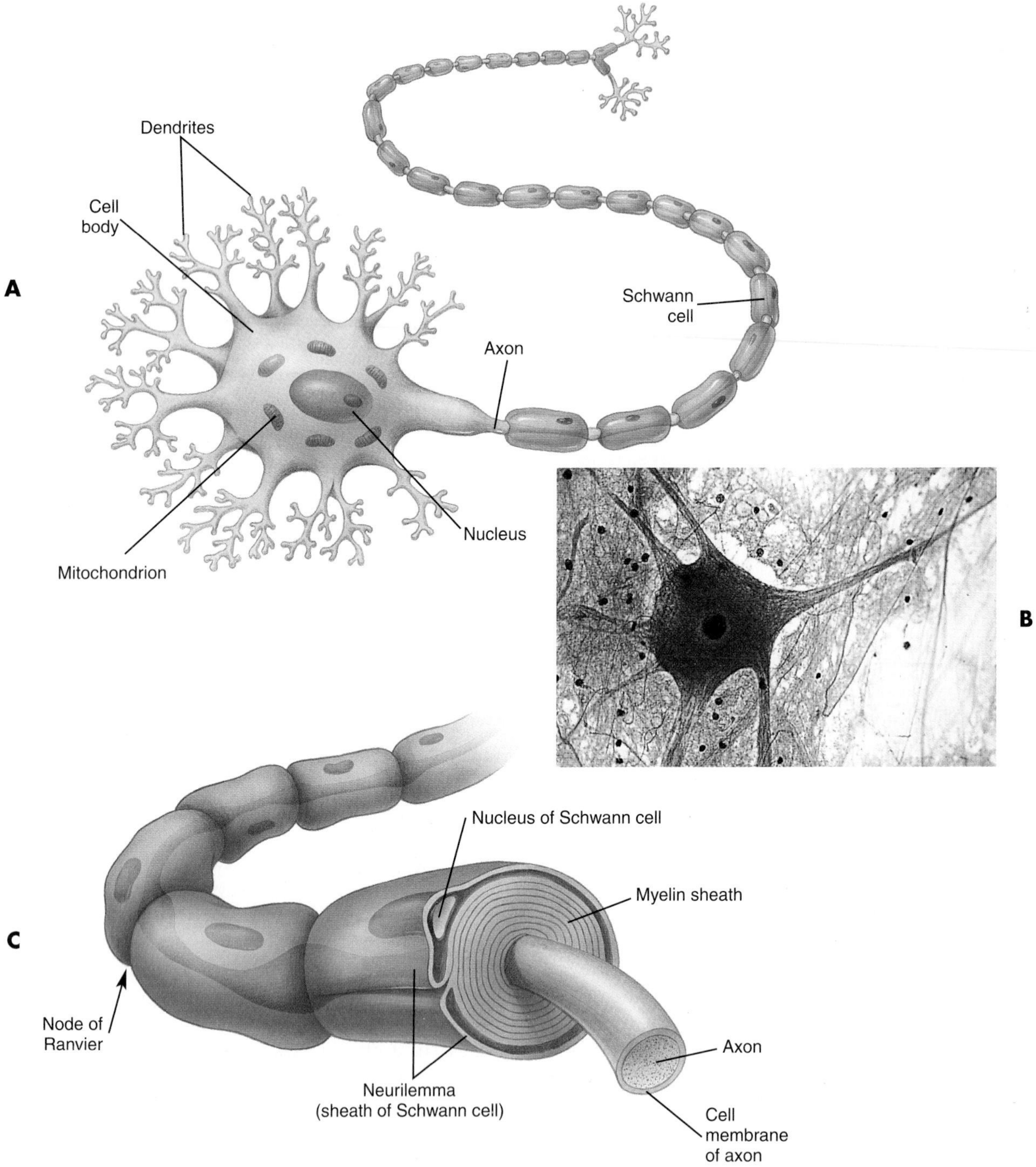

FIGURE 8-3

Glia. A, Astrocytes have extensions attached to blood vessels in the brain. **B,** Microglia within the central nervous system can enlarge and consume microbes by phagocytosis. **C,** Oligodendrocytes have extensions that form myelin sheaths around axons in the central nervous system.

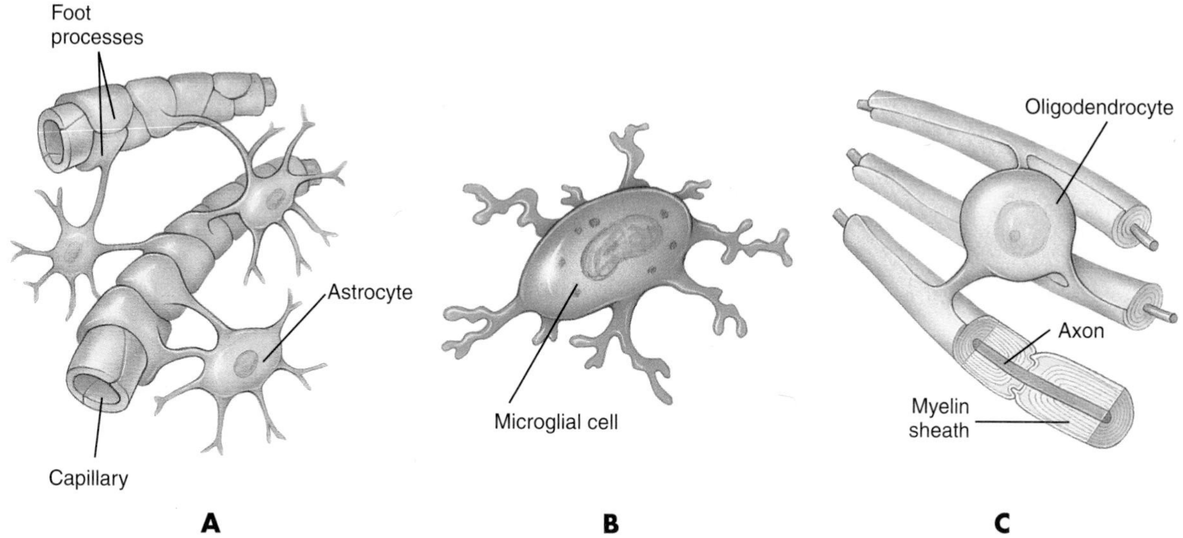

blood-brain barrier (BBB). As its name implies, the BBB separates the blood tissue and nervous tissue to protect vital brain tissue from harmful chemicals that might be in the blood.

Microglia (my-KROG-lee-ah) are smaller than astrocytes. They usually remain stationary, but in inflamed or degenerating brain tissue, they enlarge, move about, and act as microbe-eating scavengers. They surround the microbes, draw them into their cytoplasm, and digest them. Recall from Chapter 3 that phagocytosis is the scientific name for this important cellular process.

The **oligodendrocytes** (AHL-ih-go-DEN-droh-sites) help to hold nerve fibers together and also serve another and probably more important function; they produce the fatty myelin sheath that envelops nerve fibers located in the brain and spinal cord. Recall that Schwann cells also form myelin sheaths but do so only in the peripheral nervous system.

Quick Check

1. What is the difference between the central nervous system and the peripheral nervous system?
2. Can you name the major features of a neuron?
3. How are glia different from neurons?

NERVES

A **nerve** is a group of peripheral nerve fibers (axons) bundled together like the strands of a cable. Because nerve fibers usually have a myelin sheath and myelin is white, nerves are called the **white matter** of the PNS. Bundles of axons in the CNS, called **tracts,** may also be myelinated and thus form this system's white matter. Tissue composed of cell bodies and unmyelinated axons and dendrites is called **gray matter** because of its characteristic gray appearance.

Figure 8-4 shows that each axon in a nerve is surrounded by a thin wrapping of fibrous connective

FIGURE 8-4

The nerve. Each nerve contains axons bundled into fascicles. A connective tissue epineurium wraps the entire nerve. Perineurium surrounds each fascicle. Inset shows a scanning electron micrograph of a cross section of a nerve.

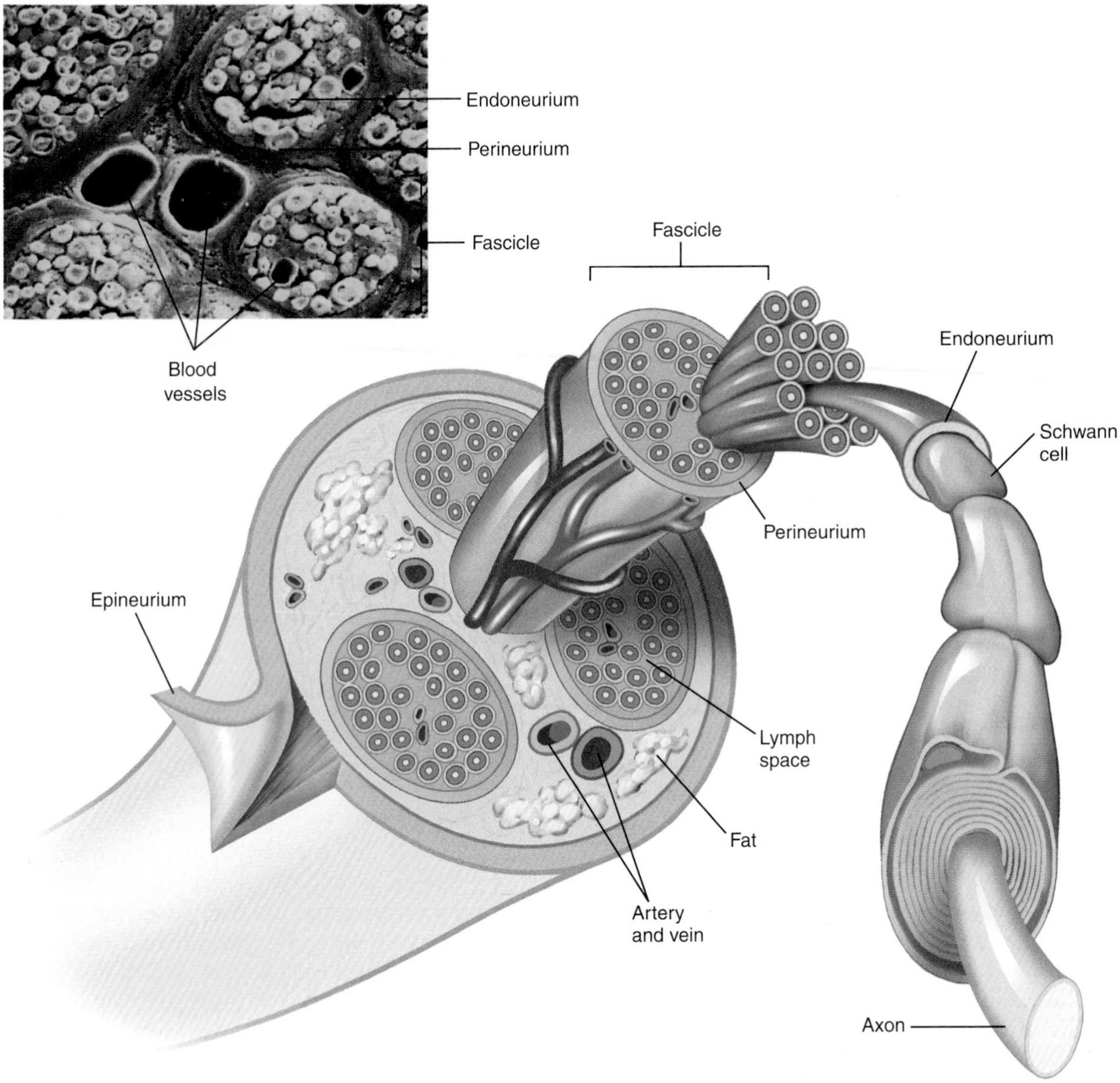

tissue called the **endoneurium** (en-doe-NOO-ree-um). Groups of these wrapped axons are called **fascicles.** Each fascicle is surrounded by a thin, fibrous **perineurium** (pair-i-NOO-ree-um). A tough, fibrous sheath called the **epineurium** (ep-i-NOO-ree-um) covers the whole nerve.

REFLEX ARCS

During every moment of our lives, nerve impulses speed over neurons to and from our spinal cords and brains. If all impulse conduction ceases, life itself ceases. Only neurons can provide the rapid

FIGURE 8-5

Patellar reflex. The neural pathway involved in the patellar ("knee-jerk") reflex.

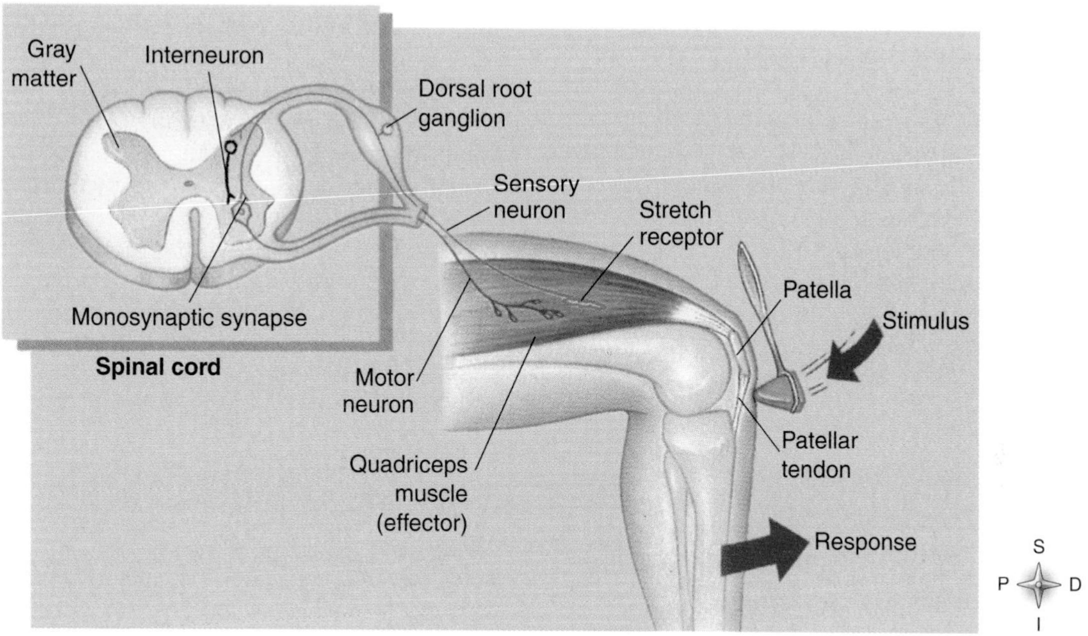

communication between cells that is necessary for maintaining life. Hormonal messages are the only other kind of communications the body can send, and they travel much more slowly than impulses. They can move from one part of the body to another only via circulating blood. Compared with impulse conduction, circulation is a very slow process.

Nerve impulses, sometimes called *action potentials*, can travel over trillions of routes—routes made up of neurons because they are the cells that conduct impulses. Hence the routes traveled by nerve impulses are sometimes spoken of as *neuron pathways*. A specialized type of neuron pathway, called a **reflex arc,** is important to nervous system functioning. The simplest kind of reflex arc is a two-neuron arc, so-called because it consists of only two types of neurons: sensory neurons and motor neurons. Three-neuron arcs are the next simplest kind. They, of course, consist of all three kinds of neurons: sensory neurons, interneurons, and motor neurons. Reflex arcs are like one-way streets; they allow impulse conduction in only one direction. The next paragraph describes this direction in detail. Look frequently at Figure 8-5 as you read it.

Impulse conduction normally starts in receptors. **Receptors** are the beginnings of dendrites of sensory neurons. They are often located at some distance from the spinal cord (in tendons, skin, or mucous membranes, for example). In Figure 8-5 the sensory receptors are located in the quadriceps muscle group and in the patellar tendon. In the reflex that is illustrated there, stretch receptors are stimulated as a result of a tap on the patellar tendon from a rubber hammer used by a physician to elicit a reflex during a physical examination. The nerve impulse that is generated, its neurologic pathway, and its ultimate "knee-jerk" effect is an example of the simplest form of a two-neuron reflex arc. In this reflex, only sensory and motor neurons are involved. The nerve impulse that is generated by stimulation of the stretch receptors travels along the length of the sensory neuron's dendrite to its cell body located in the **posterior (dorsal) root ganglion** (GANG-lee-on). A **ganglion** is a group of nerve-cell bodies located in the PNS. This ganglion is located near the spinal cord. Each spinal ganglion contains not one sensory neuron cell body as shown in Figure 8-5, but hundreds of them. The axon of the sensory neuron travels from the cell body in the dorsal root ganglion and ends near the dendrites of another neuron located in the gray matter of the spinal cord. A microscopic space separates the axon ending of one neuron from the dendrites of another neuron. This space is called a **synapse.** The nerve impulse stops at the synapse, chemical signals are sent across the gap, and the impulse then continues along the dendrites, cell body, and axon of the motor neuron. The motor neuron axon forms a synapse with a structure called an *effector*, an organ that puts nerve signals "into effect."

Effectors are muscles or glands, and muscle contractions and gland secretion are the only kinds of reflexes. The response to impulse conduction over a reflex arc is called a **reflex.** In short, impulse conduction by a reflex arc causes a reflex to occur. In a patellar reflex, the nerve impulses that reach the quadriceps muscle (the effector) result in the "knee-jerk" response.

Now turn your attention to the *interneuron* shown in Figure 8-5. Some reflexes involve three rather than two neurons. In these more complex types of responses, an interneuron, in addition to a sensory and motor neuron, is involved. In

Clinical Application

Multiple Sclerosis (MS)

Many diseases are associated with disorders of the oligodendrocytes. Because these glia cells are involved in myelin formation, these diseases are called **myelin disorders.** The most common primary disease of the CNS is a myelin disorder called **multiple sclerosis,** or **MS.** It is characterized by myelin loss and destruction accompanied by varying degrees of oligodendrocyte cell injury and death. The result is demyelination of the white matter of the CNS. Hard, plaquelike lesions replace the destroyed myelin, and affected areas are invaded by inflammatory cells. As the myelin around axons is lost, nerve conduction is impaired, and weakness, incoordination, visual impairment, and speech disturbances occur. Although the disease occurs in both sexes and all age groups, it is most common in women between 20 and 40 years.

The cause may be related to autoimmunity and viral infections in some individuals. It is relapsing and chronic in nature, but some cases of acute and unremitting disease have been reported. In most cases, MS is prolonged, with remissions and relapses occurring over many years. There is no known cure.

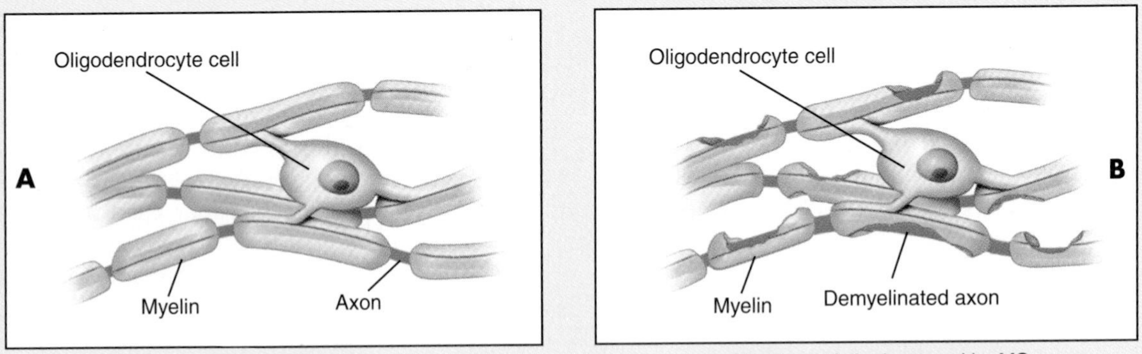

Normal myelin — Myelin partially destroyed by MS

Effects of multiple sclerosis (MS). A, A normal myelin sheath allows rapid conduction. **B,** In MS, the myelin sheath is damaged, disrupting nerve conduction.

three-neuron reflexes, the end of the sensory neuron's axon synapses first with an interneuron before chemical signals are sent across a second synapse, resulting in conduction through the motor neuron. For example, application of an irritating stimulus to the skin of the thigh initiates a three-neuron reflex response that causes contraction of muscles to pull the leg away from the irritant—a three-neuron arc reaction called the *withdrawal reflex*. All interneurons lie entirely within the gray matter of the brain or spinal cord. Gray matter forms the H-shaped inner core of the spinal cord. Because of the presence of an interneuron, three-neuron reflex arcs have two synapses. A two-neuron reflex arc, however, has only a sensory neuron and a motor neuron with one synapse between them.

Identify the motor neuron in Figure 8-5. Observe that its dendrites and cell body, like those of an interneuron, are located in the spinal cord's gray matter. The axon of this motor neuron, however, runs through the anterior (ventral) root of the spinal nerve and terminates in a muscle.

Quick Check

1. How is white matter different from gray matter?
2. Can you explain the function of a reflex arc?
3. What is a sensory receptor? How does it relate to the reflex arc?
4. What is an effector? How does it relate to the reflex arc?

NERVE IMPULSES

What are nerve impulses? Here is one widely accepted definition: a nerve impulse is a self-propagating wave of electrical disturbance that travels along the surface of a neuron's plasma membrane. You might visualize this as a tiny spark sizzling its way along a fuse. Nerve impulses do not continually race along every nerve cell's surface. First they have to be initiated by a stimulus, a change in the neuron's environment. Pressure, temperature, and chemical changes are the usual stimuli. The membrane of each resting neuron has a slight positive charge on the outside and a negative charge on the inside, as shown in Figure 8-6. This occurs because there is normally an excess of sodium ions (Na^+) on the outside of the membrane. When a section of the membrane is stimulated, its Na^+ channels suddenly open, and Na^+ rushes inward. The inside of the membrane temporarily becomes positive, and the outside becomes negative. Although this section of the membrane immediately recovers, the electrical disturbance stimulates Na^+ channels in the next section of the membrane to open. Thus a self-propagating wave of disturbance—a nerve impulse—travels in one direction across the neuron's surface (Figure 8-6, *A*). If the traveling impulse encounters a section of membrane covered with insulating myelin, it simply "jumps" around the myelin. Called **saltatory conduction,** this type of impulse travel is much faster than is possible in nonmyelinated sections. Saltatory conduction is illustrated in Figure 8-6, *B*.

THE SYNAPSE

Transmission of signals from one neuron to the next—across the synapse—is an important part of the nerve conduction process. By definition, a synapse is the place where impulses are transmitted from one neuron, called the **presynaptic neuron,** to another neuron, called the **postsynaptic neuron.** Three structures make up a synapse: a synaptic knob, a synaptic cleft, and the plasma membrane of a postsynaptic neuron. A **synaptic knob** is a tiny bulge at the end of a terminal branch of a presynaptic neuron's axon (Figure 8-7). Each synaptic knob contains many small sacs or vesicles. Each vesicle contains a very small quantity of a chemical compound called a **neurotransmitter.** When a nerve impulse arrives at the synaptic knob, neurotransmitter molecules are released from the vesicles into the **synaptic cleft.** The synaptic cleft is the space between a synaptic knob and the plasma membrane of a *postsynaptic neuron*. It is an incredibly narrow space—only about two millionths of a centimeter in width. Identify the synaptic cleft in Figure 8-7. The plasma membrane of a postsynaptic neuron has protein molecules embedded in it opposite each synaptic knob. These serve as receptors to which neurotransmitter molecules bind. This binding can initiate an impulse in the postsynaptic

FIGURE 8-6

Conduction of nerve impulses. A, In an unmyelinated fiber, a nerve impulse (action potential) is a self-propagating wave of electrical disturbance. **B,** In a myelinated fiber, the action potential "jumps" around the insulating myelin in a rapid type of conduction called *saltatory conduction*.

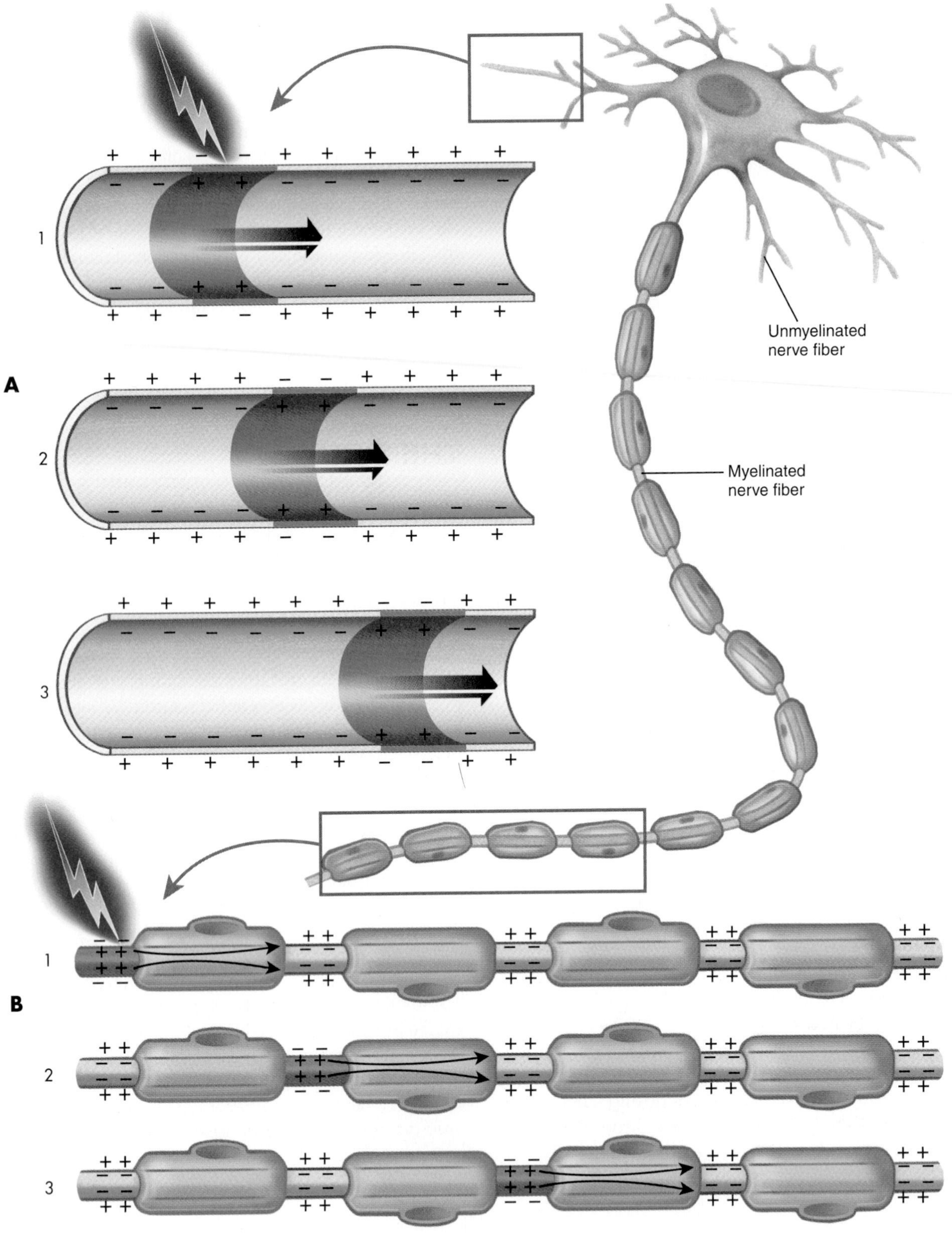

FIGURE 8-7

Components of a synapse. Diagram shows synaptic knob or axon terminal of presynaptic neuron, the plasma membrane of a postsynaptic neuron, and a synaptic cleft. On the arrival of an action potential at a synaptic knob, neurotransmitter molecules are released from vesicles in the knob into the synaptic cleft. The combining of neurotransmitter and receptor molecules in the plasma membrane of the postsynaptic neuron opens ion channels and thereby initiates impulse conduction in the postsynaptic neuron.

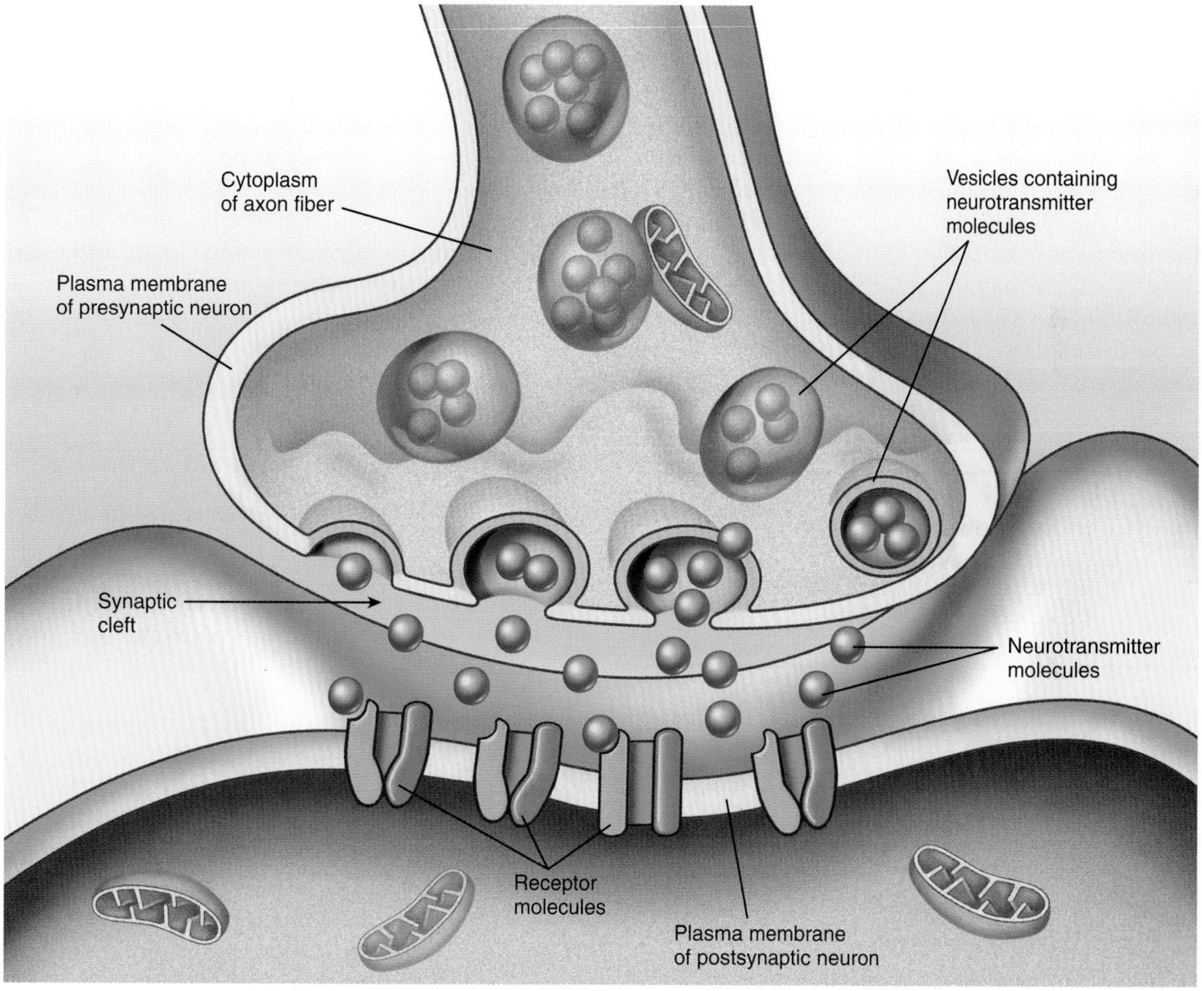

neuron by opening ion channels in the postsynaptic membrane.

After impulse conduction by postsynaptic neurons is initiated, neurotransmitter activity is rapidly terminated. Either one or both of two mechanisms cause this. Some neurotransmitter molecules diffuse out of the synaptic cleft back into synaptic knobs. Other neurotransmitter molecules are metabolized into inactive compounds by specific enzymes.

Neurotransmitters are chemicals by which neurons communicate. As previously noted, at trillions of synapses in the CNS, presynaptic neurons release neurotransmitters that assist, stimulate, or inhibit postsynaptic neurons. At least 30 different compounds have been identified as neurotransmitters. They are not distributed randomly through the spinal cord and brain. Instead, specific neurotransmitters are localized in discrete groups of neurons and released in specific pathways.

For example, the substance named **acetylcholine** (as-e-til-KO-leen) is released at some of the synapses in the spinal cord and at neuromuscular (nerve-muscle) junctions. Other well-known neurotransmitters include **norepinephrine** (nor-ep-i-NEF-rin), **dopamine** (DOE-pa-meen), and **serotonin** (sair-o-TOE-nin). They belong to a group of compounds called **catecholamines** (kat-e-kol-AM-eens), which may play a role in sleep, motor function, mood, and pleasure recognition.

Two morphinelike neurotransmitters called **endorphins** (en-DOR-fins) and **enkephalins** (en-KEF-a-lins) are released at various spinal cord and brain synapses in the pain conduction pathway. These neurotransmitters inhibit conduction of pain impulses. They are natural pain killers. Very small molecules such as **nitric oxide (NO)** have also been recently discovered to have an important role as neurotransmitters.

Quick

1. How does myelin increase the speed of nerve impulse conduction?
2. What is a synapse?
3. How do neurotransmitters transmit signals across the synapse?
4. What is a postsynaptic neuron?

Health & Well-Being

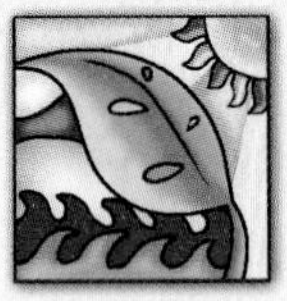

Suppressing Pain During Exercise

Research shows that the release of endorphins increases during heavy exercise. Endorphins inhibit pain, so it is no wonder that pain associated with muscle fatigue decreases when endorphins are present. Normally, pain is a warning signal that calls attention to injuries or dangerous circumstances. However, it is better to inhibit severe pain if it stops us from continuing an activity that may be necessary for survival. Athletes and others who exercise heavily have even reported a unique feeling of well-being or euphoria associated with elevated endorphin levels.

CENTRAL NERVOUS SYSTEM

The CNS, as its name implies, is centrally located. Its two major structures, the brain and spinal cord, are found along the midsagittal plane of the body (Figure 8-8). The brain is protected in the cranial cavity of the skull, and the spinal cord is surrounded in the spinal cavity by the vertebral column. In addition, the brain and spinal cord are covered by protective membranes called **meninges** (me-NIN-jeez), which are discussed in a later section of the chapter.

Divisions of the Brain

The brain, one of our largest organs, consists of the following major divisions, named in ascending order beginning with most inferior part:

I. **Brainstem**
   A. **Medulla oblongata**
   B. **Pons**
   C. **Midbrain**
II. **Cerebellum**
III. **Diencephalon**
   A. **Hypothalamus**
   B. **Thalamus**
IV. **Cerebrum**

Observe in Figure 8-9 the location and relative sizes of the medulla, pons, cerebellum, and cerebrum. Also identify the midbrain.

Brainstem

The lowest part of the brainstem is the medulla oblongata. Immediately above the medulla lies the pons and above that the midbrain. Together these three structures are called the *brainstem* (see Figure 8-9).

The **medulla oblongata** (ob-long-gah-tah) is an enlarged, upward extension of the spinal cord. It lies just inside the cranial cavity above the large hole in the occipital bone called the *foramen magnum.* As with the spinal cord, the medulla consists of gray and white matter, but the arrangement differs in the two organs. In the medulla, bits of gray matter mix closely and intricately with white matter to form the *reticular formation* (*reticular* means "netlike"). In the spinal cord, gray and white matter do not intermingle; gray matter forms the interior core of the cord, and white matter surrounds it.

The **pons** and **midbrain,** like the medulla, consist of white matter and scattered bits of gray matter.

All three parts of the brainstem function as two-way conduction paths. Sensory fibers conduct impulses up from the cord to other parts of the brain, and motor fibers conduct impulses down from the brain to the cord. In addition, many important reflex centers lie in the brainstem. The cardiac, respiratory, and vasomotor centers (collectively called the *vital centers*), for example, are located in the medulla. Impulses from these centers control heartbeat, respirations, and blood vessel diameter (which is important in regulating blood pressure).

Diencephalon

The **diencephalon** (dye-en-SEF-ah-lon) is a small but important part of the brain located between the midbrain below and the cerebrum above. It consists of two major structures: the hypothalamus and the thalamus.

Hypothalamus. The **hypothalamus** (hye-po-THAL-ah-mus), as its name suggests, is located below the thalamus. The posterior pituitary gland, the stalk that attaches it to the undersurface of the brain, and areas of gray matter located in the side walls of a fluid-filled space called the *third ventricle* are extensions of the hypothalamus. Identify the pituitary gland and the hypothalamus in Figure 8-9.

The old adage, "Don't judge by appearances," applies well to appraising the importance of the hypothalamus. Measured by size, it is one of the least significant parts of the brain, but measured by its contribution to healthy survival, it is one of the most important brain structures. Impulses from neurons whose dendrites and cell bodies lie in the hypothalamus are conducted by their axons to neurons located in the spinal cord, and many of these impulses are then relayed to muscles and glands all over the body. Thus the hypothalamus exerts a major control over virtually all internal organs. Among

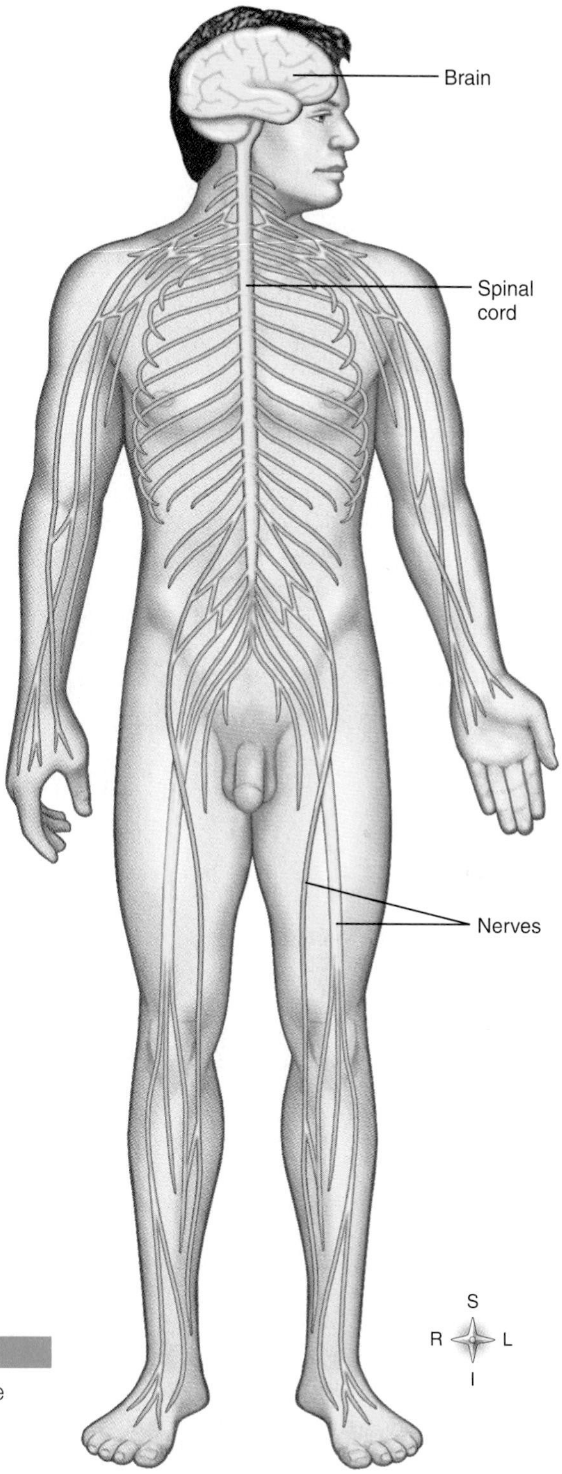

FIGURE 8-8

The nervous system. The brain and spinal cord constitute the *central nervous system* (CNS), and the nerves make up the *peripheral nervous system* (PNS).

FIGURE 8-9

Major regions of the central nervous system. A, Sagittal sections of the brain and spinal cord. **B,** Section of preserved brain.

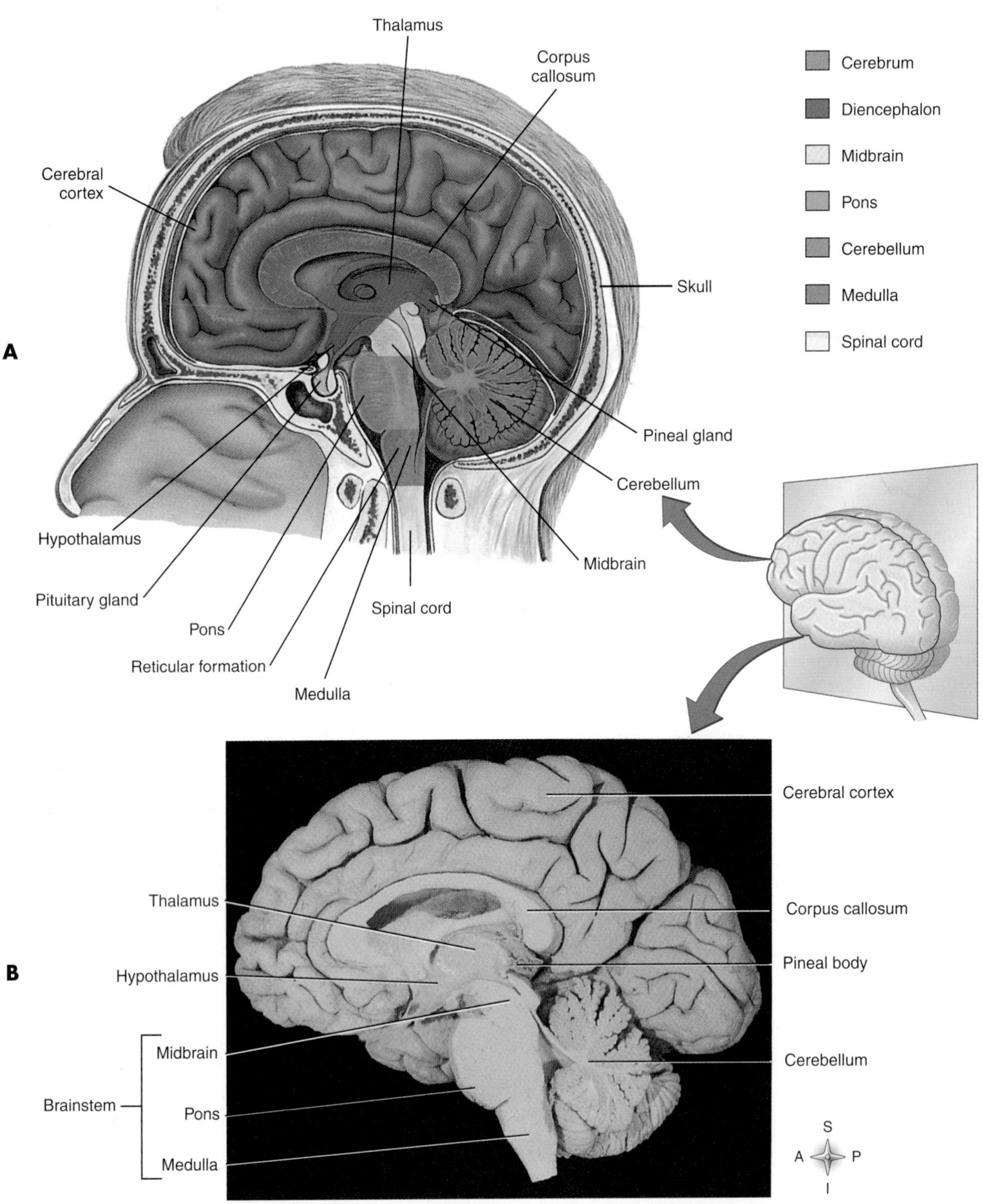

the vital functions that it helps control are the heartbeat, constriction and dilation of blood vessels, and contractions of the stomach and intestines.

Some neurons in the hypothalamus function in a surprising way; they make the hormones that the posterior pituitary gland secretes into the blood. Because one of these hormones (called *antidiuretic hormone* or *ADH*) affects the volume of urine excreted, the hypothalamus plays an essential role in maintaining the body's water balance.

Some of the neurons in the hypothalamus function as endocrine (ductless) glands. Their axons secrete chemicals called *releasing hormones* into the blood, which then carries them to the anterior pituitary gland. Releasing hormones, as their name suggests, control the release of certain anterior pituitary hormones. These in turn influence the hormone secretion of other endocrine glands. Thus the hypothalamus indirectly helps control the functioning of every cell in the body.

The hypothalamus is a crucial part of the mechanism for maintaining body temperature. Therefore marked elevation in body temperature in the absence of disease frequently characterizes injuries or other abnormalities of the hypothalamus. In addition, this important center is involved in functions such as the regulation of water balance, sleep cycles, and the control of appetite and many emotions involved in pleasure, fear, anger, sexual arousal, and pain.

Thalamus. Just above the hypothalamus is a dumbbell-shaped section of gray matter called the **thalamus** (THAL-ah-mus). Each enlarged end of the dumbbell lies in a lateral wall of the third ventricle. The thin center section of the thalamus passes from left to right through the third ventricle. The thalamus is composed chiefly of dendrites and cell bodies of neurons that have axons extending up toward the sensory areas of the cerebrum. The thalamus performs the following functions:

1. It helps produce sensations. Its neurons relay impulses to the cerebral cortex from the sense organs of the body.
2. It associates sensations with emotions. Almost all sensations are accompanied by a feeling of some degree of pleasantness or unpleasantness. The way that these pleasant and unpleasant feelings are produced is unknown except that they seem to be associated with the arrival of sensory impulses in the thalamus.
3. It plays a part in the so-called arousal or alerting mechanism.

Cerebellum

Structure. Look at Figure 8-9 to find the location, appearance, and size of the cerebellum. The cerebellum is the second largest part of the human brain. It lies under the occipital lobe of the cerebrum. In the cerebellum, gray matter composes the outer layer, and white matter composes the bulk of the interior.

Function. Most of our knowledge about cerebellar functions has come from observing patients who have some sort of disease of the cerebellum and from animals who have had the cerebellum removed. From such observations, we know that the cerebellum plays an essential part in the production of normal movements. Perhaps a few examples will make this clear. A patient who has a tumor of the cerebellum frequently loses his balance and topples over; he may feel like a drunken man when he walks. He cannot coordinate his muscles normally. He may complain, for instance, that he is clumsy about everything he does—that he cannot even drive a nail or draw a straight line. With the loss of normal cerebellar functioning, he has lost the ability to make precise movements. The general functions of the cerebellum, then, are to produce smooth coordinated movements, maintain equilibrium, and sustain normal postures.

Cerebrum

The **cerebrum** (SAIR-e-brum) is the largest and uppermost part of the brain. If you were to look at the outer surface of the cerebrum, the first features you would notice might be its many ridges and grooves. The ridges are called *convolutions* or *gyri* (JYE-rye), and the grooves are called *sulci* (SUL-kye). The deepest sulci are called *fissures;* the longitudinal fissure divides the cerebrum into right and left halves or hemispheres. These halves are almost separate structures except for their lower midportions, which are connected by a structure called the **corpus callosum** (COR-pus kal-LO-sum) (Figure 8-9). Two deep sulci subdivide each cerebral hemisphere into four major lobes and each lobe into numerous convolutions. The lobes are named for the bones that lie over them: the frontal lobe, the parietal lobe, the temporal lobe, and the occipital lobe. Identify these in Figure 8-10, *A*.

FIGURE 8-10

The cerebrum. A, The lobes of the cerebrum. **B,** Functional regions of the cerebral cortex. *Association areas* are so named because they put together (associate) information from many different parts of the brain.

A

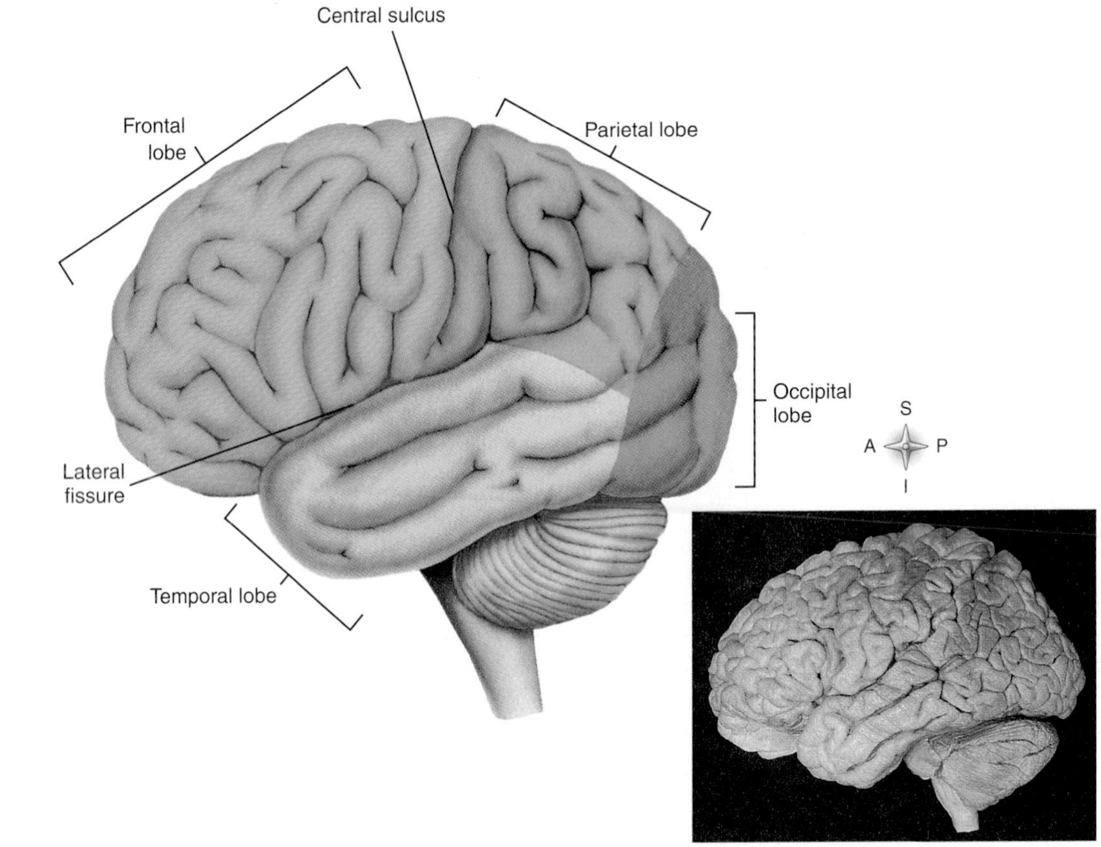

B

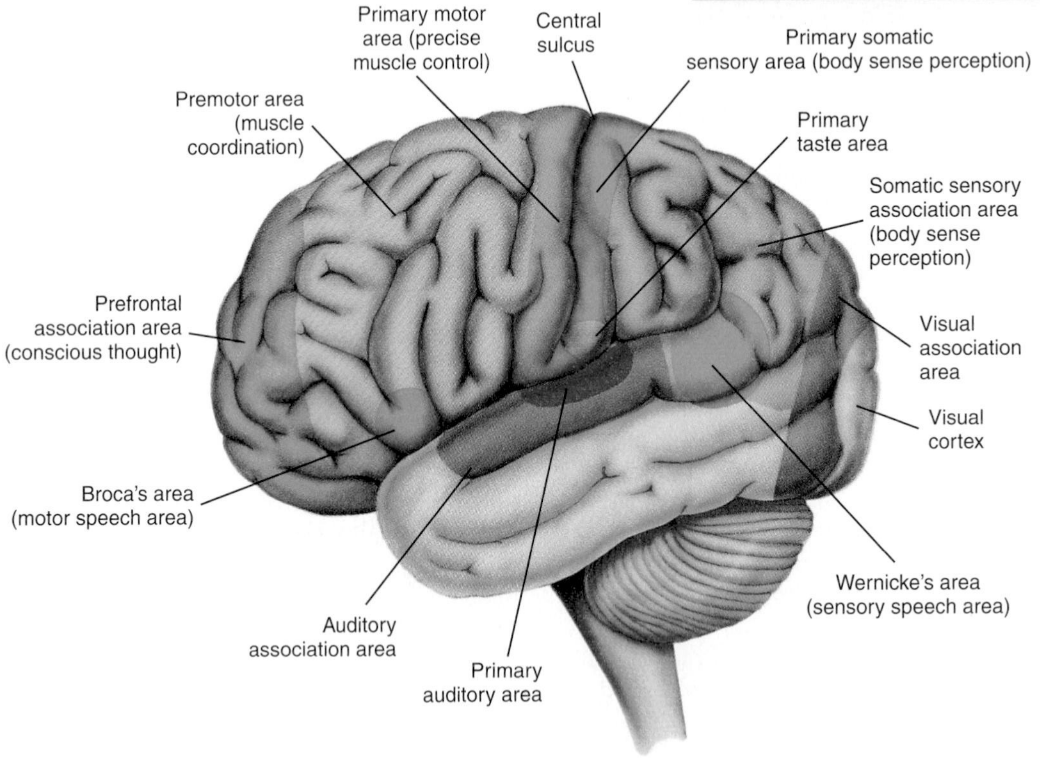

A thin layer of gray matter, made up of neuron dendrites and cell bodies, composes the surface of the cerebrum. Its name is the *cerebral cortex*. White matter, made up of bundles of nerve fibers (tracts), composes most of the interior of the cerebrum. Within this white matter, however, are a few islands of gray matter known as the **cerebral nuclei** or *basal ganglia*, whose functioning is essential for producing automatic movements and postures.

What functions does the cerebrum perform? This is a hard question to answer briefly because the neurons of the cerebrum do not function alone. They function with many other neurons in many other parts of the brain and in the spinal cord. Neurons of these structures continually bring impulses to cerebral neurons and continually transmit impulses away from them. If all other neurons were functioning normally and only cerebral neurons were not functioning, here are some of the things that you could not do. You could not think or use your will. You could not remember anything that has ever happened to you. You could not decide to make the smallest movement, nor could you make it. You would neither see nor hear. You could not experience any of the sensations that make life so rich and varied. Nothing would anger or frighten you, and nothing would bring you joy or sorrow. You would, in short, be unconscious. These terms sum up cerebral functions: consciousness, thinking, memory, sensations, emotions, and willed movements. Figure 8-10, *B*, shows the areas of the cerebral cortex essential for willed movements, general sensations, vision, hearing, and normal speech.

Injury or disease can destroy neurons. A common example is the destruction of neurons of the motor area of the cerebrum that results from a **cerebrovascular accident (CVA),** which is a hemorrhage from or cessation of blood flow through cerebral blood vessels. When this happens, the victim can no longer voluntarily move the parts of the body on the side opposite to the side on which the CVA occurred. In nontechnical language, he or she has suffered a stroke. Note in Figure 8-10, *B*, the location of the motor area in the frontal lobe of the cerebrum.

It is important to understand that very specific areas of the cortex have very specific functions. For example, the temporal lobe's auditory areas interpret incoming nervous signals from the ear as very specific sounds. The visual area of the cortex in the occipital lobe helps you identify and understand specific images. Localized areas of the cortex are directly related to specific functions, as shown in Figure 8-10, *B*. This explains the very specific symptoms associated with an injury to localized areas of the cerebral cortex after a stroke or traumatic injury to the head. Table 8-1 summarizes the major components of the brain and their main functions.

TABLE 8-1

Functions of Major Divisions of the Brain

BRAIN AREA	FUNCTION
Brainstem	
Medulla	Two-way conduction pathway oblongata between the spinal cord and higher brain centers; cardiac, respiratory, and vasomotor control center
Pons	Two-way conduction pathway between areas of the brain and other regions of the body; influences respiration
Midbrain	Two-way conduction pathway; relay for visual and auditory impulses
Diencephalon	
Hypothalamus	Regulation of body temperature, water balance, sleep-cycle control, appetite, and sexual arousal
Thalamus	Sensory relay station from various body areas to cerebral cortex; emotions and alerting or arousal mechanisms
Cerebellum	Muscle coordination; maintenance of equilibrium and posture
Cerebrum	Sensory perception, emotions, willed movements, consciousness, and memory

Research, Issues & Trends

Parkinson Disease

Parkinson disease is a chronic nervous disorder resulting from a deficiency of the neurotransmitter *dopamine* in the cerebral nuclei of the cerebrum. The group of signs associated with this disorder is a syndrome called *parkinsonism*. Parkinsonism is characterized by rigidity and trembling of the head and extremities, a forward tilt of the trunk, and shuffling manner of walking, as you can see in the figure. You may have noticed these characteristics in former boxing champion Muhammed Ali, the actor Michael J. Fox, or in others you may know with Parkinson disease. All of these characteristics result from a lack of dopamine, leading to misinformation in the part of the brain that normally prevents the skeletal muscles from being overstimulated.

Dopamine injection into the blood and dopamine pills are not effective treatments because dopamine cannot cross the blood-brain barrier. A breakthrough in the treatment of Parkinson disease came when the drug *levodopa* or *L-dopa* was found to increase the dopamine levels in afflicted patients. Neurons use L-dopa, which can cross the blood-brain barrier, to make dopamine. For some reason, L-dopa does not always have the desired effects in individual patients, so a number of alternatives have been developed. One option that has had some success is the surgical grafting of normal dopamine-secreting cells into the brains of individuals with Parkinson disease. Another experimental option is an artificial implant that gives electrical stimulation to the cerebral nuclei, causing them to produce more dopamine.

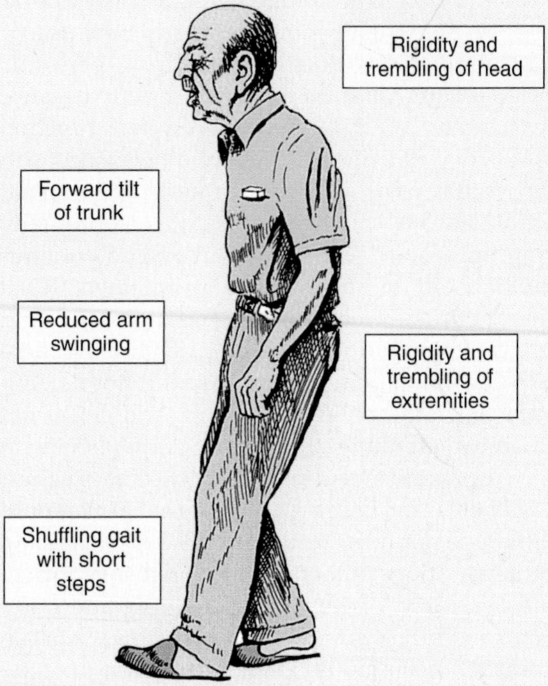

Quick Check

1. What are the four main divisions of the brain? Where is each division?
2. What regions make up the brainstem?
3. Why is the hypothalamus said to be a link between the nervous system and endocrine system?
4. In which part of your brain do you do your thinking?

Spinal Cord

Structure

If you are of average height, your spinal cord is about 17 or 18 inches long (Figure 8-11). It lies inside the spinal column in the spinal cavity and extends from the occipital bone down to the bottom of the first lumbar vertebra. Place your hands on your hips, and they will line up with your fourth lumbar vertebra. Your spinal cord ends just above this level.

Look now at Figure 8-12. Notice the H-shaped core of the spinal cord. It consists of gray matter and so is composed mainly of dendrites and cell bodies of neurons. Columns of white matter form the outer portion of the spinal cord, and bundles of myelinated nerve fibers—the **spinal tracts**—make up the white columns.

Spinal cord tracts provide two-way conduction paths to and from the brain. **Ascending tracts** conduct impulses up the cord to the brain. **Descending tracts** conduct impulses down the cord from

FIGURE 8-11

Spinal cord and spinal nerves. Inset is a dissection of the cervical segment of the spinal cord showing emerging cervical nerves. The spinal cord is viewed from behind (posterior aspect).

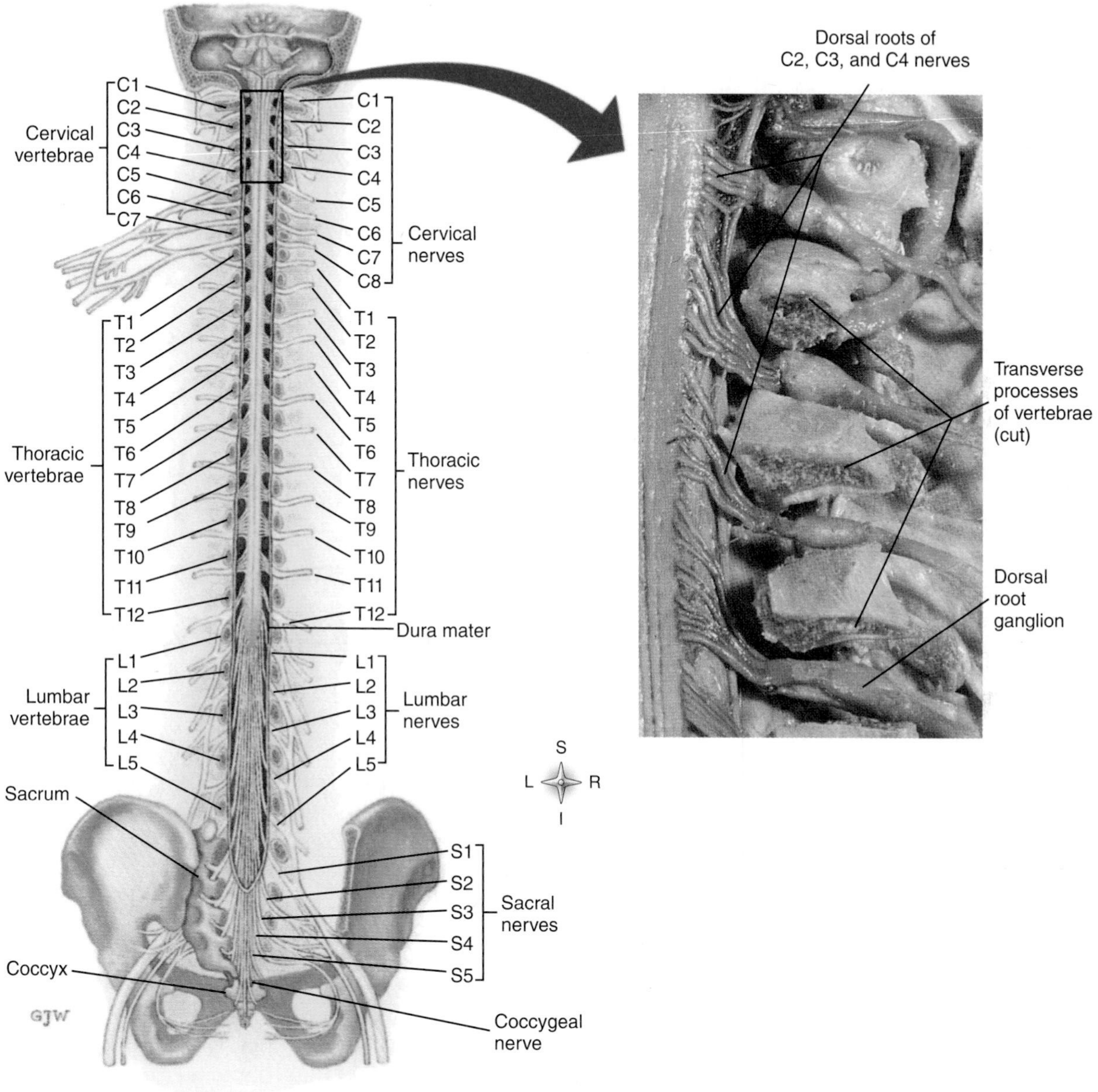

the brain. Tracts are functional organizations in that all axons composing one tract serve one general function. For instance, fibers of the spinothalamic tracts serve a sensory function. They transmit impulses that produce sensations of crude touch, pain, and temperature. Other ascending tracts shown in Figure 8-12 include the gracilis and cuneatus tracts, which transmit sensations of touch

FIGURE 8-12

Spinal cord. Cross section of the spinal cord showing the horns, pathways (nerve tracts), and roots.

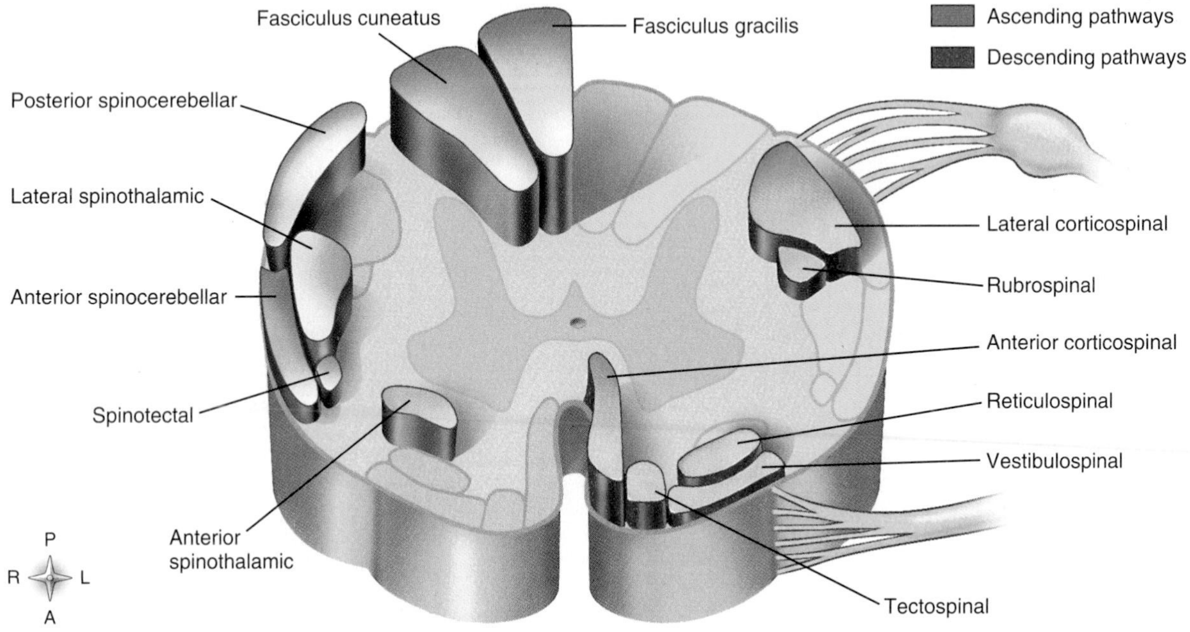

and pressure up to the brain, and the anterior and posterior spinocerebellar tracts, which transmit information about muscle length to the cerebellum. Descending tracts include the lateral and ventral corticospinal tracts, which transmit impulses controlling many voluntary movements.

Functions

To try to understand spinal cord functions, think about a hotel telephone switching system. Suppose a guest in Room 108 calls the switching system and keys in the extension number for Room 520, and in a second or so, someone in that room answers. Very briefly, three events took place: a message traveled into the switching system, the system routed the message along the proper path, and the message traveled out from the switching system toward Room 520. The telephone switching system provided the network of connections that made possible the completion of the call. We might say that the switching system transferred the incoming call to an outgoing line. The spinal cord functions similarly. It contains the centers for thousands and thousands of reflex arcs. Look back at Figure 8-5. The interneuron shown there is an example of a spinal cord reflex center. It switches or transfers incoming sensory impulses to outgoing motor impulses, thereby making it possible for a reflex to occur. Reflexes that result from conduction over arcs whose centers lie in the spinal cord are called *spinal cord reflexes*. Two common kinds of spinal cord reflexes are withdrawal and jerk reflexes. An example of a withdrawal reflex is pulling one's hand away from a hot surface. The familiar knee jerk is an example of a jerk reflex.

In addition to functioning as the primary reflex center of the body, the spinal cord tracts, as previously noted, carry impulses to and from the brain. Sensory impulses travel up to the brain in ascending tracts, and motor impulses travel down from the brain in descending tracts. Therefore if an injury cuts the cord all the way across, impulses can no longer travel to the brain from any part of the body located below the injury, nor can they travel from

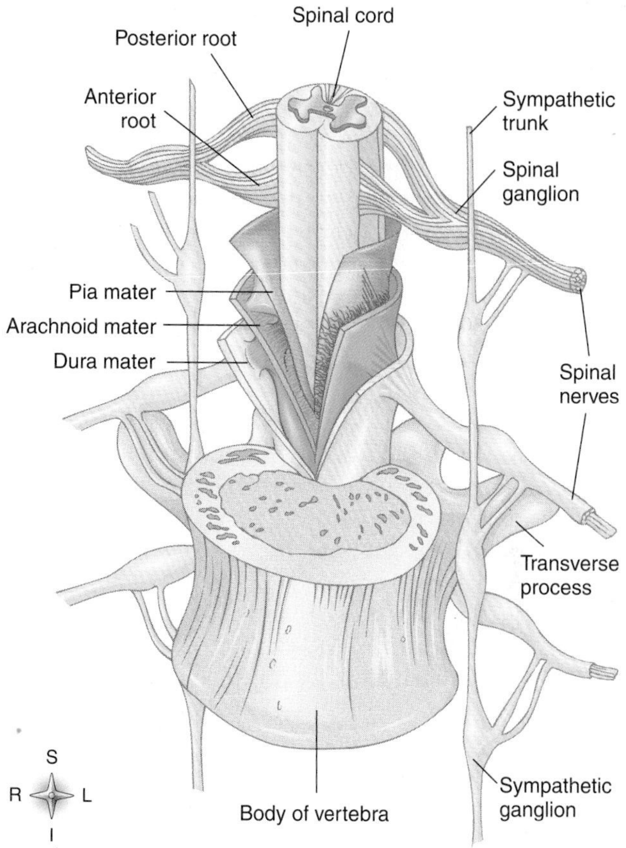

FIGURE 8-13

Spinal cord. The meninges, spinal nerves, and sympathetic trunk are visible.

the brain down to these parts. In short, this kind of spinal cord injury produces a loss of sensation, which is called **anesthesia** (an-es-THEE-zee-ah), and a loss of the ability to make voluntary movements, which is called **paralysis** (pah-RAL-i-sis).

Coverings and Fluid Spaces of the Brain and Spinal Cord

Nervous tissue is not a sturdy tissue. Even moderate pressure can kill nerve cells, so nature safeguards the chief organs made of this tissue—the spinal cord and the brain—by surrounding them with a tough, fluid-containing membrane called the **meninges** (me-NIN-jeez). The meninges are then surrounded by bone. The spinal meninges form a tubelike covering around the spinal cord and line the bony vertebral foramen of the vertebrae that surround the cord. Look at Figure 8-13, and you can identify the three layers of the spinal meninges. They are the **dura mater** (DOO-rah MA-ter), which is the tough outer layer that lines the vertebral canal, the **pia** (PEE-ah) **mater,** which is the innermost membrane covering the spinal cord itself, and the **arachnoid** (ah-RAK-noyd) **mater,** which is the membrane between the dura and the pia mater. The arachnoid mater resembles a cobweb with fluid in its spaces. The word *arachnoid* means "cobweblike." It comes from *arachne*, the Greek word for spider. Arachne is the name of the girl who was changed into a spider by Athena because she boasted of the fineness of her weaving—at least, so an ancient Greek myth tells us.

The meninges that form the protective covering around the spinal cord also extend up and around the brain to enclose it completely. Fluid fills the subarachnoid spaces between the pia mater and arachnoid in the brain and spinal cord. This fluid is called **cerebrospinal fluid (CSF).**

Cerebrospinal (ser-e-bro-SPI-nal) **fluid** also fills spaces in the brain called cerebral **ventricles.** In Figure 8-14, you can see the irregular shapes of the ventricles of the brain. These illustrations can also help you visualize the location of the ventricles if you remember that these large spaces lie deep inside the brain and that there are two lateral ventricles. One lies inside the right half of the cerebrum (the largest part of the human brain), and the other lies inside the left half.

CSF is one of the body's circulating fluids. It forms continually from fluid filtering out of the blood in a network of brain capillaries known as the **choroid plexus** (KO-royd PLEK-sus) and into the ventricles. CSF seeps from the lateral ventricles into the third ventricle and flows down through the cerebral aqueduct (find this in Figures 8-14 and 8-15) into the fourth ventricle. Most of the CSF moves through tiny openings from the fourth ventricle into the subarachnoid space near the cerebellum. Some of it moves into the small, tubelike central canal of the cord and then out into the subarachnoid spaces. Then it moves leisurely down and around the cord and up and around the brain (in the subarachnoid spaces of their meninges) and returns to the blood (in the veins of the brain).

Remembering that this fluid forms continually from blood, circulates, and is resorbed into blood can be useful. It can help you understand certain abnormalities. Suppose a person has a brain tumor that presses on the cerebral aqueduct. This blocks the way for the return of CSF to the blood. Because the fluid continues to form but cannot drain away, it accumulates in the ventricles or in the meninges. Other conditions can cause an accumulation of CSF in the ventricles. An example is **hydrocephalus** (hye-dro-SEF-ah-lus) or "water on the brain." One form of treatment involves surgical placement of a hollow tube or catheter through the blocked channel so that CSF can drain into another location in the body.

FIGURE 8-14

Fluid spaces of the brain. A, The ventricles highlighted within the brain in a left lateral view. **B,** The ventricles from above.

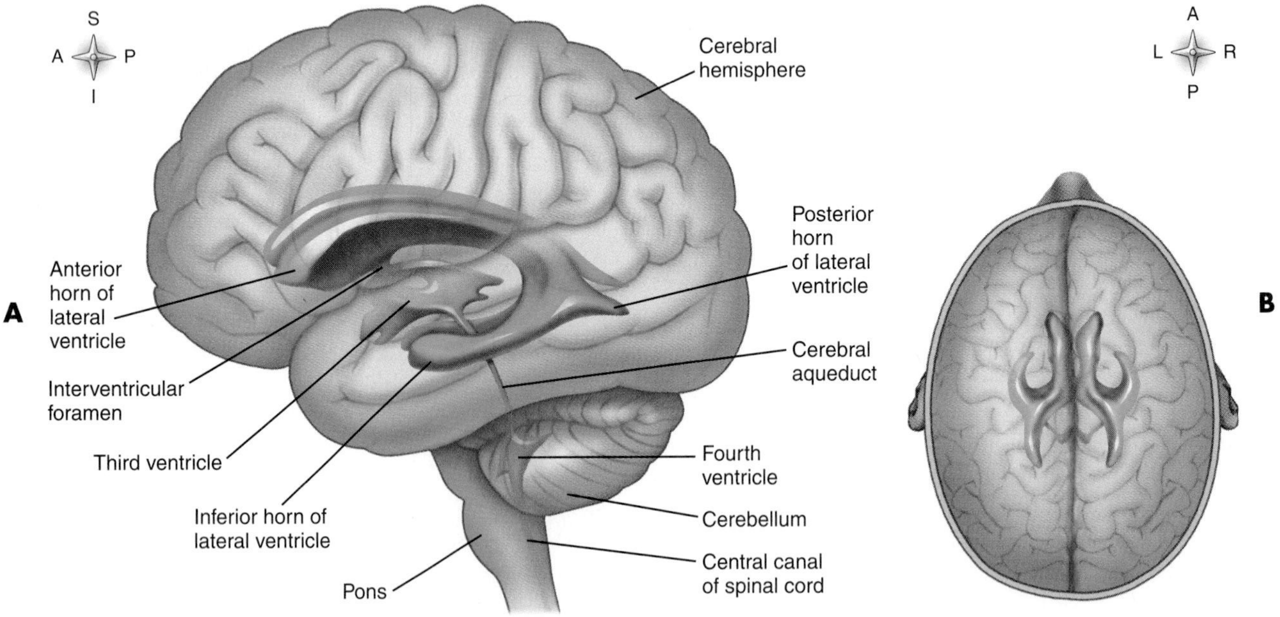

FIGURE 8-15

Flow of cerebrospinal fluid. The fluid produced by filtration of blood by the choroid plexus of each ventricle flows inferiorly through the lateral ventricles, interventricular foramen, third ventricle, cerebral aqueduct, fourth ventricle, and subarachnoid space and to the blood.

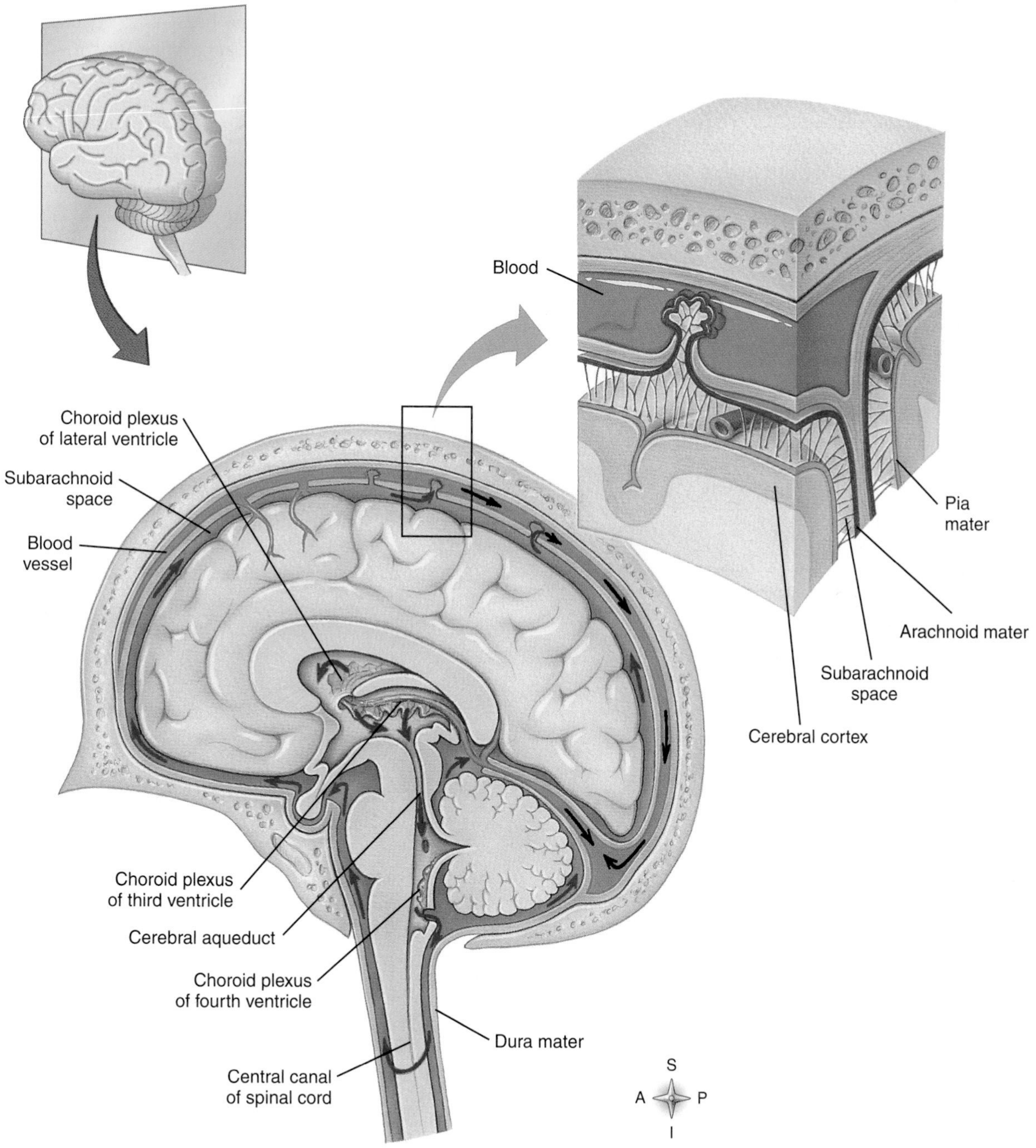

Clinical Application

Lumbar Puncture

The extension of the meninges beyond the spinal cord is convenient for performing lumbar punctures without danger of injuring the spinal cord. A **lumbar puncture** is the withdrawal of some CSF from the subarachnoid space in the lumbar region of the spinal cord. The physician inserts a needle just above or below the fourth lumbar vertebra, knowing that the spinal cord ends an inch or more above the level. The fourth lumbar vertebra can be easily located because it lies on a line with the iliac crest. Placing a patient on his side and arching his back by drawing the knees and chest together separates the vertebrae sufficiently to introduce the needle. Lumbar punctures are often performed to withdraw CSF for analysis or to reduce pressure caused by swelling of the brain or spinal cord after injury or disease.

Quick Check

1. What are the major functions of the spinal cord?
2. What are spinal tracts?
3. Can you name the three meninges that cover the brain and spinal cord?
4. What is cerebrospinal fluid?

PERIPHERAL NERVOUS SYSTEM

The nerves connecting the brain and spinal cord to other parts of the body constitute the peripheral nervous system (PNS). This system includes **cranial** and **spinal nerves** that connect the brain and spinal cord, respectively, to peripheral structures such as the skin surface and the skeletal muscles. In addition, other structures in the autonomic nervous system (ANS) are considered part of the PNS. These connect the brain and spinal cord to various glands in the body and to the cardiac and smooth muscle in the thorax and abdomen.

Cranial Nerves

Twelve pairs of cranial nerves are attached to the undersurface of the brain, mostly from the brainstem. Figure 8-16 shows the attachments of these nerves. Their fibers conduct impulses between the brain and structures in the head and neck and in the thoracic and abdominal cavities. For instance, the second cranial nerve (optic nerve) conducts impulses from the eye to the brain, where these impulses produce vision. The third cranial nerve (oculomotor nerve) conducts impulses from the brain to muscles in the eye, where they cause contractions that move the eye. The tenth cranial nerve (vagus nerve) conducts impulses between the medulla oblongata and structures in the neck and thoracic and abdominal cavities. The names of each cranial nerve and a brief description of their functions are listed in Table 8-2.

Spinal Nerves

Structure

Thirty-one pairs of nerves are attached to the spinal cord in the following order: 8 pairs are attached to the cervical segments, 12 pairs are attached to the thoracic segments, 5 pairs are attached to the lumbar segments, 5 pairs are attached to the sacrospinal segments, and 1 pair is attached to the coccygeal segment (see Figure 8-11). Unlike cranial nerves, spinal nerves have no special names; instead, a letter and number identify each one. C1, for example, indicates the pair of spinal nerves attached to the first segment of the cervical part of the cord, and T8 indicates nerves attached to the eighth segment of the thoracic part of the spinal cord. In Figure 8-11 the cervical area of the spine has been dissected to show the emerging spinal nerves in that area. After spinal nerves exit from the spinal cord, they branch to form the many peripheral nerves of the trunk and limbs. Sometimes, nerve fibers from several spinal nerves are reorganized to form a single peripheral nerve. This reorganization can be seen as a network of intersecting or "braided" branches called a **plexus.** Figure 8-11 shows several plexuses.

FIGURE 8-16

Cranial nerves. View of the undersurface of the brain shows attachments of the cranial nerves.

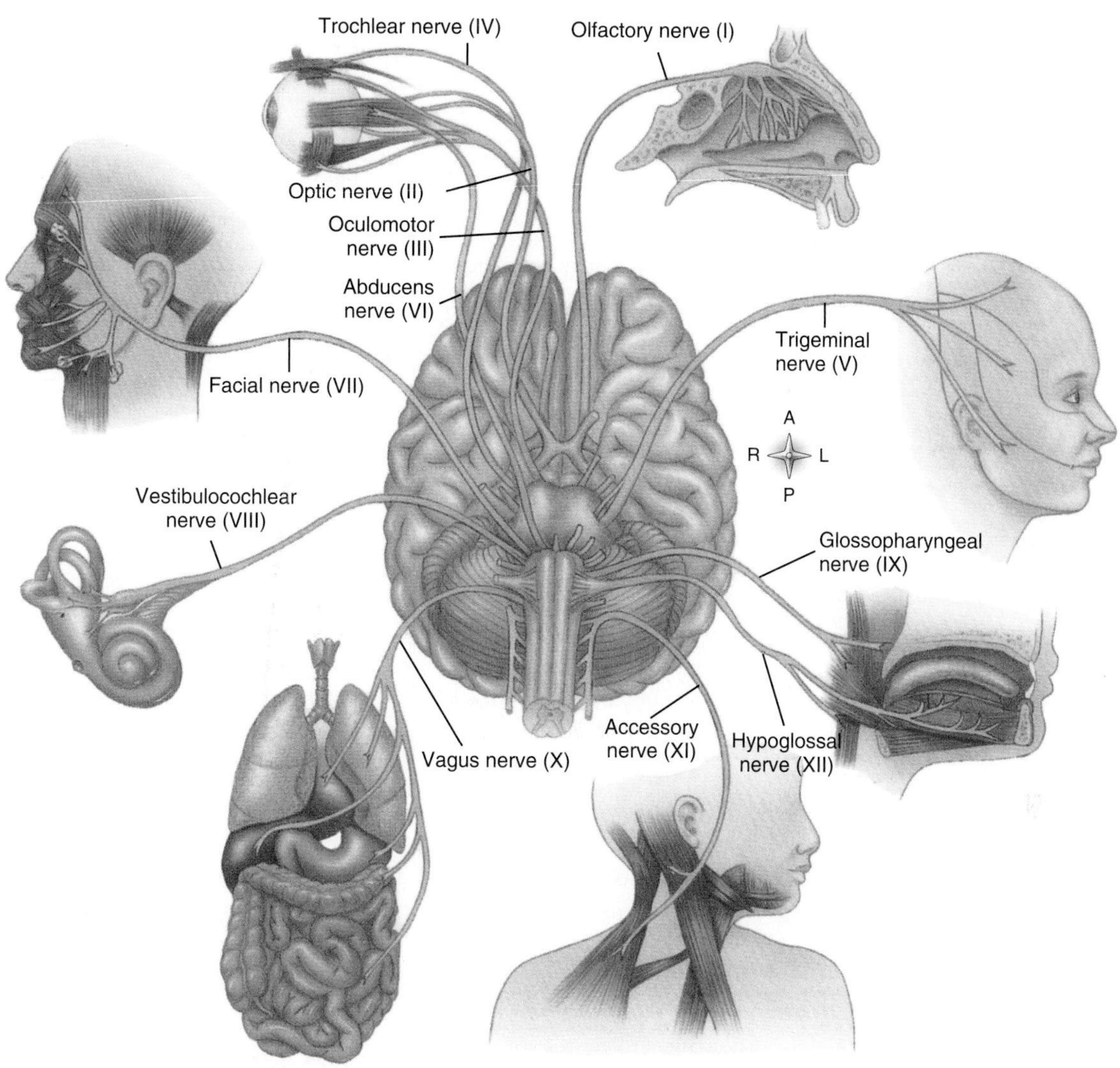

Functions

Spinal nerves conduct impulses between the spinal cord and the parts of the body not supplied by cranial nerves. The spinal nerves shown in Figure 8-11 contain, as do all spinal nerves, sensory and motor fibers. Spinal nerves therefore function to make possible sensations and movements. A disease or injury that prevents conduction by a spinal nerve thus results in a loss of feeling and a loss of movement in the part supplied by that nerve.

Detailed mapping of the skin's surface reveals a close relationship between the source on the spinal cord of each spinal nerve and the part of the body that it innervates (Figure 8-17). Knowledge of the segmental arrangement of spinal nerves is useful to physicians. For instance, a neurologist can identify

TABLE 8-2
Cranial Nerves

NERVE*		CONDUCT IMPULSES	FUNCTIONS
I	Olfactory	From nose to brain	Sense of smell
II	Optic	From eye to brain	Vision
III	Oculomotor	From brain to eye muscles	Eye movements
IV	Trochlear	From brain to external eye muscles	Eye movements
V	Trigeminal	From skin and mucous membrane of head and from teeth to brain; also from brain to chewing muscles	Sensations of face, scalp, and teeth; chewing movements
VI	Abducens	From brain to external eye muscles	Eye movements
VII	Facial	From taste buds of tongue to brain; from brain to face muscles	Sense of taste; contraction of muscles of facial expression
VIII	Vestibulocochlear	From ear to brain	Hearing; sense of balance
IX	Glossopharyngeal	From throat and taste buds of tongue to brain; also from brain to throat muscles and salivary glands	Sensations of throat, taste, swallowing movements, secretion of saliva
X	Vagus	From throat, larynx, and organs in thoracic and abdominal cavities to brain; also from brain to muscles of throat and to organs in thoracic and abdominal cavities	Sensations of throat and larynx and of thoracic and abdominal organs; swallowing, voice production, slowing of heartbeat, acceleration of peristalsis (gut movements)
XI	Accessory	From brain to certain shoulder and neck muscles	Shoulder movements; turning movements of head
XII	Hypoglossal	From brain to muscles of tongue	Tongue movements

*The first letter of the words in the following sentence are the first letters of the names of the cranial nerves, in the correct order. Many anatomy students find that using this sentence, or one like it, helps in memorizing the names and numbers of the cranial nerves. It is "**O**n **O**ld **O**lympus' **T**iny **T**ops, **A** **F**riendly **V**iking **G**rew **V**ines **A**nd **H**ops."

the site of a spinal cord or nerve abnormality from the area of the body that is insensitive to a pinprick. Skin surface areas that are supplied by a single spinal nerve are called **dermatomes** (DER-mah-tomes). A dermatome "map" of the body is shown in Figure 8-17.

Quick Check

1. How many cranial nerves does a person have? How many spinal nerves?
2. What is a spinal nerve *plexus*?
3. What are *dermatomes*?

AUTONOMIC NERVOUS SYSTEM

The autonomic nervous system consists of certain motor neurons that conduct impulses from the spinal cord or brainstem to the following kinds of tissues:

1. Cardiac muscle tissue
2. Smooth muscle tissue
3. Glandular epithelial tissue

The ANS consists of the parts of the nervous system that regulate involuntary functions (for exam-

FIGURE 8-17

Dermatomes. Segmental dermatome distribution of spinal nerves to the front, back, and side of the body. *C*, Cervical segments; *T*, thoracic segments; *L*, lumbar segments; *S*, sacral segments; *CX*, coccygeal segment.

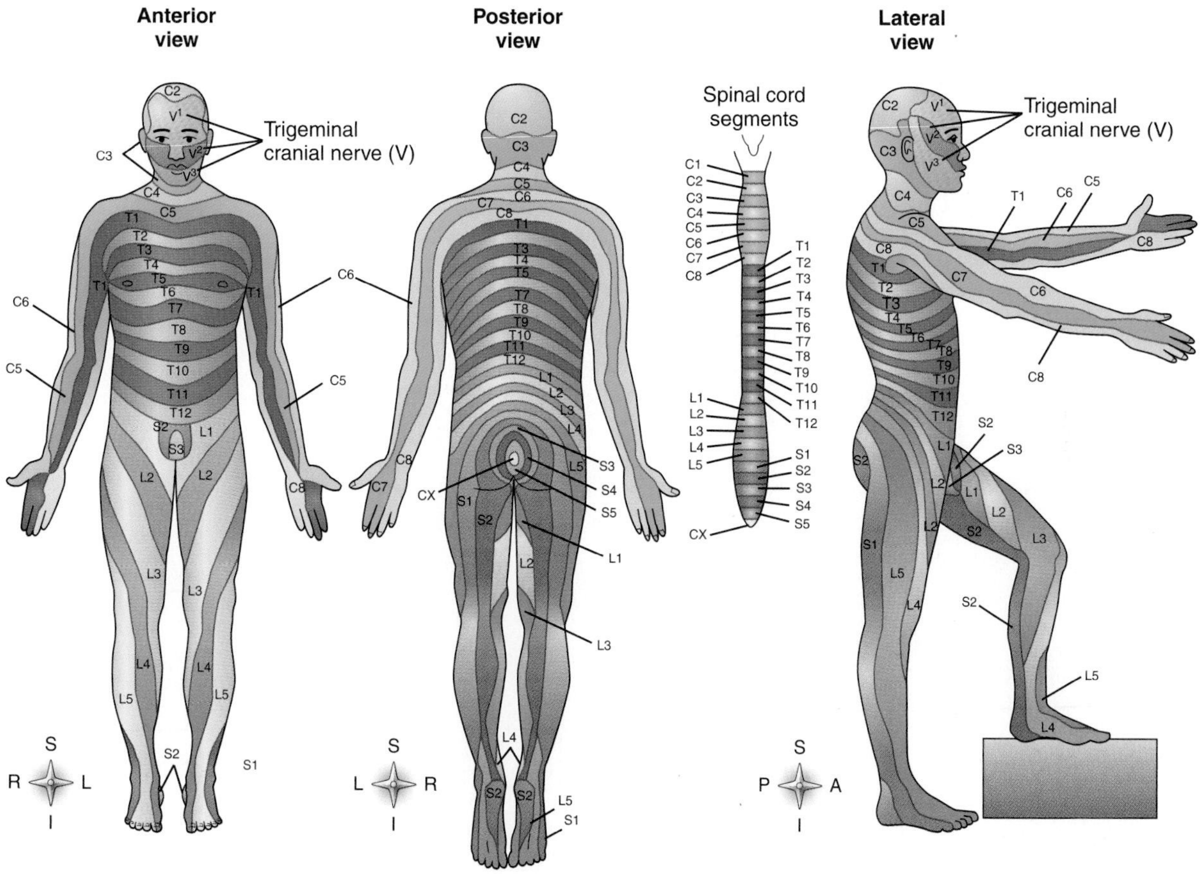

ple, the heartbeat, contractions of the stomach and intestines, and secretions by glands). On the other hand, motor nerves that control the voluntary actions of skeletal muscles are sometimes called the *somatic nervous system.*

The autonomic nervous system consists of two divisions called the **sympathetic nervous system** and the **parasympathetic nervous system** (Figure 8-18).

Functional Anatomy

Autonomic neurons are the motor neurons that make up the ANS. The dendrites and cell bodies of some autonomic neurons are located in the gray matter of the spinal cord or brainstem. Their axons extend from these structures and terminate in peripheral "junction boxes" called **ganglia** (GANG-lee-ah). These autonomic neurons are called **preganglionic neurons** because they conduct impulses between the spinal cord and a ganglion. In the ganglia the axon endings of preganglionic neurons synapse with the dendrites or cell bodies of postganglionic neurons. **Postganglionic neurons,** as their name suggests, conduct impulses from a ganglion to cardiac muscle, smooth muscle, or glandular epithelial tissue.

Autonomic or **visceral effectors** are the tissues to which autonomic neurons conduct impulses. Specifically, visceral effectors are cardiac muscle

FIGURE 8-18

Innervation of the major target organs by the autonomic nervous system. The sympathetic pathways are highlighted with orange, and the parasympathetic pathways are highlighted with green.

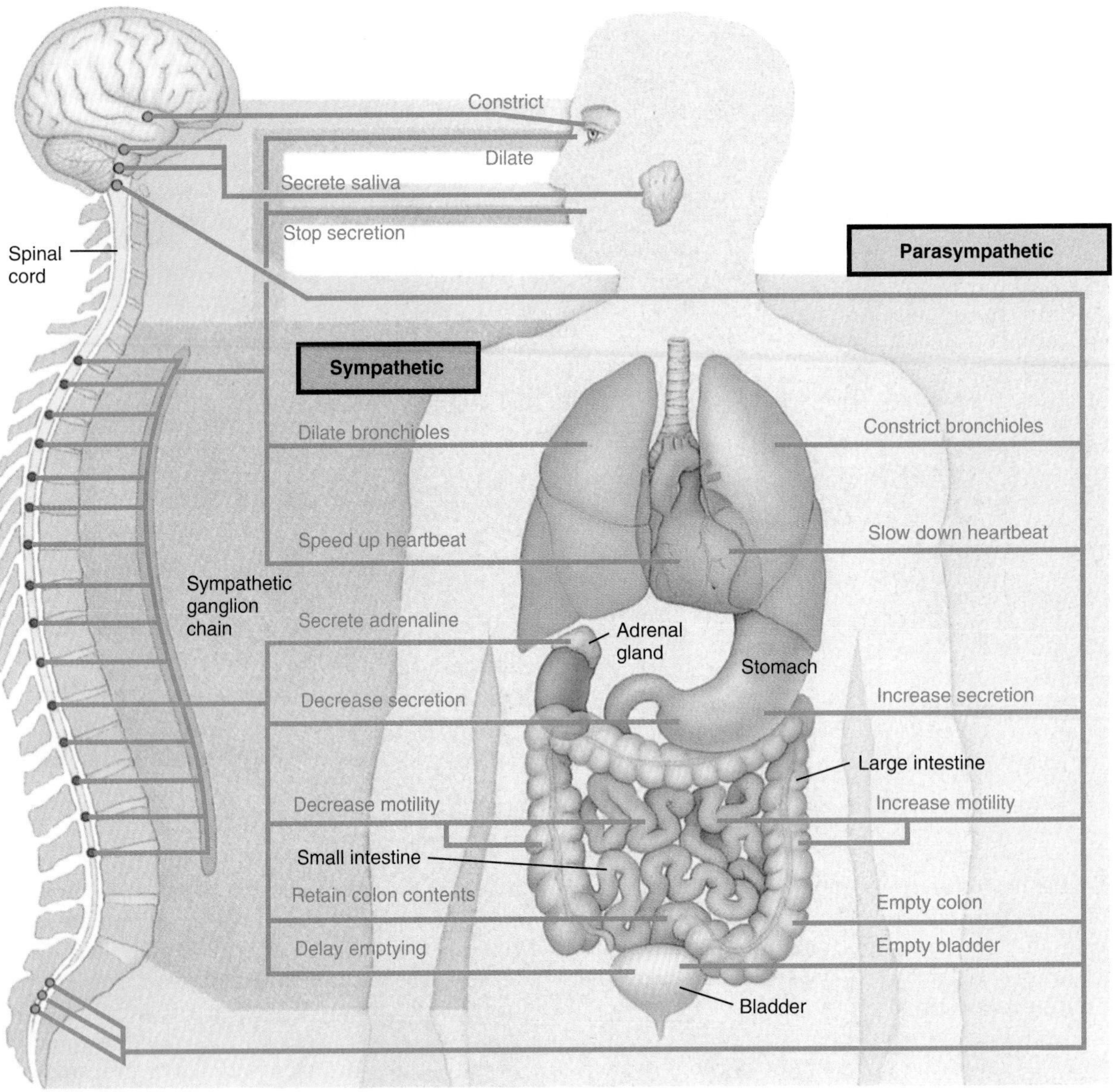

FIGURE 8-19

Autonomic conduction paths. The left side of the diagram shows that one somatic motor neuron conducts impulses all the way from the spinal cord to a somatic effector. Conduction from the spinal cord to any visceral effector, however, requires a relay of at least two autonomic motor neurons—a preganglionic and a postganglionic neuron, shown on the right side of the diagram.

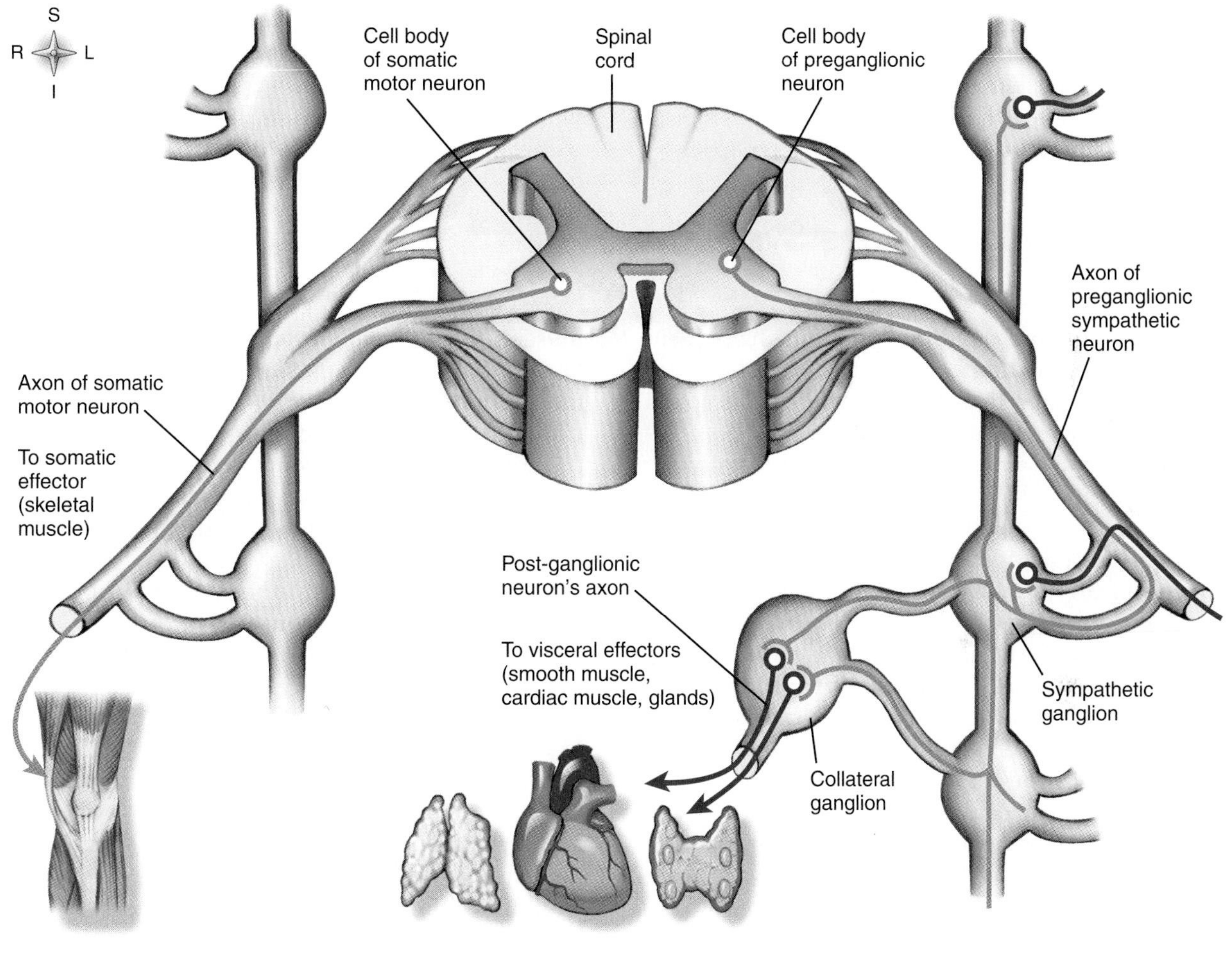

that makes up the wall of the heart, smooth muscle that partially makes up the walls of blood vessels and other hollow internal organs, and glandular epithelial tissue that makes up the secreting part of glands.

Autonomic Conduction Paths

Conduction paths to visceral and somatic effectors from the CNS (spinal cord or brainstem) differ somewhat. Autonomic paths to visceral effectors, as the right side of Figure 8-19 shows, consist of two-neuron relays. Impulses travel over preganglionic neurons from the spinal cord or brainstem to autonomic ganglia. There, they are relayed across synapses to postganglionic neurons, which then conduct the impulses from the ganglia to visceral effectors. Compare the autonomic conduction path with the somatic conduction path illustrated on the left side of Figure 8-19. Somatic motor neurons, like the ones shown here, conduct all the way from the spinal cord or brainstem to somatic effectors with no intervening synapses.

Sympathetic Nervous System

Structure

Sympathetic preganglionic neurons have dendrites and cell bodies in the gray matter of the thoracic and upper lumbar segments of the spinal cord. The sympathetic system has also been referred to as the *thoracolumbar system*. Look now at the right side of Figure 8-19. Follow the course of the axon of the sympathetic preganglionic neuron shown there. It leaves the spinal cord in the anterior (ventral) root of a spinal nerve. It next enters the spinal nerve but soon leaves it to extend to and through a sympathetic ganglion and terminate in a collateral ganglion. There, it synapses with several postganglionic neurons whose axons extend to terminate in visceral effectors. Also shown in Figure 8-19, branches of the preganglionic axon may ascend or descend to terminate in ganglia above and below their point of origin. All sympathetic preganglionic axons therefore synapse with many postganglionic neurons, and these frequently terminate in widely separated organs. Hence sympathetic responses are usually widespread, involving many organs rather than just one.

Sympathetic postganglionic neurons have dendrites and cell bodies in sympathetic ganglia. Sympathetic ganglia are located in front of and at each side of the spinal column. Because short fibers extend between the sympathetic ganglia, they look a little like two chains of beads and are often referred to as the *sympathetic chain ganglia*. Axons of sympathetic postganglionic neurons travel in spinal nerves to blood vessels, sweat glands, and arrector pili hair muscles all over the body. Separate autonomic nerves distribute many sympathetic postganglionic axons to various internal organs.

Functions of the Sympathetic Nervous System

The sympathetic nervous system functions as an emergency system. Impulses over sympathetic fibers take control of many internal organs when we exercise strenuously and when strong emotions—anger, fear, hate, anxiety—are elicited. In short, when we must cope with stress of any kind, sympathetic impulses increase to many visceral effectors and rapidly produce widespread changes within our bodies. The middle column of Table 8-3 indicates many sympathetic responses. The heart beats faster. Most blood vessels constrict, causing blood pressure to increase. Blood vessels in skeletal muscles dilate, supplying the muscles with more blood. Sweat glands and adrenal glands secrete more abundantly. Salivary and other digestive glands secrete more sparingly. Digestive tract contractions (peristalsis) become sluggish, hampering digestion. Together, these sympathetic responses make us ready for strenuous muscular work, or they prepare us for *fight or flight*. The group of changes induced by sympathetic control is known as the **fight-or-flight response.**

Parasympathetic Nervous System

Structure

The dendrites and cell bodies of parasympathetic preganglionic neurons are located in the gray matter of the brainstem and the sacral segments of the spinal cord. The parasympathetic system has also been referred to as the *craniosacral system*. The preganglionic parasympathetic axons extend some distance before terminating in the parasympathetic ganglia located in the head and in the thoracic and abdominal cavities close to the visceral effectors that they control. The dendrites and cell bodies of parasympathetic postganglionic neurons lie in these outlying parasympathetic ganglia, and their short axons extend into the nearby structures. Therefore each parasympathetic preganglionic neuron synapses only with postganglionic neurons to a single effector. For this reason, parasympa-

TABLE 8-3

Autonomic Functions

VISCERAL EFFECTORS	SYMPATHETIC CONTROL	PARASYMPATHETIC CONTROL
Heart muscle	Accelerates heartbeat	Slows heartbeat
Smooth muscle		
Of most blood vessels	Constricts blood vessels	None
Of blood vessels in skeletal muscles	Dilates blood vessels	None
Of the digestive tract	Decreases peristalsis; inhibits defecation	Increases peristalsis
Of the anal sphincter	Stimulates—closes sphincter	Inhibits—opens sphincter for defecation
Of the urinary bladder	Inhibits—relaxes bladder	Stimulates—contracts bladder
Of the urinary sphincters	Stimulates—closes sphincter	Inhibits—opens sphincter for urination
Of the eye		
Iris	Stimulates radial fibers—dilation of pupil	Stimulates circular fibers—contraction of pupil
Ciliary	Inhibits—accommodation for far vision (flattening of lens)	Stimulates—accommodation for near vision (bulging of lens)
Of hairs (arrector pili)	Stimulates—"goose pimples"	No parasympathetic fibers
Glands		
Adrenal medulla	Increases epinephrine secretion	None
Sweat glands	Increases sweat secretion	None
Digestive glands	Decreases secretion of digestive juices	Increases secretion of digestive juices

thetic stimulation frequently involves response by only one organ. This is not true of sympathetic responses; as noted, sympathetic stimulation usually results in responses by numerous organs.

Functions of the Parasympathetic Nervous System

The parasympathetic system dominates control of many visceral effectors under normal, everyday conditions. Impulses over parasympathetic fibers, for example, tend to slow heartbeat, increase peristalsis, and increase secretion of digestive juices and insulin (see Table 8-3).

Autonomic Neurotransmitters

Turn your attention now to Figure 8-20. It reveals information about autonomic neurotransmitters, the chemical compounds released from the axon terminals of autonomic neurons. Observe that three of the axons shown in Figure 8-20—the sympathetic preganglionic axon, the parasympathetic preganglionic axon, and the parasympathetic postganglionic axon—release acetylcholine. These axons are therefore classified as **cholinergic fibers.** Only one type of autonomic axon releases the neurotransmitter norepinephrine (noradrenaline). This is the axon of a sympathetic postganglionic neuron, and such neurons are classified as **adrenergic fibers.** That each division of the ANS signals its effectors with a different neurotransmitter explains how an organ can tell which division is stimulating it. The heart, for example, responds to acetylcholine from the parasympathetic division by slowing down. The presence of norepinephrine at the heart, on the other hand, is a signal from the sympathetic division, and the response is an increase in heart activity.

FIGURE 8-20

Autonomic neurotransmitters. Three of the four fiber types are cholinergic, secreting the neurotransmitter acetylcholine (Ach) into a synapse. Only the sympathetic postganglionic fiber is adrenergic, secreting norepinephrine (NE) into a synapse.

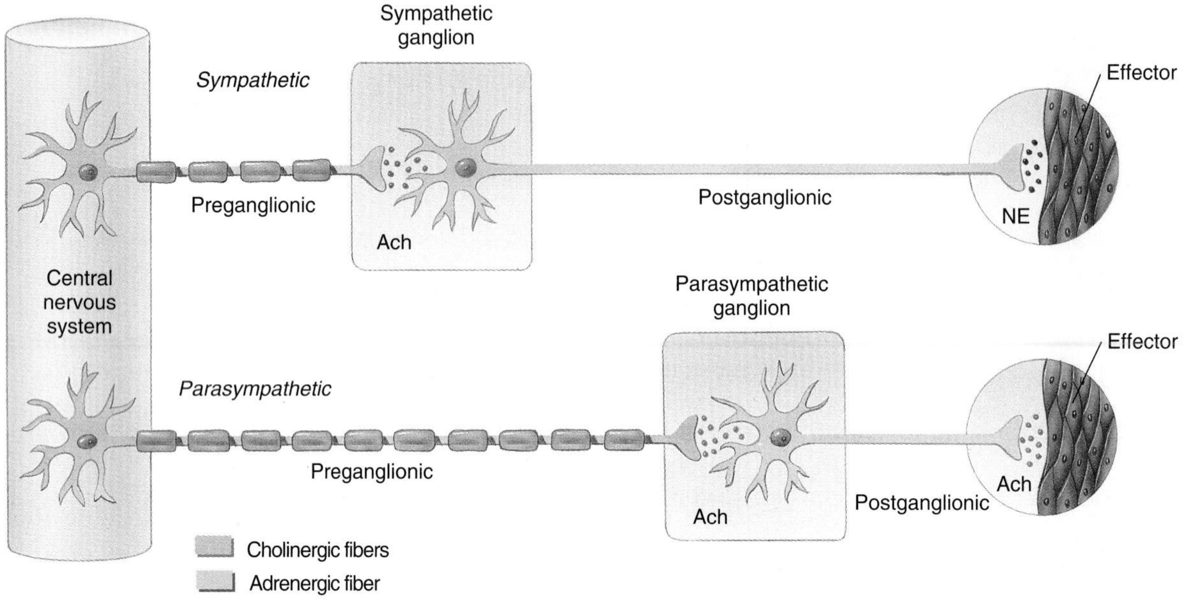

Autonomic Nervous System as a Whole

The function of the autonomic nervous system is to regulate the body's automatic, involuntary functions in ways that maintain or quickly restore homeostasis. Many internal organs are doubly innervated by the ANS. In other words, they receive fibers from parasympathetic and sympathetic divisions. Parasympathetic and sympathetic impulses continually bombard them and, as Table 8-3 indicates, influence their function in opposite or antagonistic ways. For example, the heart continually receives sympathetic impulses that make it beat faster and parasympathetic impulses that slow it down. The ratio between these two antagonistic forces, determined by the ratio between the two different autonomic neurotransmitters, determines the actual heart rate.

The name *autonomic nervous system* is something of a misnomer. It seems to imply that this part of the nervous system is independent from other parts. This is not true. Dendrites and cell bodies of preganglionic neurons are located, as observed, in the spinal cord and brainstem. They are continually influenced directly or indirectly by impulses from neurons located above them, notably by some in the hypothalamus and in the parts of the cerebral cortex called the **limbic system** or *emotional brain*. Through conduction paths from these areas, emotions can produce widespread changes in the automatic functions of our bodies, in cardiac and smooth muscle contractions, and in secretion by glands. Anger and fear, for example, lead to increased sympathetic activity and the fight-or-flight response. According to some physiologists, the altered state of consciousness known as *meditation* leads to decreased sympathetic activity and a group of changes opposite to those of the fight-or-flight response.

Quick

1. What kinds of tissues are controlled by the autonomic nervous system?
2. What are the two main divisions of the autonomic nervous system (ANS)?
3. Which division of the ANS produces the *fight-or-flight response*?
4. Which two neurotransmitters are used by autonomic nerve pathways?

Clinical Application

Herpes Zoster or Shingles

Herpes zoster or **shingles** is a unique viral infection that almost always affects the skin of a single dermatome. It is caused by a varicella zoster virus of chickenpox. About 3% of the population will suffer from shingles at some time in their lives. In most cases the disease results from reactivation of the varicella virus. The virus probably traveled through a cutaneous nerve and remained dormant in a dorsal root ganglion for years after an episode of the chickenpox. If the body's immunological protective mechanism becomes diminished in the elderly after stress, or in individuals undergoing radiation therapy or taking immunosuppressive drugs, the virus may reactivate. If this occurs, the virus travels over the sensory nerve to the skin of a single dermatome. The result is a painful eruption of red, swollen plaques or vesicles that eventually rupture and crust before clearing in 2 to 3 weeks. In severe cases, extensive inflammation, hemorrhagic blisters, and secondary bacterial infection may lead to permanent scarring. In most cases, the eruption of vesicles is preceded by 4 to 5 days of preeruptive pain, burning, and itching in the affected dermatome. Unfortunately, an attack of herpes zoster does not confer lasting immunity. Many individuals suffer three or four episodes in a lifetime.

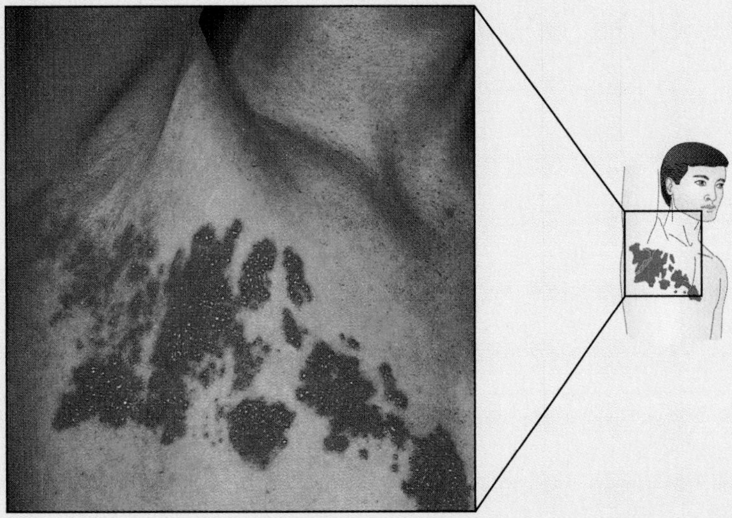

Science Applications

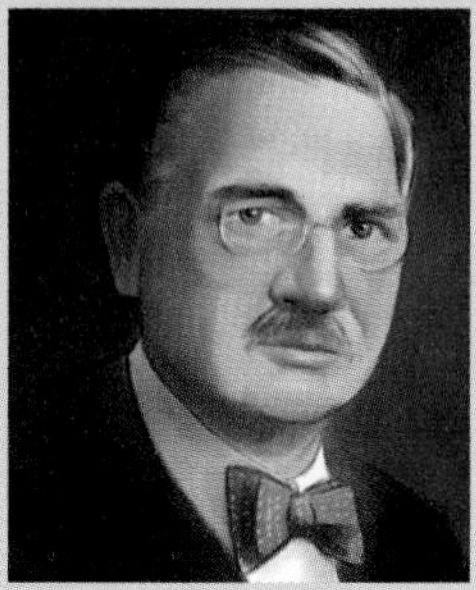

Neuroscience

Otto Loewi (1873-1961).

The Austrian scientist Otto Loewi started his studies in the humanities, not science. When he did begin university studies in medicine, he often skipped his science classes to attend lectures in philosophy. But after Dr. Loewi did turn his attention to human biology, he was brilliant. In 1921, when trying to design an experiment to find out how neurons communicate with other cells, he had a dream in which the answer came to him. He rushed to his lab and performed a now famous experiment in which he discovered what we now know as acetylcholine. For his work that showed that it is neurotransmitters that carry signals from neurons, Loewi shared a Nobel Prize in 1936. Not surprisingly, Loewi later spent some of his time studying how dreams may help us understand subconscious thoughts.

Many professions depend on neuroscience researchers like Otto Loewi to provide the information needed to help improve our lives. For example, neurologists, psychiatrists, and other medical professionals use this information to treat disorders of the nervous system. Pharmacologists and pharmacy professionals use these ideas to develop drug treatments that affect the nervous system. Mental health professionals such as psychologists and counselors use concepts of neuroscience to understand human emotions and behavior. Even people who specialize in business and marketing use some of the discoveries in neuroscience to help entice buyers to buy certain products or to predict the behavior of crowds.

OUTLINE SUMMARY

ORGANS AND DIVISIONS OF THE NERVOUS SYSTEM (Figure 8-1)
A. Central nervous system (CNS)—brain and spinal cord
B. Peripheral nervous system (PNS)—all nerves
C. Autonomic nervous system (ANS)

CELLS OF THE NERVOUS SYSTEM
A. Neurons
 1. Consist of three main parts—dendrites: conduct impulses to cell body of neuron; cell body of neuron; and axon: conducts impulses away from cell body of neuron (Figure 8-2)
 2. Neurons classified according to function—sensory: conduct impulses to the spinal cord and brain; motor: conduct impulses away from brain and spinal cord to muscles and glands; and interneurons: conduct impulses from sensory neurons to motor neurons
B. Glia (neuroglia)
 1. Support cells, bringing the cells of nervous tissue together structurally and functionally
 2. Three main types of glial cells of the CNS (Figure 8-3)
  a. Astrocytes—star-shaped cells that anchor small blood vessels to neurons
  b. Microglia—small cells that move in inflamed brain tissue carrying on phagocytosis
  c. Oligodendrocytes—form myelin sheaths on axons in the CNS
 3. Schwann cells form myelin sheaths on axons of the PNS (Figure 8-2)

NERVES (Figure 8-4)
A. Nerve—bundle of peripheral axons
 1. Tract—bundle of central axons
 2. White matter—tissue composed primarily of myelinated axons (nerves or tracts)
 3. Gray matter—tissue composed primarily of cell bodies and unmyelinated fibers
B. Nerve coverings—fibrous connective tissue
 1. Endoneurium—surrounds individual fibers within a nerve
 2. Perineurium—surrounds a group (fascicle) of nerve fibers
 3. Epineurium—surrounds the entire nerve

REFLEX ARCS
A. Nerve impulses are conducted from receptors to effectors over neuron pathways or reflex arcs; conduction by a reflex arc results in a reflex (that is, contraction by a muscle or secretion by a gland)
B. The simplest reflex arcs are two-neuron arcs—consisting of sensory neurons synapsing in the spinal cord with motor neurons; three-neuron arcs consist of sensory neurons synapsing in the spinal cord with interneurons that synapse with motor neurons (Figure 8-5)

NERVE IMPULSES
A. Definition—self-propagating wave of electrical disturbance that travels along the surface of a neuron membrane
B. Mechanism
 1. A stimulus triggers the opening of Na^+ channels in the plasma membrane of the neuron
 2. Inward movement of positive sodium ions leaves a slight excess of negative ions outside at a stimulated point; marks the beginning of a nerve impulse

THE SYNAPSE
A. Definition—chemical compounds released from axon terminals (of a presynaptic neuron) into a synaptic cleft
B. Neurotransmitters bind to specific receptor molecules in the membrane of a postsynaptic neuron, opening ion channels and thereby stimulating impulse conduction by the membrane
C. Names of neurotransmitters—acetylcholine, catecholamines (norepinephrine, dopamine, and serotonin), and other compounds

Continued

OUTLINE SUMMARY—*cont'd*

CENTRAL NERVOUS SYSTEM

A. Divisions of the brain (Figure 8-9 and Table 8-1)
   1. Brainstem
      a. Consists of three parts of brain; named in ascending order: the medulla oblongata, pons, and midbrain
      b. Structure—white matter with bits of gray matter scattered through it
      c. Function—gray matter in the brainstem functions as reflex centers (for example, for heartbeat, respirations, and blood vessel diameter); sensory tracts in the brainstem conduct impulses to the higher parts of the brain; motor tracts conduct from the higher parts of the brain to the spinal cord
   2. Diencephalon
      a. Structure and function of the hypothalamus
         (1) Consists mainly of the posterior pituitary gland, pituitary stalk, and gray matter
         (2) Acts as the major center for controlling the ANS; therefore, it helps control the functioning of most internal organs
         (3) Controls hormone secretion by anterior and posterior pituitary glands; therefore, it indirectly helps control hormone secretion by most other endocrine glands
         (4) Contains centers for controlling appetite, wakefulness, and pleasure
      b. Structure and function of the thalamus
         (1) Dumbbell-shaped mass of gray matter in each cerebral hemisphere
         (2) Relays sensory impulses to cerebral cortex sensory areas
         (3) In some way produces the emotions of pleasantness or unpleasantness associated with sensations
   3. Cerebellum
      a. Second largest part of the human brain
      b. Helps control muscle contractions to produce coordinated movements so that we can maintain balance, move smoothly, and sustain normal postures
   4. Cerebrum
      a. Largest part of the human brain
      b. Outer layer of gray matter is the cerebral cortex; made up of lobes; composed mainly of dendrites and cell bodies of neurons
      c. Interior of the cerebrum composed mainly of white matter (that is nerve fibers arranged in bundles called *tracts*)
      d. Functions of the cerebrum—mental processes of all types, including sensations, consciousness, memory, and voluntary control of movements

B. Spinal cord (Figure 8-11)
   1. Outer part is composed of white matter made up of many bundles of axons called tracts; interior composed of gray matter made up mainly of neuron dendrites and cell bodies
   2. Functions as the center for all spinal cord reflexes; sensory tracts conduct impulses to the brain, and motor tracts conduct impulses from the brain

C. Coverings and fluid spaces of the brain and spinal cord
   1. Coverings
      a. Cranial bones and vertebrae
      b. Cerebral and spinal meninges—the dura mater, the pia mater, and the arachnoid mater (Figure 8-13)
   2. Fluid spaces—subarachnoid spaces of meninges, central canal inside cord, and ventricles in brain (Figure 8-14)

OUTLINE SUMMARY—*cont'd*

PERIPHERAL NERVOUS SYSTEM

A. Cranial nerves (Figure 8-16 and Table 8-2)
   1. Twelve pairs—attached to undersurface of the brain
   2. Connect brain with the neck and structures in the thorax and abdomen
B. Spinal nerves
   1. Structure—contain dendrites of sensory neurons and axons of motor neurons
   2. Functions—conduct impulses necessary for sensations and voluntary movements

AUTONOMIC NERVOUS SYSTEM

A. Autonomic nervous system—motor neurons that conduct impulses from the central nervous system to cardiac muscle, smooth muscle, and glandular epithelial tissue; regulates the body's automatic or involuntary functions (Figure 8-18)
B. Autonomic neurons—preganglionic autonomic neurons conduct from spinal cord or brainstem to an autonomic ganglion; postganglionic neurons conduct from autonomic ganglia to cardiac muscle, smooth muscle, and glandular epithelial tissue
C. Autonomic or visceral effectors—tissues to which autonomic neurons conduct impulses (that is, cardiac and smooth muscle and glandular epithelial tissue)
D. Composed of two divisions—the sympathetic system and the parasympathetic system
E. Autonomic conduction paths
   1. Consist of two-neuron relays (that is, preganglionic neurons from the central nervous system to autonomic ganglia, synapses, postganglionic neurons from ganglia to visceral effectors)
   2. In contrast, somatic motor neurons conduct all the way from the CNS to somatic effectors with no intervening synapses
F. Sympathetic nervous system
   1. Structure
      a. Dendrites and cell bodies of sympathetic preganglionic neurons are located in the gray matter of the thoracic and upper lumbar segments of the spinal cord
      b. Axons leave the spinal cord in the anterior roots of spinal nerves, extend to sympathetic or collateral ganglia, and synapse with several postganglionic neurons whose axons extend to spinal or autonomic nerves to terminate in visceral effectors
      c. A chain of sympathetic ganglia is in front of and at each side of the spinal column
   2. Functions
      a. Serves as the emergency or stress system, controlling visceral effectors during strenuous exercise and strong emotions (anger, fear, hate, or anxiety)
      b. Group of changes induced by sympathetic control is called the *fight-or-flight response*
G. Parasympathetic nervous system
   1. Structure
      a. Parasympathetic preganglionic neurons have dendrites and cell bodies in the gray matter of the brainstem and the sacral segments of the spinal cord
      b. Parasympathetic preganglionic neurons terminate in parasympathetic ganglia located in the head and the thoracic and abdominal cavities close to visceral effectors
      c. Each parasympathetic preganglionic neuron synapses with postganglionic neurons to only one effector

Continued

OUTLINE SUMMARY—*cont'd*

2. Function—dominates control of many visceral effectors under normal, everyday conditions

H. Autonomic neurotransmitters
   1. Cholinergic fibers—preganglionic axons of parasympathetic and sympathetic systems and parasympathetic postganglionic axons release acetylcholine
   2. Adrenergic fibers—axons of sympathetic postganglionic neurons release norepinephrine (noradrenaline)

I. Autonomic nervous system as a whole
   1. Regulates the body's automatic functions in ways that maintain or quickly restore homeostasis
   2. Many visceral effectors are doubly innervated (that is, they receive fibers from parasympathetic and sympathetic divisions and are influenced in opposite ways by the two divisions)

NEW WORDS

acetylcholine
anesthesia
arachnoid
astrocytes
axon
catecholamines
dendrite
dopamine
dura mater
effectors
endorphins
enkephalins
fight-or-flight response
ganglia
ganglion
glia
hydrocephalus
interneuron
limbic system
meninges
microglia
motor neuron
multiple sclerosis
myelin
neurons
neurotransmitter
node of Ranvier
norepinephrine
oligodendrocyte
parasympathetic system
pia mater
postganglionic neurons
postsynaptic neuron
preganglionic neuron
presynaptic neuron
receptors
reflex arc
saltatory conduction
sensory neuron
serotonin
sympathetic system
synapse
synaptic cleft
tract

REVIEW QUESTIONS

1. Draw and label the three parts of the neuron and explain the function of the dendrite and axon.
2. Name the three types of neurons classified according to the direction in which the impulse is transmitted. Define and explain each of them.
3. Define or explain the following terms: *myelin*, *nodes of Ranvier*, and *neurolemma*.
4. Name and give the function of the three types of glia cells.
5. Define or explain the following terms: *epineurium*, *perineurium*, and *endoneurium*.
6. What is the physical difference between gray matter and white matter?
7. Explain how a reflex arc functions. What are the two types of reflex arc?
8. Explain what occurs during a nerve impulse. What is *saltatory conduction*?
9. Explain fully what occurs at a synapse. Explain the two ways in which neurotransmitter activity is terminated.
10. Describe and list the functions of the medulla oblongata.
11. Describe and list the functions of the hypothalamus.
12. Describe and list the functions of the thalamus.
13. Describe and list the functions of the cerebellum.
14. Give the general functions of the cerebrum. What are the specific functions of the occipital and temporal lobes?
15. Describe and list the functions of the spinal cord.
16. Name and explain the three layers of the meninges.
17. What is the function of cerebrospinal fluid? Where and how is it produced?
18. How many nerve pairs are generated from the spinal cord? How many nerve pairs are generated from each section of the spinal cord and how are they named? What is a plexus?
19. Explain the structure and function of the sympathetic nervous system.
20. Explain the structure and function of the parasympathetic nervous system.

CRITICAL THINKING

21. Compare the functional regions of the frontal, parietal, occipital and temporal lobes.
22. Which of the cranial nerves deals primarily with motor function? Which deal primarily with sensory function?
23. There is a type of medication that inhibits the functioning of acetylcholinesterase (the enzyme that deactivates acetylcholine). Explain the side effects the medication would have on the visceral effectors.

★★ 9/16/05

CHAPTER TEST

1. PNS is the name of the nervous system division that includes the nerves that extend to the outlying parts of the body.
2. CNS is the name of the nervous system division that includes the brain and spinal cord.
3. A group of peripheral axons bundled together in an epineurium is called a fascicle.
4. The two types of cells found in the nervous system are neurons and neuroglia.
5. The knee jerk is of a type of neural pathway called a reflex.
6. __________ is a self-propagating wave of electrical disturbance that travels along the surface of a neuron's plasma membrane.
7. The exterior of a resting neuron has a slight positive charge, whereas the interior has a slight negative charge.
8. During a nerve impulse, sodium is the ion that rushes into the neuron.
9. The axon is the place where impulses are passed from one neuron to another.
10. Acetylcholine and dopamine are examples of neurotransmitters which are chemicals used by neurons to communicate.
11. Duramater, Pia Mater, and Choradnoid Mater are the three membranes that make up the meninges.
12. There are __________ pairs of cranial nerves and __________ pairs of nerves that come from the spinal cord.
13. __________ are skin surface areas supplied by a single spinal nerve.
14. __________ is the part of the autonomic nervous system that regulates effectors during nonstress conditions.
15. Sympathetic is the part of the autonomic nervous system that regulates the "fight-or-flight" response.
16. The preganglionic axons of the sympathetic nervous system release the neurotransmitter __________. The postganglionic axons release __________.
17. The preganglionic axons of the parasympathetic nervous system release the neurotransmitter __________; the postganglionic axons release __________.
18. The autonomic nervous system consists of neurons that conduct impulses from the brain or spinal cord to __________ tissue, __________ tissue, and __________ tissue.

Match the function or description in Column B with the correct term in Column A.

COLUMN A

19. G Dendrite
20. C Axon
21. E Myelin
22. A Schwann cells
23. B Astrocytes
24. F Microglia
25. D Oligodendrocyte

COLUMN B

a. cells that make myelin for axons outside the CNS
b. glia cells that help form the blood-brain barrier
c. a single projection that carries nerve impulses away from the cell body
d. cells that make myelin for axons inside the CNS
e. a white fatty substance that surrounds and insulates the axon
f. cells that act as microbe-eating scavengers in the CNS
g. a highly branched part of the neuron that carries impulses toward the cell body

CHAPTER TEST—*cont'd*

Match the functions in Column B with parts of the central nervous system in Column A.

COLUMN A	COLUMN B
26. __D__ Medulla oblongota	a. part of the brainstem that is a conduction pathway between areas of the brain and body; influences respiration
27. __A__ Pons	b. sensory relay station from various body areas to the cerebral cortex; also involved with emotions and alerting and arousal mechanisms
28. __H__ Midbrain	c. carries messages to and from the brain to the rest of the body; also mediates reflexes
29. __F__ Hypothalamus	d. part of the brainstem that contains cardiac, respiratory, and vasomotor centers
30. __B__ Thalamus	e. sensory perception, willed movements, consciousness, and memory are mediated here
31. __G__ Cerebellum	f. regulates body temperature, water balance, sleep-wake cycles, appetite, and sexual arousal
32. __E__ Cerebrum	g. regulates muscle coordination, maintenance of equilibrium, and posture
33. __C__ Spinal cord	h. part of the brainstem that contains relays for visual and auditory impulses

STUDY TIPS

Before starting Chapter 8, review the synopsis of the nervous system in Chapter 4. There is a great deal of material in Chapter 8. It can be made somewhat easier if you divide the chapter into three parts: the microscopic structure and function of the nervous system, the central nervous system, and the peripheral nervous system. Keep in mind that the nervous system functions as one organized system. The divisions in the system are a way to simplify the system, but they are not separate entities. It may help to learn the terminology if you remember that *neuro* refers to nerves, *dendro-* means "branch," and *oligo-* means "few" or "little." So *oligodendrocyte*, a glia cell means "a cell with few branches." The function of the nervous system is accomplished by two processes: the conduction of nerve impulses and the passing of the nerve impulses across a synapse. Nerve impulses are an exchange of ions between the interior and exterior of the neuron. The synapse requires the production, release, and deactivation of neurotransmitters. Neurotransmitters function by stimulating receptors in the neuron on the other side of the synapse. The material on the central nervous system can best be learned by using flash cards to match the structure and the function. When studying the autonomic nervous system, remember the basic function of each part. The parasympathetic nervous system tries to maintain a quiet homeostasis. The sympathetic nervous system prepares the body for emergency situations—the "fight-or-flight" response.

In your study groups, you should go over the terms from the first part of the chapter. Discuss the processes of nerve impulse transmission and what occurs at the synapse. Go over the flash cards with the names and functions of the parts of the central nervous system. Remember that most of the structures in the central nervous system have more than one function. If you remember the general functions of the sympathetic and parasympathetic nervous system, the specific effects of the systems will be easier to remember. Go over the questions at the end of the chapter and discuss possible test questions.

9 The Senses

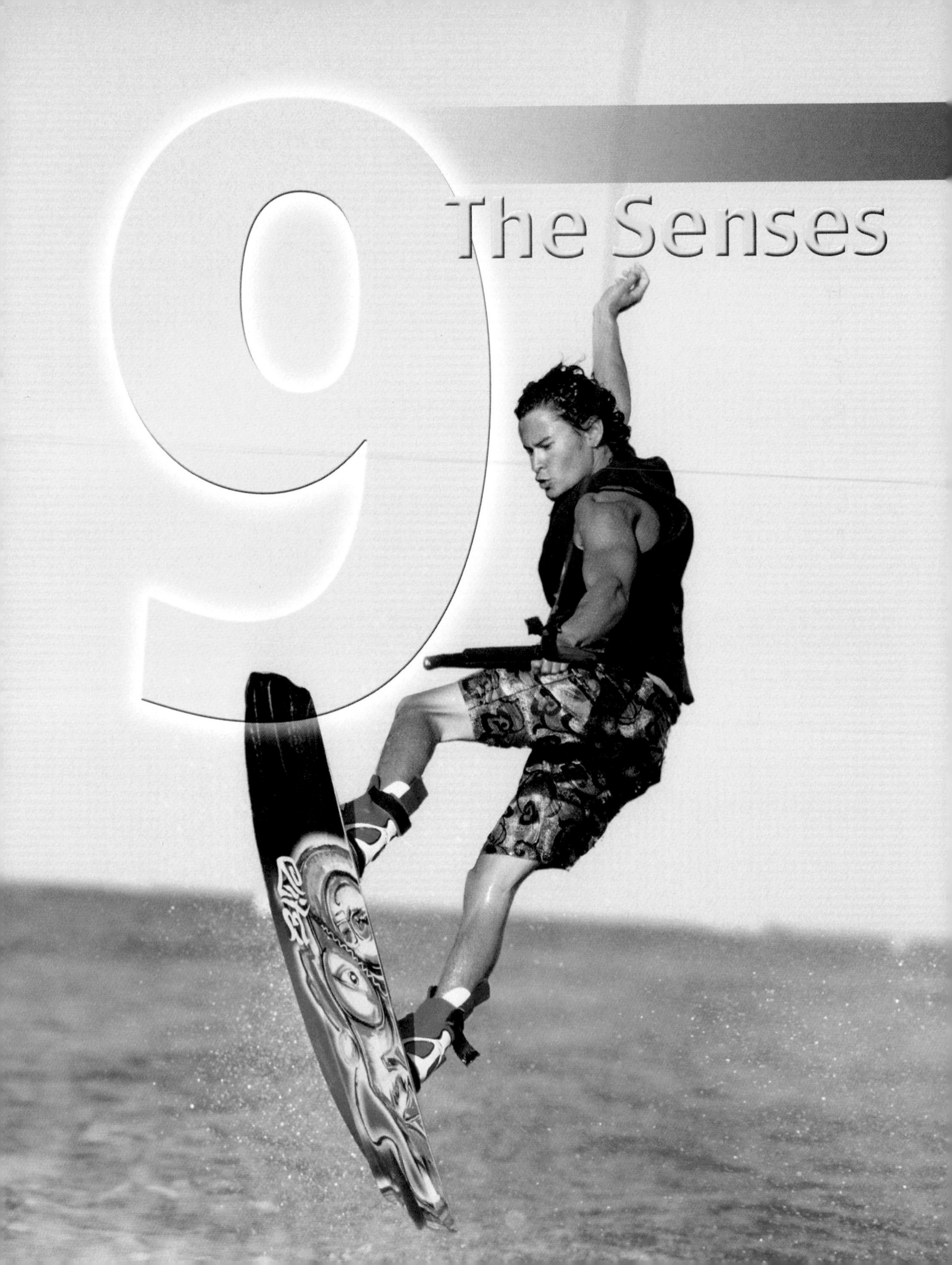

• Outline

• Objectives

AFTER YOU HAVE COMPLETED THIS CHAPTER, YOU SHOULD BE ABLE TO:

1. Classify sense organs as special or general and explain the basic differences between the two groups.
2. Discuss how a stimulus is converted into a sensation.
3. Discuss the general sense organs and their functions.
4. Describe the structure of the eye and the functions of its components.
5. Discuss the anatomy of the ear and its sensory function in hearing and equilibrium.
6. Discuss the chemical receptors and their functions.

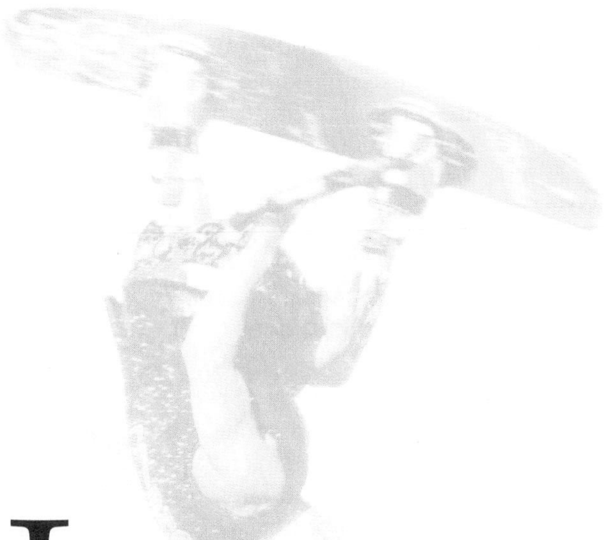

I*f you were* asked to name the sense organs, what organs would you name? Can you think of any besides the eyes, ears, nose, and taste buds? Actually there are millions of other sense organs throughout the body in our skin, internal organs, and muscles. They constitute the many **sensory receptors** that allow us to respond to stimuli such as touch, pressure, temperature, and pain. These microscopic receptors are located at the tips of dendrites of sensory neurons.

Our ability to "sense" changes in our external and internal environments is a requirement for maintaining homeostasis and for survival itself. We can initiate protective reflexes important to homeostasis only if we can sense a change or danger. External dangers may be detected by sight or hearing. If the danger is internal, such as overstretching a muscle, detecting an increase in body temperature (fever), or sensing the pain caused by an ulcer, other receptors make us aware of the problem and permit us to take appropriate action to maintain homeostasis.

CLASSIFICATION OF SENSE ORGANS

The sense organs are often classified as either **general** sense organs or **special** sense organs. The *general sense organs* consist of microscopic receptors widely distributed throughout the body in the skin, muscles, tendons, joints, and other internal organs of the body. They are responsible for such sensations as pain, temperature, touch, and pressure. The *special sense organs* are responsible for the special senses of smell, taste, vision, hearing, and equilibrium and are grouped into localized areas such as the nasal mucosa and tongue or into such complex organs as the eye and ear.

In addition to classification as either general or special sense organs, individual receptor cells are often identified according to whether or not they are: (1) *encapsulated* or *unencapsulated,* that is, whether they are covered by some sort of capsule or are "free" or "naked" of any such covering and by (2) the types of stimuli that activate them. Table 9-1 identifies the general sense organs as either free nerve endings or one of the six types of encapsulated nerve endings, whereas Table 9-2 identifies the type of receptor cells in the special sense organs that are stimulated by specific types of stimuli.

CONVERTING A STIMULUS INTO A SENSATION

All sense organs, regardless of size, type, or location, have in common some important functional characteristics. First, they must be able to sense or detect a stimulus or a change in the intensity of a particular stimulus in their environment. Of course, different sense organs detect different types of stimuli. Whether it is light, sound, temperature change, mechanical pressure, or the presence of chemicals ultimately identified as taste or smell, the stimulus must be changed into an electrical signal or nerve impulse. This signal is then transmitted over a nervous system "pathway" to the brain, where the sensation is actually perceived.

GENERAL SENSE ORGANS

The microscopic general sense organ receptors are found in almost every part of the body but they are concentrated in the skin (Figure 9-1). However, these receptors are not evenly distributed over the body surface or in the internal organs. And they do not all respond to the same type of stimulus. To demonstrate this, try touching any point of your skin over a fingertip with the tip of a toothpick. You can hardly miss stimulating at least one receptor and almost instantaneously experiencing a sensation of touch. It is the specialized form and function of the different receptor cells that allow them to respond to different stimuli. This specialized response capability of receptor cells allows us to experience different types of sensations. For example, so-called *mechanoreceptors* are activated by mechanical stimuli that "deform" or change the position or shape of the receptor. A good example is the Pacinian corpuscle, which senses pressure. Stimulation of some receptors leads to the sensation of vibration, and stimulation of still others gives the sensation of touch. The important and numerous free nerve endings respond to stimuli that permit us to sense pain, temperature, and a number of other sensations. Table 9-1 identifies the general sense receptors showing type, main location, and the sensation produced. Receptors associated with the skin are illustrated in Figure 9-1.

Some specialized receptors found near the point of junction between tendons and muscles and others found deep within skeletal muscle tissue are called *proprioceptors*. When stimulated, they provide us with information concerning the position or movement of the different parts of the body as well as the length and the extent of contraction and tension in our muscles. The Golgi tendon receptors and muscle spindles identified in Table 9-1 are important proprioceptors.

Later in the chapter you will study about specialized photoreceptors, found only in the eye, that allow us to see, and chemoreceptors, that detect chemicals responsible for our senses of taste and smell.

TABLE 9-1

General Sense Organs

TYPE	MAIN LOCATION	GENERAL SENSES	
FREE NERVE ENDINGS (NAKED NERVE ENDINGS)			
	Skin and mucosa (epithelial layers)	Pain, crude touch, temperature, itch, tickle	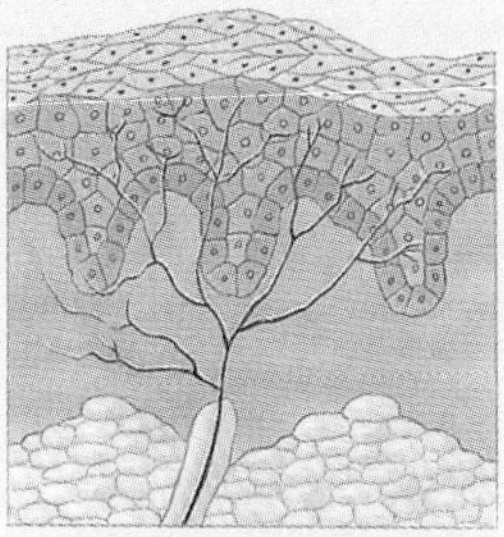
ENCAPSULATED NERVE ENDINGS			
Meissner's corpuscles	Skin (in papillae of dermis) and fingertips and lips (numerous)	Fine touch and low-frequency vibration	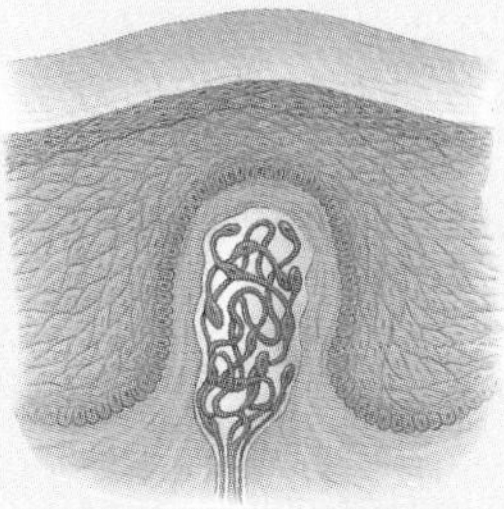
Ruffini's corpuscles	Skin (dermal layer) and subcutaneous tissue of fingers	Touch and pressure	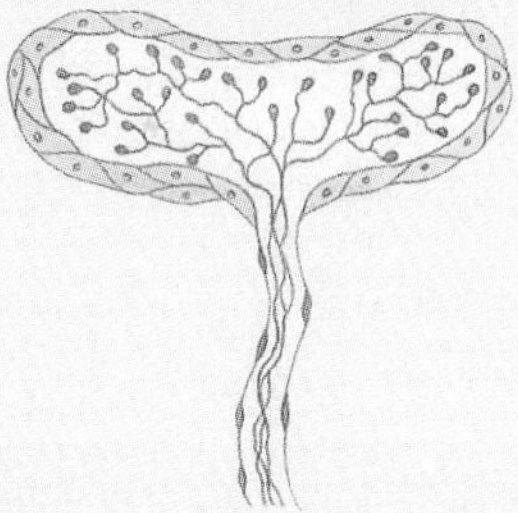
Pacinian corpuscles	Subcutaneous, submucous, and subserous tissues; around joints, in mammary glands and external genitals of both sexes	Pressure and high-frequency vibration	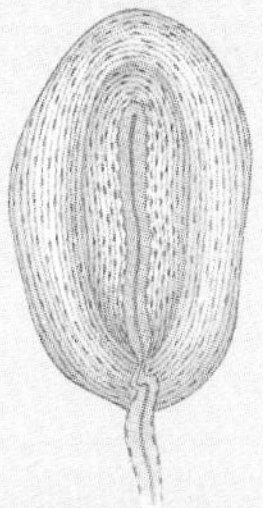

Continued

TABLE 9-1

General Sense Organs—cont'd

TYPE	MAIN LOCATION	GENERAL SENSES	
ENCAPSULATED NERVE ENDINGS—cont'd			
Krause's end-bulbs	Skin (dermal layer), subcutaneous tissue, mucosa of lips and eyelids, and external genitals	Touch and possibly cold	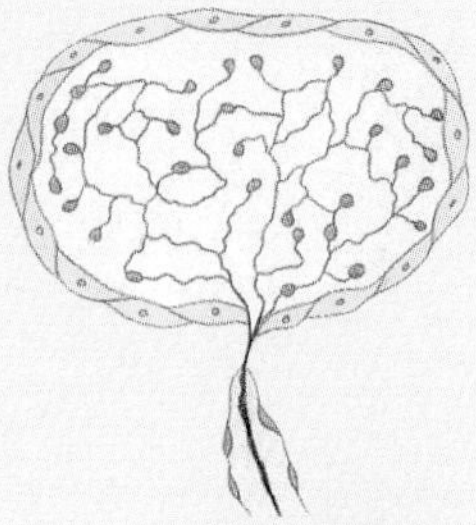
Golgi tendon receptors	Near junction of tendons and muscles	Proprioception (sense of muscle tension)	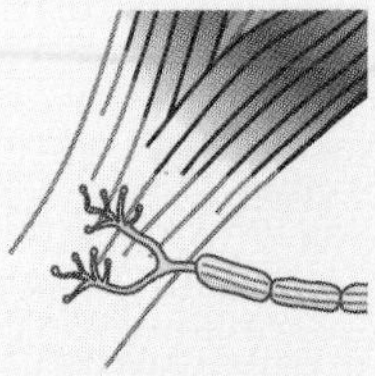
Muscle spindles	Skeletal muscles	Proprioception (sense of muscle length)	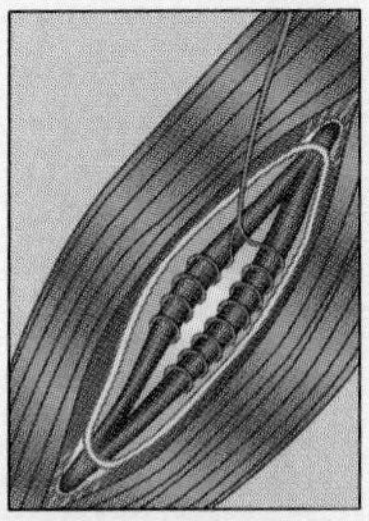

TABLE 9-2

Special Sense Organs

SENSE ORGAN	SPECIFIC RECEPTOR	TYPE OF RECEPTOR	SENSE
Eye	Rods and cones	Photoreceptor	Vision
Ear	Organ of Corti	Mechanoreceptor	Hearing
	Cristae ampullares	Mechanoreceptor	Balance
Nose	Olfactory cells	Chemoreceptor	Smell
Taste buds	Gustatory cells	Chemoreceptor	Taste

FIGURE 9-1

General sense receptors. This section of skin shows the placement of a number of receptors described in Table 9-1.

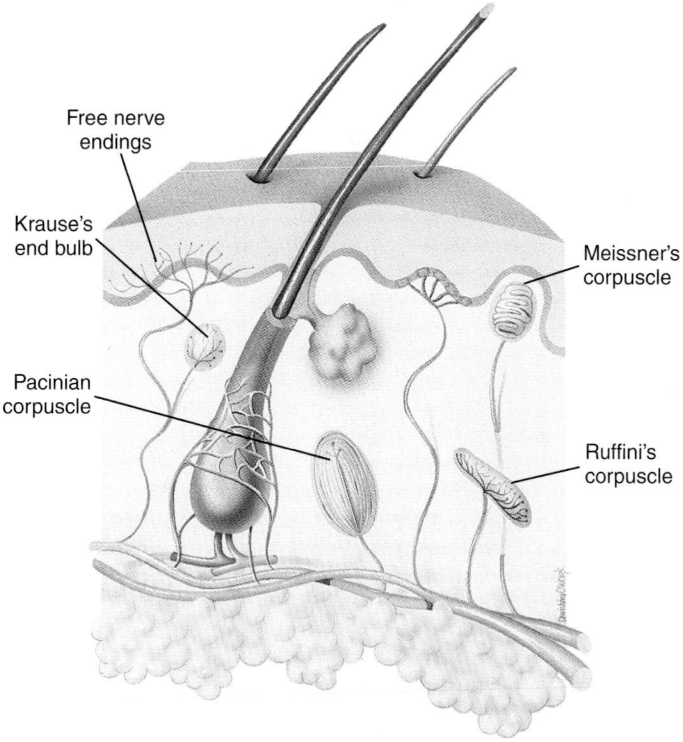

Quick

1. What are different ways that sense organs can be classified into types?
2. Where is a sensation actually perceived?
3. What is the function of a *proprioceptor*?

SPECIAL SENSE ORGANS

The Eye

When you look at a person's eye, you see only a small part of the whole eye. Three layers of tissue form the eyeball: the **sclera** (SKLE-rah), the **choroid** (KO-royd), and the **retina** (RET-i-nah) (Figure 9-2). The outer layer of sclera consists of tough fibrous tissue. The "white" of the eye is part of the front surface of the sclera. The other part of the front surface of the sclera is called the *cornea* and is sometimes spoken of as the window of the eye because of its transparency. At a casual glance, however, it does not look transparent but appears blue, brown, gray, or green because it lies over the **iris,** the colored part of the eye. A mucous membrane known as the **conjunctiva** (kon-junk-TEE-vah) lines the eyelids and covers the sclera in front. The conjunctiva is kept moist by tears formed in the **lacrimal gland.**

The middle layer of the eyeball, the *choroid*, contains a dark pigment to prevent the scattering of incoming light rays. Two involuntary muscles make up the front part of the choroid. One is the iris, the colored structure seen through the cornea, and the other is the *ciliary muscle* (Figure 9-2). The

FIGURE 9-2

Horizontal section through the left eyeball. The eye is viewed from above.

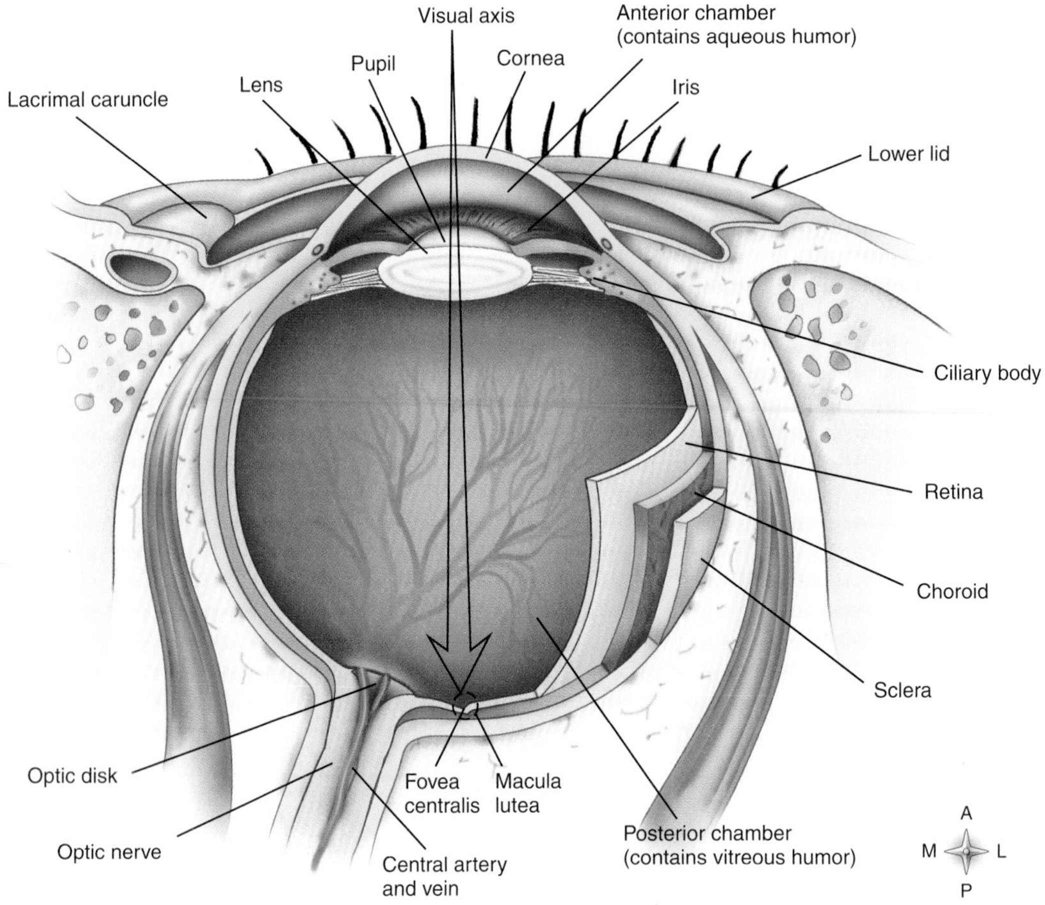

black center of the iris is really a hole in this doughnut-shaped muscle; it is the **pupil** of the eye. Some of the fibers of the iris are arranged like spokes in a wheel. When they contract, the pupils dilate, letting in more light rays. Other fibers are circular. When they contract, the pupils constrict, letting in fewer light rays. Normally, the pupils constrict in bright light and dilate in dim light.

The **lens** of the eye lies directly behind the pupil. It is held in place by a ligament attached to the ciliary muscle. When we look at distant objects, the ciliary muscle is relaxed, and the lens has only a slightly curved shape. To focus on near objects, the ciliary muscle must contract. As it contracts, it pulls the choroid coat forward toward the lens, thus causing the lens to bulge and curve even more. Most of us become more farsighted as we grow older and lose the ability to focus on close objects because our lenses lose at least some of their elasticity and can no longer bulge enough to bring near objects into focus. **Presbyopia** (pres-be-O-pe-ah) or "oldsightedness" is the name for this condition.

In most young people, the lens is both transparent and somewhat elastic so that it is capable of changing shape. Unfortunately, in some individuals, long-time exposure to ultraviolet (UV) radia-

Clinical Application

Refractive Eye Surgery

A surgical technique to treat myopia (nearsightedness) without the use of eyeglasses or contact lenses became available almost 25 years ago. The procedure, called **radial keratotomy (RK),** involves surgical placement of six or more radial slits (incisions) in a spokelike pattern around the cornea. As a result, the cornea flattens and the ability to focus improves. Other incisional types of refractory eye surgery include **astigmatic keratotomy (AK),** which involves treatment of astigmatism by placement of transverse cuts across the corneal surface; and **automated lamellar keratoplasty (ALK).** The ALK technique uses a special surgical device called a *microkeratome* to cut a thin cap off the corneal surface and then shave and reshape the underlying tissue. At the end of the procedure the corneal cap is replaced and will heal without the need for sutures. ALK is used to treat both myopia and hyperopia (farsightedness).

More recent advances in refractory eye surgery involve the use of surgical lasers. **Excimer laser surgery,** also called **photorefractive keratectomy (PRK),** uses a "cool" excimer laser beam to vaporize corneal tissue. It is used to flatten the cornea to correct mild to moderate nearsightedness. A recent refractive eye surgery procedure to correct myopia is called **laser-assisted in situ keratomileusis (LASIK).** This procedure employs both PRK and ALK techniques. First, a microkeratome is used to create a hinged cap of tissue, which is lifted off the corneal surface (*A*). An excimer laser is then used to vaporize and reshape the underlying tissue (*B*). At the end of the procedure, the cap is replaced (*C*). Another laser surgery recently approved by the U.S. Food and Drug Administration for treating hyperopia (farsightedness) is laser thermal keratoplasty (LTK). Ultra-short bursts of laser energy (lasting 3 seconds) are used to reshape the surface of the cornea, with no surgical cutting involved. Yet another recently approved treatment for correction of farsightedness is called **conductive keratoplasty (CK).** Instead of a scalpel or laser, it employs radiofrequency energy to heat hair-thin probes that are then used to change the shape of the cornea.

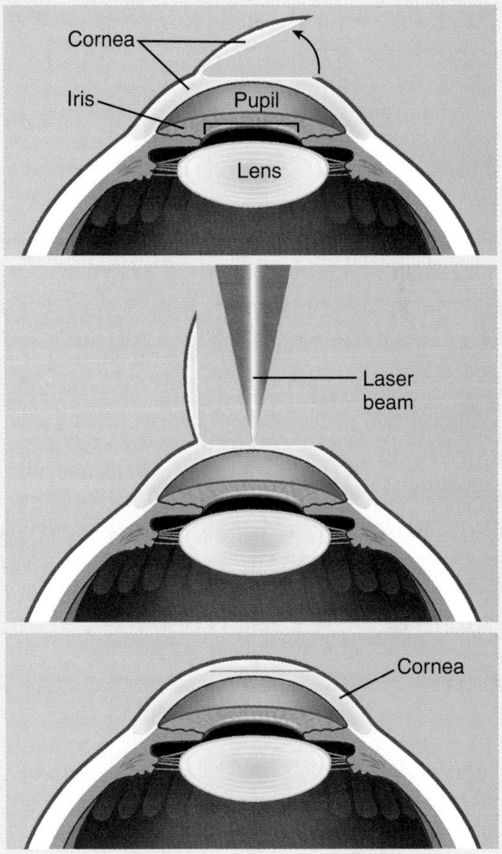

tion in sunlight may cause the lens to become hard, lose its transparency, and become "milky" in appearance. This condition is called a **cataract.** Cataract formation may occur in one or both eyes, tends to be progressive, and may result in blindness. Cataracts can be removed surgically and the defective lens replaced with an artificial implant.

The *retina* or innermost layer of the eyeball contains microscopic photoreceptor cells, called *rods* and *cones* because of their shapes. Dim light can stimulate the rods, but fairly bright light is necessary to stimulate the cones. In other words, **rods** are the receptors for night vision and **cones** are the receptors for daytime vision. There are three kinds of cones; each is sensitive to a different color: red, green, or blue. Scattered throughout the central portion of the retina, these three types of cones allow us to distinguish between different colors.

Clinical Application

Visual Acuity

Visual acuity is the clearness or sharpness of visual perception. Acuity is affected by our focusing ability, the efficiency of the retina, and the proper function of the visual pathway and processing centers in the brain.

One common way to measure visual acuity is to use the familiar test chart on which letters or other objects of various sizes and shapes are printed. The subject is asked to identify the smallest object that he or she can see from a distance of 20 feet (6.1 m). The resulting determination of visual acuity is expressed as a double number such as "20-20." The first number represents the distance (in feet) between the subject and the test chart—the standard being 20. The second number represents the number of feet a person with normal acuity would have to stand to see the same objects clearly. Thus a finding of 20-20 is normal because the subject can see at 20 feet what a person with normal acuity can see at 20 feet. A person with 20-100 vision can see objects at 20 feet that a person with normal vision can see at 100 feet.

People whose acuity is worse than 20-200 after correction are considered to be legally blind. Legal blindness is the designation used to identify the severity of a wide variety of visual disorders so that laws that involve visual acuity can be enforced. For example, laws that govern the awarding of driving licenses require that drivers have a minimum level of visual acuity.

Research, Issues & Trends

Corneal Ring Implants

One of the most recent advances in treatment of mild to moderate nearsightedness (myopia) involves implantation of tiny plastic rings around the edge of the cornea. These transparent rings, called *Intacs*, flatten the cornea without any actual cutting or shaving of the corneal surface or underlying tissue that occurs during incisional or laser-based refractive eye surgery techniques.

Clinical Application

Finding Your Blind Spot

Demonstrate the location of the blind spot in your visual field by covering your left eye and looking at the objects below. While staring at the square, begin about 35 cm (12 in) from objects and slowly bring the figures closer to your eye. At one point, the circle will seem to disappear because its image has fallen on the blind spot.

■ ●

There is a yellowish area near the center of the retina called the *macula lutea.* It surrounds a small depression, called the **fovea centralis,** which contains the greatest concentration of cones of any area of the retina (see Figure 9-2). In good light, greater *visual acuity*, or sharpness of visual perception, can be obtained if we look directly at an object and focus the image on the fovea. But in dim light or darkness, we see an object better if we look slightly to the side of it, thereby focusing the image nearer the periphery of the retina, where the rods are more plentiful.

Fluids fill the hollow inside of the eyeball. They maintain the normal shape of the eyeball and help refract light rays; that is, the fluids bend light rays to bring them to focus on the retina. **Aqueous humor** is the name of the watery fluid in front of the lens (in the anterior chamber of the eye), and **vitreous humor** is the name of the jellylike fluid behind the lens (in the posterior chamber). Aqueous humor is constantly being formed, drained, and replaced in the anterior chamber. If drainage is blocked for any reason, the internal pressure within the eye will increase, and damage that could lead to blindness will occur. This condition is called **glaucoma** (glaw-KO-mah).

FIGURE 9-3

Cells of the retina. Photoreceptors called rods and cones (notice their shapes) detect changes in light and relay the information to bipolar neurons. The bipolar cells, in turn, conduct the information to ganglion cells. The information eventually leaves the eye by way of the optic nerve.

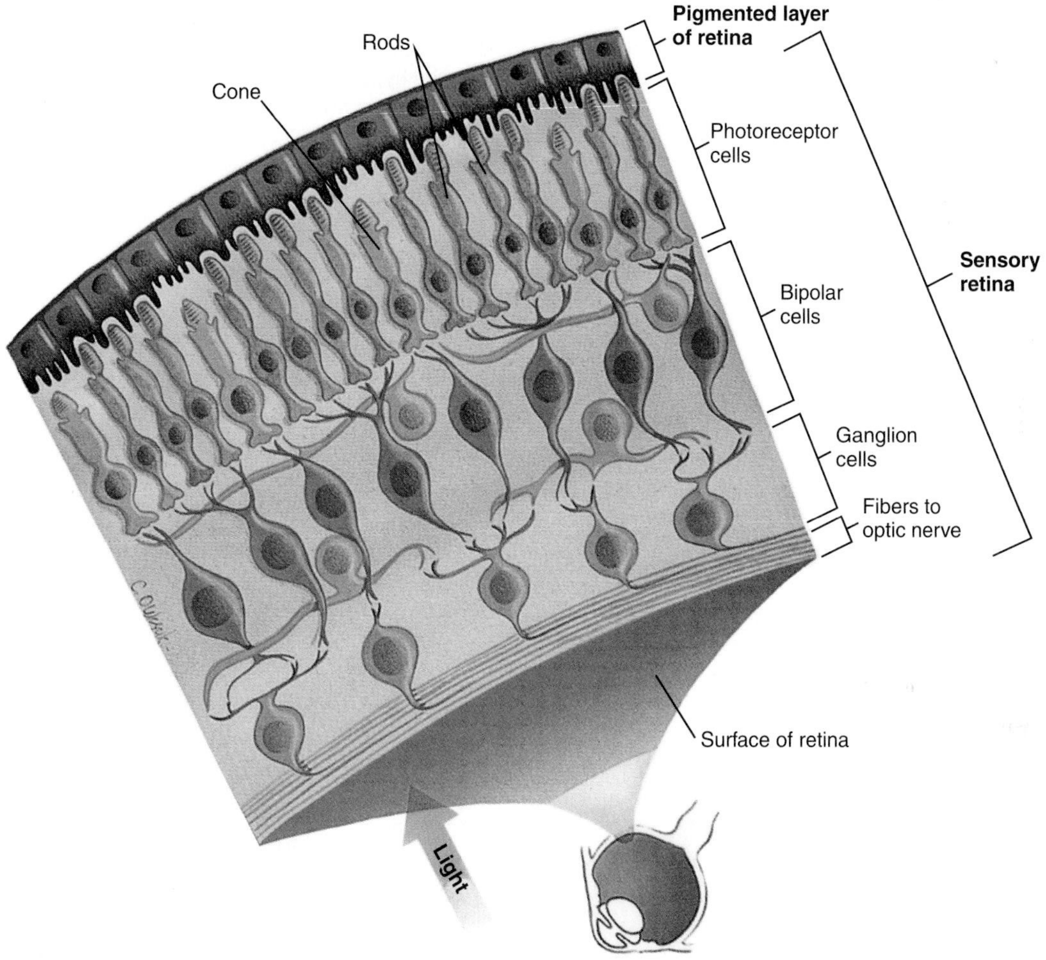

Visual Pathway

Light is the stimulus that results in vision (that is, our ability to see objects as they exist in our environment). Light enters the eye through the pupil and is *refracted*, or bent, so that it is focused on the retina. Refraction occurs as light passes through the cornea, the aqueous humor, the lens, and the vitreous humor on its way to the retina.

The innermost layer of the retina contains the rods and cones, which are the *photoreceptor* cells of the eye (Figure 9-3). They respond to a light stimulus by producing a nervous impulse. The rod and cone photoreceptor cells synapse with neurons in the bipolar and ganglionic layers of the retina. Nervous signals eventually leave the retina and exit the eye through the optic nerve on the posterior surface of the eyeball. No rods or cones are present in the area of the retina where the optic nerve fibers exit. The result is a "blind spot" known as the *optic disc* (see Figure 9-2).

Clinical Application

Focusing Problems

Focusing a clear image on the retina is essential for good vision. In the normal eye (*A*), light rays enter the eye and are focused into a clear, upside-down image on the retina. The brain can easily right the upside-down image in our conscious perception but cannot fix an image that is not sharply focused. If our eyes are elongated (*B*), the image focuses in front of the retina rather than on it. The retina receives only a fuzzy image. This condition, called **myopia** or *nearsightedness*, can be corrected by using contact lenses, glasses (*C*), or refractive eye surgery. If our eyes are shorter than normal (*D*), the image focuses behind the retina, also producing a fuzzy image. This condition, called **hyperopia** or *farsightedness*, can also be corrected by lenses (*E*) or refractive surgery. *Astigmatism* is an abnormal eye condition resulting in blurred vision. It is caused by an irregular curvature of the lens.

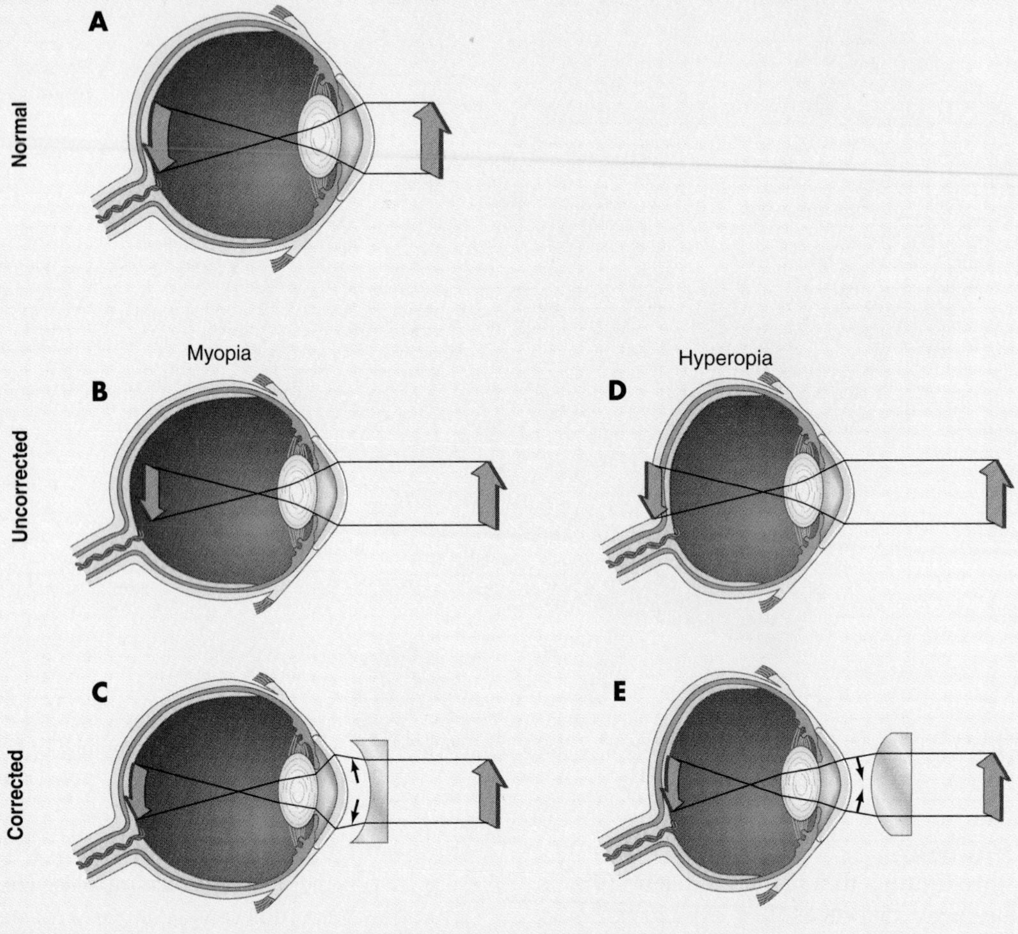

Clinical Application

Color Blindness

Color blindness, usually an inherited condition, is caused by mistakes in producing three chemicals called *photopigments* in the cones. Each photopigment is sensitive to one of the three primary colors of light: green, blue, and red. In many cases, the green-sensitive photopigment is missing or deficient; other times, the red-sensitive photopigment is abnormal. (Deficiency of the blue-sensitive photopigment is very rare.) Color-blind individuals see colors, but they cannot distinguish between them normally.

Figures such as those shown here are often used to screen individuals for color blindness. A person with red-green blindness cannot see the 74 in Figure A, whereas a person with normal vision can. To determine which photopigment is deficient, a color-blind person may try a figure similar to B. Persons with a deficiency of red-sensitive photopigment can distinguish only the 2; those deficient in green-sensitive photopigment can only see the 4.

A

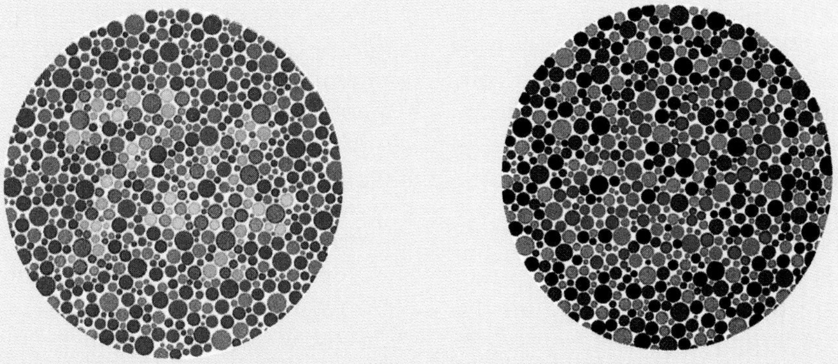

B

Research, Issues & Trends

Corneal Stem Cell Transplants

A new treatment for individuals who may be totally blind because of certain eye diseases, or because of scarring caused by abrasion or chemical burns to their corneas may make it possible for them to see again. If, because of accident or disease, the clear membrane covering the cornea is permanently destroyed and cannot be regenerated, blindness results. In these cases, traditional corneal transplants are not possible because a clear membrane formed by the eye of the recipient is necessary for survival of the transplanted tissue. Research now indicates that **corneal stem cell transplants** can restore and maintain the clear covering membrane of the cornea that may have been destroyed by disease or injury.

In this procedure, stem cells that have the ability to develop into the clear covering membrane of the cornea are first harvested from the corneas of cadavers and then transplanted into and around the edges of the diseased or damaged corneas of the blind recipient. The new stem cells then produce the clear corneal surface membrane required for normal vision. This technique is in the research stage and has limited applications, and problems associated with rejection of the foreign stem cells and suppression of the immune system of the recipient must still be resolved. However, this exciting new development in clinical medicine can effectively treat blindness that was considered permanent in the past.

After leaving the eye, the optic nerves enter the brain and travel to the visual cortex of the occipital lobe. In this area, *visual interpretation* of the nervous impulses generated by light stimuli in the rods and cones of the retina result in "seeing."

Quick

1. What are the three layers of the eyeball?
2. What are the *humors* of the eye?
3. How are rods and cones used in vision? How are they alike? How are they different?

The Ear

In addition to its role in hearing, the ear also functions as the sense organ of equilibrium and balance. As we shall later see, the stimulation or "trigger" that activates receptors involved with hearing and equilibrium is mechanical, and the receptors themselves are called *mechanoreceptors* (mek-an-o-ree-SEP-tors). Physical forces that involve sound vibrations and fluid movements are responsible for initiating nervous impulses eventually perceived as sound and balance.

The ear is more than an appendage on the side of the head. A large part of the ear and its most important functional part lies hidden from view deep inside the temporal bone. The ear is divided into the following anatomical areas (Figure 9-4):

1. External ear
2. Middle ear
3. Inner (internal) ear

External Ear

The external ear has two parts: the **auricle** (AW-ri-kul) or pinna and the **external auditory canal.** The auricle is the appendage on the side of the head surrounding the opening of the external auditory canal. The canal itself is a curving tube about 2.5 cm (1 inch) in length. It extends into the temporal bone and ends at the **tympanic** (tim-PAN-ik) **membrane** or **eardrum,** which is a partition between the external and middle ear. The skin of the auditory canal, especially in its outer one third, contains many short hairs and **ceruminous** (se-ROO-mi-nus) **glands** that produce a waxy substance called *cerumen* that may collect in the canal and impair hearing by absorbing or blocking the passage of sound waves. Sound waves traveling through the external auditory canal strike the tympanic membrane and cause it to vibrate.

Middle Ear

The middle ear is a tiny and very thin epithelium-lined cavity hollowed out of the temporal bone. It houses three very small bones. The names of these ear bones, called **ossicles** (OS-si-kuls), describe their shapes: **malleus** (hammer), **incus** (anvil), and **stapes** (stirrup). The "handle" of the malleus attaches to the inside of the tympanic membrane, and the "head" attaches to the incus. The incus attaches to the stapes, and the stapes presses against a membrane that covers a small opening, the *oval window.* The oval window separates the middle ear from the inner ear. When sound waves cause the eardrum to vibrate, that movement is transmitted and amplified by the ear ossicles as it passes through the middle ear. Movement of the stapes against the oval window causes movement of fluid in the inner ear.

A point worth mentioning, because it explains the frequent spread of infection from the throat to the ear, is the fact that a tube—the auditory or **eustachian** (yoo-STAY-shen) **tube**—connects the throat with the middle ear. The epithelial lining of the middle ears, auditory tubes, and throat are extensions of one continuous membrane. As a consequence, a sore throat may spread to produce a middle ear infection called *otitis* (o-TIE-tis) *media* (ME-dee-ah).

Inner Ear

The activation of specialized mechanoreceptors in the inner ear generates nervous impulses that result in hearing and equilibrium. Anatomically, the inner ear consists of three spaces in the temporal bone, assembled in a complex maze called the **bony labyrinth** (LAB-i-rinth). This odd-shaped bony space is filled with a watery fluid called **perilymph** (PAIR-i-limf) and is divided into the following parts: **vestibule** (VES-ti-byool), **semicircular canals,** and **cochlea** (KOK-lee-ah). The vestibule is adjacent to the oval window between the semicircular canals and the cochlea (Figure 9-5). Note in Figure 9-5 that a balloonlike

FIGURE 9-4

The ear. External, middle, and inner ears.

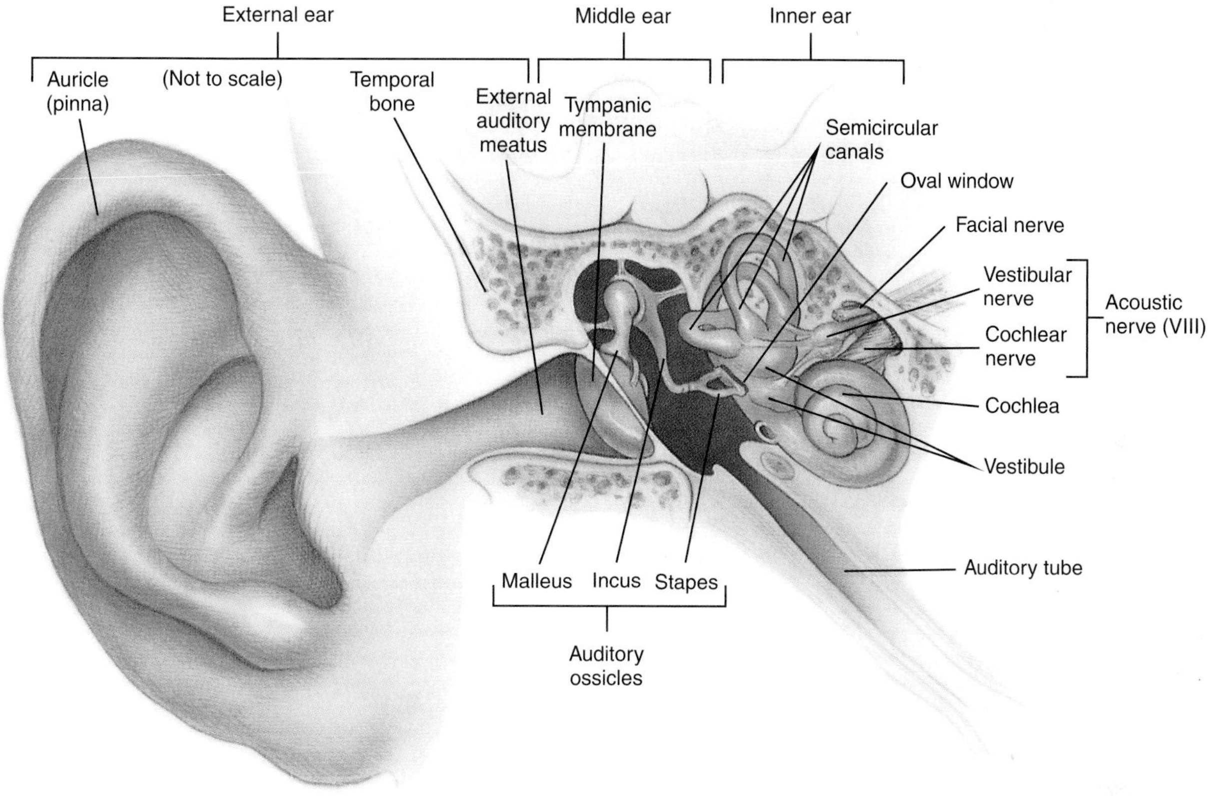

membranous sac is suspended in the perilymph and follows the shape of the bony labyrinth much like a "tube within a tube." This is the **membranous labyrinth,** and it is filled with a thicker fluid called **endolymph** (EN-doe-limf).

The specialized mechanoreceptors for balance and equilibrium are located in the three semicircular canals and the vestibule. The three half-circle semicircular canals are oriented at right angles to one another (see Figure 9-5). Within each canal is a dilated area called the *ampulla* that contains a specialized receptor called a **crista** (KRIS-tah) **ampullaris** (am-pyoo-LAIR-is), which generates a nerve impulse when you move your head. The sensory cells in the cristae ampullares have hair-like extensions that are suspended in the endolymph. The sensory cells are stimulated when movement of the head causes the endolymph to move, thus causing the hairs to bend. Nerves from other receptors in the vestibule join those from the semicircular canals to form the **vestibular nerve,** which joins with the cochlear nerve to form the acoustic nerve or cranial nerve VIII (see Figure 9-5). Eventually, nervous impulses passing through this nerve reach the cerebellum and medulla. Other connections from these areas result in impulses reaching the cerebral cortex.

The organ of hearing, which lies in the snail-shaped cochlea, is the **organ of Corti** (KOR-tie). It is surrounded by endolymph, filling the membranous cochlea or **cochlear duct,** which is the membranous tube within the bony cochlea. Specialized hair cells

FIGURE 9-5

The inner ear. The bony labyrinth (orange) is the hard outer wall of the entire inner ear, and includes semicircular canals, vestibule, and cochlea. Within the bony labyrinth is the membranous labyrinth (purple), which is surrounded by perilymph and filled with endolymph. Each ampulla in the vestibule contains a crista ampullaris that detects changes in head position and sends sensory impulses through the vestibular nerve to the brain. The inset shows a section of the membranous cochlea. Hair cells in the organ of Corti detect sound and send the information through the cochlear nerve. The vestibular and cochlear nerves join to form the eighth cranial nerve.

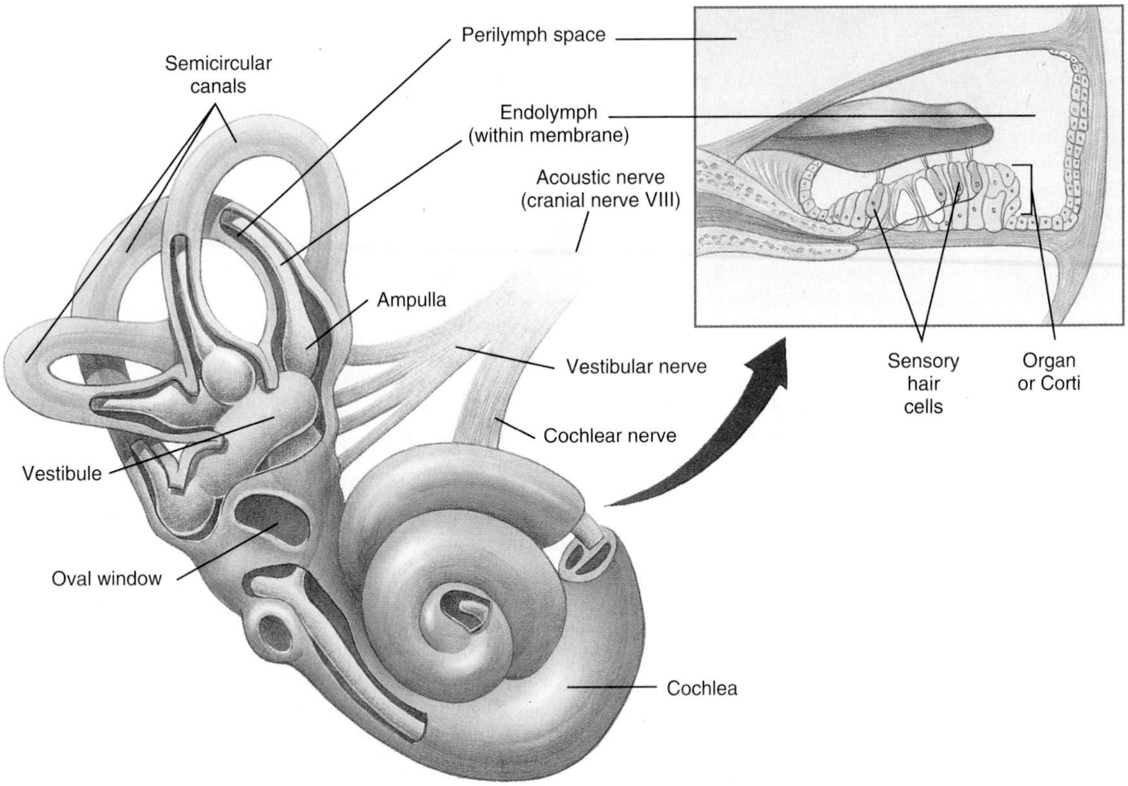

on the organ of Corti generate nerve impulses when they are bent by the movement of endolymph set in motion by sound waves (Figures 9-5 and 9-6).

Quick

1. What senses are detected in the ear?
2. Can you describe the three main parts of the ear?
3. How do the ossicles work in helping a person to hear?
4. Where are the receptor cells for hearing?

Health & Well-Being

Swimmer's Ear

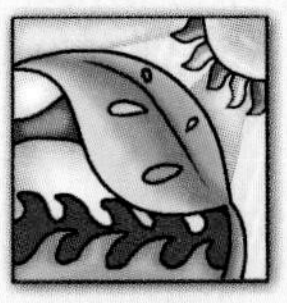

External otitis or *swimmer's ear* is a common infection of the external ear in athletes. It can be bacterial or fungal in origin and is usually associated with prolonged exposure to water. The infection generally involves, at least to some extent, the auditory canal and auricle. The ear as a whole is tender, red, and swollen. Treatment of swimmer's ear usually involves antibiotic therapy and prescription analgesics.

FIGURE 9-6

Effect of sound waves on cochlear structures. Sound waves strike the tympanic membrane and cause it to vibrate. This vibration causes the membrane of the oval window to vibrate. This vibration causes the perilymph in the bony labyrinth of the cochlea to move, which causes the endolymph in the membranous labyrinth of the cochlea or cochlear duct to move. This movement of endolymph stimulates hair cells on the organ of Corti to generate a nerve impulse. The nerve impulse travels over the cochlear nerve, which becomes a part of the eighth cranial nerve. Eventually, nerve impulses reach the auditory cortex and are interpreted as sound.

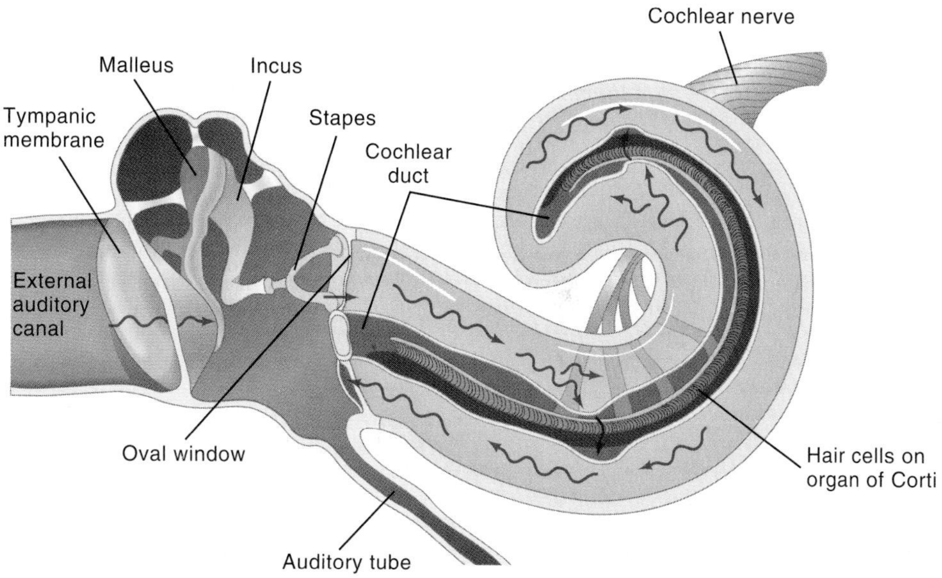

Clinical Application

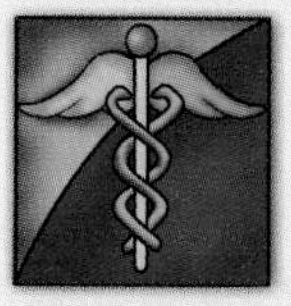

Cochlear Implants

Advances in electronic circuitry are now being used to correct some forms of nerve deafness. If the hairs on the organ of Corti are damaged, nerve deafness results—even if the vestibulocochlear nerve is healthy. A surgically implanted device can improve this form of hearing loss by eliminating the need for the sensory hairs. As you can see in the figure, a transmitter just outside the scalp sends external sound information to a receiver under the scalp (behind the auricle). The receiver translates the information into an electrical code that is relayed down an electrode to the cochlea. The electrode, wired to the organ of Corti, stimulates the vestibulocochlear nerve endings directly. Thus even though the cochlear hair cells are damaged, sound can still be perceived.

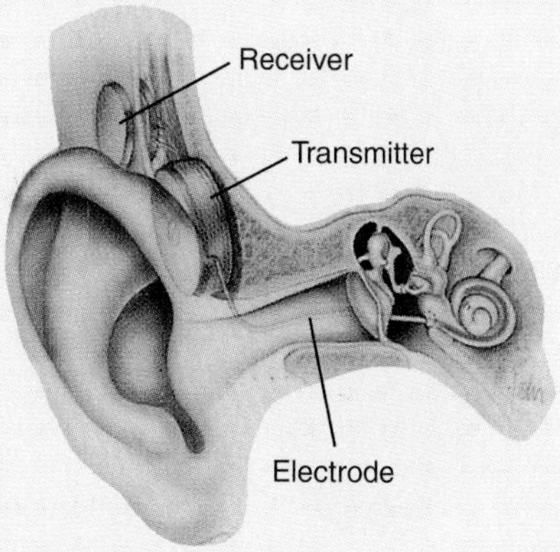

The Taste Receptors

The **taste buds** are the sense organs of taste. They contain both supporting cells and the chemoreceptors, called *gustatory* (GUS-tah-toe-ree) *cells,* which generate the nervous impulses ultimately interpreted by the brain as taste (Figure 9-7). Although a few taste buds are located in the lining of the mouth and on the soft palate, most are located on the sides of much larger and differing shaped bumps scattered across the tongue called **papillae** (pa-PIL-e). About 10-15 large *circumvallate papillae,* that form an inverted "V" pattern at the back of the tongue, contain the most taste buds. Each taste bud, as you can see in Figure 9-7, opens through an opening into a trenchlike moat that surrounds the papilla and is filled with saliva. Chemicals dissolved in the saliva stimulate the chemoreceptor gustatory cells.

Although current research suggests that we may be able to sense a large number of discrete tastes, most physiologists continue to list four kinds of "primary" taste sensations—sweet, sour, bitter, and salty—that result from stimulation of taste buds. In addition, lists of "primary" tastes sometimes include metallic and a meaty flavor discovered by Japanese researchers called umami (O-mommy). Most other flavors result from a combination of taste bud and olfactory receptor stimulation. In other words, the myriad tastes we recognize are not tastes alone but tastes plus odors. For this reason a cold that interferes with the stimulation of the olfactory receptors by odors from foods in the mouth markedly dulls taste sensations. Nervous impulses that are generated by stimulation of taste buds travel primarily through two cranial nerves (VII and IX) to end in the specialized taste area of the cerebral cortex.

FIGURE 9-7

The tongue. A, Dorsal surface of tongue showing circumvallate papillae. **B,** Section through a papilla with taste buds on the side. **C,** Enlarged view of a section through a taste bud. **D,** Scanning electron micrograph of tongue surface showing the papillae in detail.

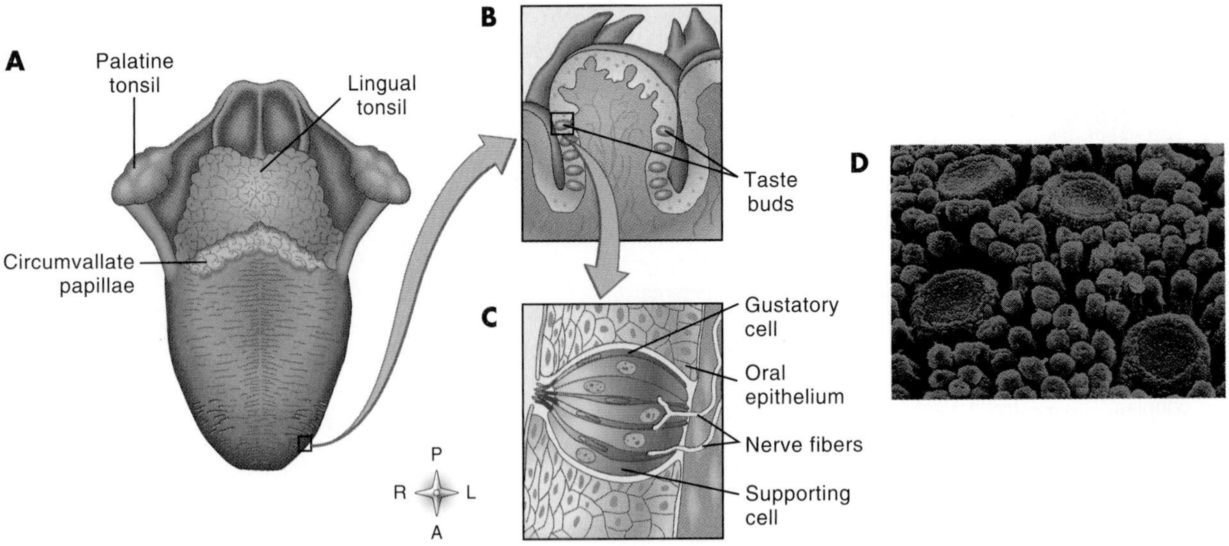

The Smell Receptors

The chemoreceptors responsible for the sense of smell are located in a small area of epithelial tissue in the upper part of the nasal cavity (Figure 9-8). The location of the **olfactory receptors** is somewhat hidden, and we must often forcefully sniff the air to smell delicate odors. Each olfactory cell has a number of specialized cilia that sense different chemicals and cause the cell to respond by generating a nervous impulse. To be detected by olfactory receptors, chemicals must be dissolved in the watery mucus that lines the nasal cavity.

Although the olfactory receptors are extremely sensitive (that is, stimulated by even very slight odors), they are also easily adapted and lose their ability to respond—a fact that explains why odors that are at first very noticeable are not sensed at all after a short time. After the olfactory cells are stimulated by odor-causing chemicals, the resulting nerve impulse travels through the olfactory nerves in the olfactory bulb and tract and then enters the thalamic and olfactory centers of the brain, where the nervous impulses are interpreted as specific odors. The pathways taken by olfactory nerve impulses and the areas where these impulses are interpreted are closely associated with areas of the brain important in memory and emotion. For this reason, we may retain vivid and long-lasting memories of particular smells and odors. The pleasant smell of bread or cookies baking in a grandmother's kitchen may be part of a memory that lasts a lifetime.

Quick Check

1. Where are taste receptors located?
2. Can you name the primary tastes that humans can perceive?
3. What is the job of olfactory receptors?

FIGURE 9-8

Olfactory structures. Gas molecules stimulate olfactory cells in the nasal epithelium. Sensory information is then conducted along nerves in the olfactory bulb and olfactory tract to sensory processing centers in the brain.

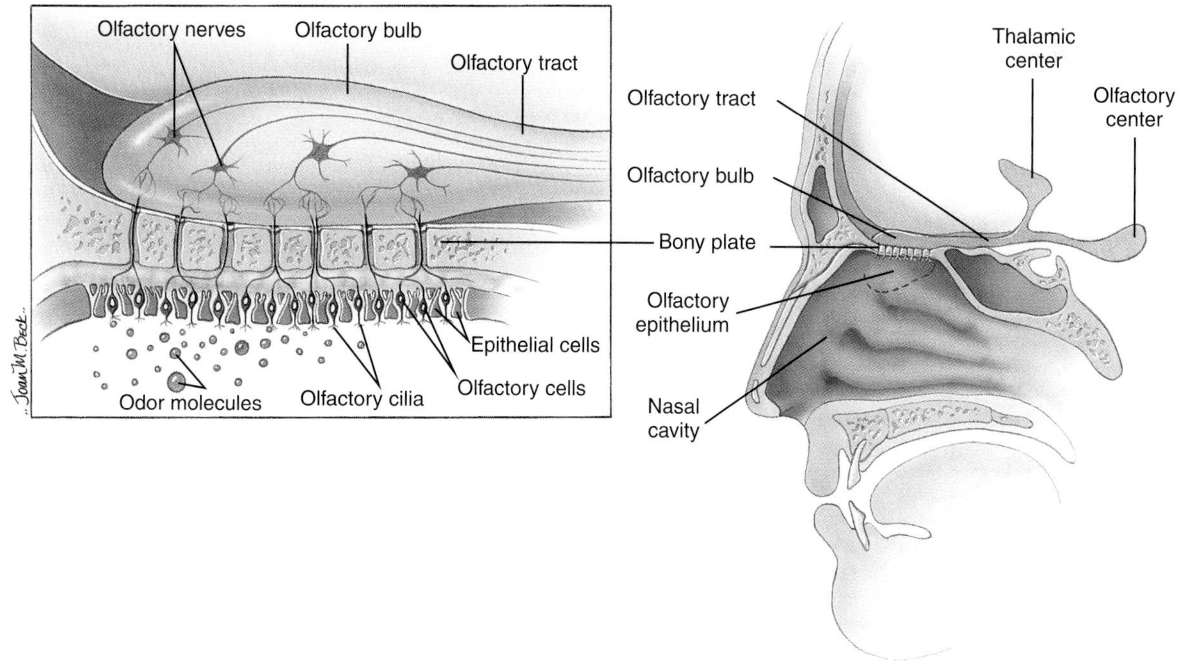

Science Applications

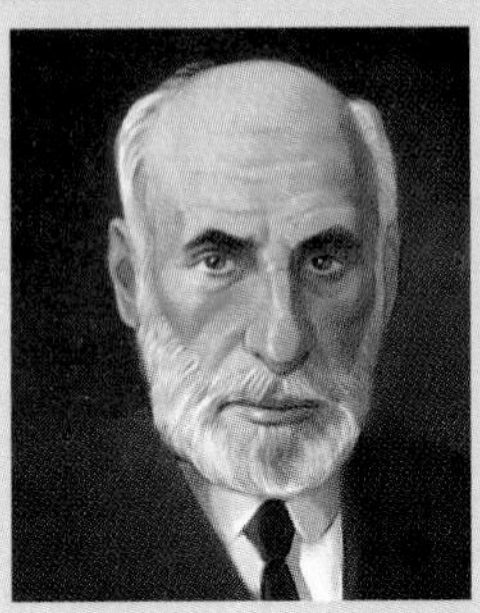

The Senses

Santiago Ramón y Cajal (1852-1934).

Santiago Ramón y Cajal is considered by many to be the originator of the modern view of the nervous system's organization. He not only uncovered much about sensory centers of the cortex and the structure of the retina, but made important discoveries about nearly every part of the nervous system. Most of this Spanish researcher's ideas about the nervous system are intact today. Although Santiago wanted to be an artist, his father convinced him to follow in his footsteps as an anatomist—a choice that led to a Nobel Prize in 1906.

The study of the sensory part of the nervous system and its relationships with the rest of the body is useful in many different fields. For example, the ideas used by optometrists and ophthalmologists, otologists and audiologists, and other professionals who assess and treat sensory disorders are based on neuroscience. Many other fields can make indirect use of neuroscience as well. For example, artists use what we know of visual perception in creating their works, musicians and architects make use of our knowledge of sound perception when performing in or designing concert halls, and aerospace professionals can use what we know of equilibrium and how it is perceived in the brain to understand motion sickness.

OUTLINE SUMMARY

CLASSIFICATION OF SENSE ORGANS

A. General sense organs (Table 9-1)
   1. Often exist as individual cells or receptor units
   2. Widely distributed throughout the body
B. Special sense organs (Table 9-2)
   1. Large and complex organs
   2. Localized grouping of specialized receptors
C. Classification by presence or absence of covering capsule
   1. Encapsulated
   2. Unencapsulated ("free" or "naked")
D. Classification by type of stimuli required to activate receptors
   1. Photoreceptors (light)
   2. Chemoreceptors (chemicals)
   3. Pain receptors (injury)
   4. Thermoreceptors (temperature change)
   5. Mechanoreceptors (movement or deforming of capsule)
   6. Proprioceptors (position of body parts or changes in muscle length or tension)

CONVERTING A STIMULUS INTO A SENSATION

A. All sense organs have common functional characteristics
   1. All are able to detect a particular stimulus
   2. A stimulus is converted into a nerve impulse
   3. A nerve impulse is perceived as a sensation in the central nervous system

GENERAL SENSE ORGANS (Table 9-1)

A. Distribution is widespread; single-cell receptors are common
B. Examples (Figure 9-1, Table 9-1)
   1. Free nerve endings—pain, temperature, and crude touch
   2. Meissner's corpuscles—fine touch and vibration
   3. Ruffini's corpuscles—touch and pressure
   4. Pacinian corpuscles—pressure and vibration
   5. Krause's end-bulbs—touch
   6. Golgi tendon receptors—proprioception
   7. Muscle spindles—proprioception

SPECIAL SENSE ORGANS

A. The eye (Figure 9-2)
   1. Layers of eyeball
      a. Sclera—tough outer coat; "white" of eye; cornea is transparent part of sclera over iris
      b. Choroid—pigmented vascular layer prevents scattering of light; front part of this layer made of ciliary muscle and iris, the colored part of the eye; the pupil is the hole in the center of the iris; contraction of iris muscle dilates or constricts pupil
      c. Retina (Figure 9-3)—innermost layer of the eye; contains rods (receptors for night vision) and cones (receptors for day vision and color vision)
   2. Conjunctiva—mucous membrane covering the front surface of the sclera and lining the eyelid; kept moist by tears found in the lacrimal gland
   3. Lens—transparent body behind the pupil; focuses light rays on the retina
   4. Eye fluids
      a. Aqueous humor—in the anterior chamber in front of the lens
      b. Vitreous humor—in the posterior chamber behind the lens
   5. Visual pathway
      a. Innermost layer of retina contains rods and cones
      b. Impulse travels from the rods and cones through the bipolar and ganglionic layers of retina (Figure 9-3)
      c. Nerve impulse leaves the eye through the optic nerve; the point of exit is free of receptors and is therefore called a *blind spot*
      d. Visual interpretation occurs in the visual cortex of the cerebrum

Continued

OUTLINE SUMMARY—*cont'd*

B. The ear
  1. The ear functions in hearing and in equilibrium and balance
    a. Receptors for hearing and equilibrium are mechanoreceptors
  2. Divisions of the ear (Figure 9-4)
    a. External ear
      (1) Auricle (pinna)
      (2) External auditory canal
        (a) Curving canal 2.5 cm (1 inch) in length
        (b) Contains ceruminous glands
        (c) Ends at the tympanic membrane
    b. Middle ear
      (1) Houses ear ossicles—malleus, incus, and stapes
      (2) Ends in the oval window
      (3) The auditory (eustachian) tube connects the middle ear to the throat
      (4) Inflammation called *otitis media*
    c. Inner ear (Figure 9-5)
      (1) Bony labyrinth filled with perilymph
      (2) Subdivided into the vestibule, semicircular canals, and cochlea
      (3) Membranous labyrinth filled with endolymph
      (4) The receptors for balance in the semicircular canals are called *cristae ampullaris*
      (5) Specialized hair cells on the organ of Corti respond when bent by the movement of surrounding endolymph set in motion by sound waves (Figure 9-6)

C. The taste receptors (Figure 9-7)
  1. Receptors are chemoreceptors called *taste buds*
  2. Cranial nerves VII and IX carry gustatory impulses
  3. Most pathologists list four kinds of "primary" taste sensations—sweet, sour, bitter, and salty
    a. Metallic and umami (meaty) tastes are also unique and may soon be added to the list of "primary" taste sensations
  4. Gustatory and olfactory senses work together to permit creation of many other taste sensations

D. The smell receptors (Figure 9-8)
  1. Receptors for fibers of olfactory or cranial nerve I lie in olfactory mucosa of nasal cavity
  2. Olfactory receptors are extremely sensitive but easily adapted (fatigued)
  3. Odor-causing chemicals initiate a nervous signal that is interpreted as a specific odor by the brain

NEW WORDS

aqueous humor
auricle
cataract
chemoreceptor
choroid
cochlea
conjunctiva
crista ampullaris
endolymph
glaucoma
gustatory cells
lacrimal gland
lens
mechanoreceptor
organ of Corti
ossicles
papillae
perilymph
photoreceptor
presbyopia
proprioception
pupil
retina
sclera
semicircular canals
tympanic membrane
vitreous humor

REVIEW QUESTIONS

1. Name the general senses found in the skin or subcutaneous tissue and list the type of stimuli to which each of them respond. Which of these are unencapsulated?
2. Name the two general senses of proprioception and give the location of each.
3. With what type of information do proprioceptors provide us?
4. Explain how the iris changes the size of the pupil.
5. Explain how the ciliary muscles allow the eye to focus on near and far objects.
6. What is *presbyopia*, and what is its cause?
7. Name the two types of receptor cells in the retina. Explain the difference between these two receptors.
8. What is *glaucoma*, and what is its cause?
9. What are *cataracts*, how are they caused, and what can be done to prevent them?
10. What is meant by the visual pathway? Where is the blind spot, and what causes it?
11. Briefly explain the structure of the external ear.
12. Explain how sound waves are transmitted through the middle ear.
13. Explain how sound waves are converted to an auditory impulse.
14. Explain how the structures in the inner ear help maintain balance or equilibrium.
15. Where are gustatory cells located, and to what four "primary" tastes do they respond?
16. Explain how the sense of smell is stimulated.

CRITICAL THINKING

17. Explain why food loses some of its taste when you have a bad cold with a stuffy nose.
18. Explain why the longer you are in a newly painted room, the less able you are to smell the paint.
19. Where in the eye is light sensed? Where is it perceived? (Be specific.)
20. Explain why the smell of a "doctor's office" or the smell of a turkey cooking on Thanksgiving can easily generate an emotional response.

CHAPTER TEST

1. The eye can be classified as a photoreceptor. Taste and smell can be classified as __________, and Golgi tendon receptors and muscle spindles can be classified as __________.
2. The specific mechanoreceptor for hearing is the __________.
3. The specific mechanoreceptor for balance is the __________.
4. The gustatory cells are involved with the sense of __________.
5. Four "primary" kinds of taste sensations that result from the stimulation of the taste buds are __________, __________, __________, and __________.
6. Taste buds can be found on much larger structures on the tongue called __________.
7. The chemoreceptors responsible for the sense of smell are the __________.

Continued

CHAPTER TEST—*cont'd*

Match the function or description in Column B with the structure of the eye in Column A.

COLUMN A	COLUMN B
8. ______Sclera	**a.** tears are formed in this gland
9. ______Cornea	**b.** the hole in the eye that lets light in
10. ______Iris	**c.** the receptors for night or dim light vision
11. ______Pupil	**d.** the thick jellylike fluid or humor of the eye
12. ______Lacrimal	**e.** the tough white outer layer of the eye
13. ______Lens	**f.** the receptors for red, blue, and green color vision
14. ______Rods	**g.** the ciliary muscles pull on this to help the eye focus
15. ______Cones	**h.** the dark pigmented middle layer of the eye that prevents the scattering of incoming light
16. ______Choroid coat	**i.** the transparent part of the sclera, the window of the eye
17. ______Vitreous	**j.** the colored part of the front of the eye
18. ______Aqueous	**k.** the thin watery humor of the eye

Match the function or description in Column B with the structure of the ear in Column A.

COLUMN A	COLUMN B
19. ______Tympanic membrane	**a.** the tube connecting the middle ear and the throat
20. ______Ossicles	**b.** the watery fluid that fills the bony labyrinth
21. ______Auditory tube	**c.** the snail-shaped structure in the inner ear
22. ______Perilymph	**d.** this is the organ of hearing
23. ______Endolymph	**e.** the thick fluid in the membranous labyrinth
24. ______Cochlea	**f.** this is another term for eardrum
25. ______Organ of Corti	**g.** the collective name for incus, malleus, and stapes

STUDY TIPS

Each sense must go through the following processes to perform its function: it must detect the physical stimulus to which it responds and it must convert that stimulus into a nerve impulse. For example, the eye must let light in and focus it on a specific point; the receptors must convert that stimulus to a nerve impulse and send it to the brain. When you study structures and their specific functions in a sensory system, try to see how they contribute to one of the two processes.

Use flash cards to learn the specific structures and functions of the sensory systems.

In your study group, discuss how each of the sensory systems detects and responds to a stimulus. Photocopy the figures of the sense organs, blacken out the labels, and quiz each other on the names, locations, and functions of the structures. Go over the questions at the back of the chapter and discuss possible test questions.

10 The Endocrine System

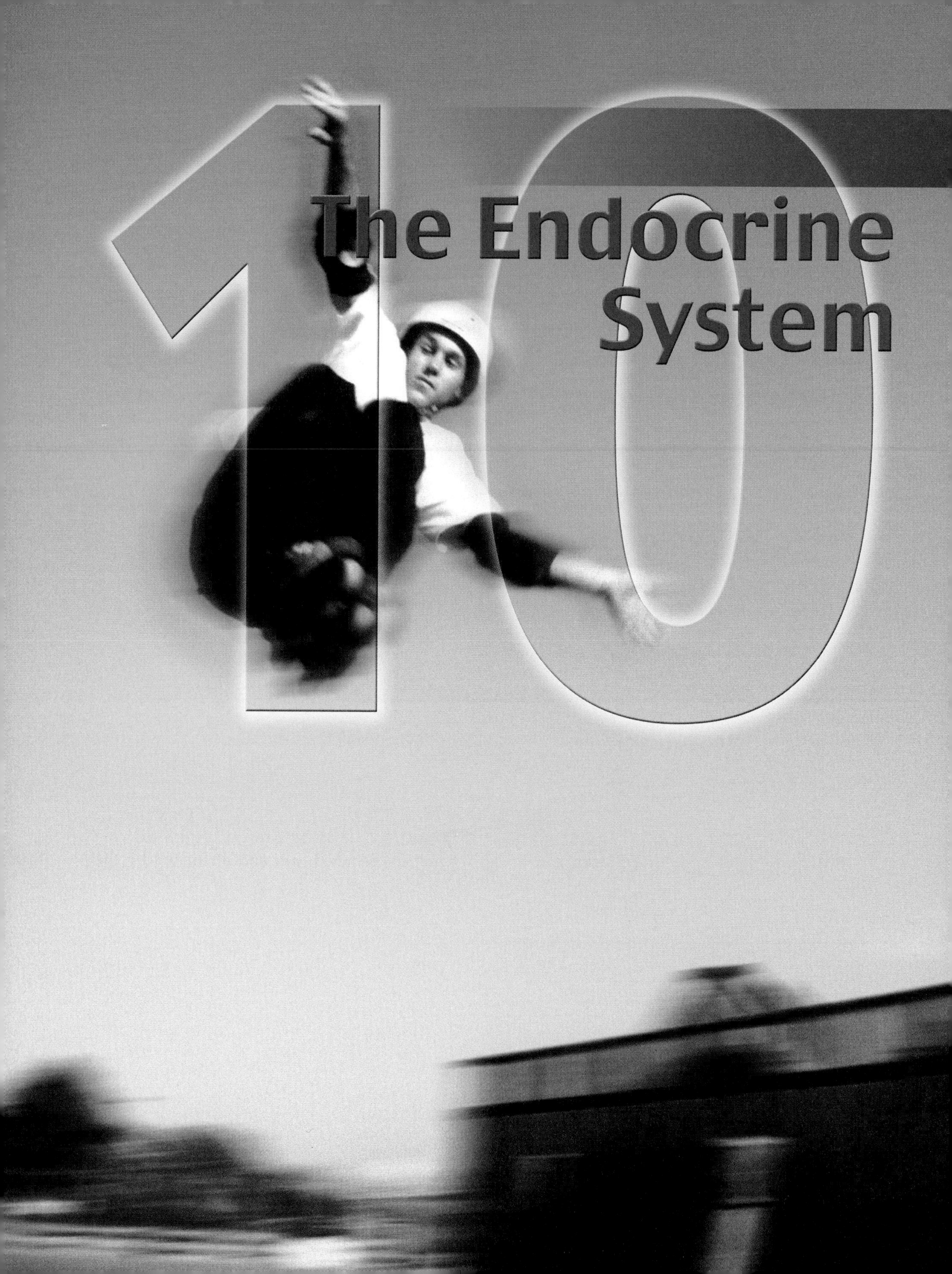

Outline

Objectives

AFTER YOU HAVE COMPLETED THIS CHAPTER, YOU SHOULD BE ABLE TO:

1. Distinguish between endocrine and exocrine glands and define the terms *hormone* and *prostaglandin.*
2. Identify and locate the primary endocrine glands and list the major hormones produced by each gland.
3. Describe the mechanisms of steroid and nonsteroid hormone action.
4. Explain how negative and positive feedback mechanisms regulate the secretion of endocrine hormones.
5. Identify the principal functions of each major endocrine hormone and describe the conditions that may result from hyposecretion or hypersecretion.
6. Define *diabetes insipidus, diabetes mellitus, gigantism, goiter, cretinism,* and *glycosuria.*

H*ave you ever* known anyone with thyroid problems or diabetes? Surely you've seen the dramatic changes that happen to a person's body as they go through puberty. These are all proof of the importance of the endocrine system for normal development and health.

The **endocrine system** performs the same general functions as the nervous system: communication and control. The nervous system provides rapid, brief control by fast-traveling nerve impulses. The endocrine system provides slower but longer-lasting control by **hormones** (chemicals) secreted into and circulated by the blood.

The organs of the endocrine system are located in widely separated parts of the body—in the neck; the cranial, thoracic, abdominal, and pelvic cavities; and outside of the body cavities. Note the names and locations of the endocrine glands shown in Figure 10-1.

All organs of the endocrine system are glands, but not all glands are organs of the endocrine system. Of the two types of glands in the body—**exocrine glands** and **endocrine glands**—only endocrine glands belong to this system. Exocrine

FIGURE 10-1

Location of the endocrine glands. Thymus gland is shown at maximum size at puberty.

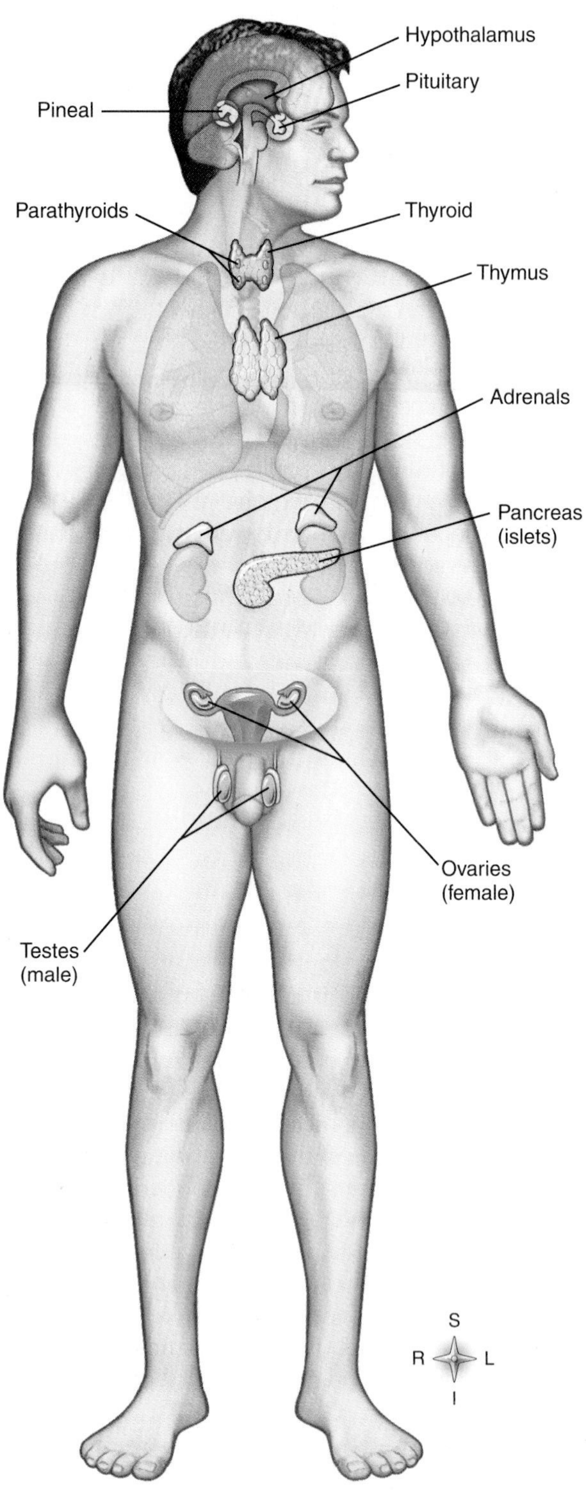

glands secrete their products into ducts that empty onto a surface or into a cavity. For example, sweat glands produce a watery secretion that empties onto the surface of the skin. Salivary glands are also exocrine glands, secreting saliva that flows into the mouth. Endocrine glands are ductless glands. They secrete chemicals known as **hormones** into intercellular spaces. From there, the hormones diffuse directly into the blood and are carried throughout the body. Each hormone molecule may then bind to a cell that has specific receptors for that hormone, triggering a reaction in the cell. Such a cell is called a **target organ cell.** The list of endocrine glands and their target organs continues to grow. The names, locations, and functions of the well-known endocrine glands are given in Figure 10-1 and Table 10-1.

In this chapter you will read about the functions of the main endocrine glands and discover why their importance is almost impossible to exaggerate. Hormones are the main regulators of metabolism, growth and development, reproduction, and many other body activities. They play important roles in maintaining homeostasis—fluid and electrolyte, acid-base, and energy balances, for example. Hormones make the difference between normalcy and many kinds of abnormalities such as dwarfism, gigantism, and sterility. They are important not only for the healthy survival of each one of us but also for the survival of the human species.

Diseases of the endocrine glands are numerous, varied, and sometimes spectacular. Tumors or other abnormalities frequently cause a gland to secrete too much or too little hormone. Production of too much hormone by a diseased gland is called **hypersecretion.** If too little hormone is produced, the condition is called **hyposecretion.**

MECHANISMS OF HORMONE ACTION

A hormone causes its target cells to respond in particular ways; this has been the subject of intense interest and research. The two major classes of hormones—**nonsteroid hormones** and **steroid hormones**—differ in the mechanisms by which they influence target organ cells.

TABLE 10-1

Endocrine Glands, Hormones, and Their Functions

GLAND/HORMONE	FUNCTION
ANTERIOR PITUITARY	
Thyroid-stimulating hormone (TSH)	Tropic hormone Stimulates secretion of thyroid hormones
Adrenocorticotropic hormone (ACTH)	Tropic hormone Stimulates secretion of adrenal cortex hormones
Follicle-stimulating hormone (FSH)	Tropic hormone Female: stimulates development of ovarian follicles and secretion of estrogens Male: stimulates seminiferous tubules of testes to grow and produce sperm
Luteinizing hormone (LH)	Tropic hormone Female: stimulates maturation of ovarian follicle and ovum; stimulates secretion of estrogen; triggers ovulation; stimulates development of corpus luteum (luteinization) Male: stimulates interstitial cells of the testes to secrete testosterone
Growth hormone (GH)	Stimulates growth in all organs; mobilizes food molecules, causing an increase in blood glucose concentration
Prolactin (lactogenic hormone)	Stimulates breast development during pregnancy and milk secretion (milk let-down) after pregnancy
POSTERIOR PITUITARY*	
Antidiuretic hormone (ADH)	Stimulates retention of water by the kidneys
Oxytocin	Stimulates uterine contractions at the end of pregnancy; stimulates the release of milk into the breast ducts
HYPOTHALAMUS	
Releasing hormones (several)	Stimulate the anterior pituitary to release hormones
Inhibiting hormones (several)	Inhibit the anterior pituitary's secretion of hormones
THYROID	
Thyroxine (T4) and triiodothyronine (T3)	Stimulate the energy metabolism of all cells
Calcitonin	Inhibits the breakdown of bone; causes a decrease in blood calcium concentration
PARATHYROID	
Parathyroid hormone (PTH)	Stimulates the breakdown of bone; causes an increase in blood calcium concentration

*Posterior pituitary hormones are synthesized in the hypothalamus but released from axon terminals in the posterior pituitary.

Continued

TABLE 10-1

Endocrine Glands, Hormones, and Their Functions—*cont'd*

GLAND/HORMONE	FUNCTION
ADRENAL CORTEX	
Mineralocorticoids: aldosterone	Regulate electrolyte and fluid homeostasis
Glucocorticoids: cortisol (hydrocortisone)	Stimulate gluconeogenesis, causing an increase in blood glucose concentration; also have antiinflammatory and anti-immunity, antiallergy effects
Sex hormones (androgens)	Stimulate sexual drive in the female but have negligible effects in the male
ADRENAL MEDULLA	
Epinephrine (adrenaline) and norepinephrine	Prolong and intensify the sympathetic nervous response during stress
PANCREATIC ISLETS	
Glucagon	Stimulates liver glycogenolysis, causing an increase in blood glucose concentration
Insulin	Promotes glucose entry into all cells, causing a decrease in blood glucose concentration
OVARY	
Estrogens	Promotes development and maintenance of female sexual characteristics (see Chapter 20)
Progesterone	Promotes conditions required for pregnancy (see Chapter 20)
TESTIS	
Testosterone	Promotes development and maintenance of male sexual characteristics (see Chapter 20)
THYMUS	
Thymosin	Promotes development of immune-system cells
PLACENTA	
Chorionic gonadotropin, estrogens, progesterone	Promote conditions required during early pregnancy
PINEAL GLAND	
Melatonin	Inhibits tropic hormones that affect the ovaries; may be involved in the body's internal clock
HEART (ATRIA)	
Atrial natriuretic hormone (ANH)	Regulates fluid and electrolyte homeostasis
FAT-STORING CELLS	
Leptin	Controls how hungry or full we feel

Research, Issues & Trends

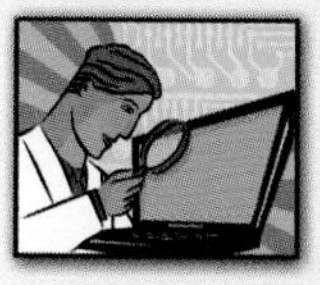

Second Messenger Systems

Rapid and revolutionary discoveries about how nonsteroid hormones act on their target cells began with the pioneering work of Earl Sutherland, who received the 1971 Nobel Prize for formulating the second messenger hypothesis, and continue right up until today. Later, the important role of the so-called G protein in getting the signal from the receptor to the enzyme that forms cyclic AMP (cAMP) was discovered. Look for the G protein in Figure 10-2. More recently, a role for nitric oxide (NO) in second messenger systems has been worked out. All of these discoveries resulted in Nobel Prizes, which shows the importance the scientific community has placed on them. Why? By working out the details of how hormones work, we can more clearly see how and why things can go wrong in endocrine disorders. Perhaps we may even see this in disorders that we previously did not even know involved hormone mechanisms. Once disease mechanisms are worked out, then we hope that scientists can find or design tests that screen for such problems. Or perhaps they can develop drugs that will fix the broken mechanisms and cure the disease. Although it seems like too much detail for you now, you will find that understanding how hormones act on target cells **(signal transduction)** will prepare you for the revolution in medicine that is now upon us.

FIGURE 10-2

Mechanism of nonsteroid hormone action. The hormone acts as "first messenger," delivering its message via the bloodstream to a membrane receptor in the target organ cell much like a key fits into a lock. The "second messenger" causes the cell to respond and perform its specialized function.

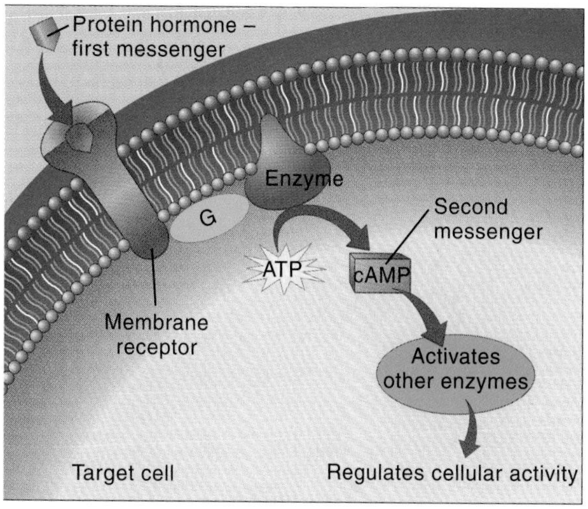

Nonsteroid Hormones

Nonsteroid hormones are whole proteins, shorter chains of amino acids, or simply versions of single amino acids. Nonsteroid hormones work according to the **second messenger mechanism.** According to this concept, a protein hormone, such as thyroid-stimulating hormone, acts as a "first messenger" (that is, it delivers its chemical message from the cells of an endocrine gland to highly specific membrane receptor sites on the cells of a target organ). This interaction between a hormone and its specific receptor site on the cell membrane of a target organ cell is often compared with the fitting of a unique key into a lock. (This idea is the *lock-and-key model* of chemical activity.) After the hormone is attached to its specific receptor site, a number of chemical reactions occur. These reactions activate molecules within the cell called *second messengers*. One example of this mechanism occurs when the hormone-receptor interaction changes energy-rich ATP molecules inside the cell into **cyclic AMP** (adenosine monophosphate). Cyclic AMP serves as the second messenger, delivering information inside the cell that regulates the cell's activity. For example, cyclic AMP causes thyroid cells to respond to thyroid-stimulating hormone by secreting a thyroid hormone such as thyroxine. Cyclic AMP is only one of several second messengers that have been discovered.

In summary, nonsteroid hormones serve as first messengers, providing communication between endocrine glands and target organs. Another molecule, such as cyclic AMP, then acts as the second messenger, providing communication within a hormone's target cells. Figure 10-2 summarizes the mechanism of nonsteroid hormone action as explained by the second messenger hypothesis.

FIGURE 10-3

Mechanism of steroid hormone action. Steroid hormones pass through the plasma membrane and enter the nucleus to form a hormone receptor complex that acts on DNA. As a result, a new protein is formed in the cytoplasm that produces specific effects in the target cell.

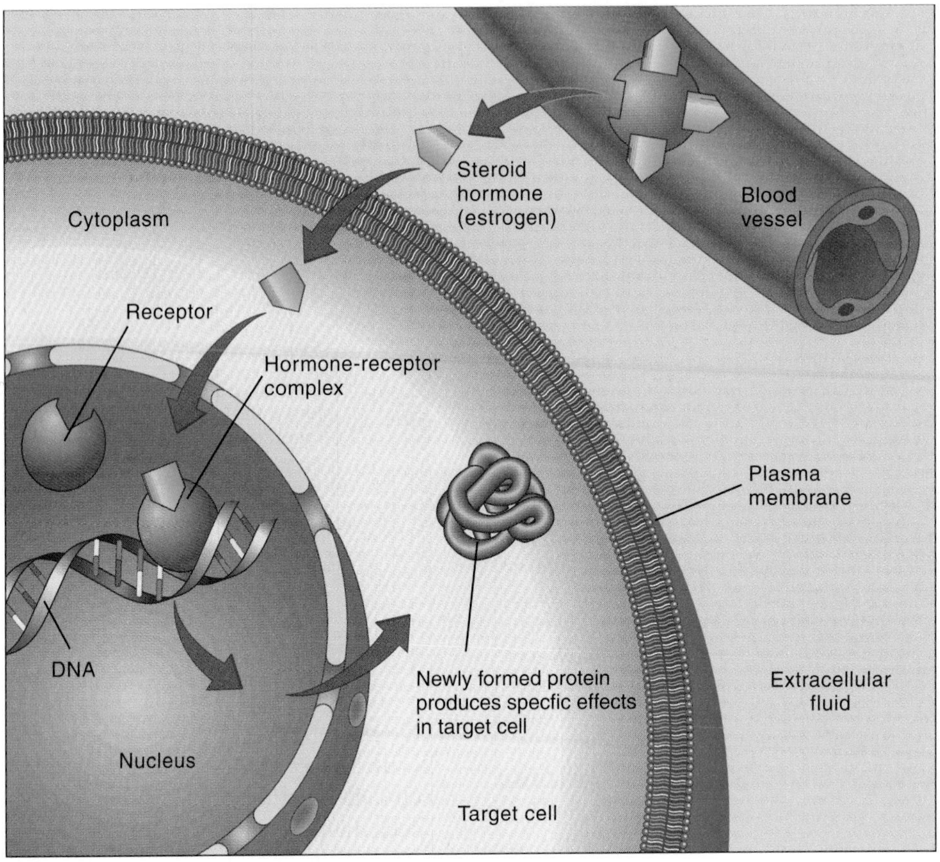

Steroid Hormones

The action of small, lipid-soluble steroid hormones such as estrogen does not occur by the second messenger system. Because they are lipid soluble, steroid hormones can pass intact directly through the cell membrane of the target organ cell. Once inside the cell, steroid hormones pass through the cytoplasm and enter the nucleus where they bind with a receptor (according to the lock-and-key model) to form a hormone-receptor complex. This complex acts on DNA, which ultimately causes the formation of a new protein in the cytoplasm that then produces specific effects in the target cell. In the case of estrogen, for example, that effect might be breast development in the female adolescent. Figure 10-3 summarizes the mechanism of steroid hormone action.

Quick

1. What is the chemical messenger used by the endocrine system?
2. How do nonsteroid hormones and steroid hormones differ? How are they alike?
3. What is a *second messenger* system?

FIGURE 10-4

Negative feedback. The secretion of most hormones is regulated by negative feedback mechanisms that tend to reverse any deviations from normal. In this example, an increase in blood glucose triggers secretion of insulin. Because insulin promotes glucose uptake by cells, the blood glucose level is restored to its lower, normal level.

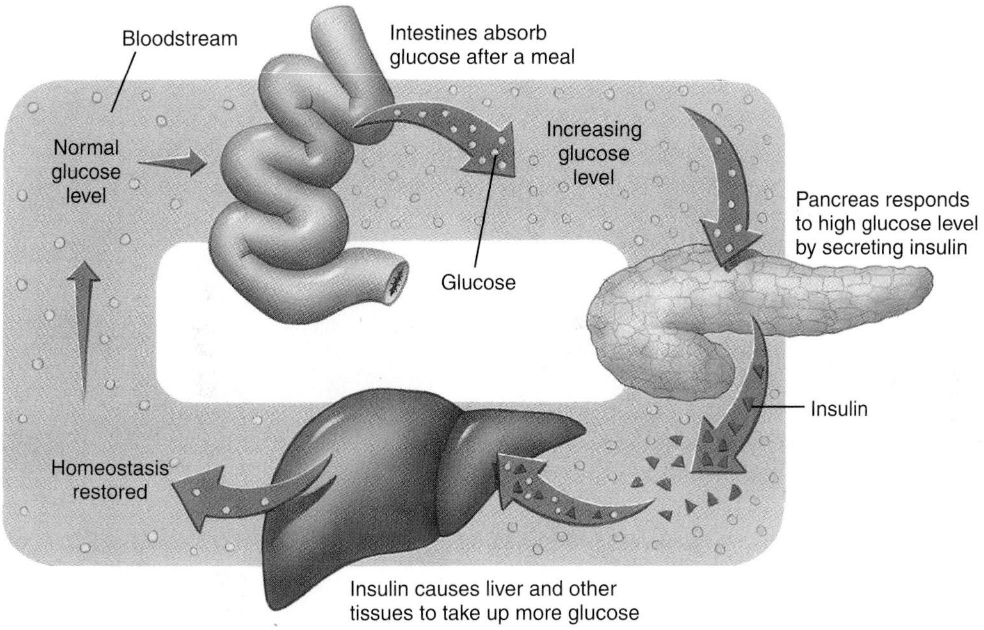
Bloodstream
Intestines absorb glucose after a meal
Normal glucose level
Increasing glucose level
Pancreas responds to high glucose level by secreting insulin
Glucose
Insulin
Homeostasis restored
Insulin causes liver and other tissues to take up more glucose

REGULATION OF HORMONE SECRETION

The regulation of hormone levels in the blood depends on a highly specialized homeostatic mechanism called *negative feedback* (see Chapter 1, p. 14). The principle of **negative feedback** can be illustrated by using the hormone insulin as an example. When released from endocrine cells in the pancreas, insulin lowers blood sugar levels. Normally, elevated blood sugar levels occur after a meal, after the absorption of sugars from the digestive tract takes place. The elevated blood sugar stimulates the release of insulin from the pancreas. Insulin then assists in the transfer of sugar from the blood into cells, and blood sugar levels drop. Low blood sugar levels then cause endocrine cells in the pancreas to cease the production and release of insulin. These responses are *negative*. Therefore the homeostatic mechanism is called a negative feedback control mechanism because it reverses the change in blood sugar level (Figure 10-4).

Positive feedback mechanisms, which are uncommon, amplify changes rather than reverse them. Usually, such amplification threatens homeostasis, but in some situations it can help the body maintain its stability. For example, during labor, the muscle contractions that push the baby through the birth canal become stronger and stronger by means of a positive feedback mechanism that regulates secretion of the hormone oxytocin.

PROSTAGLANDINS

Prostaglandins (PGs) or tissue hormones are important and extremely powerful substances found in a wide variety of tissues. They play an important role in communication and the control of

Clinical Application

Growth Hormone Abnormalities

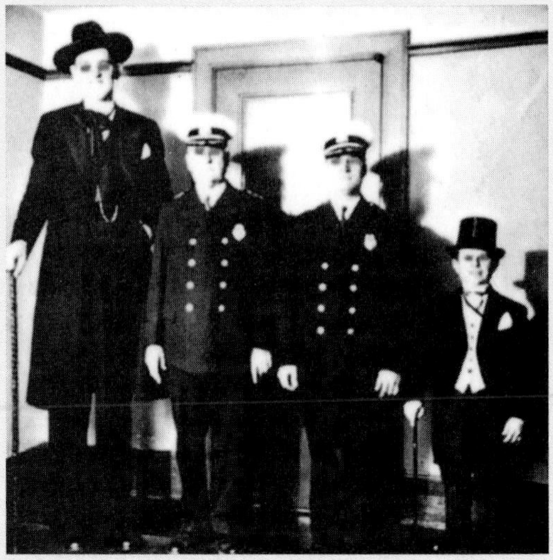

Hypersecretion of growth hormone during the early years of life produces a condition called **gigantism** (jye-GAN-tizm) *(left side of photo)*. The name suggests the obvious characteristics of this condition. The child grows to giant size. Hyposecretion of the growth hormone produces pituitary **dwarfism** (DWARF-izm) *(right side of photo)*.

If the anterior pituitary gland secretes too much growth hormone after the normal growth years, then the disease called **acromegaly** (ak-ro-MEG-ah-lee) develops. Characteristics of this disease are enlargement of the bones of the hands, feet, jaws, and cheeks. The facial appearance typical of acromegaly results from the combination of bone and soft tissue overgrowth. A prominent forehead and large nose are characteristic. In addition, the skin is characterized by large, widened pores, and the mandible grows in length so that separation of the lower teeth commonly occurs.

many body functions but do not meet the definition of a typical hormone. The term *tissue hormone* is appropriate because in many instances a prostaglandin is produced in a tissue and diffuses only a short distance to act on cells within that tissue. Typical hormones influence and control activities of widely separated organs; typical prostaglandins influence activities of neighboring cells.

The prostaglandins in the body can be divided into several groups. Three classes of prostaglandins—prostaglandin A (PGA), prostaglandin E (PGE), and prostaglandin F (PGF)—are among the best known. PGs have profound effects on many body functions. They influence respiration, blood pressure, gastrointestinal secretions, inflammation, and the reproductive system. Researchers believe that most PGs regulate cells by influencing the production of cyclic AMP. Although much research is yet to be done, PGs are already playing an important role in the treatment of conditions such as high blood pressure, asthma, and ulcers. In fact, many common treatments such as aspirin have their effects by altering the functions of PGs in the body.

Quick Check

1. How does negative feedback affect hormone levels in the blood?
2. Why are prostaglandins called *tissue hormones*?

PITUITARY GLAND

The **pituitary** (pi-TOO-i-tair-ee) **gland** is a small but mighty structure. Although no larger than a pea, it is really two endocrine glands. One is called the **anterior pituitary gland** or *adenohypophysis* (ad-e-no-hye-POF-i-sis), and the other is called the **posterior pituitary gland** or *neurohypophysis* (noo-ro-hye-POF-i-sis). Differences between the two glands are indicated by their names—*adeno* means "gland," and *neuro* means "nervous." The adenohypophysis has the structure of an endocrine gland, whereas the neurohypophysis has the structure of nervous tissue. Hormones secreted by the adenohypophysis serve very different functions from those released from the neurohypophysis.

The protected location of this dual gland suggests its importance. The pituitary gland lies buried deep in the cranial cavity, in the small depression of the sphenoid bone that is shaped like a saddle and called the *sella turcica* (Turkish saddle). A stemlike structure, the pituitary stalk, attaches the gland to the undersurface of the brain. More specifically, the stalk attaches the pituitary body to the hypothalamus.

Anterior Pituitary Gland Hormones

The anterior pituitary gland secretes several major hormones. Each of the four hormones listed as a **tropic** (TRO-pik) **hormone** in Table 10-1 stimulates another endocrine gland to grow and secrete its hormones. Because the anterior pituitary gland exerts this control over the structure and function of the thyroid gland, the adrenal cortex, the ovarian follicles, and the corpus luteum, it was sometimes called the *master gland*. However, because its secretions are in turn controlled by the hypothalamus and other mechanisms, the anterior pituitary is hardly the master of body function it was once thought to be.

Thyroid-stimulating hormone (TSH) acts on the thyroid gland. As its name suggests, it stimulates the thyroid gland to increase secretion of thyroid hormone.

The **adrenocorticotropic** (ad-re-no-kor-ti-ko-TRO-pik) **hormone (ACTH)** acts on the adrenal cortex. It stimulates the adrenal cortex to increase in size and to secrete larger amounts of its hormones, especially larger amounts of cortisol (hydrocortisone).

Follicle-stimulating hormone (FSH) stimulates the primary ovarian follicles in an ovary to start growing and to continue developing to maturity (that is, to the point of ovulation). FSH also stimulates follicle cells to secrete estrogens. In the male, FSH stimulates the seminiferous tubules to grow and form sperm.

Luteinizing (LOO-te-nye-zing) **hormone (LH)** acts with FSH to perform several functions. It stimulates a follicle and ovum to complete their growth to maturity, it stimulates follicle cells to secrete estrogens, and it causes ovulation (rupturing of the mature follicle with expulsion of its ripe ovum). Because of this function, LH is sometimes called the *ovulating hormone.* Finally, LH stimulates the formation of a golden body, the corpus luteum, in the ruptured follicle; the process is called *luteinization.* This function, of course, is the one that earned LH its title of *luteinizing hormone.* As it promotes luteinization, LH stimulates the corpus luteum to produce the hormone progesterone. The male pituitary gland also secretes LH; it was formerly called *interstitial cell-stimulating hormone (ICSH)* because it stimulates interstitial cells in the testes to develop and secrete testosterone, the male sex hormone.

Another important hormone secreted by the anterior pituitary gland is **growth hormone.** Growth hormone (GH) speeds up the movement of digested proteins (amino acids) out of the blood and into the cells, and this accelerates the cells' anabolism (build up) of amino acids to form tissue proteins; hence, this action promotes normal growth. Growth hormone also affects fat and carbohydrate metabolism; it accelerates fat catabolism (breakdown) but slows glucose catabolism. This means that less glucose leaves the blood to enter cells, and therefore the amount of glucose in the blood increases. Thus growth hormone and insulin have opposite effects on blood glucose. Insulin decreases blood glucose, and growth hormone increases it. Too much insulin in the blood produces **hypoglycemia** (hye-po-glye-SEE-me-ah) (lower than normal blood glucose concentration). Too much growth hormone produces **hyperglycemia** (higher than normal blood glucose concentration).

The anterior pituitary gland also secretes **prolactin** (pro-LAK-tin) or lactogenic hormone. During pregnancy, prolactin stimulates the breast development necessary for eventual lactation (milk secretion). Also, soon after delivery of a baby, a woman's prolactin stimulates the breasts to start secreting milk, a function suggested by prolactin's other name, lactogenic hormone.

FIGURE 10-5

Pituitary hormones. Principal anterior and posterior pituitary hormones and their target organs.

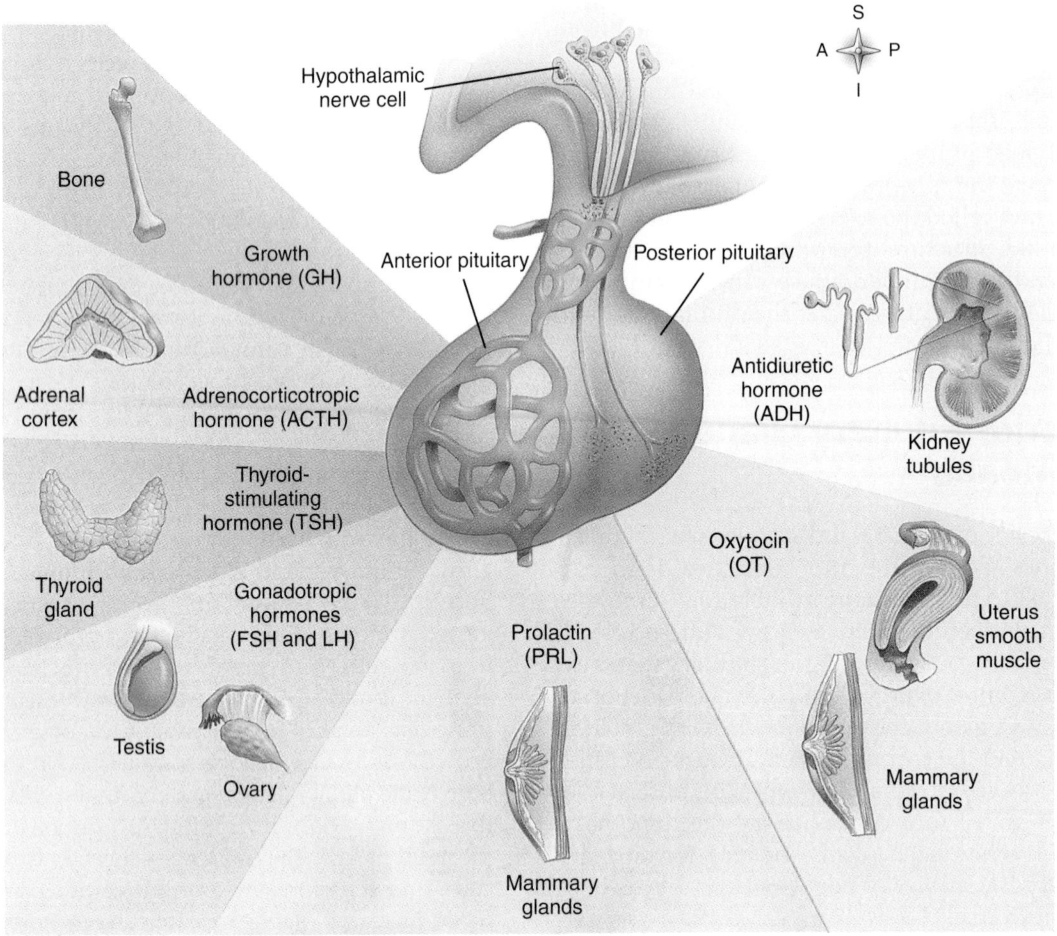

For a brief summary of anterior pituitary hormone target organs and functions, see Figure 10-5.

Posterior Pituitary Gland Hormones

The posterior pituitary gland releases two hormones—**antidiuretic** (an-tie-dye-yoo-RET-ik) **hormone (ADH)** and **oxytocin** (ok-see-TOE-sin). ADH accelerates the reabsorption of water from urine in kidney tubules back into the blood. With more water moving out of the tubules into the blood, less water remains in the tubules, and therefore less urine leaves the body. The name *antidiuretic hormone* is appropriate because *anti-* means "against" and *diuretic* means "increasing the volume of urine excreted." Therefore *antidiuretic* means "acting against an increase in urine volume"; in other words, ADH acts to decrease urine volume. Hyposecretion of ADH results in **diabetes insipidus** (dye-ah-BEE-tes in-SIP-i-dus), a condition in which large volumes of urine are formed. Dehydration and electrolyte imbalances may cause serious problems unless the sufferer is treated with injections or nasal sprays containing ADH.

The posterior pituitary hormone oxytocin is secreted by a woman's body before and after she has a baby. Oxytocin stimulates contraction of the smooth muscle of the pregnant uterus and is believed to initiate and maintain labor. This is why physicians sometimes prescribe oxytocin injections to induce or increase labor. Oxytocin also performs a function important to a newborn baby. It causes the glandular cells of the breast to release milk into ducts from which a baby can obtain it by sucking. In short, oxytocin stimulates "milk letdown." The right side of Figure 10-5 summarizes posterior pituitary functions.

HYPOTHALAMUS

In discussing ADH and oxytocin, we noted that these hormones were *released* from the posterior lobe of the pituitary. Actual production of these two hormones occurs in the hypothalamus. Two groups of specialized neurons in the hypothalamus synthesize the posterior pituitary hormones, which then pass down along axons into the pituitary gland. Release of ADH and oxytocin into the blood is controlled by nervous stimulation.

In addition to oxytocin and ADH, the hypothalamus also produces substances called **releasing** and **inhibiting hormones.** These substances are produced in the hypothalamus and then travel directly through a specialized blood capillary system to the anterior pituitary gland, where they cause the release of anterior pituitary hormones or, in a number of instances, inhibit their production and their release into the general circulation.

The combined nervous and endocrine functions of the hypothalamus allow it to play a dominant role in the regulation of many body functions related to homeostasis. Examples include the regulation of body temperature, appetite, and thirst.

Quick Check

1. How are the anterior pituitary and posterior pituitary different? How are they alike?
2. What makes a hormone a *tropic* hormone?
3. Can you name the hormones produced by the pituitary gland?
4. How does the hypothalamus control the pituitary gland?

THYROID GLAND

Earlier in this chapter, we mentioned that some endocrine glands are not located in a body cavity. The thyroid is one of these. It lies in the neck just below the larynx (Figure 10-6).

The thyroid gland secretes two thyroid hormones, **thyroxine** (thye-ROK-sin) or $\mathbf{T_4}$ and **triiodothyronine** (try-eye-o-doe-THY-ro-neen) or $\mathbf{T_3}$. It also secretes the hormone **calcitonin** (kal-si-TOE-nin). Of the two thyroid hormones, T_4 is the more abundant; however, T_3 is the more potent and is considered by physiologists to be the principal thyroid hormone. One molecule of T_4 contains four atoms of iodine, and one molecule of T_3, as its name suggests, contains three iodine atoms. For T_4 to be produced in adequate amounts, the diet must contain sufficient iodine.

Most endocrine glands do not store their hormones but secrete them directly into the blood as they are produced. The thyroid gland is different in that it stores considerable amounts of the thyroid hormones in the form of a colloid compound seen in Figure 10-7. The colloid material is stored in the follicles of the gland, and when the thyroid hormones are needed, they are released from the colloid and secreted into the blood.

T_4 and T_3 influence every one of the trillions of cells in our bodies. They make them speed up their release of energy from foods. In other words, these thyroid hormones stimulate cellular metabolism. This has far-reaching effects. Because all body functions depend on a normal supply of energy, they all depend on normal thyroid secretion. Even normal mental and physical growth and development depend on normal thyroid functioning.

Calcitonin decreases the concentration of calcium in the blood by first acting on bone to inhibit

FIGURE 10-6

Thyroid and parathyroid glands. Note their relationship to each other and to the larynx (voice box) and trachea.

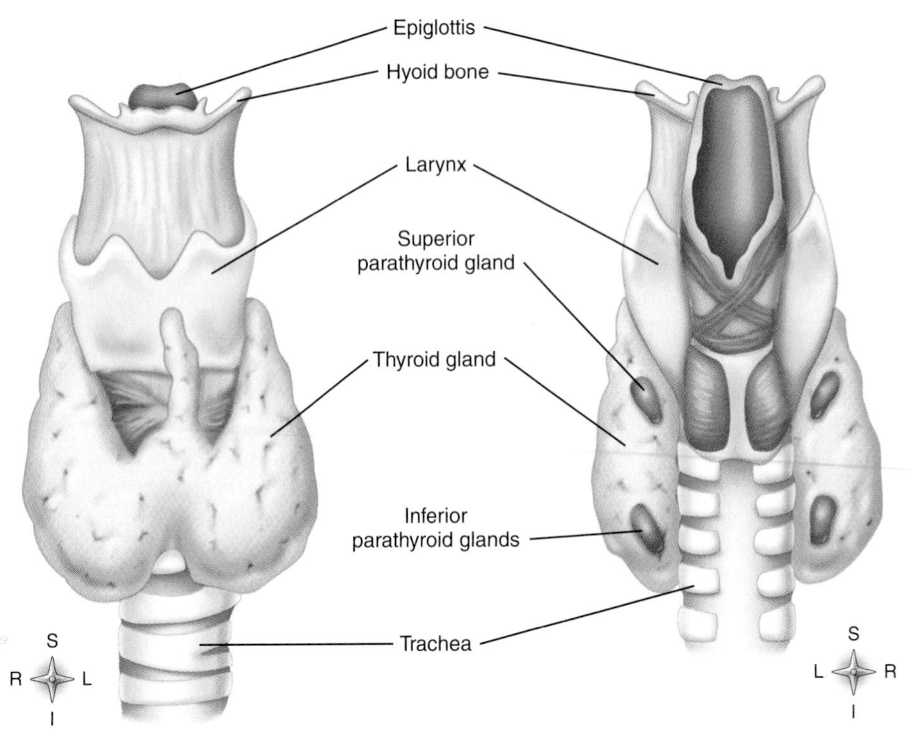

FIGURE 10-7

Thyroid gland tissue. Note that each of the follicles is filled with colloid. The colloid serves as a storage medium for the thyroid hormones.

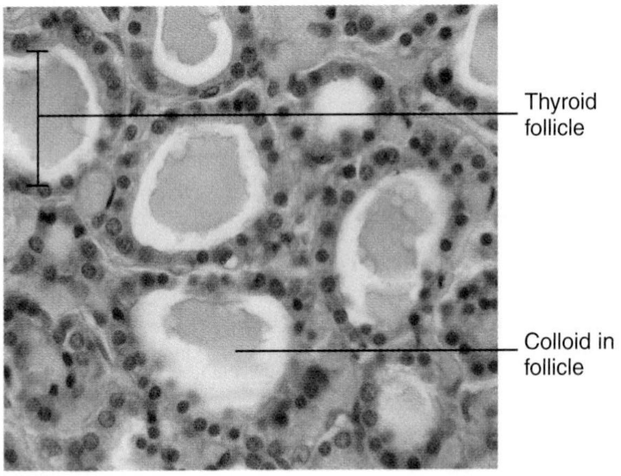

its breakdown. With less bone being resorbed, less calcium moves out of bone into blood, and, as a result, the concentration of calcium in blood decreases. An increase in calcitonin secretion quickly follows any increase in blood calcium concentration, even if it is a slight one. This causes blood calcium concentration to decrease to its normal level. Calcitonin thus helps maintain homeostasis of blood calcium. It prevents a harmful excess of calcium in the blood, a condition called **hypercalcemia** (hye-per-kal-SEE-me-ah), from developing.

PARATHYROID GLANDS

The **parathyroid glands** are small glands. There are usually four of them, and they are found on the back of the thyroid gland (see Figure 10-6). The parathyroid glands secrete **parathyroid hormone (PTH).**

FIGURE 10-8

Regulation of blood calcium levels. Calcitonin and parathyroid hormones have antagonistic (opposite) effects on calcium concentration in the blood.

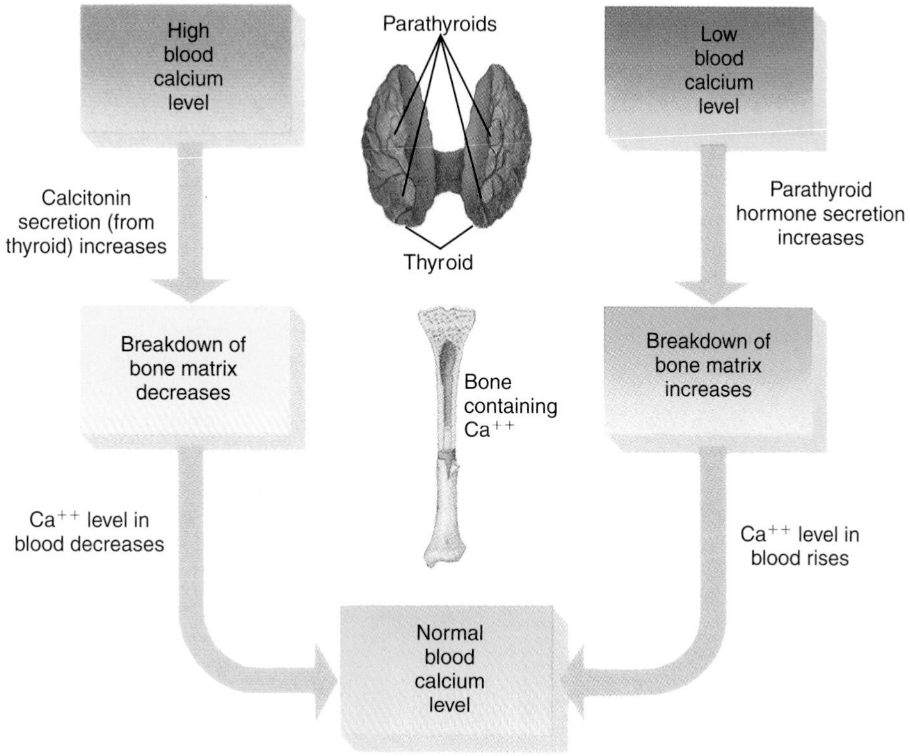

PTH increases the concentration of calcium in the blood—the opposite effect of the thyroid gland's calcitonin. Whereas calcitonin acts to decrease the amount of calcium being resorbed from bone, PTH acts to increase it. PTH stimulates bone-resorbing cells or osteoclasts to increase their breakdown of bone's hard matrix, a process that frees the calcium stored in the matrix. The released calcium then moves out of bone into blood, and this in turn increases the blood's calcium concentration. For a summary of the antagonistic effects of calcitonin and parathyroid hormone, see Figure 10-8. This is a matter of life-and-death importance because our cells are extremely sensitive to changing amounts of blood calcium. They cannot function normally with too much or too little calcium. For example, with too much blood calcium, brain cells and heart cells soon do not function normally; a person becomes mentally disturbed, and the heart may stop. However, with too little blood calcium, nerve cells become overactive, sometimes to such a degree that they bombard muscles with so many impulses that the muscles go into spasms.

Quick

1. Where are the thyroid and parathyroid glands located?
2. What gland stores its hormones for later use?
3. Calcitonin and parathyroid hormone both regulate the blood concentration what important ion?

Clinical Application

Thyroid Hormone Abnormalities

Hyperthyroidism (hye-per-THY-royd-izm) or oversecretion of the thyroid hormones dramatically increases the metabolic rate. Food material is burned by the cells at an excessive rate, and individuals who suffer from this condition lose weight, are irritable, have an increased appetite, and often show protrusion of the eyeballs due in part to edema of tissue at the back of the eye socket; see Figure A.

Hypothyroidism (hye-po-THY-royd-izm) or undersecretion of thyroid hormones can be caused by and result in a number of different conditions. Low dietary intake of iodine causes a painless enlargement of the thyroid gland called **simple goiter** (GOY-ter), shown in Figure B. This condition was once common in areas of the United States where the iodine content of the soil and water is inadequate. The use of iodized salt has dramatically reduced the incidence of simple goiter caused by low iodine intake. In simple goiter the gland enlarges to compensate for the lack of iodine in the diet necessary for the synthesis of thyroid hormones.

Hyposecretion of thyroid hormones during the formative years leads to a condition called **cretinism** (KREE-tin-izm). It is characterized by a low metabolic rate, retarded growth and sexual development, and, frequently, mental retardation. Fortunately, health screening for low thyroid function can lead to treatment before cretinism develops. Later in life, deficient thyroid hormone secretion produces the disease called **myxedema** (mik-se-DEE-mah). The low metabolic rate that characterizes myxedema leads to lessened mental and physical vigor, weight gain, loss of hair, and swelling of tissues.

A

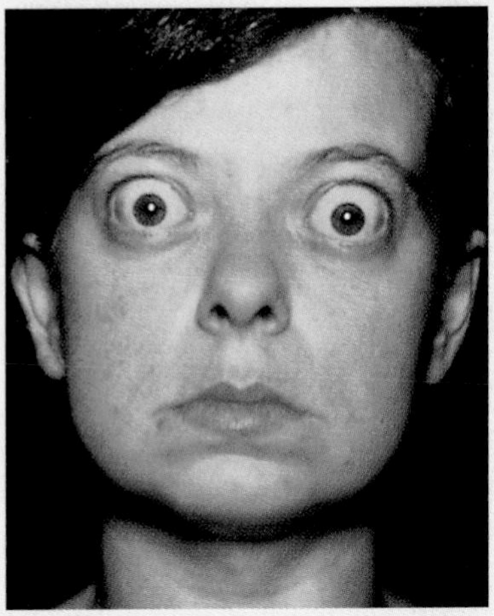

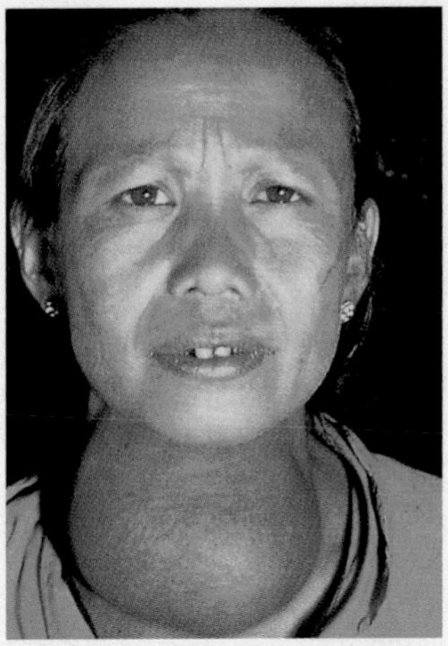

B

ADRENAL GLANDS

As you can see in Figures 10-1 and 10-9, an adrenal gland curves over the top of each kidney. From the surface an adrenal gland appears to be only one organ, but it is actually two separate endocrine glands: the **adrenal cortex** and the **adrenal medulla.** Does this two-glands-in-one structure remind you of another endocrine organ? (see pp. 258-261). The adrenal cortex is the outer part of an adrenal gland, and the medulla is its inner part. Adrenal cortex hormones have different names and quite different actions from adrenal medulla hormones.

Adrenal Cortex

Three different zones or layers of cells make up the **adrenal cortex** as you can see in Figure 10-9. Follow this diagram carefully as you read the following paragraph and you will easily see the special function of each layer of the adrenal cortex.

FIGURE 10-9

The adrenal gland. The three cell layers of the adrenal cortex are easily seen here. The outer zone cells secrete mineralocorticoids (aldosterone). The middle zone cells secrete glucocorticoids (hydrocortisone). The inner zone cells secrete sex hormones (androgens).

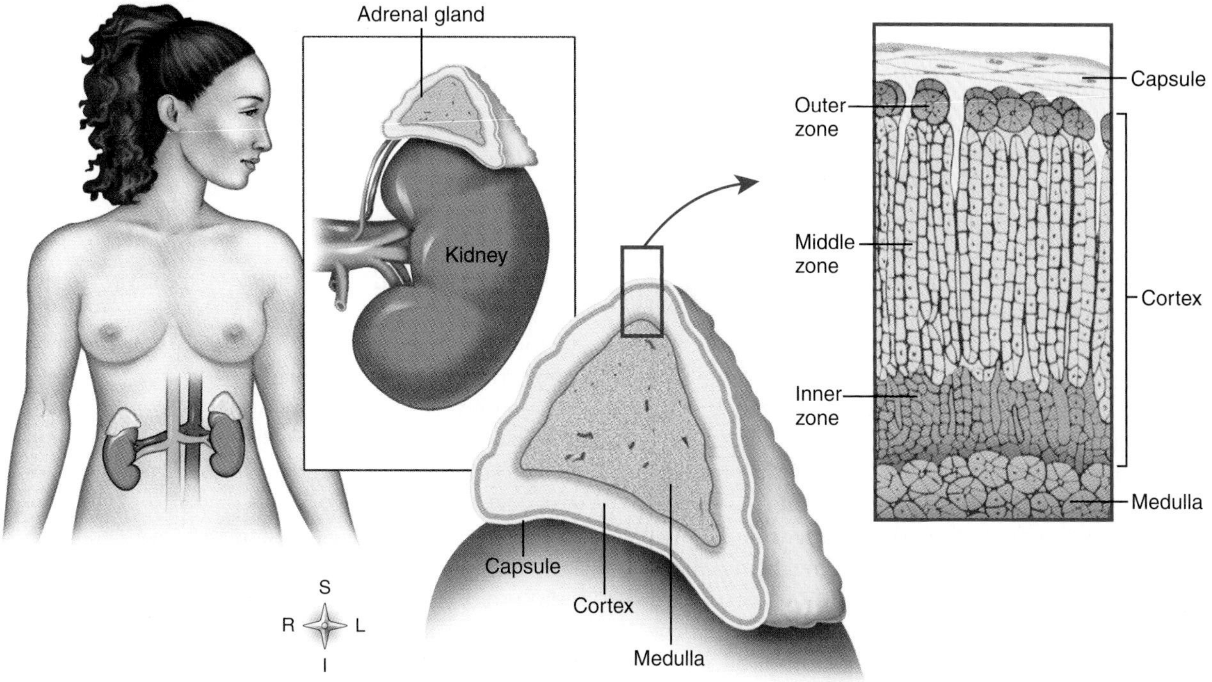

Hormones secreted by the three cell layers or zones of the adrenal cortex are called **corticoids** (KOR-ti-koyds). The outer zone of adrenal cortex cells secretes hormones called **mineralocorticoids** (min-er-al-o-KOR-ti-koyds) or **MCs** for short. The main mineralocorticoid is the hormone **aldosterone** (al-DOS-ste-rone). The middle zone secretes **glucocorticoids** (gloo-ko-KOR-ti-koyds) or **GCs. Cortisol** or **hydrocortisone** is the chief glucocorticoid. The innermost or deepest zone of the cortex secretes small amounts of **sex hormones.** Sex hormones secreted by the adrenal cortex resemble testosterone. We shall now discuss briefly the functions of these three kinds of adrenal cortical hormones.

As their name suggests, **mineralocorticoids** help control the amount of certain mineral salts (mainly sodium chloride) in the blood. Aldosterone is the chief mineralocorticoid. Remember its main functions—to increase the amount of sodium and decrease the amount of potassium in the blood—because these changes lead to other profound changes. Aldosterone increases blood sodium and decreases blood potassium by influencing the kidney tubules. It causes them to speed up their reabsorption of sodium back into the blood so that less of it will be lost in the urine. At the same time, aldosterone causes the tubules to increase their secretion of potassium so that more of this mineral will be lost in the urine. The effects of aldosterone speed up kidney reabsorption of water.

One of the important functions of glucocorticoids is to help maintain normal blood glucose concentration. Glucocorticoids increase **gluconeogenesis** (gloo-ko-nee-o-JEN-e-sis), a process that converts amino acids or fatty acids to glucose and that is performed mainly by liver cells. Glucocorticoids act in several ways to increase gluconeogenesis. They promote the breakdown of tissue proteins to amino acids, especially in muscle cells. Amino acids thus formed move out of the tissue cells into blood and circulate to the liver. Liver cells then change them to glucose by the process of gluconeogenesis. The newly formed glucose leaves the liver cells and enters the blood. This action increases blood glucose concentration.

In addition to performing these functions—which are necessary for maintaining normal blood glucose concentration—glucocorticoids also play an essential part in maintaining normal blood pressure. They act in a complicated way to make it possible for two other hormones secreted by the adrenal medulla to partially constrict blood vessels, a condition necessary for maintaining normal blood pressure. Also, glucocorticoids act with these hormones from the adrenal medulla to produce an antiinflammatory effect. They bring about a normal recovery from inflammations produced by many kinds of agents. The use of hydrocortisone to relieve skin rashes, for example, is based on the antiinflammatory effect of glucocorticoids.

Another effect produced by glucocorticoids is called their *anti-immunity, antiallergy effect.* Glucocorticoids bring about a decrease in the number of certain cells that produce antibodies, substances that make us immune to some factors and allergic to others.

When extreme stimuli act on the body, they produce an internal state or condition known as *stress.* Surgery, hemorrhage, infections, severe burns, and intense emotions are examples of extreme stimuli that bring on stress. The normal adrenal cortex responds to the condition of stress by quickly increasing its secretion of glucocorticoids. This fact is well established. What is still not known, however, is whether the increased amount of glucocorticoids helps the body cope successfully with stress. Increased glucocorticoid secretion is only one of many ways in which the body responds to stress, but it is one of the first stress responses, and it brings about many of the other stress responses. Examine Figure 10-10 to discover what stress responses are produced by a high concentration of glucocorticoids in the blood.

The sex hormones that are secreted by the inner zone are male hormones **(androgens)** similar to testosterone. These hormones are secreted in small amounts in both males and females. In females, these androgens stimulate the female sexual drive. In males, so much testosterone is secreted by the testes that adrenal androgens are physiologically insignificant.

Adrenal Medulla

The **adrenal medulla,** or inner portion of the adrenal gland shown in Figure 10-9, secretes the hormones **epinephrine** (ep-i-NEF-rin) and **norepinephrine** (nor-ep-i-NEF-rin).

Our bodies have many ways to defend themselves against enemies that threaten their well-being. A physiologist might say that the body resists stress by making many stress responses. We have just discussed increased glucocorticoid secretion. An even faster-acting stress response is increased secretion by the adrenal medulla. This occurs very rapidly because nerve impulses conducted by sympathetic nerve fibers stimulate the adrenal medulla. When stimulated, it literally squirts epinephrine and norepinephrine into the blood. As with glucocorticoids, these hormones may help the body resist or avoid stress. In other words, these hormones produce the body's "fight-or-flight" response to danger (stress). However, epinephrine and norepinephrine are not essential for maintaining life. On the other hand, glucocorticoids, the hormones from the adrenal cortex, are essential for life.

Suppose you suddenly faced some threatening situation. Imagine that a gunman threatened to kill you or that your doctor told you that you had to have a dangerous operation. Almost instantaneously, the medullas of your two adrenal glands would be galvanized into feverish activity. They would quickly secrete large amounts of epinephrine (adrenaline) into your blood. Many of your body functions would seem to be supercharged. Your heart would beat faster; your blood pressure would rise; more blood would be pumped to your skeletal

FIGURE 10-10

Stress responses induced by high concentrations of glucocorticoids in blood.

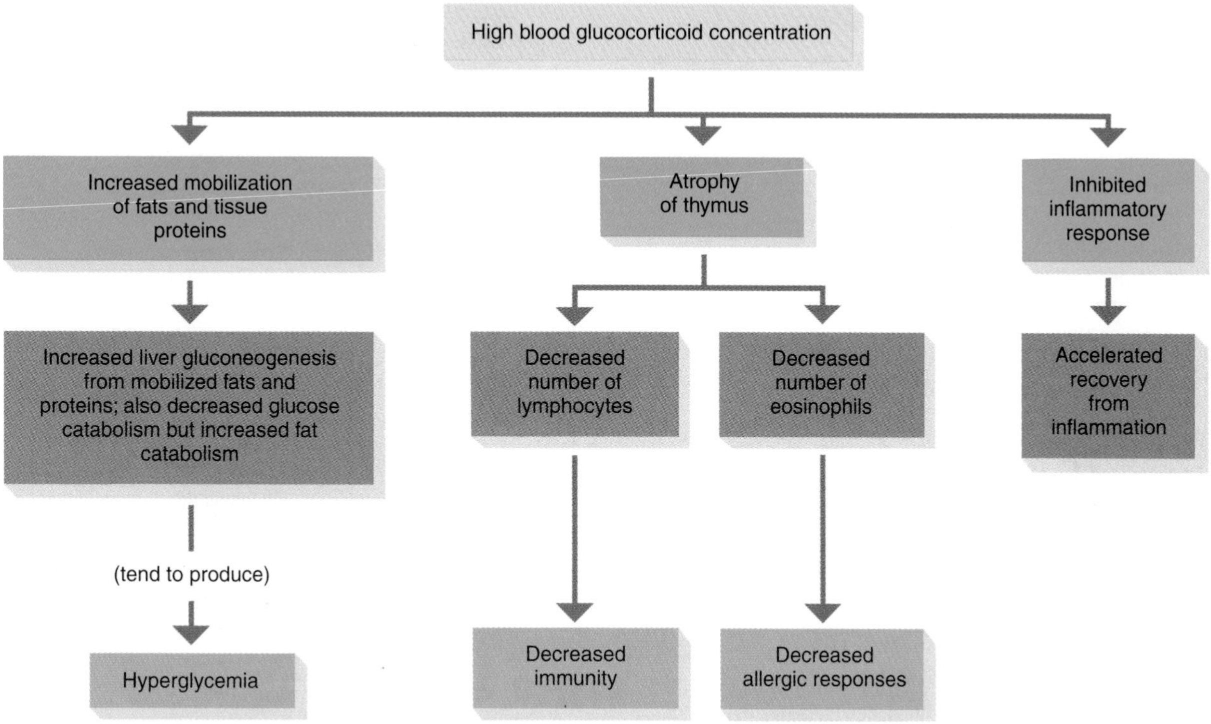

muscles; your blood would contain more glucose for more energy, and so on. In short, you would be geared for strenuous activity, for "fight or flight." Epinephrine prolongs and intensifies changes in body function brought about by the stimulation of the sympathetic subdivision of the autonomic nervous system. Recall from Chapter 8 that sympathetic or adrenergic fibers release epinephrine and norepinephrine as neurotransmitter substances.

The close functional relationship between the nervous and the endocrine systems is perhaps most noticeable in the body's response to stress. In stress conditions the hypothalamus acts on the anterior pituitary gland to cause the release of ACTH, which stimulates the adrenal cortex to secrete glucocorticoids. In addition, the sympathetic subdivision of the autonomic nervous system is stimulated with the adrenal medulla, so the release of epinephrine and norepinephrine occurs to assist the body in responding to the stressful stimulus. Unfortunately, during periods of prolonged stress, glucocorticoids may have harmful side effects because they are anti-inflammatory and cause blood vessels to constrict. For example, decreased immune activity in the body may promote the spread of infections and cancer, and prolonged blood vessel constriction may lead to increased blood pressure.

Quick Check

1. Why is the adrenal gland often thought of as two separate glands?
2. Can you name the hormones produced by the adrenal gland?
3. How does the pituitary gland influence adrenal function?

Clinical Application

Adrenal Hormone Abnormalities

Injury, disease states, or malfunction of the adrenal glands can result in hypersecretion or hyposecretion of several different hormones.

Tumors of the adrenal cortex located in the middle zone of the cortex often result in the production of abnormally large amounts of glucocorticoids. The medical name for this is **Cushing's syndrome.** Figure A shows a boy just diagnosed with Cushing's syndrome. Figure B shows the same boy 4 months later, after treatment. For some reason many more women than men develop Cushing's syndrome. Its most noticeable features are the so-called moon face and the buffalo hump on the upper back that develop because of redistribution of body fat. These individuals also have elevated blood sugar levels and suffer frequent infections. Surgical removal of a glucocorticoid-producing tumor may result in dramatic improvement of the moon-face symptom within 6 months.

Deficiency or hyposecretion of adrenal cortex hormones results in a condition called **Addison's disease.** President John F. Kennedy suffered from Addison's disease, which causes reduced cortical hormone levels result in muscle weakness, reduced blood sugar, nausea, loss of appetite, and weight loss.

A

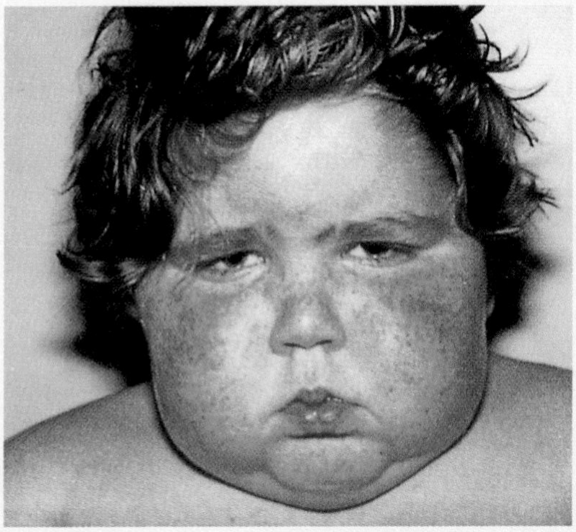

B

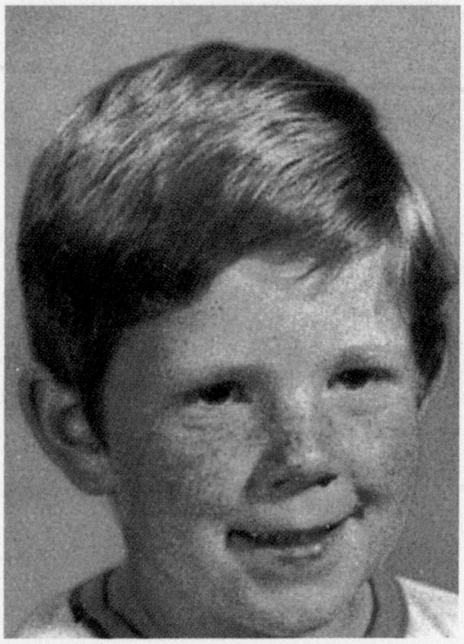

PANCREATIC ISLETS

All the endocrine glands discussed so far are big enough to be seen without a magnifying glass. The **pancreatic islets** or **islets of Langerhans,** in contrast, are too tiny to be seen without a microscope. These glands are merely little clumps of cells scattered like islands in a sea among the exocrine pancreatic cells that secrete the pancreatic digestive juice (Figure 10-11).

Two kinds of cells in the pancreatic islets are the alpha cells (or A cells) and beta cells (or B cells). Alpha cells secrete a hormone called **glucagon,** whereas beta cells secrete one of the most famous of all hormones, **insulin.** Glucagon accelerates a process called **liver glycogenolysis** (glye-ko-jen-OL-i-sis). Glycogenolysis is a chemical process by which the glucose stored in the liver cells in the form of glycogen is converted to glucose. This glucose then leaves the liver cells and enters the

FIGURE 10-11

Pancreas. A, Location and structure of the pancreas (cut open). **B,** A pancreatic islet (of Langerhans) in cross section, showing the glucagon-producing alpha cells and insulin-producing beta cells. Notice the many exocrine cells surrounding the endocrine pancreatic islet.

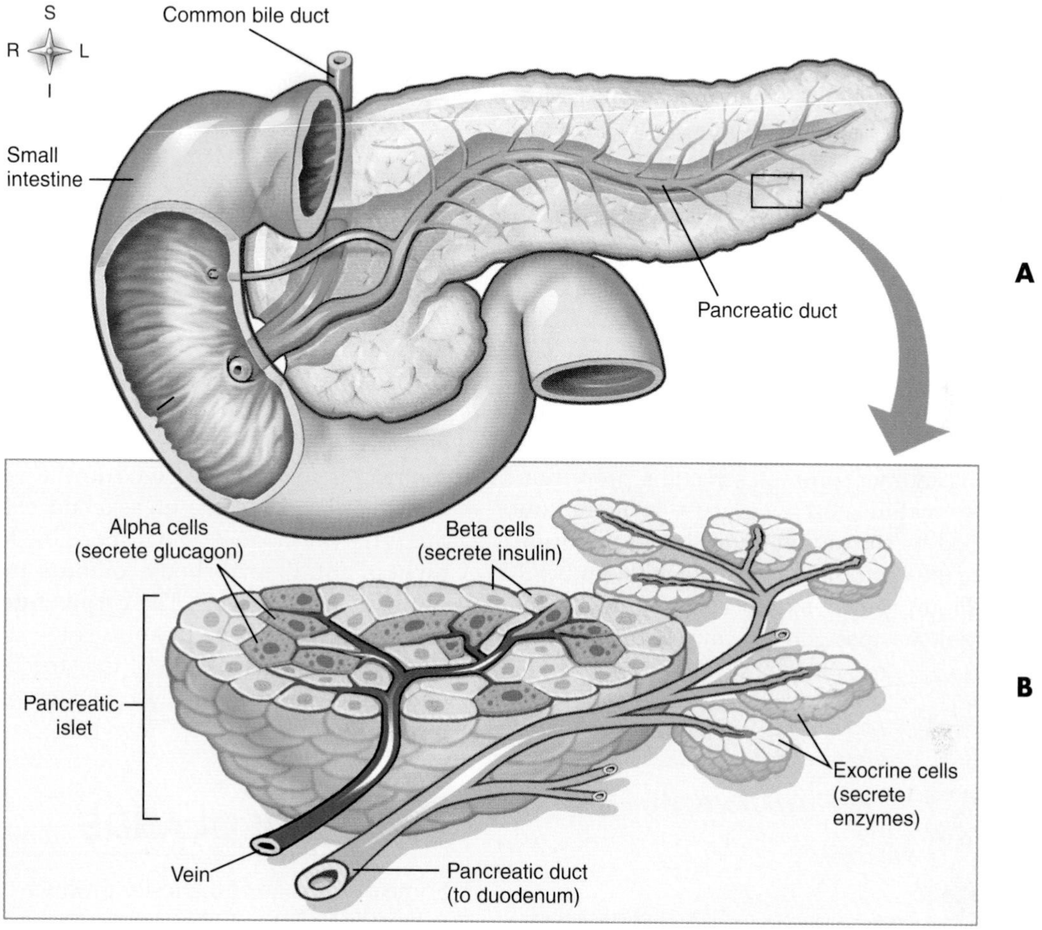

blood. Glucagon therefore increases blood glucose concentration.

Insulin and glucagon are antagonists. In other words, insulin decreases blood glucose concentration; glucagon increases it. Insulin is the only hormone that can decrease blood glucose concentration. Other hormones, however, increase its concentration, including glucocorticoids, growth hormone, and glucagon. Insulin decreases blood glucose by accelerating its movement out of the blood, through cell membranes, and into cells. As glucose enters the cells at a faster rate, the cells increase their metabolism of glucose. Briefly then, insulin decreases blood glucose and increases glucose metabolism.

If the pancreatic islets secrete a normal amount of insulin, a normal amount of glucose enters the cells, and a normal amount of glucose stays behind in the blood. ("Normal" blood glucose is about 70 to 110 mg of glucose in every 100 ml of blood.) If the pancreatic islets secrete too much insulin, as they sometimes do when a person has a tumor of the pancreas, more glucose than usual leaves the blood to enter the cells, and blood glucose decreases. If the pancreatic islets secrete too little insulin, as they do in **type 1 diabetes** (dye-ah-BEE-tes) **mellitus** (mell-EYE-tus), less glucose leaves the blood to enter the cells, so the blood glucose increases, sometimes to even three or more times the normal amount. Most cases of **type 2 diabetes mellitus** result from some decrease of insulin and an abnormality of the insulin receptors, preventing the normal effects of insulin on its target cells and thus also raising blood glucose levels.

Screening tests for all types of diabetes mellitus rely on the fact that the blood glucose level is elevated in this condition. Today, most screening is done with a simple test with a drop of blood. Subjects with a high blood glucose level are suspected of having diabetes mellitus. Testing for sugar in the urine is another common screening procedure. In diabetes mellitus, excess glucose is filtered out of the blood by the kidneys and lost in the urine, producing the condition **glycosuria** (glye-ko-SOO-ree-ah). Figure 10-12 summarizes some of the many problems that can be caused by diabetes mellitus. A quick look at these problems underscores the importance of insulin and insulin receptors in healthy bodies.

Health & Well-Being

Exercise and Diabetes Mellitus

Type 1 diabetes mellitus is characterized by high blood glucose concentration because the lack of sufficient insulin prevents glucose from entering cells. However, exercise physiologists have found that aerobic training increases the number of insulin receptors in target cells and the insulin affinity (attraction) of the receptors. This condition allows a small amount of insulin to have a greater effect than it would have otherwise had. Thus exercise reduces the severity of the diabetic condition.

All forms of diabetes benefit from properly planned exercise therapy. Not only is this form of treatment natural and cost effective, but it also helps reduce or prevent other problems such as obesity and heart disease.

Quick Check

1. Can you name the two primary hormones of the pancreatic islets?
2. What effect does insulin have on the blood's glucose concentration?
3. How does diabetes produce glucose in the urine?

FEMALE SEX GLANDS

A woman's primary sex glands are her two ovaries. Each ovary contains two different kinds of glandular structures: the ovarian follicles and the corpus luteum. **Ovarian follicles** are little pockets in which egg cells or **ova** develop. Ovarian follicles also secrete estrogen, the "feminizing hormone." Estrogen is involved in the development and maturation of the breasts and external genitals. This hormone is also responsible for development of adult female body contours and initiation of the menstrual cycle. The **corpus luteum** chiefly secretes progesterone but also some estrogen. We shall save our discussion of the structure of these endocrine glands and the functions of their hormones for Chapter 20.

MALE SEX GLANDS

Some of the cells of the testes produce the male sex cells called **sperm.** Other cells in the testes, male reproductive ducts, and glands produce the liquid portion of the male reproductive fluid called *semen*. The interstitial cells in the testes secrete the male sex hormone called **testosterone** directly into the blood. These cells of the testes are therefore the male endocrine glands. Testosterone is the "masculinizing hormone." It is responsible for the maturation of the external genitals, beard growth, changes in voice at puberty, and for the muscular development and body contours typical of the male. Chapter 20 contains more information about the structure of the testes and the functions of testosterone.

FIGURE 10-12

Diabetes mellitus. The signs and symptoms of this disorder *(highlighted in yellow)* all result from decreased insulin effects.

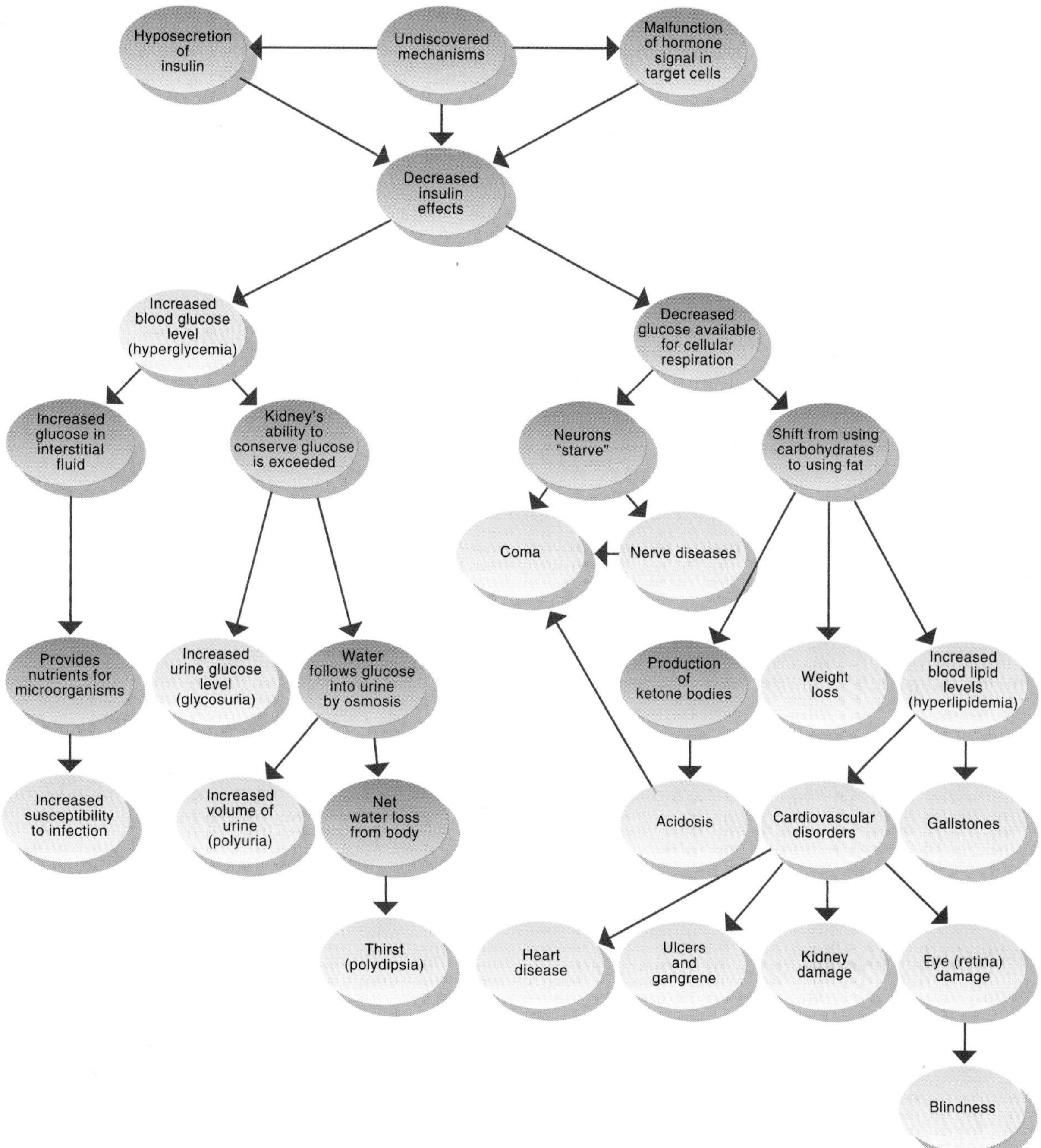

THYMUS

The thymus is located in the mediastinum (see Figure 10-1), and in infants it may extend up into the neck as far as the lower edge of the thyroid gland. Like the adrenal gland, the thymus has a cortex and medulla. Both portions are composed largely of lymphocytes (white blood cells). As part of the body's immune system, the endocrine function of the thymus is not only important but essential. This small structure (it weighs less than a gram at most) plays a critical part in the body's defenses against infections—its vital immunity mechanism.

The hormone **thymosin** (THY-mo-sin) is actually a group of several hormones that together play an important role in the development and function of the body's immune system.

PLACENTA

The placenta functions as a temporary endocrine gland. During pregnancy, it produces **chorionic** (KO-ree-on-ik) **gonadotropins** (gon-ah-doe-TRO-pins), so called because they are tropic hormones secreted by cells of the **chorion** (KO-ree-on), the outermost membrane that surrounds the baby during development in the uterus. In addition to chorionic gonadotropins, the placenta also produces estrogen and progesterone. During the earliest weeks of pregnancy, the kidneys excrete large amounts of chorionic gonadotropins in the urine. This fact, discovered more than a half century ago, led to the development of early pregnancy tests.

PINEAL GLAND

The pineal gland is a small gland near the roof of the third ventricle of the brain (see Figure 8-9). It is named "pineal" because it resembles the pine nut (which looks like a kernel of corn). The pineal gland is easily located in a child but becomes fibrous and encrusted with calcium deposits as a person ages. The pineal gland produces a number of hormones in very small quantities, with **melatonin** being the most significant. Melatonin inhibits the tropic hormones that affect the ovaries, and it is thought to be involved in regulating the onset of puberty and the menstrual cycle in women. Because the pineal gland receives and responds to sensory information from the optic nerves, it is sometimes called the *third eye*. The pineal gland uses information regarding changing light levels to adjust its output of melatonin; melatonin levels increase during the night and decrease during the day. This cyclic variation is thought to be an important timekeeping mechanism for the body's internal clock.

OTHER ENDOCRINE STRUCTURES

Continuing research into the endocrine system has shown that nearly every organ and system has an endocrine function. Tissues in the kidneys, stomach, intestines, and other organs secrete hormones that regulate a variety of essential human functions. For example, **atrial natriuretic hormone (ANH)** is secreted by cells in the wall of the heart's atria (upper chambers). ANH is an important regulator of fluid and electrolyte homeostasis and is an antagonist to aldosterone. Aldosterone stimulates the kidney to retain sodium ions and water, whereas ANH stimulates loss of sodium ions and water. A more recently discovered hormone is **leptin,** which is secreted by fat-storing cells throughout the body. Leptin seems to regulate how hungry or full we feel and how fat is metabolized by the body. Researchers are now looking at how leptin works with other hormones in the hopes of finding ways to deal with obesity, diabetes mellitus, and other disorders involving fat storage.

Quick Check

1. Which hormones are produced by the male and female sex glands?
2. Why is the placenta considered to be a gland?
3. Why is the pineal gland sometimes called a timekeeper of the body?

Science Applications

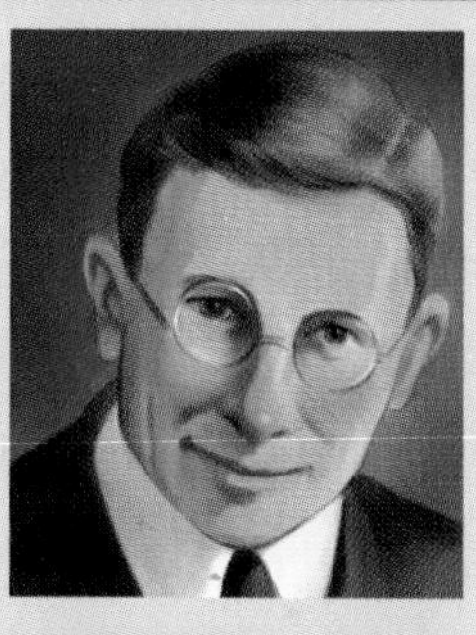

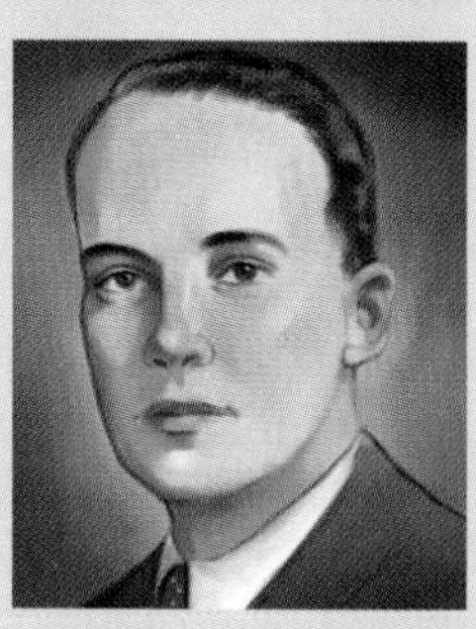

Endocrinology

Banting (1891-1941) and Best (1899-1978).

The undisputed heroes of endocrinology are Canadian surgeon Frederick Banting and his assistant Charles Best. Until the early twentieth century, children with Type 1 diabetes mellitus died a slow, horrible death from their cells literally starving to death from lack of glucose. Acting on Banting's idea for removing insulin from the pancreatic islets of dogs, the two were the first to successfully isolate this important hormone. Chemist James Collip was able to purify the insulin sufficiently so that in 1921 their colleague, Scots physiologist John Macleod, could administer the insulin to a 14-year-old boy with diabetes. It worked! The treatment not only relieved the boy's suffering, but gave him a healthy, long life. This breakthrough, for which Banting and Macleod received the 1923 Nobel Prize, was the start of a century of rapid progress in understanding and treating endocrine disorders.

Because hormones affect so many different body functions, nearly every kind of health professional, from medical doctors to nurses to dieticians, needs to be aware of their functions. Of course, hormones and chemicals that influence hormone actions are often used in treatments, so pharmacologists and pharmacists must also have an excellent knowledge of endocrinology. Some scientists have applied principles of endocrinology in a variety of unexpected ways, including the development of early pregnancy test kits and ovulation test kits to the use of synthetic hormones in healthy people to control their fertility.

OUTLINE SUMMARY

MECHANISMS OF HORMONE ACTION

A. Endocrine glands secrete chemicals (hormones) into the blood (Figure 10-1)
B. Hormones perform general functions of communication and control but a slower, longer-lasting type of control than that provided by nerve impulses
C. Cells acted on by hormones are called *target organ cells*
D. Nonsteroid hormones (first messengers) bind to receptors on the target cell membrane, triggering second messengers to affect the cell's activities (Figure 10-2)
E. Steroid hormones bind to receptors within the target cell nucleus and influence cell activity by acting on DNA (Figure 10-3)

REGULATION OF HORMONE SECRETION

A. Hormone secretion is controlled by homeostatic feedback
B. Negative feedback—mechanisms that reverse the direction of a change in a physiological system (Figure 10-4)
C. Positive feedback—(uncommon) mechanisms that amplify physiological changes

PROSTAGLANDINS

A. Prostaglandins (PGs) are powerful substances found in a wide variety of body tissues
B. PGs are often produced in a tissue and diffuse only a short distance to act on cells in that tissue
C. Several classes of PGs include prostaglandin A (PGA), prostaglandin E (PGE), and prostaglandin F (PGF)
D. PGs influence many body functions, including respiration, blood pressure, gastrointestinal secretions, and reproduction

PITUITARY GLAND (FIGURE 10-5)

A. Anterior pituitary gland (adenohypophysis)
   1. Names of major hormones
      a. Thyroid-stimulating hormone (TSH)
      b. Adrenocorticotropic hormone (ACTH)
      c. Follicle-stimulating hormone (FSH)
      d. Luteinizing hormone (LH)
      e. Growth hormone (GH)
      f. Prolactin (lactogenic hormone)
   2. Functions of major hormones
      a. TSH—stimulates growth of the thyroid gland; also stimulates it to secrete thyroid hormone
      b. ACTH—stimulates growth of the adrenal cortex and stimulates it to secrete glucocorticoids (mainly cortisol)
      c. FSH—initiates growth of ovarian follicles each month in the ovary and stimulates one or more follicles to develop to the stage of maturity and ovulation; FSH also stimulates estrogen secretion by developing follicles; stimulates sperm production in the male
      d. LH—acts with FSH to stimulate estrogen secretion and follicle growth to maturity; causes ovulation; causes luteinization of the ruptured follicle and stimulates progesterone secretion by corpus luteum; causes interstitial cells in the testes to secrete testosterone in the male
      e. GH—stimulates growth by accelerating protein anabolism; also accelerates fat catabolism and slows glucose catabolism; by slowing glucose catabolism, tends to increase blood glucose to higher than normal level (hyperglycemia)
      f. Prolactin or lactogenic hormone—stimulates breast development during pregnancy and secretion of milk after the delivery of the baby
B. Posterior pituitary gland (neurohypophysis)
   1. Names of hormones
      a. Antidiuretic hormone (ADH)
      b. Oxytocin
   2. Functions of hormones
      a. ADH—accelerates water reabsorption from urine in the kidney tubules into the blood, thereby decreasing urine secretion
      b. Oxytocin—stimulates the pregnant uterus to contract; may initiate labor; causes glandular cells of the breast to release milk into ducts

OUTLINE SUMMARY—*cont'd*

HYPOTHALAMUS

A. Actual production of ADH and oxytocin occurs in the hypothalamus
B. After production in the hypothalamus, hormones pass along axons into the pituitary gland
C. The secretion and release of posterior pituitary hormones is controlled by nervous stimulation
D. The hypothalamus controls many body functions related to homeostasis (temperature, appetite, and thirst)

THYROID GLAND (FIGURE 10-6)

A. Names of hormones
   1. Thyroid hormone—thyroxine (T_4) and triiodothyronine (T_3)
   2. Calcitonin
B. Functions of hormones
   1. Thyroid hormones—accelerate catabolism (increase the body's metabolic rate)
   2. Calcitonin—decreases the blood calcium concentration by inhibiting breakdown of bone, which would release calcium into the blood

PARATHYROID GLAND (FIGURE 10-6)

A. Name of hormone—parathyroid hormone (PTH)
B. Function of hormone—increases blood calcium concentration by increasing the breakdown of bone with the release of calcium into the blood

ADRENAL GLANDS (FIGURE 10-9)

A. Adrenal cortex
   1. Names of hormones (corticoids)
      a. Glucocorticoids (GCs)—chiefly cortisol (hydrocortisone)
      b. Mineralocorticoids (MCs)—chiefly aldosterone
      c. Sex hormones—small amounts of male hormones (androgens) secreted by adrenal cortex of both sexes
   2. Three cell layers (zones)
      a. Outer layer, secretes mineralocorticoids
      b. Middle layer, secretes glucocorticoids
      c. Inner layer, secretes sex hormones
   3. Mineralocorticoids—increase blood sodium and decrease body potassium concentrations by accelerating kidney tubule reabsorption of sodium and excretion of potassium
   4. Functions of glucocorticoids
      a. Help maintain normal blood glucose concentration by increasing gluconeogenesis—the formation of "new" glucose from amino acids produced by the breakdown of proteins, mainly those in muscle tissue cells; also the conversion to glucose of fatty acids produced by the breakdown of fats stored in adipose tissue cells
      b. Play an essential part in maintaining normal blood pressure—make it possible for epinephrine and norepinephrine to maintain a normal degree of vasoconstriction, a condition necessary for maintaining normal blood pressure
      c. Act with epinephrine and norepinephrine to produce an antiinflammatory effect, to bring about normal recovery from inflammations of various kinds
      d. Produce anti-immunity, antiallergy effect; bring about a decrease in the number of lymphocytes and plasma cells and therefore a decrease in the amount of antibodies formed
      e. Secretion of glucocorticoid quickly increases when the body is thrown into a condition of stress; high blood concentration of glucocorticoids, in turn, brings about many other stress responses (Figure 10-10)

Continued

OUTLINE SUMMARY—*cont'd*

B. Adrenal medulla
   1. Names of hormones—epinephrine (adrenaline) and norepinephrine
   2. Functions of hormones—help the body resist stress by intensifying and prolonging the effects of sympathetic stimulation; increased epinephrine secretion is the first endocrine response to stress

PANCREATIC ISLETS (FIGURE 10-11)

A. Names of hormones
   1. Glucagon—secreted by alpha cells
   2. Insulin—secreted by beta cells
B. Functions of hormones
   1. Glucagon increases the blood glucose level by accelerating liver glycogenolysis (conversion of glycogen to glucose)
   2. Insulin decreases the blood glucose by accelerating the movement of glucose out of the blood into cells, which increases glucose metabolism by cells

FEMALE SEX GLANDS

The ovaries contain two structures that secrete hormones—the ovarian follicles and the corpus luteum; see Chapter 20

A. Effects of estrogen (feminizing hormone)
   1. Development and maturation of breasts and external genitals
   2. Development of adult female body contours
   3. Initiation of menstrual cycle

MALE SEX GLANDS

The interstitial cells of testes secrete the male hormone testosterone; see Chapter 19

A. Effects of testosterone (masculinizing hormone)
   1. Maturation of external genitals
   2. Beard growth
   3. Voice changes at puberty
   4. Development of musculature and body contours typical of the male

THYMUS

A. Name of hormone—thymosin
B. Function of hormone—plays an important role in the development and function of the body's immune system

PLACENTA

A. Name of hormones—chorionic gonadotropins, estrogens, and progesterone
B. Functions of hormones—maintain the corpus luteum during pregnancy

PINEAL GLAND

A. A small gland near the roof of the third ventricle of the brain
   1. Glandular tissue predominates in children and young adults
   2. Becomes fibrous and calcified with age
B. Called *third eye* because its influence on secretory activity is related to the amount of light entering the eyes
C. Secretes melatonin, which
   1. Inhibits ovarian activity
   2. Regulates the body's internal clock

OTHER ENDOCRINE STRUCTURES

A. Many organs (for example, the stomach, intestines, and kidney) produce endocrine hormones
B. The atrial wall of the heart secretes atrial natriuretic hormone (ANH), which stimulates sodium loss from the kidneys
C. Fat-storing cells secrete leptin, which controls how full or hungry we feel

NEW WORDS

corticoids
cretinism
Cushing's syndrome
diabetes insipidus
diabetes mellitus
diuresis
endocrine
exocrine
gigantism
glucocorticoids
gluconeogenesis
glycogenolysis
goiter
hormone
hypercalcemia
hyperglycemia
hypoglycemia
luteinization
mineralocorticoids
myxedema
negative feedback
prostaglandins
second messenger
steroids
stress
target organ cell

REVIEW QUESTIONS

1. Differentiate between endocrine and exocrine glands.
2. Define or explain *hormone, target organ, hypersecretion*, and *hyposecretion*.
3. Explain the mechanism of action of nonsteroid hormones.
4. Explain the mechanism of action of steroid hormones.
5. Explain and give an example of a negative feedback loop for the regulation of hormone secretion.
6. Explain and give an example of a positive feedback loop for the regulation of hormone secretion.
7. Explain the difference between prostaglandins and hormones. List some of the body functions that can be influenced by prostaglandins.
8. Describe the structure of the pituitary gland and where it is located.
9. Name the four tropic hormones released by the anterior pituitary gland and briefly explain their function.
10. Explain the function of growth hormone.
11. Explain the function of ADH.
12. Explain the function of prolactin and oxytocin.
13. Explain the function of the hypothalamus in the endocrine system.
14. Explain the difference between T_3 and T_4. What is unique about the thyroid gland?
15. Name the hormones produced by the zones or areas of the adrenal cortex.
16. Explain the function of aldosterone.
17. Explain the function of glucocorticoids.

CRITICAL THINKING

18. Explain why a second messenger system is necessary for nonsteroid hormones but not for steroid hormones.
19. Pick a body function (regulation of glucose or calcium levels in the blood) and explain how the interaction of hormones is used to help maintain homeostasis.
20. What would be the effect on the body if the thyroid gland were removed?
21. A doctor discovered a patient had very low levels of thyroxine but high levels of TSH. Is the patient's problem in the thyroid gland or the pituitary gland? Explain your answer.

CHAPTER TEST

1. Exocrine glands secrete their products into ducts that empty onto a surface or into a cavity.
2. Endocrine glands are ductless and secrete their products, called hormones, into intercellular spaces where they diffuse into the blood.
3. The two major classes of hormones are Protein hormones and Steroid hormones.
4. A cell or body organ that has receptors for a hormone that triggers a reaction is called a Target organ
5. One example of a second messenger system involves the conversion of ATP into Cyclic AMP.
6. The hormone receptors for nonsteroid hormones are located on the membrane whereas the receptors for steroid hormones are located in the nucleus
7. "Tissue hormones" is another name for Prostaglandins
8. This part of the pituitary gland is made of nervous tissue: Posterior. Pituitary
9. This part of the pituitary gland is made of glandular tissue: Anterior Pituitary
10. The hormone oxytocin is released by the Posterior Pituitary but is made in the hypothalmus.
11. A tropic hormone secreted by the anterior pituitary gland is:
    a. thyroid-stimulating hormone
    b. adrenocorticotropic hormone
    c. luteinizing hormone
    d. all of the above
12. Antidiuretic hormone (ADH):
    a. is made in the posterior pituitary gland
    b. accelerates water reabsorption in the kidney
    c. in high concentrations causes diabetes insipidus
    d. all of the above
13. This hormone is released by the anterior pituitary and stimulates breast development during pregnancy necessary for eventual milk production:
    a. estrogen
    b. oxytocin
    c. prolactin
    d. progesterone
14. This hormone is released by the posterior pituitary and stimulates the contraction of the pregnant uterus:
    a. estrogen
    b. oxytocin
    c. prolactin
    d. progesterone
15. Thyroxine:
    a. is symbolized by T_3
    b. is made in the thyroid gland
    c. contains less iodine then triiodothyronine
    d. all of the above
16. Calcitonin:
    a. decreases the level of calcium in the blood
    b. increases the level of calcium in the blood
    c. stimulates the release of calcium from bone tissue
    d. both b and c

CHAPTER TEST—*cont'd*

25/25

Match the function or source in Column B with the hormone in Column A.

COLUMN A	COLUMN B
17. __D__ Parathyroid hormone	**a.** released by the adrenal medulla; prolongs the effect of the sympathetic nervous system
18. __F__ Mineralocorticoids	**b.** made in the heart; helps regulate blood sodium
19. __I__ Glucocorticoids	**c.** made in the islets of Langerhans; decreases blood glucose levels
20. __A__ Epinephrine	**d.** has the opposite effect of calcitonin
21. __E__ Glucagon	**e.** made by alpha cells in the pancreatic islets
22. __C__ Insulin	**f.** made in the outermost layer of the adrenal cortex
23. __H__ Chorionic gonadotropins	**g.** the most significant hormone released by the pineal gland
24. __G__ Melatonin	**h.** the hormone made by the placenta and detected by home pregnancy tests
25. __B__ Atrial natriuretic hormone	**i.** made by the middle layer of the adrenal cortex

STUDY TIPS

Before studying Chapter 10, review the synopsis of the endocrine system in Chapter 4. The function of the endocrine system is the same as that of the nervous system. The differences are in the methods used and the extent of the effect. The endocrine system uses chemicals in the blood (hormones) rather than nerve impulses. Hormones can have a direct effect on almost every cell in the body, an impossible task for the nervous system. Steroid hormones can act directly since they can enter the cell; protein hormones cannot enter the cell so they need a second messenger system. Material from earlier chapters such as receptor proteins in the cell membrane, ATP, homeostasis, and negative feedback loops will help you understand the material in this chapter. Use flash cards to learn the names of the hormones, what they do, and the names and locations of the glands that produce them. Remember that hormones released by the posterior pituitary gland are made in the hypothalamus.

In your study group, discuss the hormone mechanisms and the negative feedback loops involved in hormone regulation. Go over the hormone flash cards. A photocopy of the figure with the glands may be helpful. You can quiz each other on which gland produces what hormone. Go over the questions at the end of the chapter and discuss possible test questions.

11 Blood

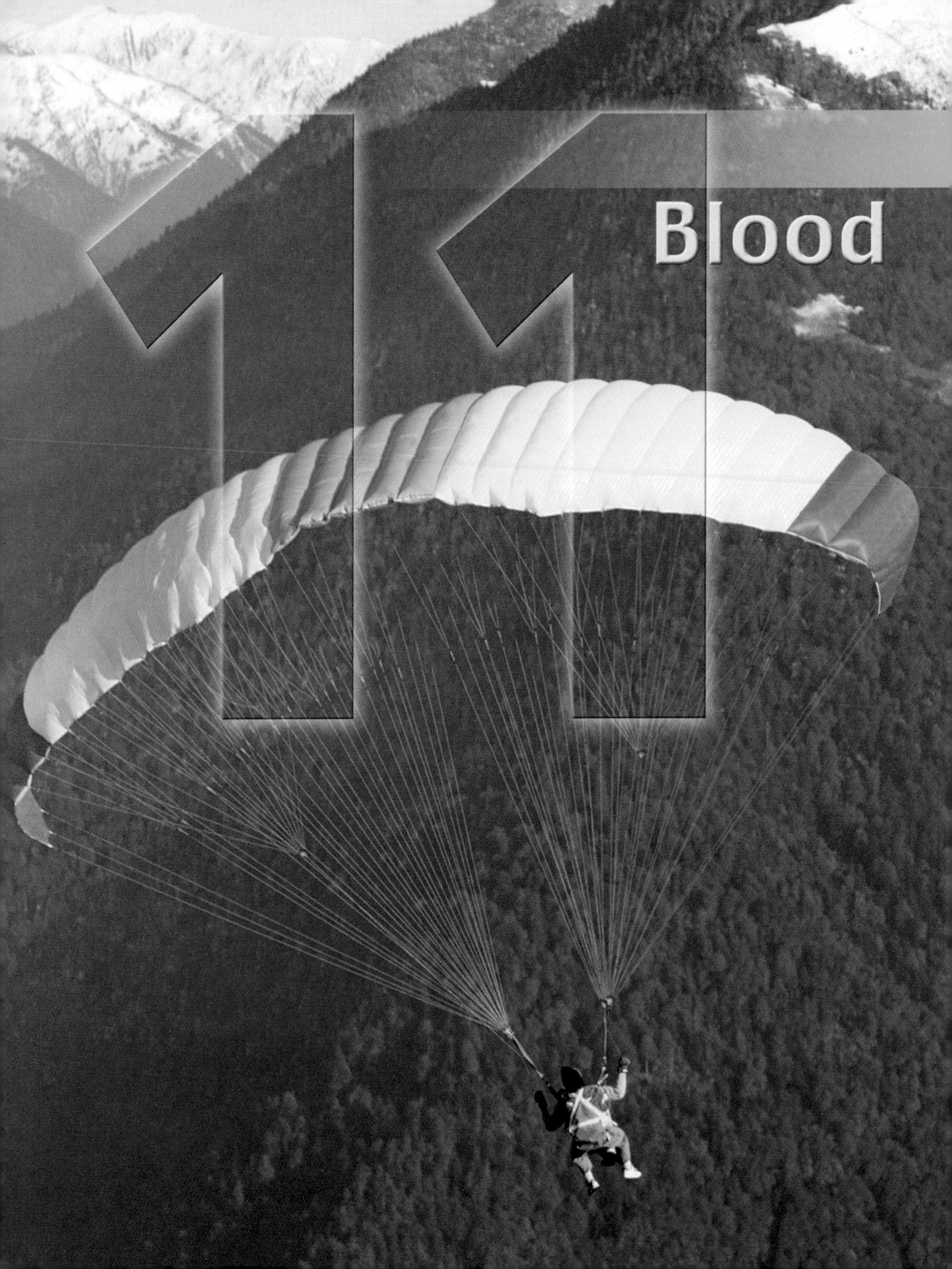

Outline

Objectives

AFTER YOU HAVE COMPLETED THIS CHAPTER, YOU SHOULD BE ABLE TO:

1. Describe the primary functions of blood.
2. Describe the characteristics of blood plasma.
3. List the formed elements of blood and identify the most important function of each.
4. Discuss anemia in terms of red blood cell numbers and hemoglobin content.
5. Explain the steps involved in blood clotting.
6. Describe ABO and Rh blood typing.
7. Define the following medical terms associated with blood: *hematocrit, leukocytosis, leukopenia, polycythemia, sickle cell, phagocytosis, acidosis, thrombosis, erythroblastosis fetalis, serum, fibrinogen, Rh factor, anemia.*

T*he next few* chapters deal with **transportation** and **protection,** two of the body's most important functions. Have you ever thought of what would happen if the transportation ceased in your city or town? Or what would happen if the police, firefighters, and armed services stopped doing their jobs? Food would become scarce, garbage would pile up, and no one would protect you or your property. Stretch your imagination just a little, and you can imagine many disastrous results. Similarly, lack of transportation and protection for the cells—the "individuals" of the body—threatens the homeostasis of the body. The systems that provide these vital services for the body are the **circulatory system** and **lymphatic system.** In this chapter, we will discuss the primary transportation fluid: blood. Blood not only performs vital pickup and delivery services, but it also provides much of the protection necessary to withstand foreign "invaders." Blood vessels and the heart are discussed in Chapter 12. The lymphatic system is discussed in Chapter 13.

BLOOD COMPOSITION

Blood is a fluid tissue that has many kinds of chemicals dissolved in it and millions upon millions of cells floating in it (Figure 11-1). The liquid (extracellular) part is called **plasma.** Suspended in the plasma are many different types of cells and cell fragments, which make up the **formed elements** of blood.

Blood Plasma

Blood plasma is the liquid part of the blood, or blood minus its formed elements. It consists of water with many substances dissolved in it. All of the chemicals needed by cells to stay alive—food, oxygen, and salts, for example—have to be brought to them by the blood. Food and salts are dissolved in plasma; so, too, is a small amount of oxygen. (Most of the oxygen in the blood is carried in the red blood cells as oxyhemoglobin.) Wastes that cells must get rid of are dissolved in plasma and transported to the excretory organs. The hormones and other regulatory chemicals that help control cells' activities are also dissolved in plasma. As Figure 11-1 shows, the most abundant type of solute in the plasma is a group of **plasma proteins.** These proteins include *albumins,* which help thicken the blood; *globulins,* which include the an-

FIGURE 11-1

Components of blood. Approximate values for the components of blood in a normal adult. Values will vary with age, sex, and nutritional status.

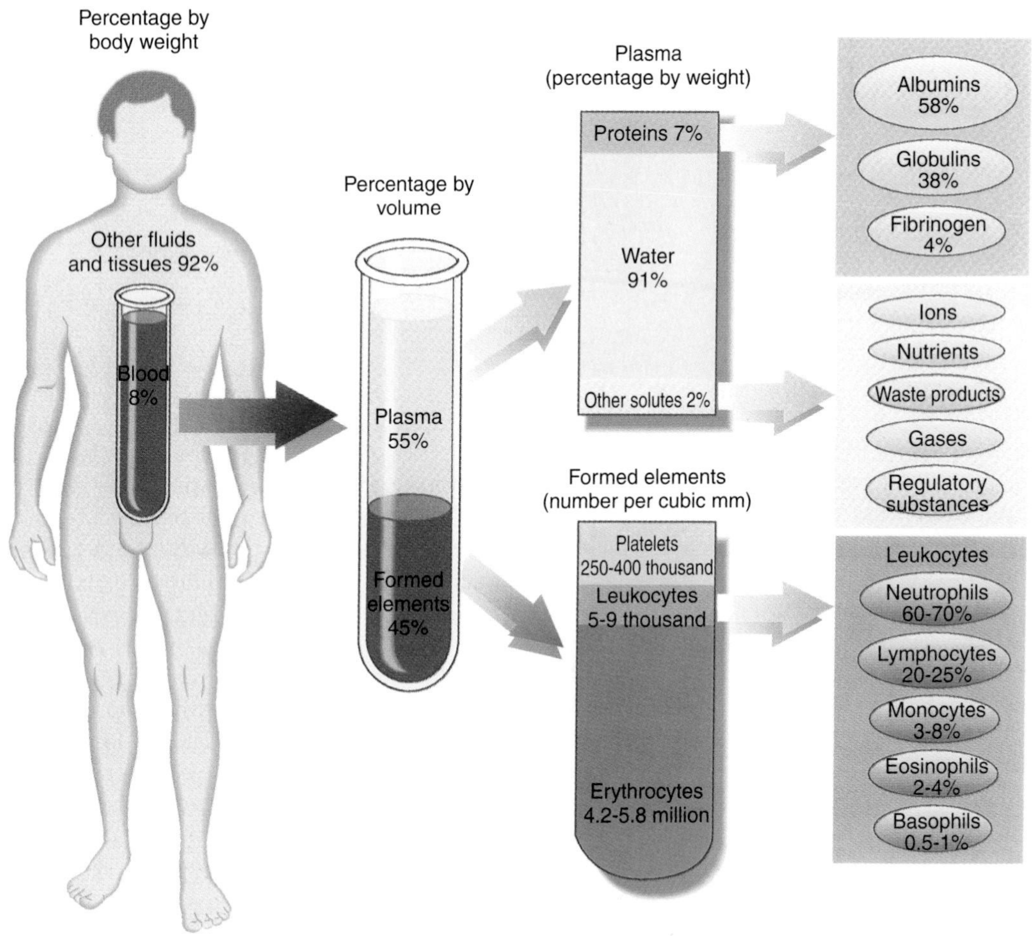

tibodies that help protect us from infections; and *fibrinogen*, which is necessary for blood clotting.

Blood **serum** is plasma minus its clotting factors, such as fibrinogen. Serum is obtained from whole blood by allowing it to clot in the bottom of a tube and then pouring off the liquid serum. Serum still contains antibodies, so it can be used to treat patients that have a need for specific antibodies.

Many people seem curious about how much blood they have. The amount depends on how big they are and whether they are male or female. A big person has more blood than a small person, and a man has more blood than a woman. But as a general rule, most adults probably have between 4 and 6 liters of blood. It normally accounts for about 7% to 9% of the total body weight.

The volume of the plasma part of blood is usually a little more than half the volume of whole blood. Examples of normal volumes are plasma: 2.6 L; blood cells: 2.4 L; and total blood: 5 L.

Formed Elements

There are three main types and several subtypes of formed elements:

1. Red blood cells (RBCs) or **erythrocytes** (e-RITH-ro-sites)
2. White blood cells (WBCs) or **leukocytes** (LOO-ko-sites)
    a. Granular leukocytes (have granules in their cytoplasm)
        (1) Neutrophils
        (2) Eosinophils
        (3) Basophils
    b. Nongranular leukocytes (do not have granules in their cytoplasm)
        (1) Lymphocytes
        (2) Monocytes
3. Platelets or **thrombocytes** (THROM-bo-sites)

Figure 11-1 shows the breakdown of numbers and percentages of the formed elements. Table 11-1 lists the functions of these different kinds of blood cells and shows what each looks like under the microscope.

It is difficult to believe how many blood cells and cell fragments there are in the body. For instance, 5,000,000 RBCs, 7500 WBCs, and 300,000 platelets in 1 cubic millimeter (mm^3) of blood (approximately 1 drop) would be considered normal RBC, WBC, and platelet counts. Because RBCs, WBCs, and platelets are continually being destroyed, the body must continually make new ones to take their place at a really staggering rate; a few million RBCs are manufactured *each second*!

Two kinds of connective tissue—**myeloid tissue** and **lymphatic tissue**—make blood cells for the body. Recall that formation of new blood cells is called *hemopoiesis*. Myeloid tissue is better known as *red bone marrow*. In the adult, it is chiefly in the sternum, ribs, and hipbones. A few other bones such as the vertebrae, clavicles, and cranial bones also contain small amounts of this important tissue. Red bone marrow forms all types of blood cells except some lymphocytes and monocytes. Most of these others are formed by lymphatic tissue, which is located chiefly in the lymph nodes, thymus, and spleen.

As blood cells mature, they move into the circulatory vessels. Erythrocytes circulate for up to 4 months before they break apart and their components are removed from the bloodstream by the liver. Granular leukocytes often have a lifespan of only a few days, but nongranular leukocytes may live for more than 6 months.

Quick Check

1. What are "formed elements" of blood?
2. What is the difference between blood *plasma* and blood *serum*?

Red Blood Cells

As you can see in Figure 11-2, RBCs have an unusual shape. The cell is "caved in" on both sides so that each one has a thin center and thicker edges. Notice also that mature RBCs have no nucleus. Figure 11-2 shows RBCs photographed with a scanning electron microscope. With this instrument, extremely small objects can be enlarged far more than is possible with a standard light microscope, and, as you can see in the illustration, objects appear more three-dimensional. Because of the large numbers of RBCs and their unique shape, their total surface area is enormous. In fact, the total surface area of the body's RBCs provides an area larger than a football field for the exchange of oxygen and carbon dioxide between the blood and the body's cells.

TABLE 11-1

Classes of Blood Cells

BODY CELL		FUNCTION	BODY CELL		FUNCTION
Erythrocyte	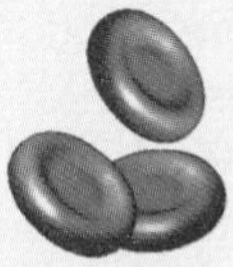	Oxygen and carbon dioxide transport	B-lymphocyte	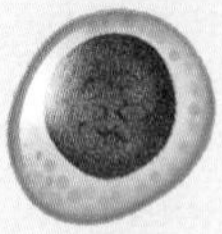	Antibody production
Neutrophil	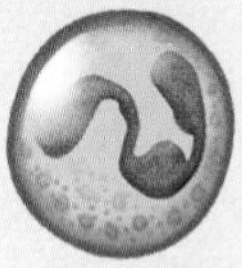	Immune defense (phagocytosis)	T-lymphocyte	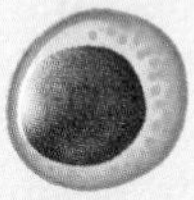	Cellular immune response
Eosinophil	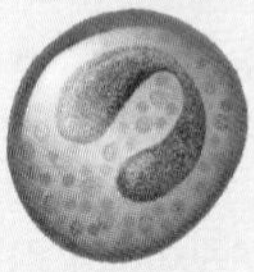	Defense against parasites	Monocyte	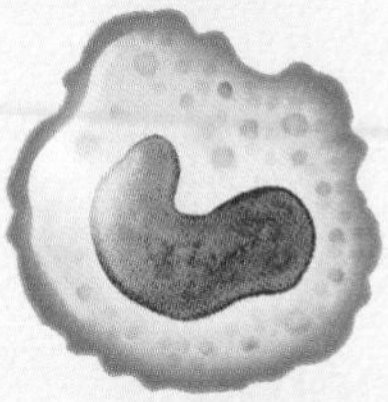	Immune defenses (phagocytosis)
Basophil	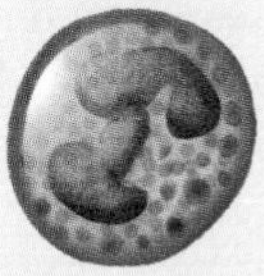	Inflammatory response	Platelet	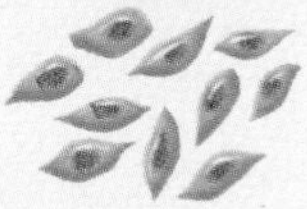	Blood clotting

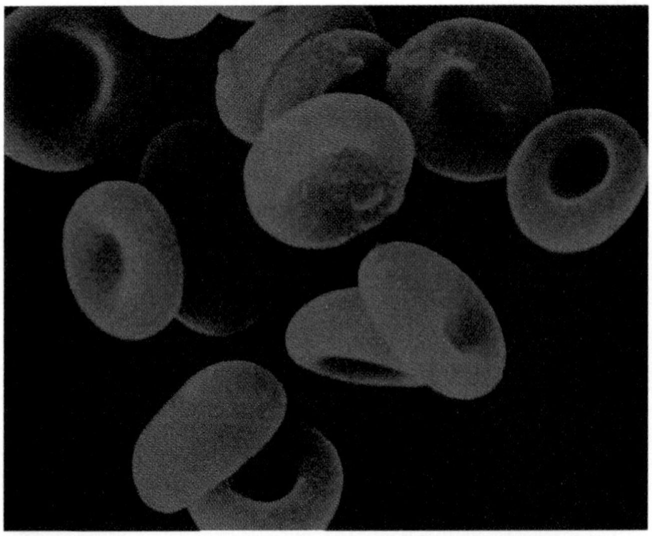

FIGURE 11-2

RBCs. Color-enhanced scanning electron micrograph shows the detailed structure of normal red blood cells.

RBCs perform several important functions. One essential function is to help transport carbon dioxide. Carbon dioxide (CO_2) is a harmful waste produced by the energy-producing processes of all living cells. It must be carried away from cells and to the lungs for disposal into the external environment. RBCs also transport oxygen from the lungs to other cells in the body. A red pigment called **hemoglobin** (hee-mo-glo-bin) in RBCs unites with oxygen to form **oxyhemoglobin** (ok-see-hee-mo-glo-bin). This combined oxygen-hemoglobin complex makes possible the efficient transport of large quantities of oxygen to body cells. Hemoglobin can also carry a small proportion of the CO_2 carried by the blood, forming **carbaminohemoglobin** (kar-bam-ee-no-hee-mo-GLO-bin).

The term **anemia** (ah-NEE-me-ah) is used to describe a number of different disease conditions caused by an inability of the blood to carry sufficient oxygen to the body cells. Anemias can result from inadequate numbers of RBCs or a deficiency of hemoglobin. Thus anemia can occur if the hemoglobin in RBCs is inadequate, even if adequate numbers of RBCs are present. Anemias caused by an actual decrease in the number of RBCs can occur if blood is lost by hemorrhage, as with accidents or bleeding ulcers, or if the blood-forming tissues cannot maintain normal numbers of blood cells. Such failures occur because of cancer, radiation (x-ray) damage, and certain types of infections. The term **pernicious** (per-NISH-us) **anemia** is used to describe a deficiency of RBCs caused by the lack of vitamin B_{12}. If bone marrow produces an excess of RBCs, the result is a condition called **polycythemia** (pol-ee-sye-THEE-me-ah). The blood in individuals suffering from this condition may contain so many RBCs that it may become too thick to flow properly.

Iron is a critical component of the hemoglobin molecule. Without adequate iron in the diet, the body cannot manufacture enough hemoglobin. The result is **iron deficiency anemia,** a worldwide medical problem. If hemoglobin falls below the normal level, as it does in this type of anemia, it starts an unhealthy chain reaction: less hemoglobin, less oxygen transported to cells, slower breakdown and use of nutrients by cells, less energy produced by cells, decreased cellular functions. If you understand this relationship between hemoglobin and energy, you can correctly guess that an anemic person's chief complaint will probably be that he or she feels "so tired all the time."

A common laboratory test called the **hematocrit** can tell a physician a great deal about the volume of RBCs in a blood sample. If whole blood is placed in a special hematocrit tube and then "spun down" in a centrifuge, the heavier formed elements will quickly settle to the bottom of the tube. During the hematocrit procedure, RBCs are forced to the bottom of the tube first. The WBCs and platelets then settle out in a layer called the **buffy coat.** In Figure 11-3 the buffy coat can be seen between the packed RBCs on the bottom of the hematocrit tube and the liquid layer of plasma above. Normally about 45% of the blood volume consists of RBCs. For a patient with anemia, the percentage of RBCs drops, and for a patient with polycythemia, it increases dramatically (see Figure 11-3).

FIGURE 11-3

Hematocrit tubes showing normal blood, anemia, and polycythemia. Note the buffy coat located between the packed RBCs and the plasma. **A,** A normal percentage of red blood cells (RBCs). **B,** Anemia (a low percentage of RBCs). **C,** Polycythemia (a high percentage of RBCs).

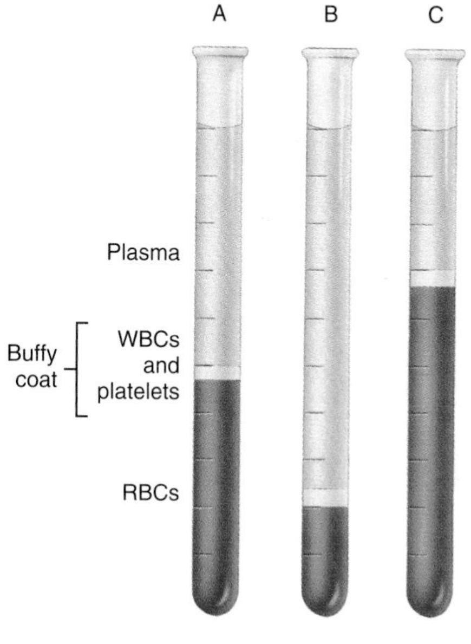

Clinical Application

Sickle Cell Anemia

Sickle cell anemia is a severe and sometimes fatal hereditary disease caused by an abnormal type of hemoglobin. A person who inherits only one defective gene develops a form of the disease called *sickle cell trait*. In this condition, RBCs contain a small amount of a type of hemoglobin that is less soluble than normal. It forms solid crystals when the blood oxygen level is low, causing distortion of the RBC. If two defective genes are inherited (one from each parent), more of the defective hemoglobin is produced, and the distortion of red blood cells becomes severe. In the United States, nearly 1 in every 500 African-American and 1 in every 1000 Hispanic newborns are affected each year.

Stroke is one of the most devastating problems associated with sickle cell anemia in children. Unfortunately, after a stroke occurs, recurrence is common. Recent studies have shown that frequent blood transfusions in addition to standard care can dramatically reduce the risk of stroke in many children suffering from sickle cell anemia.

The illustration shows the characteristic shape of many RBCs in sickle cell anemia.

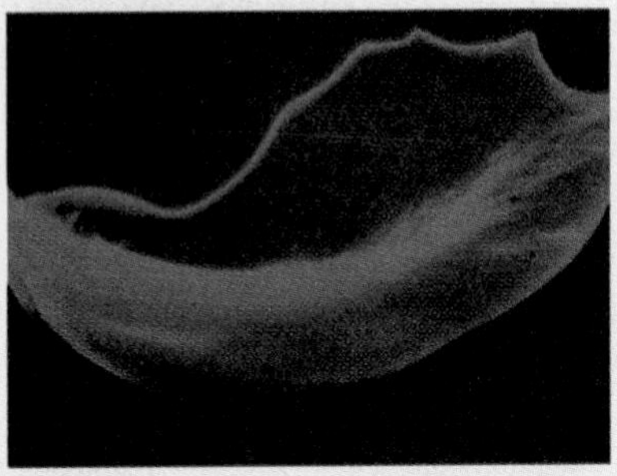

Quick
1. What protein in blood cells carries oxygen?
2. Can you give a broad definition of *anemia*?

White Blood Cells

WBCs have a function that is just as vital as that of RBCs. They defend the body from microorganisms that have succeeded in invading our body. WBCs also attack cancer cells that form inside our tissues. For example, **neutrophils** (NOO-tro-fils) (Figure 11-4, *A*) and **monocytes** (MON-o-sites) (Figure 11-4, *E*) engulf microbes. They actually take them into their own cell bodies and digest them in the process of **phagocytosis** (see p. 347), and the cells that carry on this process are called **phagocytes** (FAG-o-sites) (Figure 11-5). The neutrophils are the most numerous of the phagocytes.

WBCs of the type called **lymphocytes** (LIM-fo-sites) (Figure 11-4, *D*) also help protect us against infections, but they do it by a process different from that of phagocytosis. Lymphocytes function in the immune mechanism, the complex process that makes us immune to infectious diseases and that suppresses cancer. The immune mechanism starts to operate, for example, when microbes invade the body. In some way, their presence stimulates lymphocytes to start multiplying and become active immune cells. Lymphocytes called *B-lymphocytes* begin to actively produce specific antibodies that inhibit the microbes. Other lymphocytes, called *T-lymphocytes*, may also become involved by directly attacking the microbes or aiding in the function of B-lymphocytes. Details of the immune system are discussed in Chapter 13.

Eosinophils (ee-o-SIN-o-fils) (Figure 11-4, *B*) are granulocytic WBCs that help protect the body from parasites and the numerous irritants that cause allergies. They are also capable of phagocytosis. **Basophils** (BAY-so-fils) (Figure 11-4, C) also function in allergic reactions. These leukocytes, which are less abundant than other types, also secrete a number of important substances. For example, they secrete the potent chemical **heparin,** which helps prevent the clotting of blood as it flows through the blood vessels of the body.

The term **leukopenia** (loo-ko-PEE-nee-ah) refers to an abnormally low WBC count (less than 5000 WBCs/mm^3 of blood). A number of disease conditions may affect the immune system and decrease the amount of circulating WBCs. **Acquired immunodeficiency syndrome** or **AIDS,** which will be discussed in Chapter 13, is one example of a disease characterized by marked leukopenia. **Leukocytosis** (loo-ko-SYE-toe-sis) refers to

FIGURE 11-4

Leukocytes in human blood smears. Each light micrograph shows a different type of stained white blood cell surrounded by several smaller red blood cells.

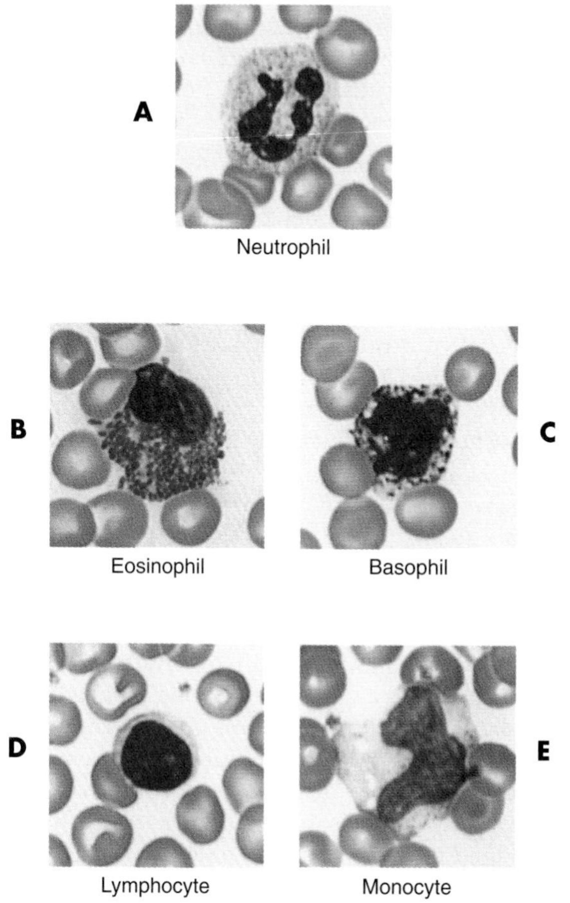

FIGURE 11-5

Phagocytosis. This transmission electron micrograph shows a phagocytic cell consuming a foreign particle in a manner similar to that used by a white blood cell. Extensions of the plasma membrane literally reach out and grab a particle and then digest the particle within an intracellular vesicle.

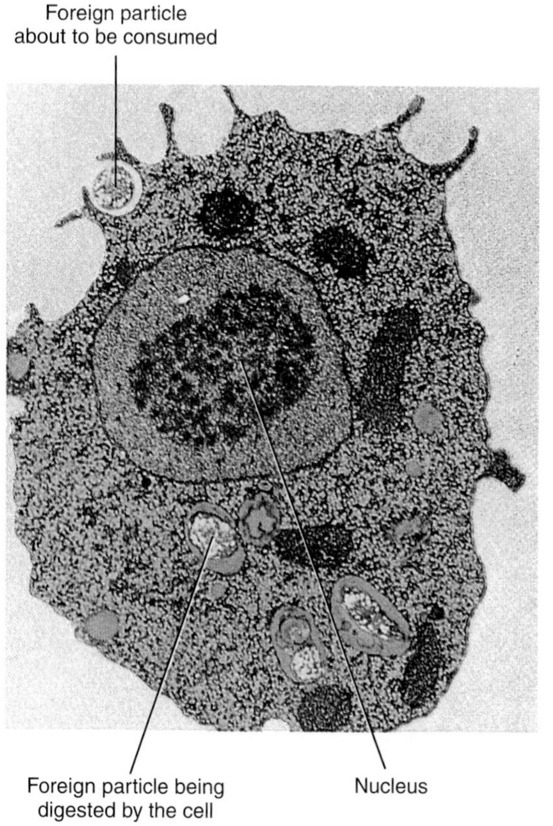

an abnormally high WBC count (more than 10,000 WBCs/mm^3 of blood). Leukocytosis is a much more common problem than leukopenia and almost always accompanies infections. There is also a malignant disease, **leukemia** (loo-KEE-mee-ah), in which the number of WBCs increases tremendously. The buffy coat is thicker and more noticeable in the hematocrit of blood from patients with leukemia because of the elevated WBC counts. You may have heard of this disease as "blood cancer." As in all cancers, the extra cells do not function properly.

Platelets and Blood Clotting

Platelets, the third main type of formed element, play an essential part in blood clotting. Your life might someday be saved just because your blood can clot. A clot plugs up torn or cut vessels and stops bleeding that otherwise might prove fatal.

The story of how blood clots is the story of a chain of rapid-fire reactions. The first step in the chain is some kind of an injury to a blood vessel that makes a rough spot in its lining. (Normally the lining of blood vessels is extremely smooth.) Almost immediately, damaged tissue cells in the injured vessel wall release certain clotting factors into the plasma. These factors rapidly react with other factors already present in the plasma to form **prothrombin activator** (pro-THROM-bin AK-tiv-ayt-or). At the same time this is happening, platelets become "sticky" at the point of injury and soon accumulate near the opening in the broken blood vessel, forming a soft, temporary *platelet plug*. As the platelets accumulate, they release additional clotting factors, forming even more prothrombin activator. If the normal amount of blood calcium is present, prothrombin activator triggers the next step of clotting by converting **prothrombin** (a protein in normal blood) to **thrombin** (THROM-bin). In the last step, thrombin reacts with **fibrinogen** (fi-BRIN-o-jen) (a normal plasma protein) to change it to a fibrous gel called **fibrin.** Under the microscope, fibrin looks like a tangle of fine threads with RBCs caught in the tangle. This meshwork is the blood clot that forms a more long-term seal of the damaged blood vessel. Figure 11-6 illustrates the steps in the blood-clotting mechanism.

The clotting mechanism contains clues for ways to stop bleeding by speeding up blood clotting. For example, you might simply apply gauze to a bleeding surface. Its slight roughness would cause more platelets to stick together and release more clotting factors. These additional factors would then make the blood clot more quickly.

Physicians sometimes prescribe vitamin K before surgery to make sure that the patient's blood will clot fast enough to prevent hemorrhage. Vitamin K stimulates liver cells to increase the synthesis of prothrombin. More prothrombin in blood allows faster production of thrombin during clotting and thus faster clot formation. A few years ago, surgeons also began using a product made of fibrinogen and thrombin which, when mixed, form a kind of "artificial clot" at the site of bleeding.

Unfortunately, clots sometimes form in unbroken blood vessels of the heart, brain, lungs, or some other organ—a dreaded thing because they may produce sudden death by shutting off the blood supply to a vital organ. When a clot stays in the place where it formed, it is called a **thrombus** (THROM-bus) and the condition is spoken of as **thrombosis** (throm-BO-sus). If part of the clot dislodges and circulates through the bloodstream, the dislodged part is then called an **embolus** (EM-bo-lus), and the condition is called an **embolism** (EM-bo-lizm). A number of drugs are now available to

Clinical Application

Anticoagulant Therapy

The anticoagulant Coumadin (warfarin sodium) acts by inhibiting the synthesis of prothrombin and other vitamin K–dependent clotting factors. By doing so, Coumadin decreases the ability of blood to clot and is effective in preventing repeat thromboses after a heart attack or the formation of clots after surgical replacement of heart valves. Heparin can also be used to prevent excessive blood clotting. Heparin inhibits the conversion of prothrombin to thrombin, thus preventing formation of a thrombus.

A laboratory test called the *prothrombin time (PT)* is often used to regulate dosage of Coumadin. In this test thromboplastin and calcium are added simultaneously to a tube of the patient's plasma and a tube containing a normal control solution, and the time required for clot formation in both tubes is determined. A patient prothrombin time in excess of the standard control value (11 to 12.5 seconds) indicates the level of anticoagulant effect caused by the administered drug. Heparin dosage is regulated with results of a similar type of test called *partial prothrombin time (PPT)*. Information from these tests allows the physician to adjust the dose required to maintain an appropriate level of anticoagulant effect.

Clinical Application

Surgical Glue

A new product developed to stop bleeding and seal wounds in surgery was approved for sale in the United States in 1999. The product, called *Tisseel*, consists of purified fibrinogen and thrombin which, when mixed, form an effective and immediate gluelike seal at the point of hemorrhage.

FIGURE 11-6

Blood clotting. **A,** The extremely complex clotting mechanism can be distilled into three basic steps: 1, release of clotting factors from both injured tissue cells and sticky platelets at the injury site (which form a temporary platelet plug); 2, series of chemical reactions that eventually result in the formation of thrombin; and 3, formation of fibrin and trapping of red blood cells to form a clot. **B,** Red and white blood cells (WBCs) entrapped in a fibrin (yellow) mesh during clot formation (WBCs are blue).

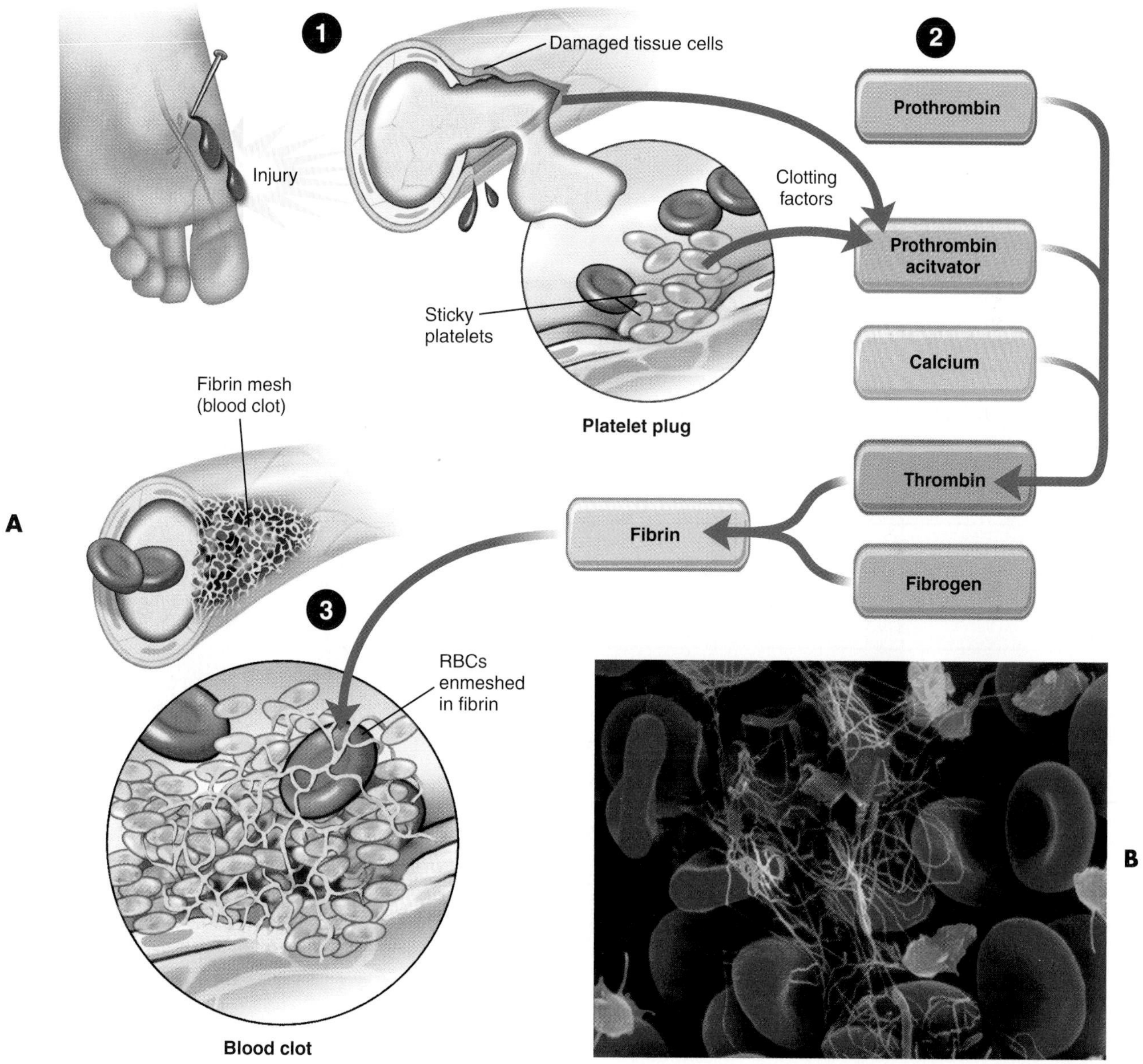

help dissolve clots. *Streptokinase* and *recombinant tissue plasminogen activator* (*t-PA*) are drugs frequently used in a variety of conditions, including treatment of clot-induced strokes, heart attacks, and other thrombus- and embolus-induced medical emergencies. Suppose that your doctor told you that you had a clot in one of your coronary arteries. Which diagnosis would he or she make—coronary thrombosis or coronary embolism—if the physician thought that the clot had formed originally in the coronary artery as a result of the accumulation of fatty material in the vessel wall? Physicians now have effective drugs that they can use to help prevent thrombosis and embolism.

Quick

1. Can you name the five major types of WBC?
2. In general, what function do the white blood cells perform?
3. What is the role of fibrin in blood clotting?

BLOOD TYPES

ABO System

Blood types are identified by certain "self-antigens" located in the plasma membrane of the RBCs (Figure 11-7). An **antigen** (AN-ti-gen) is a substance

FIGURE 11-7

Results of different combinations of donor and recipient blood. The left columns show the recipient's blood characteristics and the top row shows the donor's blood type.

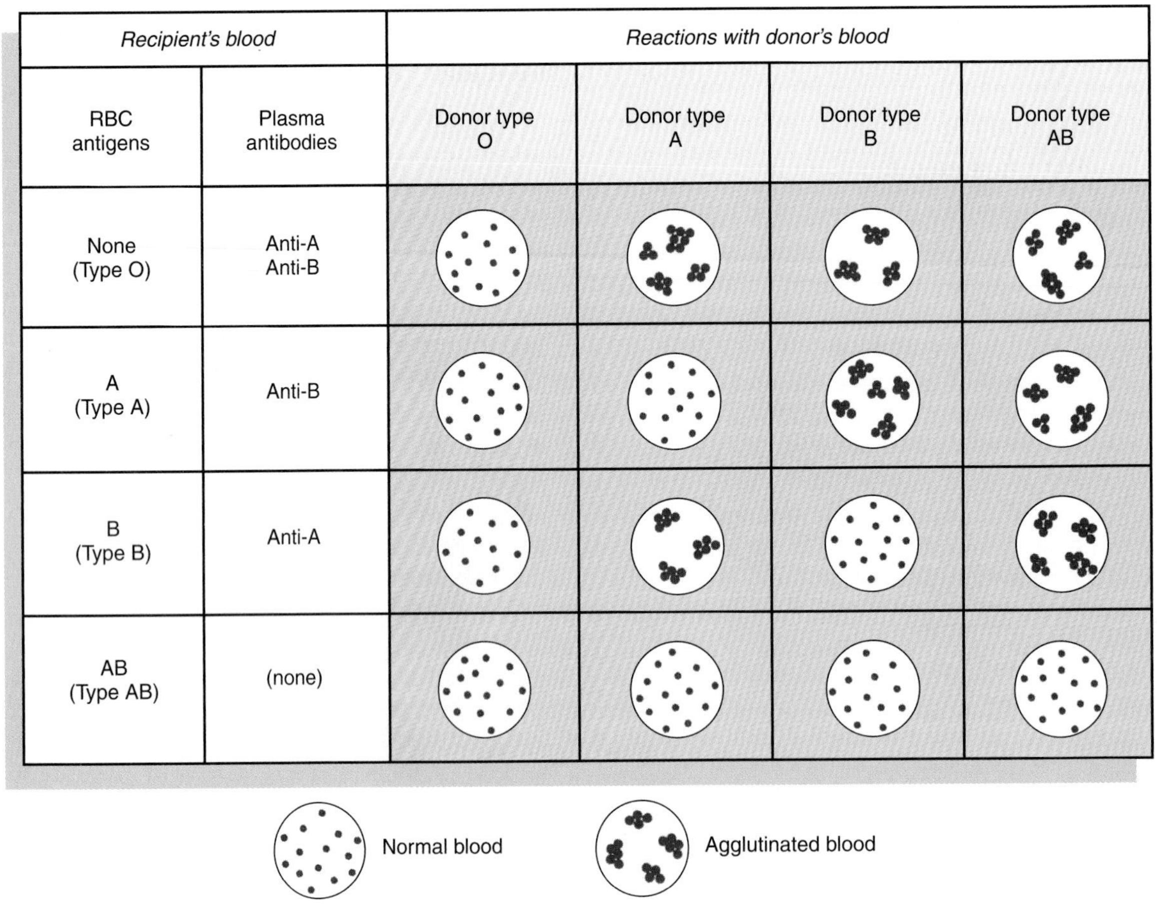
Recipient's blood
Reactions with donor's blood
RBC antigens
Plasma antibodies
Donor type O
Donor type A
Donor type B
Donor type AB
None (Type O)
Anti-A Anti-B
A (Type A)
Anti-B
B (Type B)
Anti-A
AB (Type AB)
(none)
Normal blood
Agglutinated blood

that can activate the immune system to make certain responses, including the production of antibodies. Almost all substances that act as antigens and stimulate the immune system are foreign proteins called "non-self" antigens. That is, they are not the body's own natural self-antigens, which are found on the cell membranes of normal body cells. Instead, they are generally proteins that have entered the body from the outside by infection, transfusion, or some other method.

The word *antibody* can be defined in terms of what causes its formation or in terms of how it functions. Defined the first way, an **antibody** (an-ti-bod-ee) is a substance made by the body in response to stimulation by an antigen. Defined according to its functions, an antibody is a substance that reacts with the antigen that stimulated its formation. Many antibodies react with their antigens to clump or **agglutinate** (ah-GLOO-tin-ate) them. In other words, they cause their antigens to stick together in little clusters.

Every person's blood is one of the following blood types in the ABO system of typing:

1. Type A
2. Type B
3. Type AB
4. Type O

Suppose that you have type A blood (as do about 41% of Americans). The letter A stands for a certain type of "self-antigen" (a protein) in the plasma membrane of your RBCs since birth. Because you were born with type A antigen, your body does not form antibodies to react with it. In other words, your blood plasma contains no anti-A antibodies. It does, however, contain anti-B antibodies. For some unknown reason, these antibodies are present naturally in type A blood plasma. The body did not form them in response to the presence of the B antigen. In summary, in type A blood the RBCs contain type A antigen and the plasma contains anti-B antibodies.

Similarly, in type B blood, the RBCs contain type B self-antigen, and the plasma contains anti-A antibodies. In type AB blood, as its name indicates, the RBCs contain both type A and type B self-antigens, and the plasma contains neither anti-A nor anti-B antibodies. The opposite is true of type O blood; its RBCs contain neither type A nor type B antigens, and its plasma contains both anti-A and anti-B antibodies.

Harmful effects or even death can result from a blood transfusion if the donor's RBCs become agglutinated by antibodies in the recipient's plasma. If a donor's RBCs do not contain any A or B antigen, they of course cannot be clumped by anti-A or anti-B antibodies. For this reason the type of blood that contains neither A nor B antigens—namely, type O blood—can be used in an emergency as donor blood without the danger of anti-A or anti-B antibodies clumping its RBCs. Type O blood has therefore been called **universal donor** blood. Similarly, blood type AB has been called **universal recipient** blood because it contains neither anti-A nor anti-B antibodies in its plasma. Therefore it does not clump any donor's RBCs containing A or B antigens. In a normal clinical setting, however, all blood intended for transfusion is matched carefully to the blood of the recipient for a variety of factors.

Figure 11-7 shows the results of different combinations of donor and recipient blood.

Rh System

You may be familiar with the term **Rh-positive** blood. It means that the RBCs of this type of blood contain an antigen called the Rh factor. This is the case for about 85% of the white and 88% of the African-American population in the United States. If, for example, a person has type AB, Rh-positive

Health & Well-Being

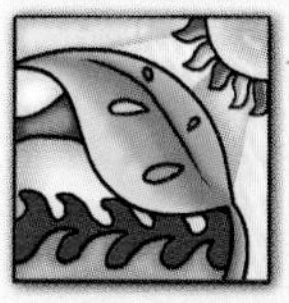

Blood Doping

A number of athletes have reportedly improved their performance by a practice called **blood doping.** A few weeks before an important event, an athlete has some blood drawn. The RBCs are separated and frozen. Just before competition, the RBCs are thawed and injected into the athlete. The increased hematocrit that results slightly improves the oxygen-carrying capacity of the blood, which theoretically improves performance. This method is judged to be an unfair and unwise practice in athletics.

blood, his red blood cells contain type A antigen, type B antigen, and the Rh factor antigen. The term *Rh* is used because this important blood cell antigen was first discovered in the blood of Rhesus monkeys.

In **Rh-negative** blood the RBCs do not contain the Rh factor. Plasma never naturally contains anti-Rh antibodies. But if Rh-positive blood cells are introduced into an Rh-negative person's body, anti-Rh antibodies soon appear in the blood plasma. In this fact lies the danger for a baby born to an Rh-negative mother and an Rh-positive father. If the baby inherits the Rh-positive trait from his father, the Rh factor on his RBCs may stimulate the mother's body to form anti-Rh antibodies. Then, if she later carries another Rh-positive fetus, he may develop a disease called **erythroblastosis** (e-rith-ro-blas-TOE-sis) **fetalis** (fe-TAL-is), caused by the mother's Rh antibodies reacting with the baby's Rh-positive cells (Figure 11-8).

All Rh-negative mothers who carry an Rh-positive baby should be treated with a protein marketed as RhoGAM. RhoGAM stops the mother's body from forming anti-Rh antibodies and thus prevents the possibility of harm to the next Rh-positive baby.

Quick

1. What is an *antigen* in blood typing?
2. What is meant when a person's blood is described as "Rh negative?"

Research, Issues & Trends

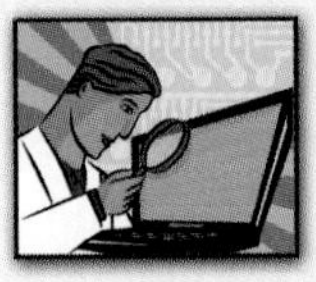

Artificial Blood

One of the primary benefits of blood transfusion is an increase in oxygen-carrying capacity caused by increases in hemoglobin levels. However, blood is a complex liquid tissue, and transfusion always carries with it certain risks. For years medical researchers have worked to develop "artificial blood" or a "blood substitute" that could duplicate one or more blood functions without subjecting a recipient to transfusion reactions, infections, or other health dangers.

A new "artificial blood" product currently in the final stages of development is called **PolyHeme.** It is produced from chemically treated hemoglobin obtained from outdated human blood. The manufacturing process used to produce PolyHeme results in an oxygen-carrying blood substitute that can be transfused into any blood-type recipient without "typing" and is free of blood-borne viruses such as HIV and hepatitis C. Another "second-generation" artificial blood product is also under development. If efforts are successful, it will be produced using recombinant hemoglobin technology. By using genetic engineering techniques, production of this type of product would not require the use of existing human blood or blood products. When available, artificial blood substitutes will be viewed as exciting and welcome developments in transfusion medicine.

Science Applications

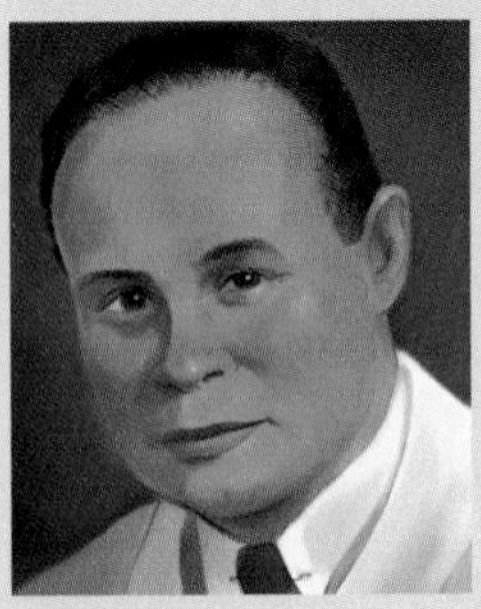

Hematology

Charles Richard Drew (1904-1950).

American physician Charles Richard Drew was a pioneer in hematology, the study of blood. During World War II, he developed the idea of blood banks and researched the best way to store blood for transfusions to wounded soldiers. In New York, he set up the first blood bank ever in 1941—one that served as the model for a network of blood banks opened by the American Red Cross.

Many hematologists continue in Drew's footsteps, refining and perfecting the practice of blood science. Many professions benefit from this research. Phlebotomists collect blood for testing or storage, clinical laboratory technicians analyze blood samples, and many different health professionals use blood analysis and blood transfusions to help their patients. Of course, military medics still rely on blood banking technology to provide immediate aid to wounded combat and terrorism victims.

FIGURE 11-8

Erythroblastosis fetalis. A, Rh-positive blood cells enter the mother's bloodstream during delivery of an Rh-positive baby. If not treated, the mother's body will produce anti-Rh antibodies. **B,** A later pregnancy involving an Rh-negative baby is normal because there are no Rh antigens in the baby's blood. **C,** A later pregnancy involving an Rh-positive baby may result in erythroblastosis fetalis. Anti-Rh antibodies enter the baby's blood supply and cause agglutination of RBCs with the Rh antigen.

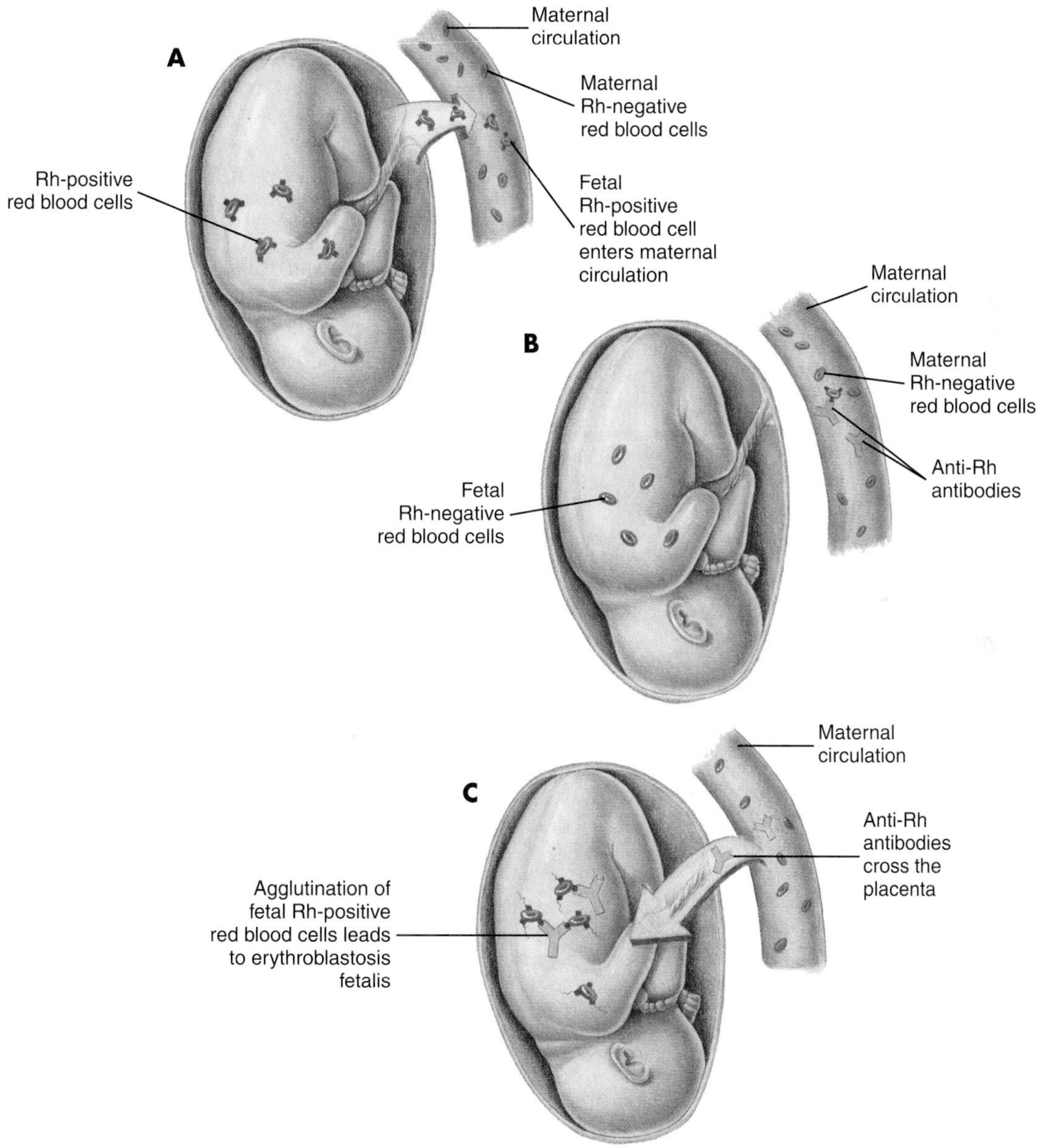

OUTLINE SUMMARY

BLOOD COMPOSITION (TABLE 11-1)

A. Blood plasma
- **1.** Definition—blood minus its cells
- **2.** Composition—water containing many dissolved substances (for example, foods, salts, and hormones)
- **3.** Amount of blood—varies with size and sex; 4 to 6 L about average; about 7% to 9% of body weight

B. Formed elements
- **1.** Kinds
  - **a.** RBCs (erythrocytes)
  - **b.** WBCs (leukocytes)
    - **(1)** Granular leukocytes—neutrophils, eosinophils, and basophils
    - **(2)** Nongranular leukocytes—lymphocytes and monocytes
  - **c.** Platelets or thrombocytes
- **2.** Numbers
  - **a.** RBCs—4.5 to 5 million per mm^3 of blood
  - **b.** WBCs—5000 to 10,000 per mm^3 of blood
  - **c.** Platelets—300,000 per mm^3 of blood
- **3.** Formation—red bone marrow (myeloid tissue) forms all blood cells except some lymphocytes and monocytes, which are formed by lymphatic tissue in the lymph nodes, thymus, and spleen

C. RBCs
- **1.** Structure—disk-shaped, without nuclei
- **2.** Functions—transport oxygen and carbon dioxide
- **3.** Anemia—inability of blood to carry adequate oxygen to tissues; caused, for example, by:
  - **a.** Inadequate RBC numbers
  - **b.** Deficiency of hemoglobin
  - **c.** Pernicious anemia—deficiency of vitamin B_{12}
- **4.** Hematocrit—medical test in which a centrifuge is used to separate whole blood into formed elements and liquid fraction (Figure 11-3)
  - **a.** Buffy coat is WBC and platelet fraction
  - **b.** Normal RBC level is about 45%
  - **c.** Polycythemia—abnormally high RBC count

D. WBCs
- **1.** General function—defense
- **2.** Neutrophils and monocytes carry out phagocytosis
- **3.** Lymphocytes produce antibodies (B-lymphocytes) or directly attack foreign cells (T-lymphocytes)
- **4.** Eosinophils protect against parasitic irritants that cause allergies
- **5.** Basophils produce heparin, which inhibits clotting
- **6.** Clinical conditions related to blood:
  - **a.** Leukopenia—abnormally low WBC count
  - **b.** Leukocytosis—abnormally high WBC count
  - **c.** Leukemia—cancer: elevated WBC count; cells do not function properly

E. Platelets and blood clotting (Figure 11-6)
- **1.** Platelets play an essential role in blood clotting
- **2.** Blot clot formation
  - **a.** Clotting factors released at the injury site produce prothrombin activator
  - **b.** Prothrombin activator and calcium convert prothrombin to thrombin
  - **c.** Thrombin triggers formation of fibrin, which traps RBC to form a clot

BLOOD TYPES

A. ABO system (Figure 11-7)
- **1.** Type A blood—type A self-antigens in RBCs; anti-B type antibodies in plasma

OUTLINE SUMMARY—*cont'd*

2. Type B blood—type B self-antigens in RBCs; anti-A type antibodies in plasma
3. Type AB blood—type A and type B self-antigens in RBCs; no anti-A or anti-B antibodies in plasma
4. Type O blood—no type A or type B self-antigens in RBCs; both anti-A and anti-B antibodies in plasma

B. Rh system
1. Rh-positive blood—Rh factor antigen present in RBCs
2. Rh-negative blood—no Rh factor present in RBCs; no anti-Rh antibodies present naturally in plasma; anti-Rh antibodies, however, appear in the plasma of Rh-negative persons if Rh-positive RBCs have been introduced into their bodies
3. Erythroblastosis fetalis—may occur when Rh-negative mother carries a second Rh-positive fetus; caused by mother's Rh antibodies reacting with baby's Rh-positive cells

NEW WORDS

anemia	erythroblastosis fetalis	leukocytosis	plasma protein
antibodies	erythrocyte	leukopenia	polycythemia
antigens	fibrin	lymphocyte	prothrombin
basophil	fibrinogen	monocyte	prothrombin activator
buffy coat	hematocrit	neutrophil	serum
carbaminohemoglobin	hemoglobin	oxyhemoglobin	thrombin
embolism	heparin	pernicious anemia	thrombocyte
embolus	leukemia	phagocyte	thrombosis
eosinophil	leukocyte	plasma	thrombus

REVIEW QUESTIONS

1. Name several substances found in blood plasma.
2. Explain the function of albumins, globulins and fibrinogen.
3. What is the difference between serum and plasma?
4. What two types of connective tissue form blood cells? Where are they found and what do each of them form?
5. Describe the structure of a red blood cell. What advantage does the unique shape of the red blood have?
6. What is anemia? Give two possible causes of anemia.
7. What is the buffy coat?
8. Explain the function of neutrophils and monocytes.
9. Explain the function of lymphocytes.

Continued

REVIEW QUESTIONS—*cont'd*

10. Explain the function of eosinophils and basophils.
11. Explain fully the process of blood clot formation.
12. Differentiate between a thrombus and an embolus.
13. Explain how type A blood differs from type B blood.
14. Explain the cause of erythroblastosis fetalis.

CRITICAL THINKING

15. Explain how heparin inhibits blood clot formation.
16. Differentiate between the process of blood clot formation and the process of blood agglutination.
17. Why is the first Rh-positive baby born to an Rh-negative mother usually unaffected?

CHAPTER TEST

1. The liquid part of the blood is called __________.
2. Three important plasma proteins are __________, __________, and __________.
3. Blood plasma without the clotting factors is called __________.
4. The three types of formed elements in the blood are __________, __________, and __________.
5. The two types of connective tissue that make blood cells are __________ and __________.
6. The red pigment in red blood cells that carries oxygen is called __________.
7. The term __________ is used to describe a number of disease conditions caused by the inability of red blood cells to carry a sufficient amount of oxygen.
8. If the body produces an excess of red blood cells, the condition is called __________.
9. These white blood cells are the most numerous of the phagocytes: __________.
10. These white blood cells produce antibodies to fight microbes: __________.
11. Prothrombin activator and the mineral __________ in the blood convert prothrombin to thrombin in blood clot formation.
12. Thrombin converts the inactive plasma protein __________ into a fibrous gel called __________.
13. Vitamin __________ stimulates the liver to increase the synthesis of prothrombin.
14. A __________ is an unneeded blood clot that stays in the place where it was formed.
15. If part of a blood clot is dislodged and circulates through the bloodstream, it is called an __________.
16. __________ is a foreign substance that can cause the body to produce an antibody.
17. A person with type AB blood has __________ antigens on the blood cell and __________ antibodies in the plasma.
18. A person with type B blood has __________ antigens on the blood cell and __________ antibodies in the plasma.
19. Type __________ blood is considered the universal donor.
20. Type __________ blood is considered the universal recipient.
21. A condition called __________ can develop if an Rh-negative mother produces antibodies against an Rh-positive fetus.

STUDY TIPS

Blood consists of a liquid portion, the plasma, and formed elements: the red blood cells, white blood cells, and platelets. The function of the blood is to carry substances from one part of the body to another. Many transported materials are dissolved in the plasma, so the composition of the plasma varies based on what is going on in the body. Because of its function, the blood plays an important role in a number of other systems such as the respiratory, digestive, urinary, and immune systems. The material in this chapter will show up again in later chapters. Flash cards will help in learning the names and functions of the blood cells. The process of blood clot formation is important and it is necessary that you get the sequence of events correct. The prefix *pro-* and the suffix *-ogen* indicate an inactive substance. When you see a term with either of these word parts, look for what activates the substance. In studying the ABO blood typing system, the things you will need to remember are what antigens are on the red blood cell and what antibodies are in the plasma. The antigens give the blood type its name: type A blood has A self-antigens. The antibodies are the opposite of the type. Type A blood has anti-B antibodies. Type O has no self-antigens and both antibodies, and type AB has both self-antigens and no antibodies.

In your study group, go over the flash cards with the function of the blood cells. Discuss the process of blood clot formation. Go through the antigens and antibodies for the various blood types. Go over the questions at the end of the chapter and discuss possible test questions.

12 The Circulatory System

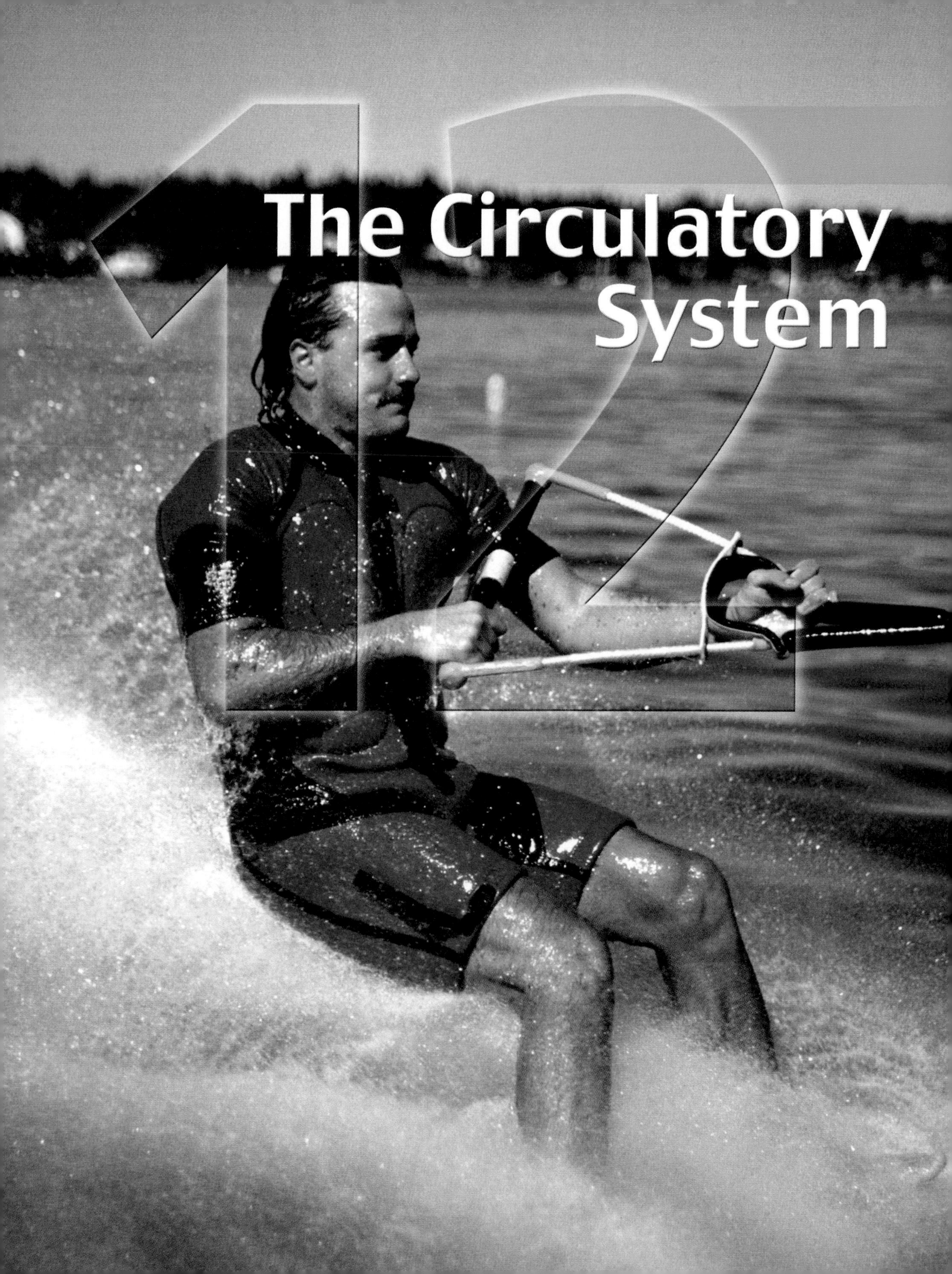

Outline

Objectives

AFTER YOU HAVE COMPLETED THIS CHAPTER, YOU SHOULD BE ABLE TO:

1. Discuss the location, size, and position of the heart in the thoracic cavity and identify the heart chambers, sounds, and valves.
2. Trace blood through the heart and compare the functions of the heart chambers on the right and left sides.
3. List the anatomical components of the heart conduction system and discuss the features of a normal electrocardiogram.
4. Explain the relationship between blood vessel structure and function.
5. Trace the path of blood through the systemic, pulmonary, hepatic portal, and fetal circulations.
6. Identify and discuss the primary factors involved in the generation and regulation of blood pressure and explain the relationships between these factors.

D*iffering amounts of* nutrients and waste products enter and leave the fluid surrounding each body cell continually. In addition, requirements for hormones, body salts, water, and other critical substances constantly change. However, homeostasis or constancy of the body fluid contents surrounding the billions of cells that make up our bodies is required for survival. The system that supplies our cells' transportation needs is the **circulatory system.** The levels of dozens of substances in the blood can remain constant even though the absolute amounts that are needed or produced may change because we have this extremely effective system that transports these substances to or from each cell as circumstances change.

We will begin the study of the circulatory system with the heart—the pump that keeps blood moving through a closed circuit of blood vessels. Details related to heart structure will be followed by a discussion of how the heart functions. This chapter concludes with a study of the vessels through which blood flows as a result of the pumping action of the heart. As a group, these vessels are multipurpose structures. Some allow for rapid movement of blood from one body area to another. Others, such as the microscopic capillaries, permit the movement or exchange of many substances between the blood and fluid surrounding body cells. Chapter 13 will cover the lymphatic system and immunity topics that relate in many ways to the structure and functions of the circulatory system.

HEART

Location, Size, and Position

No one needs to be told where the heart is or what it does. Everyone knows that the heart is in the chest, that it beats night and day to keep the blood flowing, and that if it stops, life stops.

Most of us probably think of the heart as located on the left side of the body. As you can see in Figure 12-1, the heart is located between the lungs in the lower portion of the mediastinum. Draw an imaginary line through the middle of the trachea in Figure 12-1 and continue the line down through the thoracic cavity to divide it into right and left halves. Note that about two thirds of the mass of the heart is to the left of this line and one third to the right.

The heart is often described as a triangular organ, shaped and sized roughly like a closed fist. In Figure 12-1 you can see that the **apex** or blunt point of the lower edge of the heart lies on the diaphragm, pointing toward the left. Doctors and nurses often listen to the heart sounds by placing a stethoscope on the chest wall directly over the apex of the heart. Sounds of the so-called apical beat are easily heard in this area (that is, in the space between the fifth and sixth ribs on a line even with the midpoint of the left clavicle).

The heart is positioned in the thoracic cavity between the sternum in front and the bodies of the thoracic vertebrae behind. Because of this placement, it can be compressed or squeezed by application of pressure to the lower portion of the body of the sternum using the heel of the hand. Rhythmic compression of the heart in this way can maintain blood flow in cases of cardiac arrest and, if combined with effective artificial respiration, the resulting procedure, called **cardiopulmonary resuscitation (CPR),** can be lifesaving.

Anatomy

Heart Chambers

If you cut open a heart, you can see many of its main structural features (Figure 12-2). This organ is hollow, not solid. A partition divides it into right and left sides. The heart contains four cavities or hollow chambers. The two upper chambers are called **atria** (AY-tree-ah), and the two lower chambers are called **ventricles** (VEN-tri-kuls). The atria are smaller than the ventricles, and their walls are thinner and less muscular. Atria are often called *receiving chambers* because blood enters the heart through veins that open into these upper cavities. Eventually, blood is pumped from the heart into arteries that exit from the ventricles; therefore, the ventricles are sometimes referred to as the discharging chambers of the heart. Each heart chamber is named according to its location. Thus there is a right and left atrial chamber above and a right and left ventricular chamber below. The wall of each heart chamber is composed of cardiac muscle tissue usually referred to as the **myocardium** (my-o-KAR-dee-um). The septum between the atrial chambers is called the *interatrial septum*; the *interventricular septum* separates the ventricles.

Each chamber of the heart is lined by a thin layer of very smooth tissue called the **endocardium** (en-doe-KAR-dee-um) (see Figure 12-2). Inflammation of this lining is referred to as **endocarditis** (en-doe-kar-DYE-tis). If inflamed, the endocardial lining can become rough and abrasive to RBCs passing over its surface. Blood flowing over a rough surface is subject to clotting, and a **thrombus** (THROM-bus) or clot may form (see Chapter 11). Unfortunately, rough spots caused by endocarditis or injuries to blood vessel walls often cause the release of platelet factors. The result is often the formation of a fatal blood clot.

Covering Sac or Pericardium

The heart has a covering and a lining. Its covering, called the **pericardium** (pair-i-KAR-dee-um), consists of two layers of fibrous tissue with a small space in between. The inner layer of the

FIGURE 12-1

The heart. The heart and major blood vessels viewed from the front (anterior). Inset shows the relationship of the heart to other structures in the thoracic cavity.

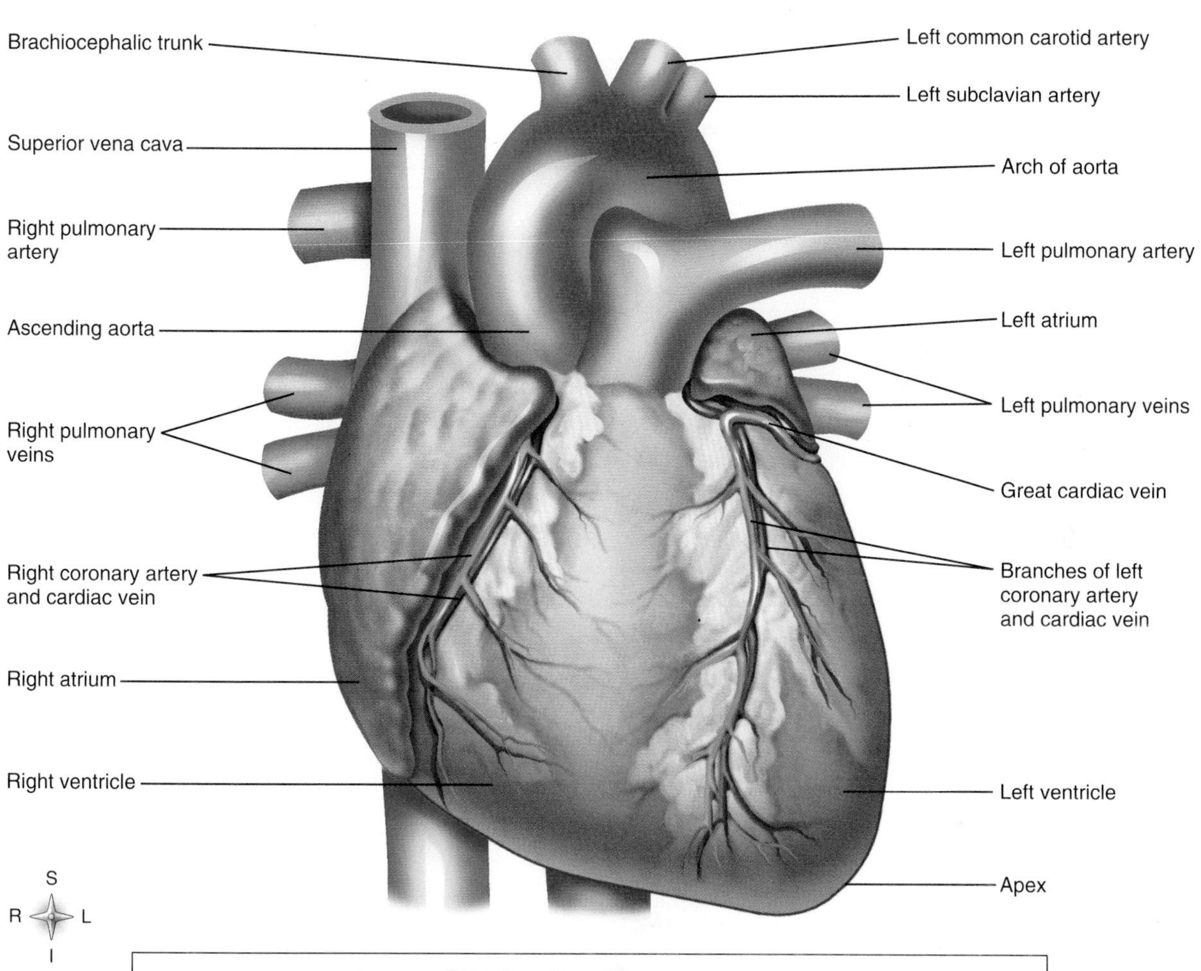

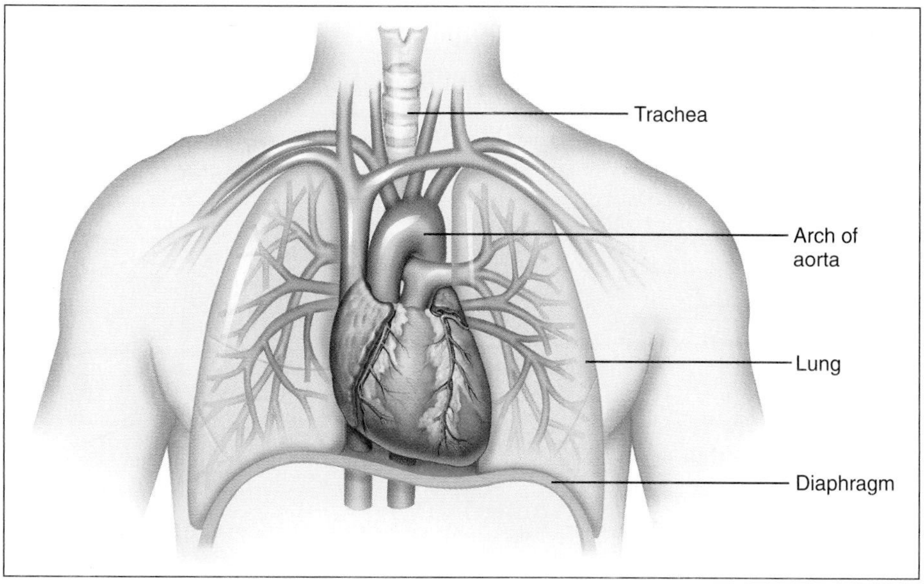

FIGURE 12-2

An internal view of the heart. The inset shows a cross section of the heart wall, including the pericardium.

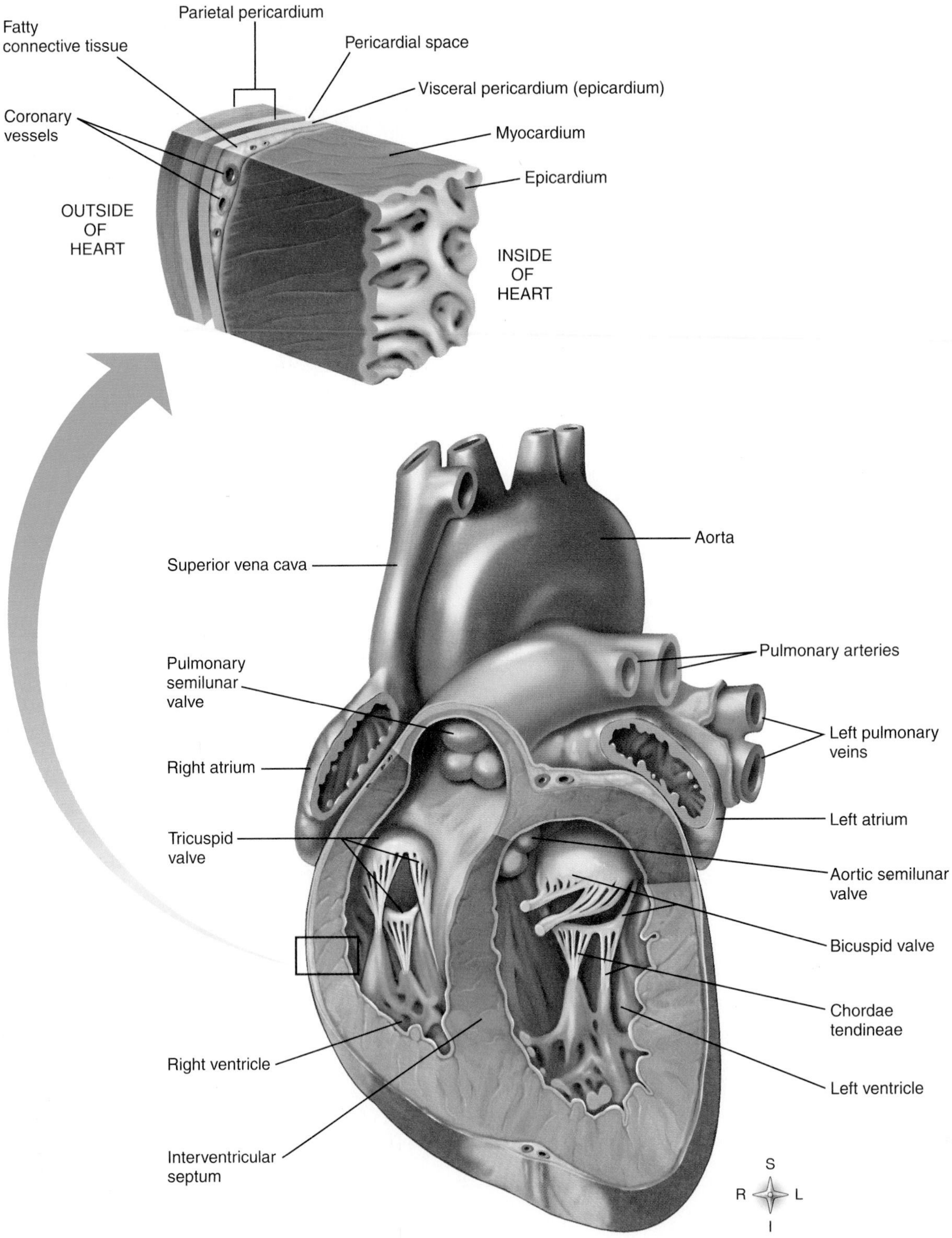

pericardium is called the **visceral pericardium** or **epicardium** (ep-i-KAR-dee-um). It covers the heart the way an apple skin covers an apple. The outer layer of pericardium is called the **parietal pericardium.** It fits around the heart like a loose-fitting sack, allowing enough room for the heart to beat. It is easy to remember the difference between the *endocardium,* which lines the heart chambers, and the *epicardium,* which covers the surface of the heart (see Figure 12-2), if you understand the meaning of the prefixes *endo-* and *epi-*. *Endo-* comes from the Greek word meaning "inside" or "within," and *epi-* comes from the Greek word meaning "upon" or "on."

The two pericardial layers slip against each other without friction when the heart beats because these are serous membranes with moist, not dry, surfaces. A thin film of pericardial fluid furnishes the lubricating moistness between the heart and its enveloping pericardial sac. If the pericardium becomes inflamed, a condition called **pericarditis** (pair-i-kar-DYE-tis) results.

Heart Action

The heart serves as a muscular pumping device for distributing blood to all parts of the body. Contraction of the heart is called **systole** (SIS-toe-lee), and relaxation is called **diastole** (dye-AS-toe-lee). When the heart beats (that is, when it contracts), the atria contract first (atrial systole), forcing blood into the ventricles. Once filled, the two ventricles contract (ventricular systole) and force blood out of the heart (Figure 12-3). For the heart to be efficient in its pumping action, more than just the rhythmic contraction of its muscular fibers is required. The direction of blood flow must be directed and controlled. This is accomplished by four sets of valves located at the entrance and near the exit of the ventricles.

Heart Valves

The two valves that separate the atrial chambers above from the ventricles below are called **AV** or **atrioventricular** (ay-tree-o-ven-TRIK-yoo-lar) **valves.** The two AV valves are called the **bicuspid** or **mitral** (MY-tral) **valve,** located between the left atrium and ventricle, and the **tricuspid valve,** located between the right atrium and ventricle. The AV valves prevent backflow of blood into the atria when the ventricles contract. Locate the AV valves in Figures 12-2 and 12-3. Note that a number of stringlike structures called **chordae tendineae** (KOR-dee ten-DIN-ee) attach the AV valves to the wall of the heart.

The **SL** or **semilunar** (sem-i-LOO-nar) **valves** are located between the two ventricular chambers and the large arteries that carry blood away from the heart when contraction occurs (see Figure 12-3). The ventricles, like the atria, contract together; therefore, the two semilunar valves open and close at the same time. The **pulmonary semilunar valve** is located at the beginning of the pulmonary artery and allows blood going to the lungs to flow out of the right ventricle but prevents it from flowing back into the ventricle. The **aortic semilunar valve** is located at the beginning of the aorta and allows blood to flow out of the left ventricle up into the aorta but prevents backflow into this ventricle.

Heart Sounds

If a stethoscope is placed on the anterior chest wall, two distinct sounds can be heard. They are rhythmical and repetitive sounds that are often described as **lub dup.**

The first or *lub* sound is caused by the vibration and abrupt closure of the AV valves as the ventricles contract. Closure of the AV valves prevents blood from rushing back up into the atria during contraction of the ventricles. This first sound is of longer duration and lower pitch than the second. The pause between this first sound and the *dup* or second sound is shorter than that after the second sound and the *lub dup* of the next systole. The second heart sound is caused by the closing of both the semilunar valves when the ventricles undergo diastole (relax).

Blood Flow Through the Heart

The heart acts as two separate pumps. The right atrium and the right ventricle perform a task quite different from the left atrium and the left ventricle. When the heart "beats," first the atria contract simultaneously. This is atrial systole. Then the ventricles fill with blood, and they, too, contract together

FIGURE 12-3

Heart action. A, During atrial systole (contraction) cardiac muscle in the atrial wall contracts, forcing blood through the atrioventricular (AV) valves and into the ventricles. Bottom illustration shows superior view of all four valves, with semilunar (SL) valves closed and AV valves open. **B,** During ventricular systole that follows, the AV valves close, and blood is forced out of the ventricles through the semilunar valves and into the arteries. Bottom illustration shows superior view of SL valves open and AV valves closed.

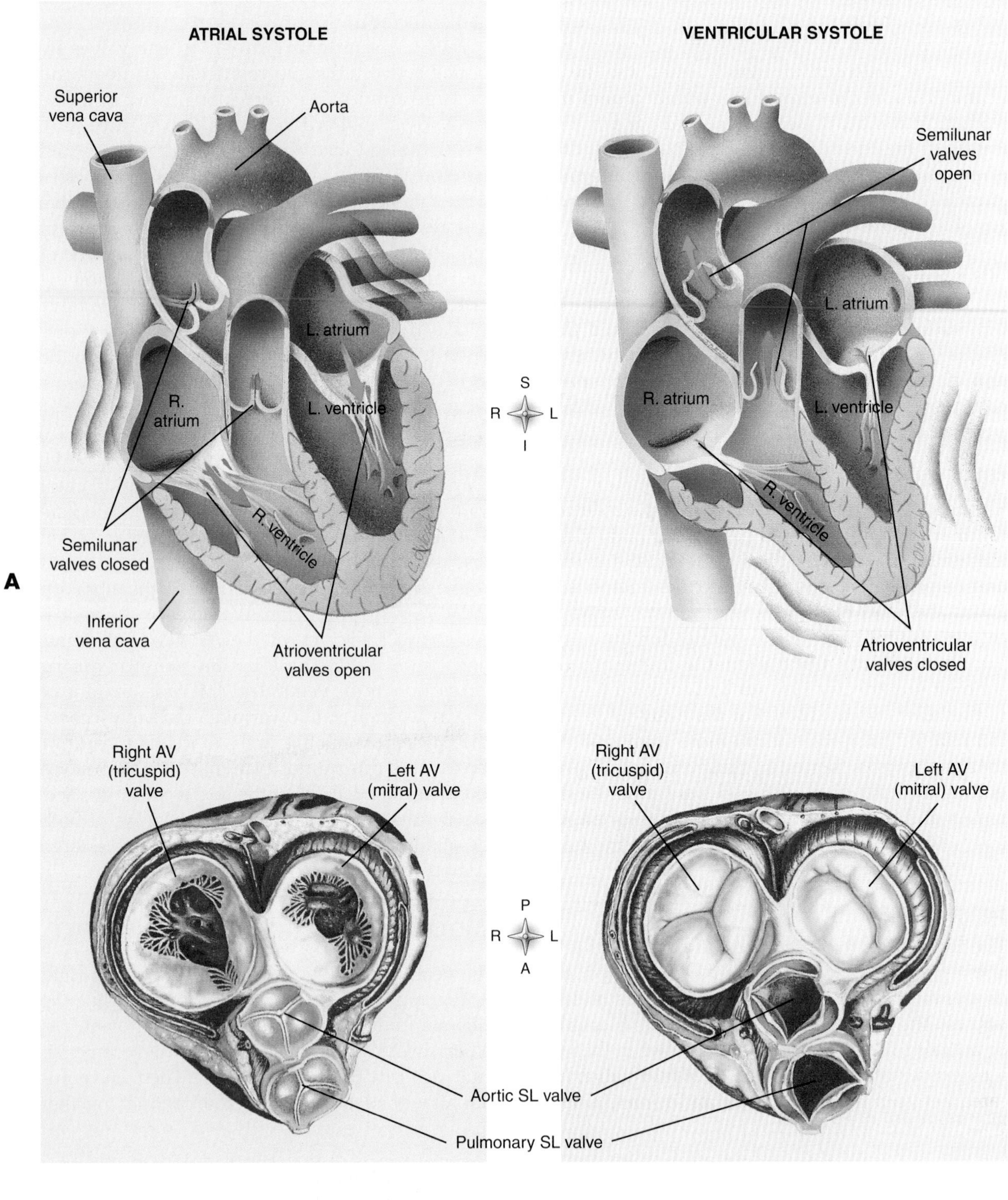

during ventricular systole. Although the atria contract as a unit followed by the ventricles below, the right and left sides of the heart act as separate pumps. As we study the blood flow through the heart, the separate functions of the two pumps will become clearer.

Note in Figure 12-3 that blood enters the right atrium through two large veins called the **superior vena** (VEE-nah) **cava** (KAY-vah) and **inferior vena cava.** The right heart pump receives oxygen-poor blood from the veins. After entering the right atrium, it is pumped through the right AV or tricuspid valve and enters the right ventricle. When the ventricles contract, blood in the right ventricle is pumped through the pulmonary semilunar valve into the **pulmonary artery** and eventually to the lungs, where oxygen is added and carbon dioxide is lost.

As you can see in Figure 12-3, blood rich in oxygen returns to the left atrium of the heart through four **pulmonary veins.** It then passes through the left AV or bicuspid valve into the left ventricle. When the left ventricle contracts, blood is forced through the aortic semilunar valve into the **aorta** (ay-OR-tah) and is distributed to the body as a whole.

As you can tell from Figure 12-4, the two sides of the heart actually pump blood through two separate "circulations" and function as two separate pumps. The **pulmonary circulation** involves movement of blood from the right ventricle to the lungs, and the **systemic circulation** involves movement of blood from the left ventricle throughout the body as a whole. The pulmonary and systemic circulations are discussed later in this chapter.

Blood Supply to the Heart Muscle

To sustain life, the heart must pump blood throughout the body on a regular and ongoing basis. As a result, the heart muscle or myocardium requires a constant supply of blood containing nutrients and oxygen to function effectively. The delivery of oxygen and nutrient-rich arterial blood to cardiac muscle tissue and the return of oxygen-poor blood from this active tissue to the venous system are called **coronary circulation.**

Blood flows into the heart muscle by way of two small vessels—the **right** and **left coronary arteries.** The coronary arteries are the aorta's first branches (Figure 12-5). The openings into these small vessels lie behind the flaps of the aortic SL valve. During ventricular diastole, blood in the aorta that backs up behind the aortic SL valve can flow into the coronary arteries.

In both coronary thrombosis and coronary **embolism** (EM-bo-lizm), a blood clot occludes or plugs up some part of a coronary artery. Blood cannot pass through the occluded vessel and so cannot reach the heart muscle cells it normally supplies. Deprived of oxygen, these cells soon die or are damaged. In medical terms, **myocardial** (my-o-KAR-dee-al) **infarction** (in-FARK-shun) or tissue death occurs. Myocardial infarction or "heart attack" is a common cause of death during middle and late adulthood. Recovery from a myocardial infarction is possible if the amount of heart tissue damaged was small enough so that the remaining undamaged heart muscle can pump blood effectively enough to supply the needs of the rest of the heart and the body. The term **angina** (an-JYE-nah) **pectoris** (PEK-tor-is) is used to describe the severe chest pain that occurs when the myocardium is deprived of adequate oxygen. It is often a warning that the coronary arteries are no longer able to supply enough blood and oxygen to the heart muscle. **Coronary bypass surgery** is a frequent treatment for those who suffer from severely restricted coronary artery blood flow. In this procedure, veins or arteries are "harvested" or removed from other areas of the body and used to bypass partial blockages in coronary arteries (Figure 12-6). Another treatment to improve coronary blood flow is *angioplasty*, a procedure in which a device is inserted into a blood vessel to open a channel for blood flow.

After blood has passed through the capillary beds in the myocardium, it flows into **cardiac veins,** which empty into the **coronary sinus** and finally into the right atrium.

Cardiac Cycle

The beating of the heart is a regular and rhythmic process. Each complete heartbeat is called a **cardiac cycle** and includes the contraction (systole) and relaxation (diastole) of atria and ventricles. Each cycle takes about 0.8 seconds to complete if

FIGURE 12-4

Blood flow through the circulatory system. In the pulmonary circulatory route, blood is pumped from the right side of the heart to the gas-exchange tissues of the lungs. In the systemic circulation, blood is pumped from the left side of the heart to all other tissues of the body.

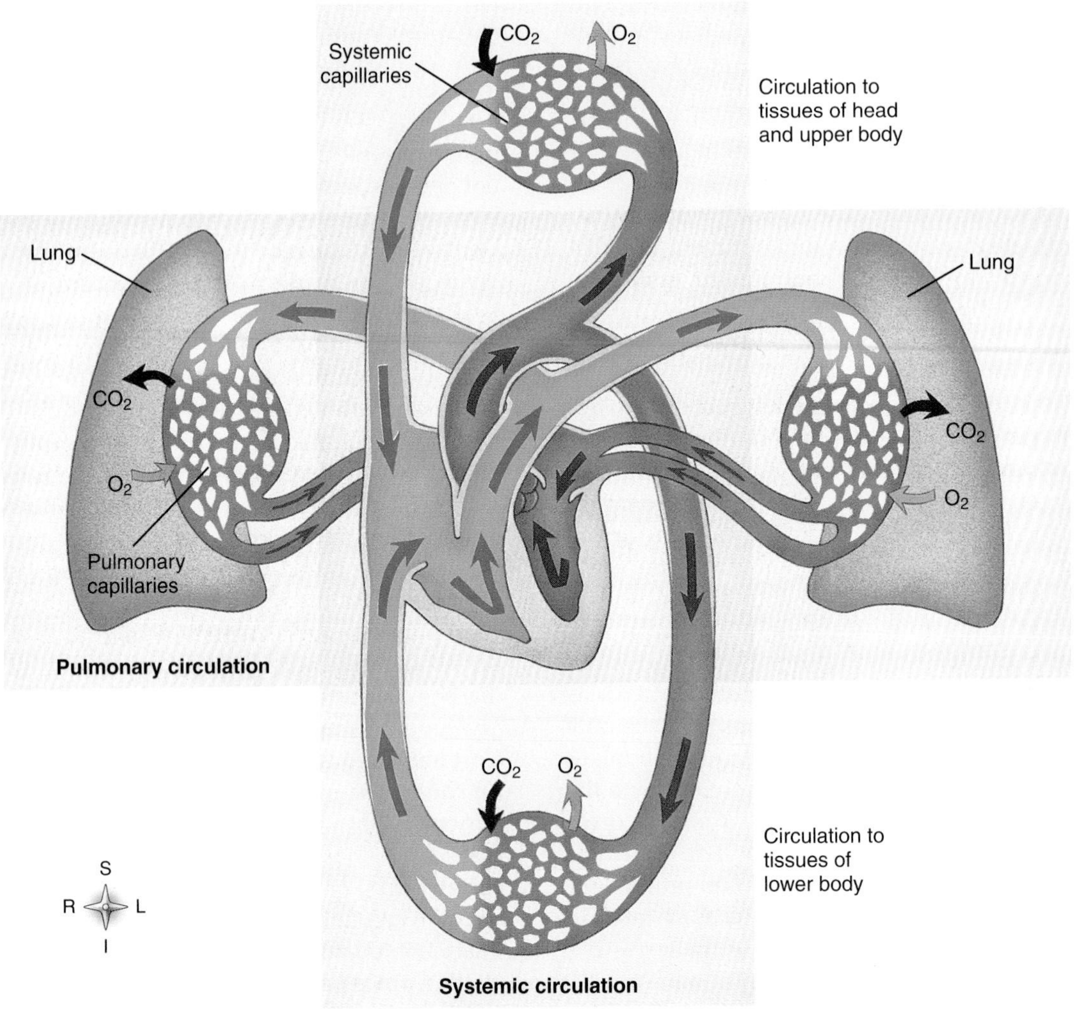

the heart is beating at an average rate of about 72 beats per minute. The term **stroke volume** refers to the volume of blood ejected from the ventricles during each beat. **Cardiac output,** or the volume of blood pumped by one ventricle per minute, averages about 5 L in a normal, resting adult.

Quick

1. What are the functions of the atria and ventricles of the heart?
2. What coverings does the heart have? What is the heart's lining called?
3. What are systole and diastole of the heart?
4. What are the two major "circulations" of the body?

FIGURE 12-5

Coronary circulation. A, Arteries. **B,** Veins. Both are anterior views of the heart. Vessels near the anterior surface are more darkly colored than those of the posterior surface seen through the heart.

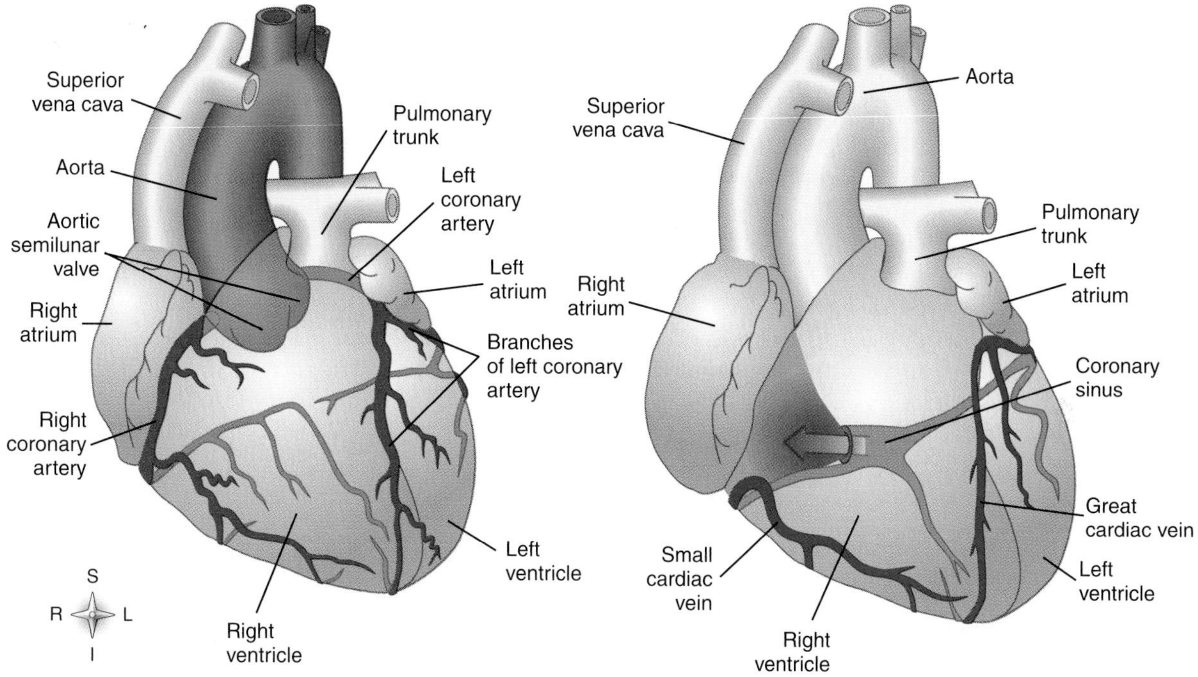

FIGURE 12-6

Coronary bypass. In coronary bypass surgery, blood vessels are "harvested" from other parts of the body and used to construct detours around blocked coronary arteries. Artificial vessels can also be used.

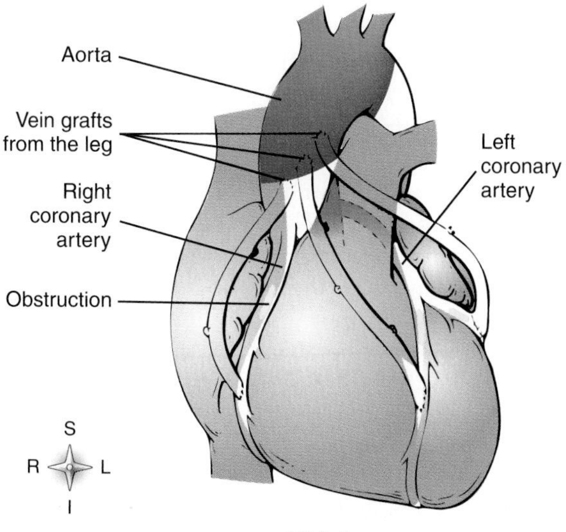

Triple bypass

Conduction System of the Heart

Cardiac muscle fibers can contract rhythmically on their own. However, they must be coordinated by electrical signals (impulses) if the heart is to pump effectively. Although the rate of the cardiac muscle's rhythm is controlled by autonomic nerve signals, the heart has its own built-in conduction system for coordinating contractions during the cardiac cycle. The most important thing to realize about this conduction system is that all of the cardiac muscle fibers in each region of the heart are electrically linked together. The *intercalated disks* that were first introduced in Chapter 3 (see Figure 3-20, p. 68) are actually electrical connectors that join muscle fibers into a single unit that can conduct an impulse through the entire wall of a heart chamber without stopping. Thus both atrial walls will contract at about the same time because all their fibers are electrically linked. Likewise, both ventricular walls will contract at about the same time.

Four structures embedded in the wall of the heart are specialized to generate strong impulses and conduct them rapidly to certain regions of the heart wall. Thus they make sure that the atria contract and then the ventricles contract in an efficient manner. The names of the structures that make up this conduction system of the heart follow:

1. **Sinoatrial** (sye-no-AY-tree-al) **node,** which is sometimes called the SA node or the *pacemaker*
2. **Atrioventricular** (ay-tree-o-ven-TRIK-yoo-lar) **node** or **AV node**
3. **AV bundle** or **bundle of His**
4. **Purkinje** (pur-KIN-jee) **fibers**

Impulse conduction normally starts in the heart's pacemaker, namely, the SA node. From there, it spreads, as you can see in Figure 12-7, in all directions through the atria. This causes the atrial fibers to contract. When impulses reach the AV node, it relays them by way of the bundle of His and Purkinje fibers to the ventricles, causing them to contract. Normally, therefore, a ventricular beat follows each atrial beat. Various conditions such as endocarditis or myocardial infarction, however, can damage the heart's conduction system and thereby disturb its rhythmic beating. One such disturbance is the condition commonly called *heart block*. Impulses are blocked from getting through to the ventricles, resulting in the heart beating at a much slower rate than normal. A physician may treat heart block by implanting in the heart an **artificial pacemaker,** an electrical device that causes ventricular contractions at a rate fast enough to maintain an adequate circulation of blood.

Electrocardiogram

The specialized structures of the heart's conduction system generate tiny electrical currents that spread through surrounding tissues to the surface of the body. This fact is of great clinical significance because these electrical signals can be picked up from the body surface and transformed into visible tracings by an instrument called an **electrocardiograph** (e-lek-tro-KAR-dee-o-graf).

The **electrocardiogram** (e-lek-tro-KAR-dee-o-gram) or **ECG** is the graphic record of the heart's electrical activity. Skilled interpretation of these ECG records may sometimes make the difference between life and death. A normal ECG tracing is shown in Figure 12-8.

A normal ECG tracing has three very characteristic deflections or waves called the **P wave,** the **QRS complex,** and the **T wave.** These deflections represent the electrical activity that regulates the contraction or relaxation of the atria or ventricles. The term *depolarization* describes the electrical activity that triggers contraction of the heart muscle. *Repolarization* begins just before the relaxation phase of cardiac muscle activity. In the normal ECG shown in Figure 12-8, the small P wave occurs with depolarization of the atria. The QRS complex occurs as a result of depolarization of the ventricles, and the T wave results from electrical activity generated by repolarization of the ventricles. You may wonder why no visible record of atrial repolarization is noted in a normal ECG. The

FIGURE 12-7

Conduction system of the heart. Specialized cardiac muscle cells in the wall of the heart rapidly conduct an electrical impulse throughout the myocardium. The signal is initiated by the SA node (pacemaker) and spreads to the rest of the atrial myocardium and to the atrioventricular (AV) node. The AV node then initiates a signal that is conducted through the ventricular myocardium by way of the AV bundle (of His) and Purkinje fibers.

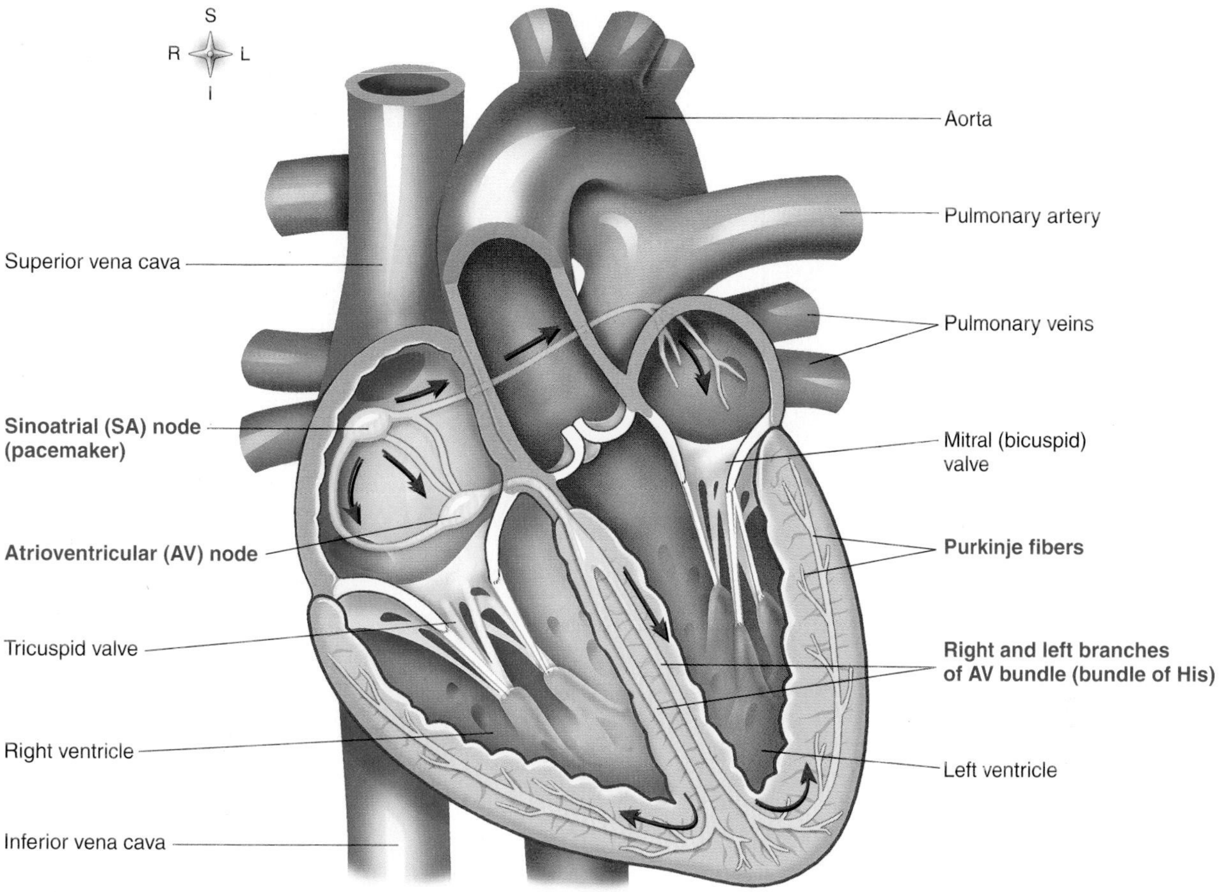

reason is simply that the deflection is very small and is hidden by the large QRS complex that occurs at the same time.

Damage to cardiac muscle tissue that is caused by a myocardial infarction or disease affecting the heart's conduction system results in distinctive changes in the ECG. Therefore ECG tracings are extremely valuable in the diagnosis and treatment of heart disease.

Quick Check

1. What structure is the natural "pacemaker" of the heart?
2. What information is in an electrocardiogram?

FIGURE 12-8

Events represented by the electrocardiogram (ECG). It is nearly impossible to illustrate the invisible, dynamic events of heart conduction in a few cartoon panels or "snapshots," but the sketches here give you an idea of what is happening in the heart as the ECG is recorded. **A,** The heart wall is completely relaxed, with no change in electrical activity, so the ECG remains constant. **B,** P wave occurs when the AV node and atrial walls depolarize. **C,** Atrial walls are completely depolarized and thus no change is recorded on the ECG. **D,** The QRS complex occurs as the atria repolarize and the ventricular walls depolarize. **E,** The atrial walls are now completely repolarized, and the ventricular walls are now completely depolarized and thus no change is recorded on the ECG. **F,** The T wave appears on the ECG when the ventricular walls repolarize. **G,** After the ventricles are completely repolarized, we are back at the baseline of the ECG—essentially back where we began in part A of this figure.

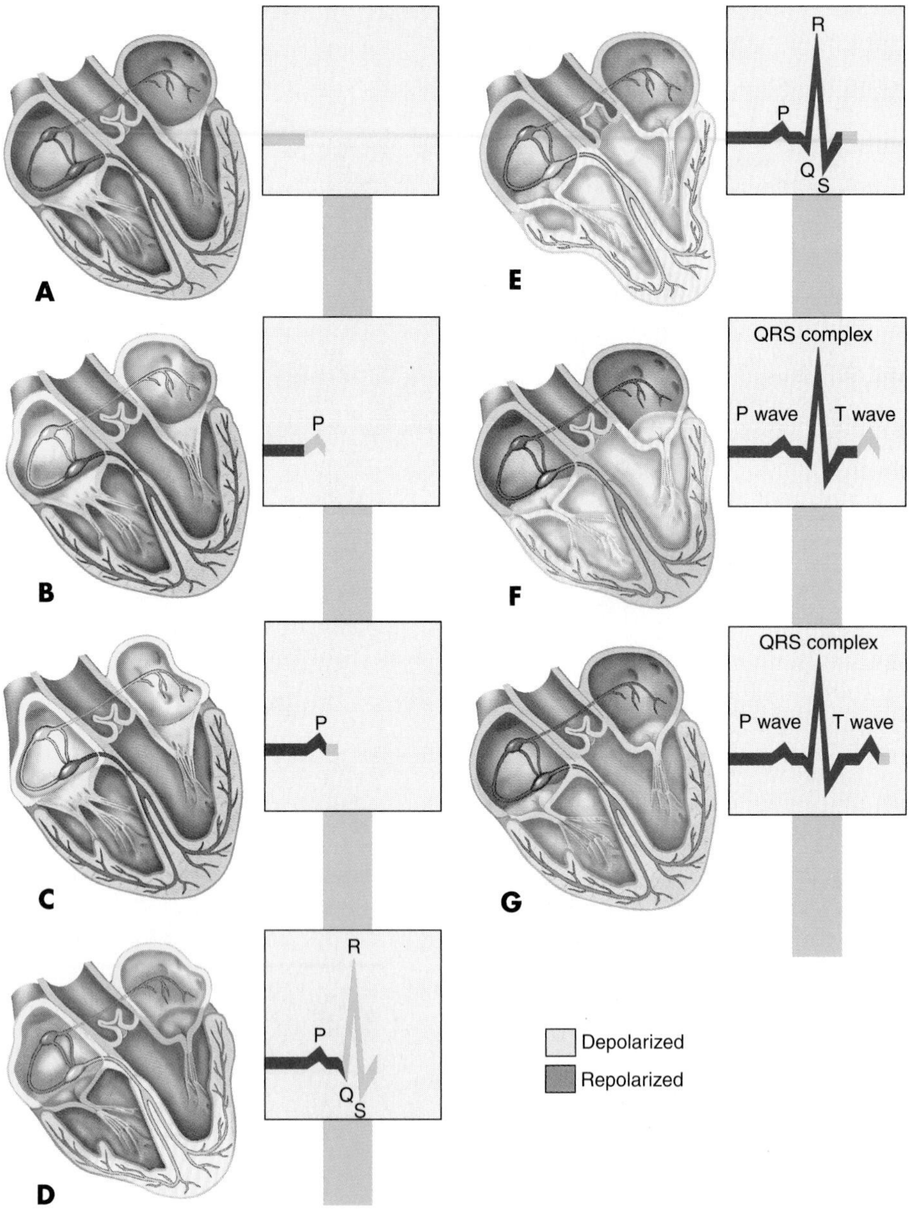

Health & Well-Being

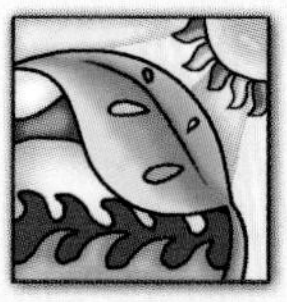

Changes in Blood Flow During Exercise

Not only does the overall rate of blood flow increase during exercise, the relative blood flow through the different organs of the body also changes. During exercise, blood is routed away from the kidneys and digestive organs and toward the skeletal muscles, cardiac muscle, and skin. Rerouting of blood is accomplished by contracting precapillary sphincters in some tissues (thus reducing blood flow) while relaxing precapillary sphincters in other tissues (thus increasing blood flow). How can homeostasis be better maintained by these changes? One reason is because glucose and oxygen levels are dropping rapidly in muscles as they use up these substances to produce energy. Increased blood flow restores normal levels of glucose and oxygen rapidly. Blood warmed up in active muscles flows to the skin for cooling. This helps keep the body temperature from getting too high. Can you think of other ways this situation helps maintain homeostasis? Typical changes in organ blood flow with exercise are shown in the illustration. The green bar in each pair shows the resting blood flow; the blue bar shows the flow during exercise.

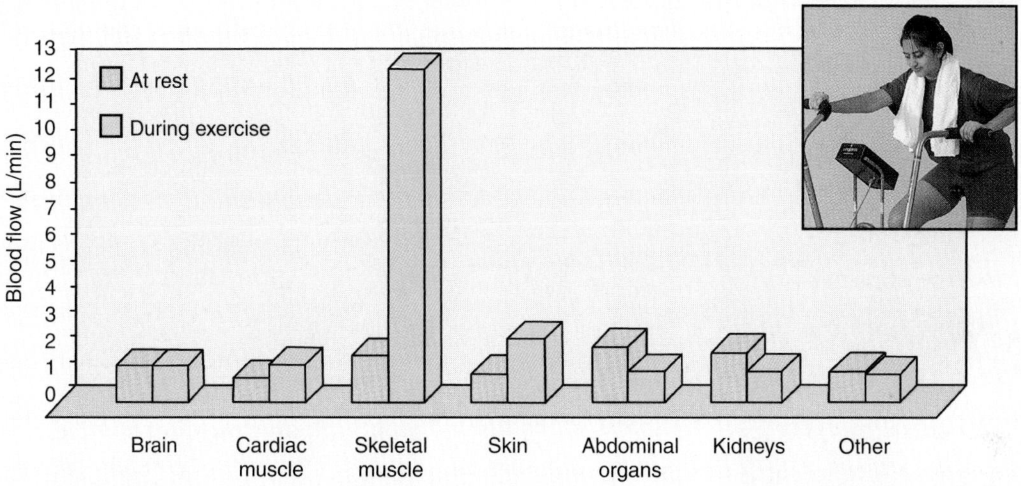

BLOOD VESSELS

Types

Arterial blood is pumped from the heart through a series of large distribution vessels—the **arteries.** The largest artery in the body is the aorta. Arteries subdivide into vessels that become progressively smaller and finally become tiny **arterioles** (ar-TEER-ee-ols) that control the flow into microscopic exchange vessels called **capillaries** (KAP-i-lair-ees). In the so-called capillary beds, the exchange of nutrients and respiratory gases occurs between the blood and tissue fluid around the cells. Blood exits or is drained from the **capillary beds** and then enters the small **venules** (VEN-yools), which join with other venules and increase in size, becoming **veins.** The largest veins are the superior vena cava and the inferior vena cava.

As noted previously (see Figure 12-4), arteries carry blood away from the heart toward capillaries. Veins carry blood toward the heart away from capillaries, and capillaries carry blood from the tiny arterioles into tiny venules. The aorta carries blood out of the left ventricle of the heart, and the venae cavae return blood to the right atrium after the blood has circulated through the body.

Structure

Arteries, veins, and capillaries differ in structure. Three coats or layers are found in both arteries and veins (Figure 12-9). The outermost layer is called the **tunica adventitia.** This outer layer is made of connective tissue fibers, which reinforce the wall of the vessel so that it will not burst under pressure. Note that smooth muscle tissue is found in the middle layer or **tunica media** of arteries and veins. However, the muscle layer is much thicker in arteries than in veins. Why is this important? Because the thicker muscle layer in the artery wall is able to resist great pressures generated by ventricular systole. In arteries, the tunica media plays a critical role in maintaining blood pressure and controlling blood distribution. This is a smooth

FIGURE 12-9

Artery and vein. Schematic drawings of an artery, **A,** and a vein, **B,** show comparative thicknesses of the three layers: the outer layer or tunica adventitia, the muscle layer or tunica media, and the tunica intima made of endothelium. Note that the muscle and outer layer are much thinner in veins than in arteries and that veins have valves.

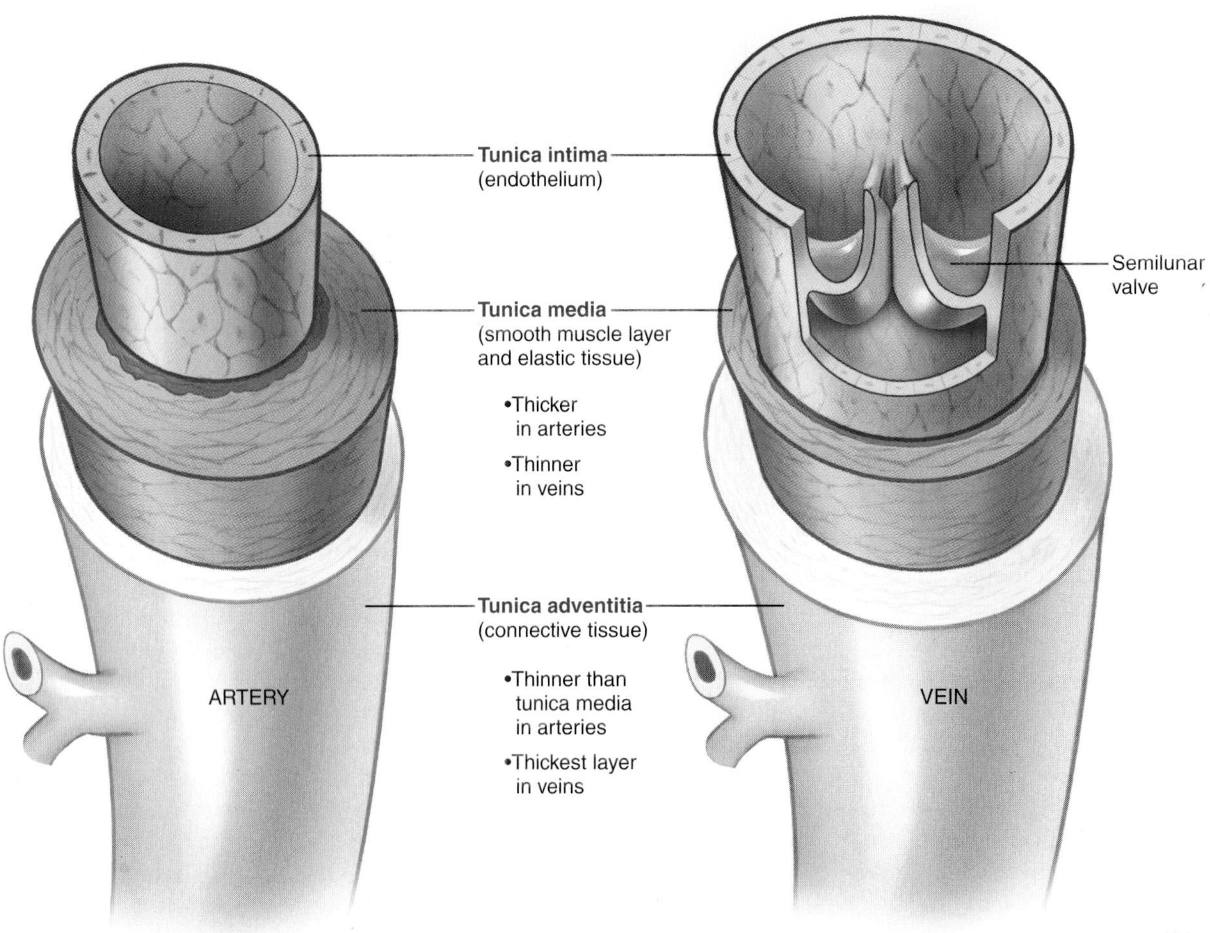

muscle, so it is controlled by the autonomic nervous system. The tunica media also includes a thin layer of elastic fibrous tissue.

An inner layer of endothelial cells called the **tunica intima** lines arteries and veins. The tunica intima is actually a single layer of squamous epithelial cells called **endothelium** (en-doe-THEE-lee-um) that lines the inner surface of the entire circulatory system.

As you can see in Figure 12-9, veins have a unique structural feature not present in arteries. They are equipped with one-way valves that prevent the backflow of blood. When a surgeon cuts into the body, only arteries, arterioles, veins, and venules can be seen. Capillaries cannot be seen because they are microscopic. The most important structural feature of capillaries is their extreme thinness—only one layer of flat, endothelial cells composes the capillary membrane. Instead of three layers or coats, the capillary wall is composed of only one—the tunica intima. Substances such as glucose, oxygen, and wastes can quickly pass through it on their way to or from cells. Smooth muscle cells called **precapillary sphincters** guard the entrance to the capillary and determine into which capillary blood will flow.

Functions

Arteries, veins, and capillaries have different functions. Arteries and arterioles distribute blood from the heart to capillaries in all parts of the body. In addition, by constricting or dilating, arterioles help maintain arterial blood pressure at a normal level. Venules and veins collect blood from capillaries and return it to the heart. They also serve as blood reservoirs because they can expand to hold a larger volume of blood or constrict to hold a much smaller amount. Capillaries function as exchange vessels. For example, glucose and oxygen move out of the blood in capillaries into interstitial fluid and on into cells. Carbon dioxide and other substances move in the opposite direction (that is, into the capillary blood from the cells). Fluid is also exchanged between capillary blood and interstitial fluid (see Chapter 18).

Study Figure 12-10 and Table 12-1 to learn the names of the main arteries of the body and Figures 12-11 and 12-12 and Table 12-2 for the names of the main veins.

Quick

1. What are the two main types of blood vessel in the body? How are they different?
2. Can you describe the three major layers of a large blood vessel?
3. What are capillaries?

CIRCULATION

Systemic and Pulmonary Circulation

The term *circulation of blood* is self-explanatory, meaning that blood flows through vessels that are arranged to form a circuit or circular pattern. Blood flow from the left ventricle of the heart through blood vessels to all parts of the body and back to the right atrium of the heart has already been described as the **systemic circulation.** The left ventricle pumps blood into the aorta. From there, it flows into arteries that carry it into the tissues and organs of the body. As indicated in Figure 12-13, within each structure, blood moves from arteries to arterioles to capillaries. There, the vital two-way exchange of substances occurs between blood and cells. Next, blood flows out of each organ by way of its venules and then its veins to drain eventually into the inferior or superior venae cavae. These two great veins return venous blood to the right atrium of the heart to complete the systemic circulation. But the blood has not quite come full circle back to its starting point in the left ventricle. To do this and start on its way again, it must first flow through another circuit, referred to earlier as the **pulmonary circulation.** Observe in Figure 12-13 that venous blood moves from the right atrium to the right ventricle to the pulmonary artery to lung arterioles and capillaries. There, the exchange of gases between the blood and air takes place, converting the deep crimson typical of venous blood to the scarlet of arterial blood. This oxygenated blood then flows through lung venules into four pulmonary veins

FIGURE 12-10

Principal arteries of the body.

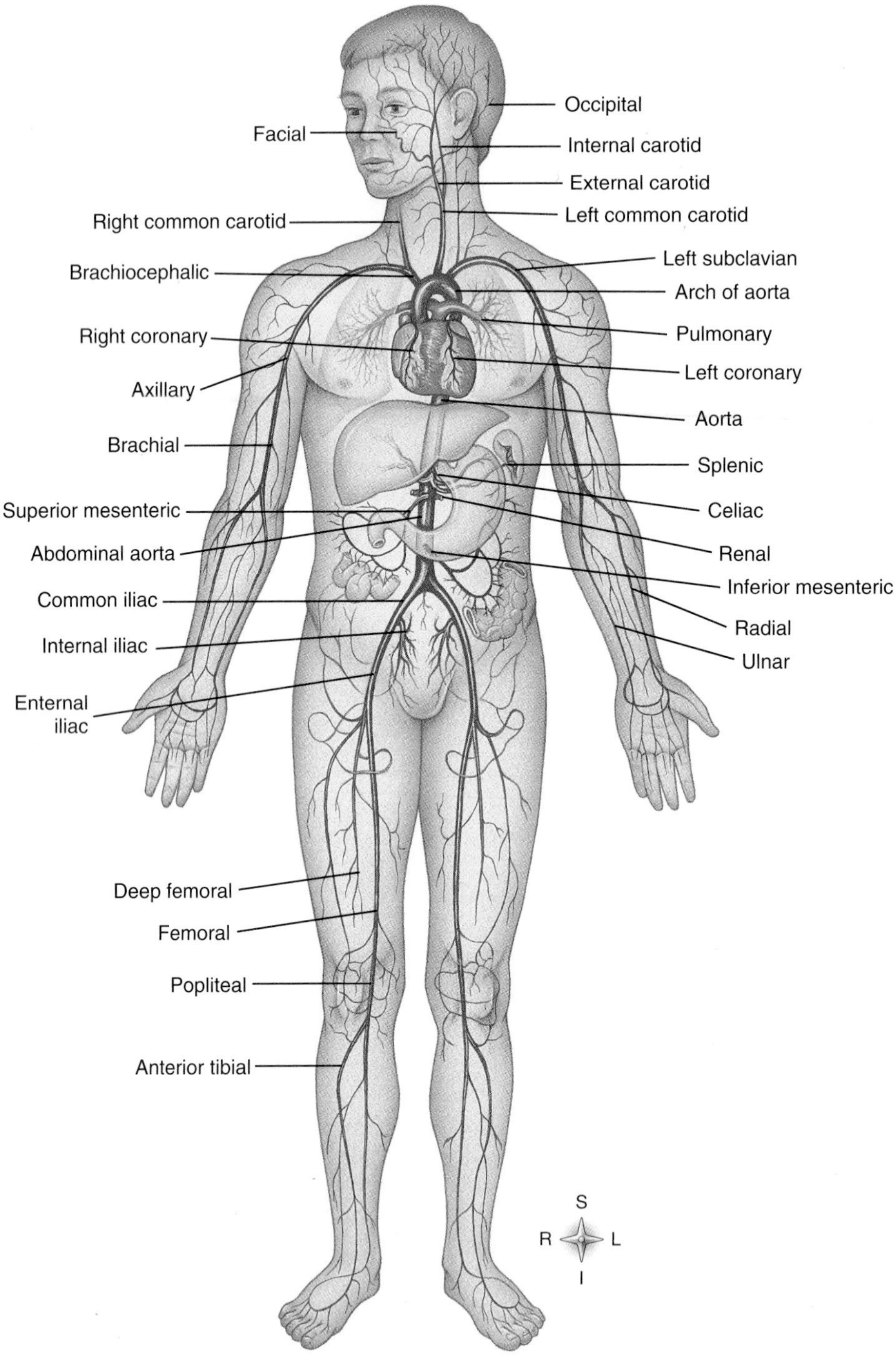
Occipital
Facial
Internal carotid
External carotid
Right common carotid
Left common carotid
Left subclavian
Brachiocephalic
Arch of aorta
Pulmonary
Right coronary
Left coronary
Axillary
Aorta
Brachial
Splenic
Superior mesenteric
Celiac
Abdominal aorta
Renal
Inferior mesenteric
Common iliac
Radial
Internal iliac
Ulnar
Enternal
iliac
Deep femoral
Femoral
Popliteal
Anterior tibial
S
R
L
I

TABLE 12-1

The Major Arteries

ARTERY	TISSUES SUPPLIED	ARTERY	TISSUES SUPPLIED
HEAD AND NECK			
Occipital	Posterior head and neck	Superior mesenteric	Small intestine; upper half of the large intestine
Facial	Mouth, pharynx, and face	Inferior mesenteric	Lower half of the large intestine
Internal carotid	Anterior brain and meninges	UPPER EXTREMITY	
External carotid	Superficial neck, face, eyes, and larynx	Axillary	Axilla (armpit)
Right common carotid	Right side of the head and neck	Brachial	Arm
Left common carotid	Left side of the head and neck	Radial	Lateral side of the hand
THORAX		Ulnar	Medial side of the hand
Left subclavian	Left upper extremity	LOWER EXTREMITY	
Brachiocephalic	Head and arm	Internal iliac	Pelvic viscera and rectum
Arch of aorta	Branches to head, neck, and upper extremities	External iliac	Genitalia and lower trunk muscles
Coronary	Heart muscle	Deep femoral	Deep thigh muscles
ABDOMEN		Femoral	Thigh
Celiac	Stomach, spleen, and liver	Popliteal	Leg and foot
Splenic	Spleen	Anterior tibial	Leg
Renal	Kidneys		

and returns to the left atrium of the heart. From the left atrium, it enters the left ventricle to be pumped again through the systemic circulation.

Hepatic Portal Circulation

The term **hepatic portal circulation** refers to the route of blood flow through the liver. Veins from the spleen, stomach, pancreas, gallbladder, and intestines do not pour their blood directly into the inferior vena cava as do the veins from other abdominal organs. Instead, they send their blood to the liver by means of the hepatic portal vein (Figure 12-14). The blood then must pass through the liver before it reenters the regular venous return to the heart. Blood leaves the liver by way of the hepatic veins, which drain into the inferior vena cava. As noted in Figure 12-13, blood normally flows from arteries to arterioles to capillaries to venules to veins and back to the heart. Blood flow in the hepatic portal circulation, however, does not follow this typical route. Venous blood, which would ordinarily return directly to the heart, is sent instead through a second capillary bed in the liver. The hepatic portal vein shown in Figure 12-14 is located between two capillary beds—one set in

FIGURE 12-11

Principal veins of the body.

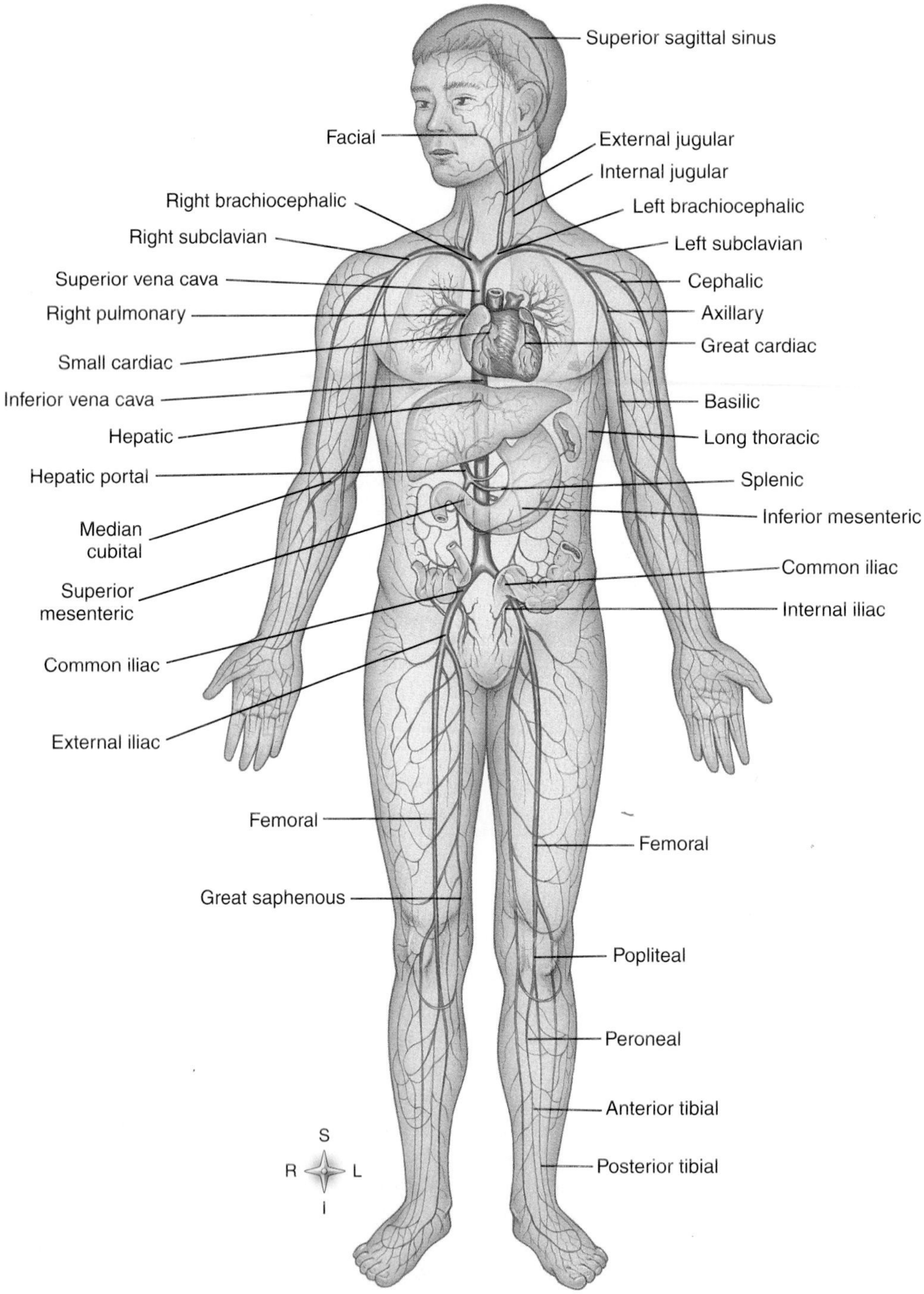
Superior sagittal sinus
Facial
External jugular
Internal jugular
Right brachiocephalic
Left brachiocephalic
Right subclavian
Left subclavian
Superior vena cava
Cephalic
Right pulmonary
Axillary
Great cardiac
Small cardiac
Inferior vena cava
Basilic
Hepatic
Long thoracic
Hepatic portal
Splenic
Inferior mesenteric
Median cubital
Common iliac
Superior mesenteric
Internal iliac
Common iliac
External iliac
Femoral
Femoral
Great saphenous
Popliteal
Peroneal
Anterior tibial
S
R
L
I
Posterior tibial

TABLE 12-2

The Major Veins

VEIN	TISSUES DRAINED	VEIN	TISSUES DRAINED
HEAD AND NECK			
Superior sagittal sinus	Brain	Superior mesenteric	Small intestine and most of the colon
Anterior facial	Anterior and superficial face	Inferior mesenteric	Descending colon and rectum
External jugular	Superficial tissues of the head and neck	**UPPER EXTREMITY**	
Internal jugular	Sinuses of the brain	Cephalic	Lateral arm
THORAX		Axillary	Axilla and arm
Brachiocephalic	Viscera of the thorax	Basilic	Medial arm
Subclavian	Upper extremities	Median cubital	Cephalic vein (to basilic vein)
Superior vena cava	Head, neck, and upper extremities	**LOWER EXTREMITY**	
Pulmonary	Lungs	External iliac	Lower limb
Cardiac	Heart	Internal iliac	Pelvic viscera
Inferior vena cava	Lower body	Femoral	Thigh
ABDOMEN		Great saphenous	Leg
Hepatic	Liver	Popliteal	Lower leg
Long thoracic	Abdominal and thoracic muscles	Peroneal	Foot
Hepatic portal	Liver and gallbladder	Anterior tibial	Deep anterior leg and dorsal foot
Splenic	Spleen	Posterior tibial	Deep posterior leg and plantar aspect of foot

the digestive organs and the other in the liver. From the liver capillary beds, the path of blood returns to its normal route.

The detour of venous blood through a second capillary bed in the liver before its return to the heart serves some valuable purposes. For example, when a meal is being absorbed, the blood in the portal vein contains a higher-than-normal concentration of glucose. Liver cells remove the excess glucose and store it as glycogen; therefore, blood leaving the liver usually has a normal blood glucose concentration. Liver cells also remove and detoxify various poisonous substances that may be present in the blood. The hepatic portal system is an excellent example of how "structure follows function" in helping the body maintain homeostasis.

FIGURE 12-12

Main superficial veins of the arm.

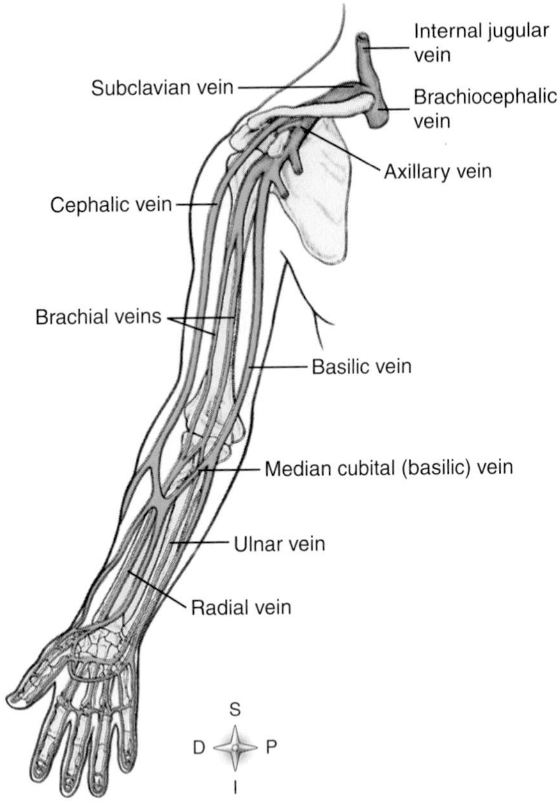

Fetal Circulation

Circulation in the body before birth differs from circulation after birth because the fetus must secure oxygen and food from maternal blood instead of from its own lungs and digestive organs. For the exchange of nutrients and oxygen to occur between fetal and maternal blood, specialized blood vessels must carry the fetal blood to the **placenta** (plah-SEN-tah), where the exchange occurs, and then return it to the fetal body. Three vessels (shown in Figure 12-15 as part of the **umbilical cord**) accomplish this purpose. They are the two small **umbilical arteries** and a single, much larger **umbilical vein.** The movement of blood in the umbilical vessels may seem unusual at first in that the umbilical vein carries oxygenated blood, and the umbilical artery carries oxygen-poor blood. Remember that arteries are vessels that carry blood away from the heart, whereas veins carry blood toward the heart, regardless of the oxygen supply they may have.

Another structure unique to fetal circulation is called the **ductus venosus** (DUK-tus ve-NO-sus). As you can see in Figure 12-15, it is actually a continuation of the umbilical vein. It serves as a shunt, allowing most of the blood returning from the placenta to bypass the immature liver of the developing baby and empty directly into the inferior vena cava. Two other structures in the developing fetus allow most of the blood to bypass the developing lungs, which remain collapsed until birth. The **foramen ovale** (fo-RAY-men o-VAL-ee) shunts blood from the right atrium directly into the left atrium, and the **ductus arteriosus** (DUK-tus ar-teer-ee-O-sus) connects the aorta and the pulmonary artery.

At birth, the baby's specialized fetal blood vessels and shunts must be rendered nonfunctional. When the newborn infant takes its first deep breaths, the circulatory system is subjected to increased pressure. The result is closure of the foramen ovale and rapid collapse of the umbilical blood vessels, the ductus venosus, and ductus arteriosus.

Quick

1. How do systemic and pulmonary circulations differ?
2. What is the hepatic portal circulation?
3. How is fetal circulation different than adult circulation?

BLOOD PRESSURE

Understanding Blood Pressure

A good way to understand blood pressure might be to try to answer a few questions about it. What is blood pressure? Just what the words say—blood pressure is the pressure or push of blood.

Where does blood pressure exist? It exists in all blood vessels, but it is highest in the arteries and lowest in the veins. In fact, if we list blood vessels in order according to the amount of blood pressure in them and draw a graph, as in Figure 12-16, the graph looks like a hill, with aortic blood pres-

FIGURE 12-13

Diagram of blood flow in the circulatory system. Blood leaves the heart through arteries, then travels through arterioles, capillaries, venules, and veins before returning to the opposite side of the heart. Compare this figure with Figure 12-4.

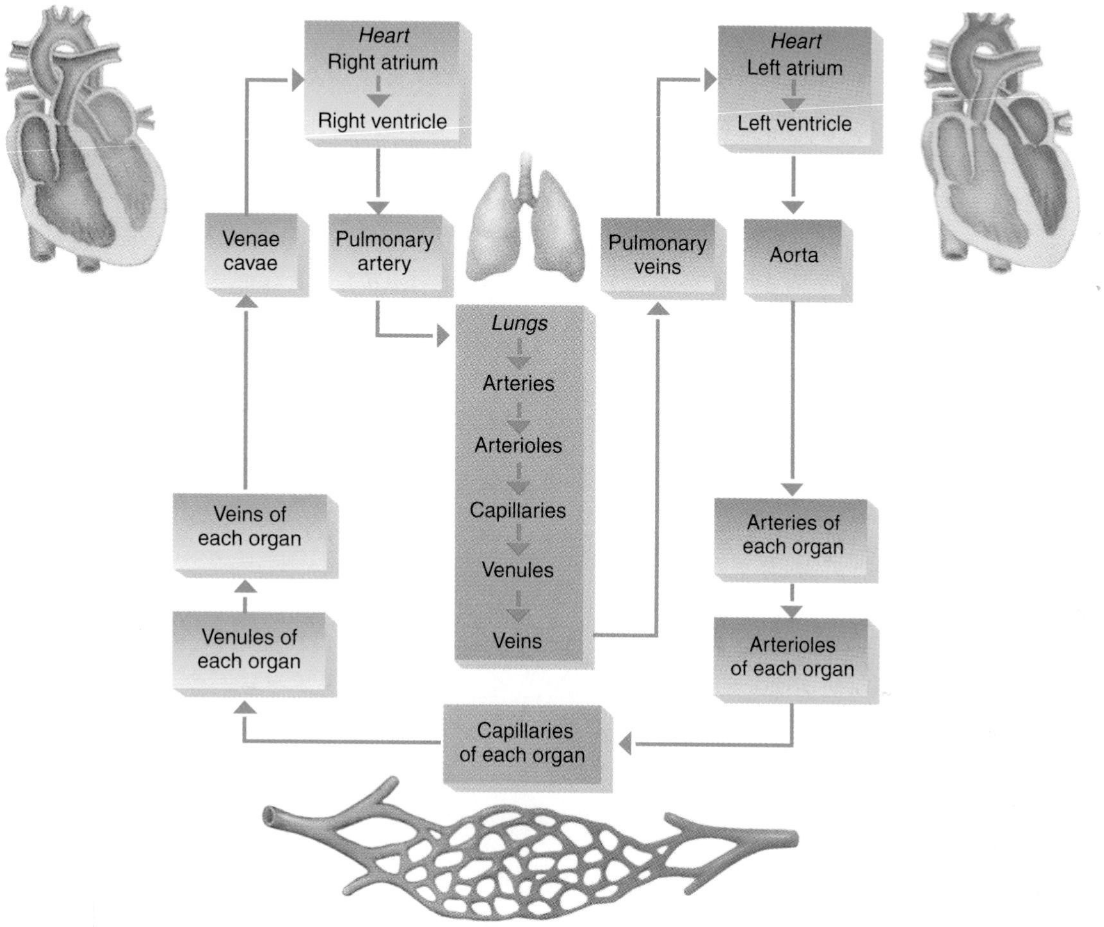

sure at the top and vena caval pressure at the bottom. This blood pressure "hill" is spoken of as the *blood pressure gradient*. More precisely, the blood pressure gradient is the difference between two blood pressures. The blood pressure gradient for the entire systemic circulation is the difference between the average or mean blood pressure in the aorta and the blood pressure at the termination of the venae cavae where they join the right atrium of the heart. The mean blood pressure in the aorta, given in Figure 12-16, is 100 mm of mercury (mm Hg), and the pressure at the termination of the venae cavae is 0. Therefore, with these typical normal figures, the systemic blood pressure gradient is 100 mm Hg (100 minus 0).

Why is it important to understand blood pressure? What is its function? The blood pressure gradient is vitally involved in keeping the blood flowing. When a blood pressure gradient is present, blood circulates; conversely, when a blood pressure gradient is not present, blood does not circulate. For example, suppose that the blood

FIGURE 12-14

Hepatic portal circulation. In this very unusual circulation, a vein is located between two capillary beds. The hepatic portal vein collects blood from capillaries in visceral structures located in the abdomen and empties it into the liver. Hepatic veins return blood to the inferior vena cava. (Organs are not drawn to scale.)

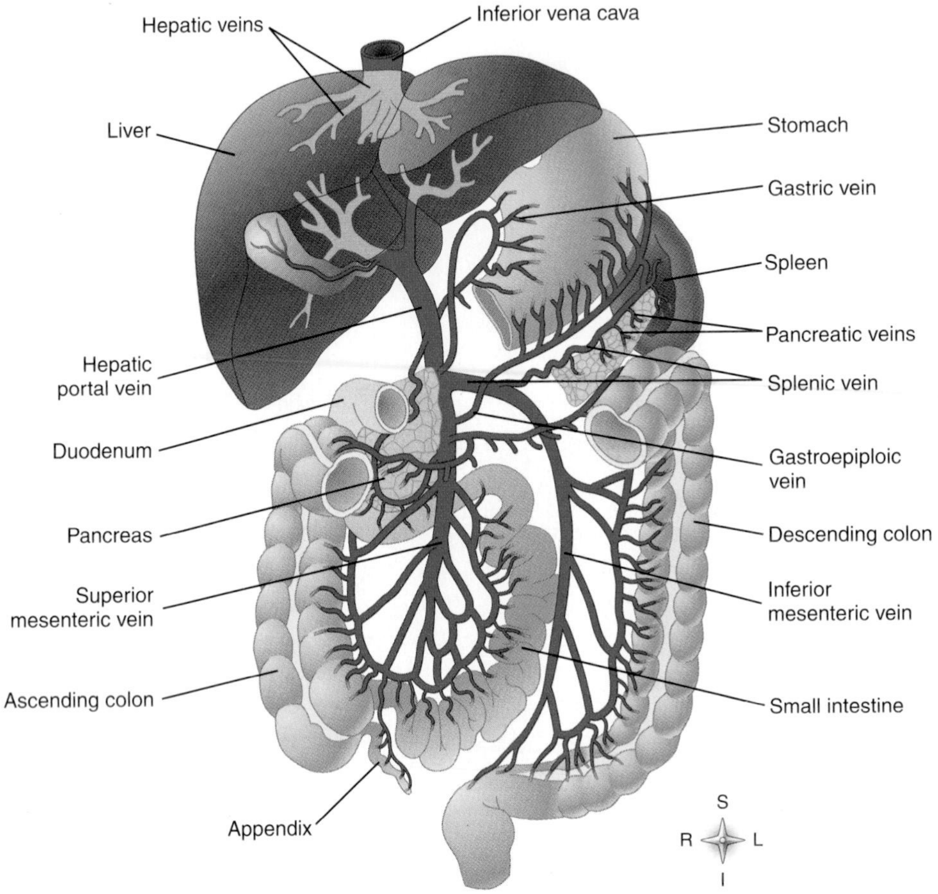

pressure in the arteries were to decrease so that it became equal to the average pressure in arterioles. There would no longer be a blood pressure gradient between arteries and arterioles, and therefore there would no longer be a force to move blood out of arteries into arterioles. Circulation would stop, in other words, and very soon life itself would cease. This is why when arterial blood pressure is observed to be falling rapidly, whether in surgery or elsewhere, emergency measures must be started quickly to try to reverse this fatal trend.

What we have just said may start you wondering about why high blood pressure (meaning, of course, high arterial blood pressure) and low blood pressure are bad for circulation. High blood pressure is bad for several reasons. For one thing, if it becomes too high, it may cause the rupture of one or more blood vessels (for example, in the brain, as happens in a stroke). But low blood pressure also can be dangerous. If arterial pressure falls low enough, circulation and life cease. Massive hemorrhage, which dramatically reduces blood pressure, kills in this way.

FIGURE 12-15

The fetal circulation.

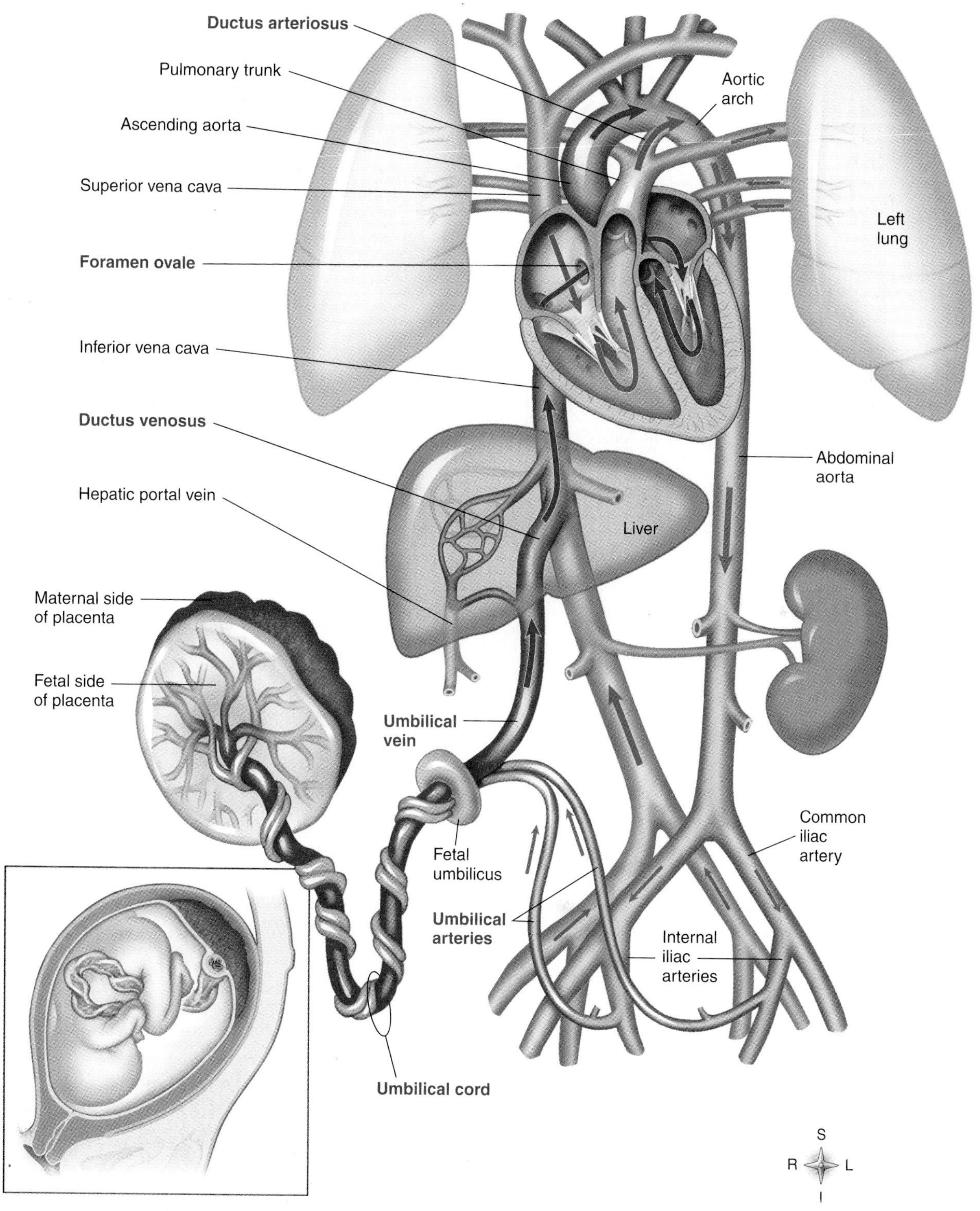
Ductus arteriosus
Pulmonary trunk
Ascending aorta
Superior vena cava
Foramen ovale
Inferior vena cava
Ductus venosus
Hepatic portal vein
Maternal side of placenta
Fetal side of placenta
Umbilical vein
Fetal umbilicus
Umbilical arteries
Umbilical cord
Aortic arch
Left lung
Abdominal aorta
Liver
Common iliac artery
Internal iliac arteries
S
R
L
I

FIGURE 12-16

Pressure gradients in blood flow. Blood flows down a "blood pressure hill" from arteries, where blood pressure is highest, into arterioles, where it is somewhat lower, into capillaries, where it is still lower, and so on. All numbers on the graph indicate blood pressure measured in millimeters of mercury. The broken line, starting at 100 mm, represents the average pressure in each part of the circulatory system.

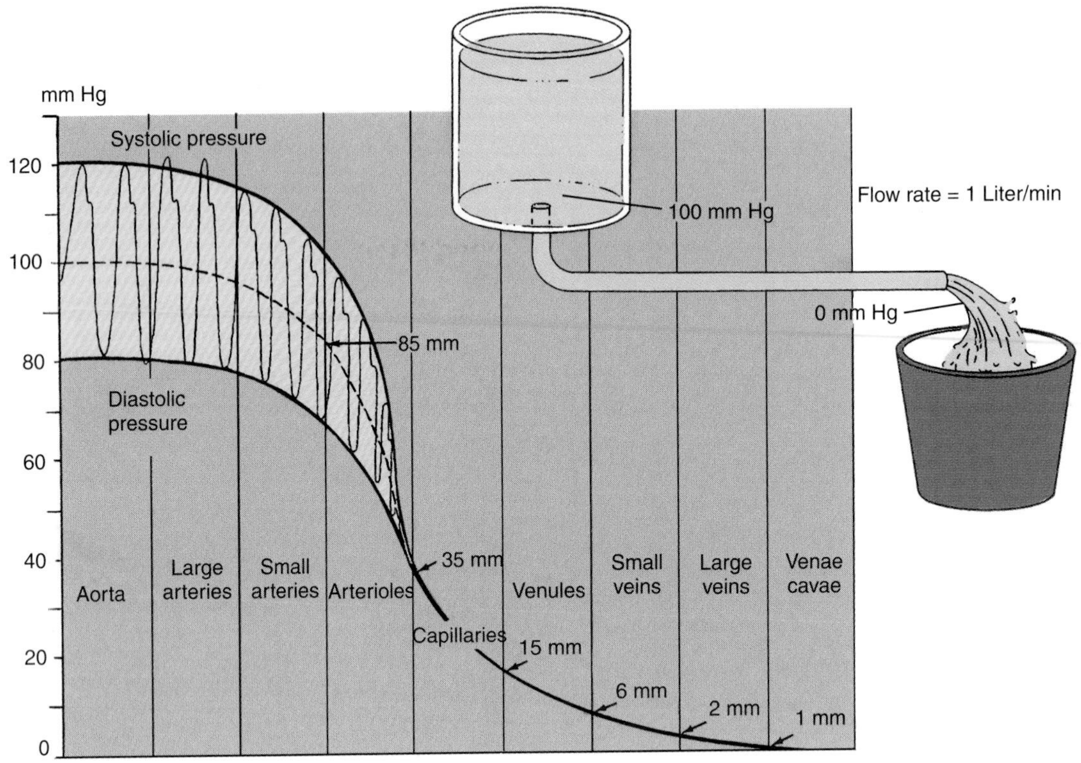

Factors That Influence Blood Pressure

What causes blood pressure, and what makes blood pressure change from time to time? Factors such as blood volume, the strength of each heart contraction, heart rate, and the thickness of blood are all discussed in the following paragraphs.

Blood Volume

The direct cause of blood pressure is the volume of blood in the vessels. The larger the volume of blood in the arteries, for example, the more pressure the blood exerts on the walls of the arteries, or the higher the arterial blood pressure.

Conversely, the less blood in the arteries, the lower the blood pressure tends to be. Hemorrhage demonstrates this relation between blood volume and blood pressure. In hemorrhage a pronounced loss of blood occurs, and this decrease in the volume of blood causes blood pressure to drop. In fact, the major sign of hemorrhage is a rapidly falling blood pressure.

The volume of blood in the arteries is determined by how much blood the heart pumps into the arteries and how much blood the arterioles drain out of them. The diameter of the arterioles plays an important role in determining how much blood drains out of arteries into arterioles.

Strength of Heart Contractions

The strength and the rate of the heartbeat affect cardiac output and therefore blood pressure. Each time the left ventricle contracts, it squeezes a certain volume of blood (the stroke volume) into the aorta and on into other arteries. The stronger that each contraction is, the more blood it pumps into the aorta and arteries. Conversely, the weaker that each contraction is, the less blood it pumps. Suppose that one contraction of the left ventricle pumps 70 ml of blood into the aorta, and suppose that the heart beats 70 times a minute; 70 ml × 70 equals 4900 ml. Almost 5 L of blood would enter the aorta and arteries every minute (the cardiac output). Now suppose that the heartbeat were to become weaker and that each contraction of the left ventricle pumps only 50 ml instead of 70 ml of blood into the aorta. If the heart still contracts 70 times a minute, it will obviously pump much less blood into the aorta—only 3500 ml instead of the more normal 4900 ml per minute. This decrease in the heart's output decreases the volume of blood in the arteries, and the decreased arterial blood volume decreases arterial blood pressure. In summary, the strength of the heartbeat affects blood pressure in this way: a stronger heartbeat increases blood pressure, and a weaker beat decreases it.

Heart Rate

The rate of the heartbeat may also affect arterial blood pressure. You might reason that when the heart beats faster, more blood enters the aorta, and therefore the arterial blood volume and blood pressure increase. This is true only if the stroke volume does not decrease sharply when the heart rate increases. Often, however, when the heart beats faster, each contraction of the left ventricle takes place so rapidly that it has little time to fill, and it squeezes out much less blood than usual into the aorta. For example, suppose that the heart rate speeded up from 70 to 100 times per minute and that, at the same time, its stroke volume decreased from 70 ml to 40 ml. Instead of a cardiac output of 70 × 70 or 4900 ml per minute, the cardiac output would have changed to 100 × 40 or 4000 ml per minute. Arterial blood volume decreases under these conditions, and therefore blood pressure also decreases, even though the heart rate has increased.

What generalization, then, can we make? We can only say that an increase in the rate of the heartbeat increases blood pressure, and a decrease in the rate decreases blood pressure. But whether a change in the heart rate actually produces a similar change in blood pressure depends on whether the stroke volume also changes and in which direction.

Blood Viscosity

Another factor that we ought to mention in connection with blood pressure is the viscosity of blood, or in plainer language, its thickness. If blood becomes less viscous than normal, blood pressure decreases. For example, if a person suffers a hemorrhage, fluid moves into the blood from the interstitial fluid. This dilutes the blood and decreases its viscosity, and blood pressure then falls because of the decreased viscosity. After hemorrhage, whole blood or plasma is preferred to saline solution for transfusions. The reason is that saline solution is not a viscous liquid and so cannot keep blood pressure at a normal level.

In a condition called *polycythemia*, the number of red blood cells increases beyond normal and thus increases blood viscosity. This in turn increases blood pressure. Polycythemia can occur when oxygen levels in the air decrease and the body attempts to increase its ability to attract oxygen to the blood, as happens in working at high altitudes.

Fluctuations in Blood Pressure

No one's blood pressure stays the same all the time. It fluctuates, even in a perfectly healthy individual. For example, it goes up when a person exercises strenuously. Not only is this normal, but the increased blood pressure serves a good purpose. It increases circulation to bring more blood to muscles each minute and thus supplies them with more oxygen and food for more energy.

A normal average arterial blood pressure is about 120/80, or 120 mm Hg systolic pressure (as the ventricles contract) and 80 mm Hg diastolic pressure (as the ventricles relax). Remember, however, that what is "normal" varies somewhat among individuals and also varies with age.

The venous blood pressure, as you can see in Figure 12-15, is very low in the large veins and falls almost to 0 by the time blood leaves the venae cavae and enters the right atrium. The venous blood pressure within the right atrium is called the **central venous pressure.** This pressure level is important because it influences the pressure that exists in the large peripheral veins. If the heart beats strongly, the central venous pressure is low as blood enters and leaves the heart chambers efficiently. However, if the heart is weakened, central venous pressure increases, and the flow of blood into the right atrium is slowed. As a result, a person suffering heart failure, who is sitting at rest in a chair, often has distended external jugular veins as blood "backs up" in the venous network.

Five mechanisms help to keep venous blood moving back through the circulatory system and into the right atrium. They include:

1. Continued beating of the heart, which pumps blood through the entire circulatory system;
2. Adequate blood pressure in the arteries, to push blood to and through the veins;
3. Semilunar valves in the veins that ensure continued blood flow in one direction (toward the heart);
4. Contraction of skeletal muscles squeezes veins, producing a kind of pumping action; and
5. Changing pressures in the chest cavity during breathing produce a kind of pumping action in the veins in the thorax.

FIGURE 12-17

Pulse points. Each pulse point is named after the artery with which it is associated.

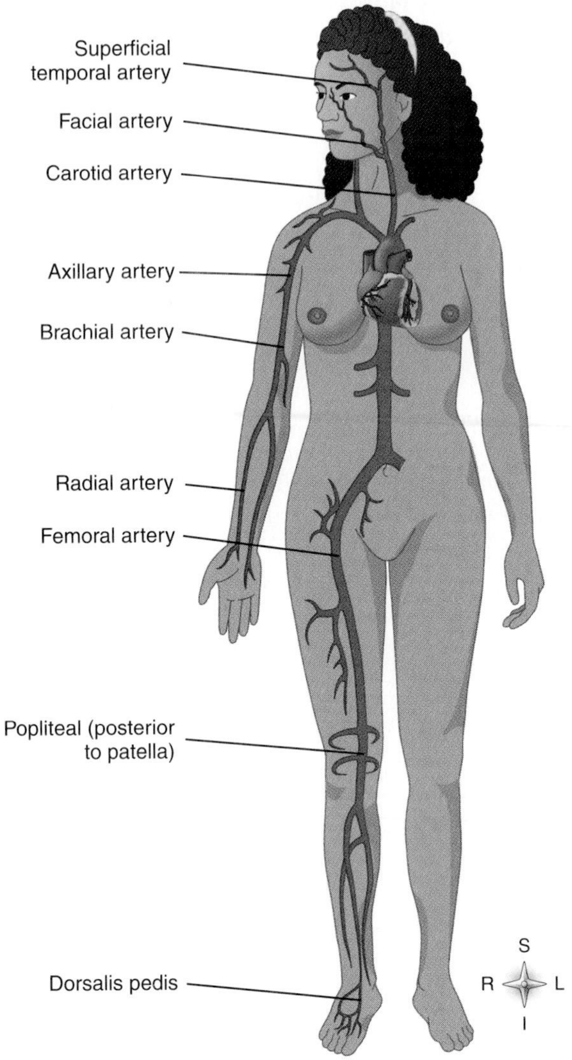

PULSE

What you feel when you take a pulse is an artery expanding and then recoiling alternately. To feel a pulse, you must place your fingertips over an artery that lies near the surface of the body and over a bone or other firm base. The pulse is a valuable clinical sign. It can provide information, for example, about the rate, strength, and rhythmicity of the heartbeat. It is also easily determined with little or no danger or discomfort. There are nine major "pulse points" named after the arteries where they are felt. Locate each pulse point on Figure 12-17 and on your own body.

Clinical Application

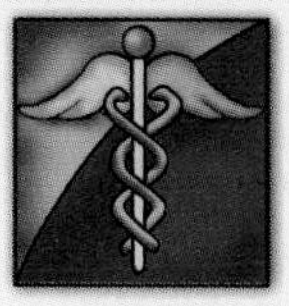

Blood Pressure Readings

A device called a **sphygmomanometer** (sfig-mo-ma-NAH-me-ter) is often used to measure blood pressures in both clinical and home health care situations. The traditional sphygmomanometer is an inverted tube of mercury (Hg) with a balloonlike air cuff attached via an air hose. The air cuff is placed around a limb, usually the subject's upper arm as shown in the figure. A stethoscope sensor is placed over a major artery (the *brachial artery* in the figure) to listen for the arterial pulse. A hand-operated pump fills the air cuff, increasing the air pressure and pushing the column of mercury higher. While listening through the stethoscope, the operator opens the air cuff's outlet valve and slowly reduces the air pressure around the limb. Loud, tapping *Korotkoff sounds* suddenly begin when the cuff pressure measured by the mercury column equals the **systolic pressure**—usually about 120 mm. As the air pressure surrounding the arm continues to decrease, the Korotkoff sounds disappear. The pressure measurement at which the sounds disappear is equal to the **diastolic pressure**—usually 70 to 80 mm. The subject's blood pressure is then expressed as systolic pressure (the maximum arterial pressure during each cardiac cycle) over the diastolic pressure (the minimum arterial pressure), such as 120/80 (read "one-twenty over eighty"). The final reading can then be compared with the expected value, which is based on the patient's age and various other individual factors. Mercury sphygmomanometers have been replaced in many clinical settings by nonmercury devices that similarly measure the maximum and minimum arterial blood pressures. In home health care settings, patients can often learn to monitor their own blood pressure.

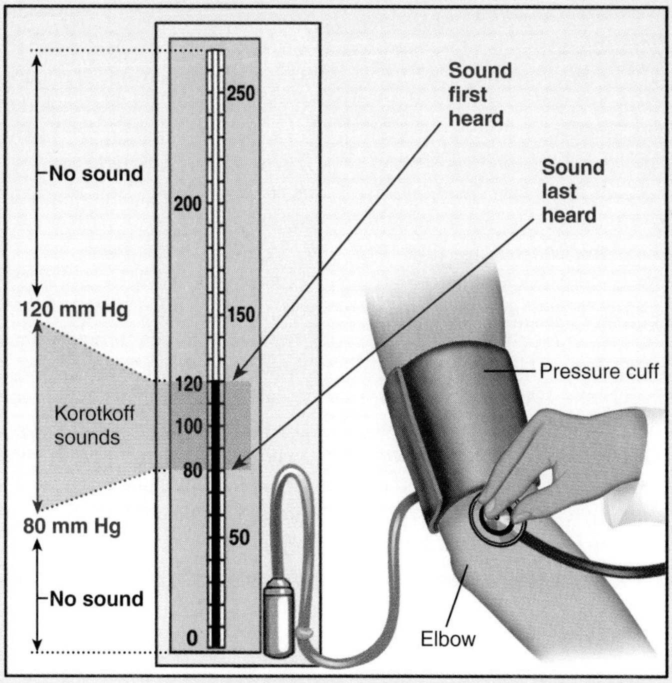

The following pulse points are located on each side of the head and neck: (1) over the superficial temporal artery in front of the ear, (2) the common carotid artery in the neck along the front edge of the sternocleidomastoid muscle, and (3) over the facial artery at the lower margin of the mandible at a point below the corner of the mouth.

A pulse is also detected at three points in the upper limb: (1) in the axilla over the axillary artery; (2) over the brachial artery at the bend of the elbow along the inner or medial margin of the biceps brachii muscle, and (3) at the radial artery at the wrist. The so-called radial pulse is the most frequently monitored and easily accessible in the body.

The pulse can also be felt at three locations in the lower extremity: (1) over the femoral artery in the groin, (2) at the popliteal artery behind and just proximal to the knee, and (3) at the dorsalis pedis artery on the front surface of the foot, just below the bend of the ankle joint.

Quick Check

1. How does the blood pressure gradient explain blood flow?
2. Can you name four factors that influence blood pressure?
3. Does a person's blood pressure stay the same all the time?
4. Where are the places on your body that you can likely feel your pulse?

Science Applications

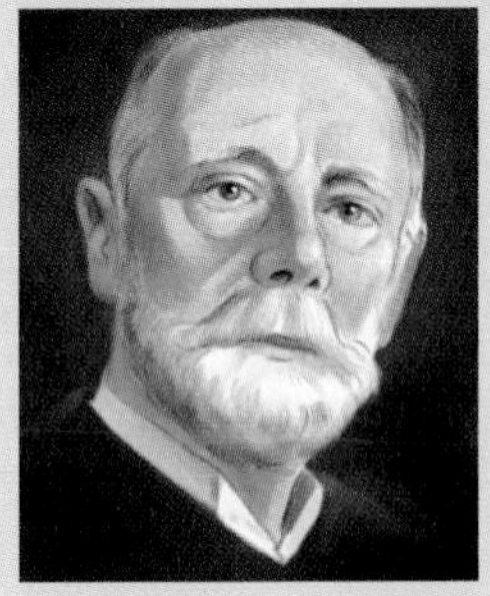

Cardiology

Willem Einthoven (1860-1927).

Cardiology, the study and treatment of the heart, owes much to Dutch physiologist Willem Einthoven and his invention of the modern electrocardiograph in 1903. Einthoven's first major contribution was the invention of a machine that could record electrocardiograms (ECGs) with far greater sensitivity than the crude machines of the 19th century. Then, with the help British physician Lewis Thomas, Einthoven demonstrated and named the P, Q, R, S, and T waves and proved that these waves precisely record the electrical activity of the heart (see Figure 12-7). In 1905, he even invented a way that ECG data could be sent from a patient over the telephone to his laboratory where they could be recorded and analyzed—a technique now called *telemetry*. His detailed studies of ECG recordings changed the practice of heart medicine forever. In fact, his invention was later applied to the study of nerve impulses and led to breakthrough discoveries in the neurosciences.

Cardiologists today still use modern versions of Einthoven's machine to diagnose heart disorders. Of course, biomedical engineers continue to develop refinements to electrocardiograph equipment and to invent new machines to monitor heart function. In fact, engineers and designers have worked with cardiologists to develop artificial heart valves, artificial pacemakers, and even artificial hearts! With all of this medical equipment being used in cardiology, and medicine in general, there are also many technicians working to keep it all in good repair.

OUTLINE SUMMARY

HEART

A. Location, size, and position
  1. Triangular organ located in mediastinum with two thirds of the mass to the left of the body midline and one third to the right; the apex on the diaphragm; shape and size of a closed fist (Figure 12-1)
  2. Cardiopulmonary resuscitation (CPR)—the heart lies between the sternum in front and the bodies of the thoracic vertebrae behind; rhythmic compression of the heart between the sternum and vertebrae can maintain blood flow during cardiac arrest; if combined with artificial respiration procedure, it can be life saving

B. Anatomy
  1. Heart chambers (Figure 12-2)
     a. Two upper chambers are called *atria* (receiving chambers)—right and left atria
     b. Two lower chambers called *ventricles* (discharging chambers)—right and left ventricles
     c. Wall of each heart chamber is composed of cardiac muscle tissue called *myocardium*
     d. Endocardium—smooth lining of heart chambers—inflammation of endocardium called *endocarditis*
  2. Covering sac or pericardium
     a. Pericardium is a two-layered fibrous sac with a lubricated space between the two layers
     b. Inner layer is called *visceral pericardium* or *epicardium*
     c. Outer layer called *parietal pericardium*
  3. Heart action
     Contraction of the heart is called *systole;* relaxation is called *diastole.*
  4. Heart valves (Figure 12-3)
     Four valves keep blood flowing through the heart; prevent backflow (two atrioventricular or AV and two semilunar valves)
     a. Tricuspid—at the opening of the right atrium into the ventricle
     b. Bicuspid (mitral)—at the opening of the left atrium into the ventricle
     c. Pulmonary semilunar—at the beginning of the pulmonary artery
     d. Aortic semilunar—at the beginning of the aorta

C. Heart sounds
  1. Two distinct heart sounds in every heartbeat or cycle—"lub-dup"
  2. First (lub) sound is caused by the vibration and closure of AV valves during contraction of the ventricles
  3. Second (dup) sound is caused by the closure of the semilunar valves during relaxation of the ventricles

D. Blood flow through the heart (Figure 12-4)
  1. The heart acts as two separate pumps—the right atrium and ventricle performing different functions from the left atrium and ventricle
  2. Sequence of blood flow: venous blood enters the right atrium through the superior and inferior venae cavae—passes from the right atrium through the tricuspid valve to the right ventricle; from the right ventricle it passes through the pulmonary semilunar valve to the pulmonary artery to the lungs—blood moves from the lungs to the left atrium, passing through the bicuspid (mitral) valve to the left ventricle; blood in the left ventricle is pumped through the aortic semilunar valve into the aorta and is distributed to the body as a whole

Continued

OUTLINE SUMMARY—*cont'd*

E. Blood supply to the heart muscle
   1. Blood, which supplies oxygen and nutrients to the myocardium of the heart, flows through the right and left coronary arteries (Figure 12-5)
   2. Blockage of blood flow through the coronary arteries is called *myocardial infarction* (*heart attack*)
   3. Angina pectoris—chest pain caused by inadequate oxygen to the heart
   4. Coronary bypass surgery—veins from other parts of the body are used to bypass blockages in coronary arteries (Figure 12-6)

F. Cardiac cycle
   1. Heartbeat is regular and rhythmic—each complete beat is called a *cardiac cycle*—average is about 72 beats per minute
   2. Each cycle, about 0.8 seconds long, is subdivided into systole (contraction phase) and diastole (relaxation phase)
   3. Stroke volume—volume of blood ejected from one ventricle with each beat
   4. Cardiac output—amount of blood that one ventricle can pump each minute; average is about 5 L per minute at rest

G. Conduction system (Figure 12-7)
   1. Intercalated disks are electrical connectors that join all the cardiac muscle fibers in a region together so that they receive their impulse, and thus contract, at about the same time
   2. SA (sinoatrial) node, the pacemaker—located in the wall of the right atrium near the opening of the superior vena cava
   3. AV (atrioventricular) node—located in the right atrium along the lower part of the interatrial septum
   4. AV bundle (bundle of His)—located in the septum of the ventricle
   5. Purkinje fibers—located in the walls of the ventricles

H. Electrocardiogram (Figure 12-8)
   1. Specialized conduction system structures generate and transmit the electrical impulses that result in contraction of the heart
   2. These tiny electrical impulses can be picked up on the surface of the body and transformed into visible tracings by a machine called an electrocardiograph
   3. The visible tracing of these electrical signals is called an *electrocardiogram* or *ECG*
   4. The normal ECG has three deflections or waves called the *P wave*, the *QRS complex*, and the *T wave*
      a. P wave—associated with depolarization of the atria
      b. QRS complex—associated with depolarization of the ventricles
      c. T wave—associated with repolarization of the ventricles

BLOOD VESSELS

A. Kinds
   1. Arteries—carry blood away from the heart
   2. Veins—carry blood toward the heart
   3. Capillaries—carry blood from the arterioles to the venules

B. Structure (Figure 12-9)
   1. Arteries
      a. Tunica intima—inner layer of endothelial cells
      b. Tunica media—smooth muscle with some elastic tissue, thick in arteries; important in blood pressure regulation
      c. Tunica adventitia—thin layer of elastic tissue
   2. Capillaries—microscopic vessels
      a. Only layer is the tunica intima

OUTLINE SUMMARY

3. Veins
   a. Tunica intima—inner layer; valves prevent retrograde movement of blood
   b. Tunica media—smooth muscle; thin in veins
   c. Tunica adventitia—heavy layer in many veins

C. Functions
1. Arteries—distribution of nutrients, gases, etc., with movement of blood under high pressure; assist in maintaining the arterial blood pressure
2. Capillaries—serve as exchange vessels for nutrients, wastes, and fluids
3. Veins—collect blood for return to the heart; low pressure vessels

D. Names of main arteries—see Figure 12-10 and Table 12-1

E. Names of main veins—see Figures 12-11 and 12-12 and Table 12-2

CIRCULATION

A. Plan of circulation—refers to the blood flow through the vessels arranged to form a circuit or circular pattern (Figure 12-13)

B. Types of circulation
1. Systemic circulation
   a. Carries blood throughout the body
   b. Path goes from left ventricle through aorta, smaller arteries, arterioles, capillaries, venules, venae cavae, to right atrium
2. Pulmonary circulation
   a. Carries blood to and from the lungs; arteries deliver deoxygenated blood to the lungs for gas exchange
   b. Path goes from right ventricle through pulmonary arteries, lungs, pulmonary veins, to left atrium
3. Hepatic portal circulation (Figure 12-14)
   a. Unique blood route through the liver
   b. Vein (hepatic portal vein) exists between two capillary beds
   c. Assists with homeostasis of blood glucose levels
4. Fetal circulation (Figure 12-15)
   a. Refers to circulation before birth
   b. Modifications required for fetus to efficiently secure oxygen and nutrients from the maternal blood
   c. Unique structures include the placenta, umbilical arteries and vein, ductus venosus, ductus arteriosus, and foramen ovale

BLOOD PRESSURE

A. Blood pressure is push or force of blood in the blood vessels

B. Highest in arteries, lowest in veins (Figure 12-16)

C. Blood pressure gradient causes blood to circulate—liquids can flow only from the area where pressure is higher to where it is lower

D. Blood volume, heartbeat, and blood viscosity are main factors that produce blood pressure

E. Blood pressure varies within normal range from time to time

F. Venous return of blood to the heart depends on five mechanisms—a strongly beating heart, adequate arterial blood pressure, valves in the veins, pumping action of skeletal muscles as they contract, and changing pressures in the chest cavity caused by breathing.

PULSE

A. Definition—alternate expansion and recoil of the blood vessel wall

B. Places where you can count the pulse easily (Figure 12-17)

NEW WORDS

angina pectoris
arteriole
artery
atrioventricular (AV) valve
atrium
bicuspid valve
capillary
cardiac output
cardiopulmonary resuscitation (CPR)
coronary bypass surgery
coronary circulation
diastolic pressure
ductus arteriosus
ductus venosus
electrocardiogram (ECG)
endocarditis
endocardium
epicardium
foramen ovale
hepatic portal circulation
mitral valve
myocardial infarction
myocardium
P wave
pacemaker
pericardium
pulmonary circulation
pulse
Purkinje fibers
QRS complex
semilunar valve
sinoatrial node
systemic circulation
T wave
tricuspid valve
umbilical
vein
ventricle
venule

REVIEW QUESTIONS

1. Describe the heart and its position in the body.
2. Name the four chambers of the heart.
3. What is the myocardium? What is the endocardium?
4. Describe the two layers of the pericardium. What is the function of pericardial fluid?
5. Define *systole* and *diastole*.
6. Name and give the location of the four heart valves.
7. Trace the flow of blood from the superior vena cava to the aorta.
8. What is angina pectoris?
9. Differentiate between stroke volume and cardiac output.
10. Trace the path and name the structures involved in the conduction system of the heart.
11. Name and describe the main types of blood vessels in the body.
12. Name the three tissue layers that make up arteries and veins.
13. Describe both systemic and pulmonary circulation.
14. Name and briefly explain the four factors that influence blood pressure.
15. List the five mechanisms that keep the venous blood moving toward the right atrium.
16. Name four locations in the body where the pulse can be felt.

CRITICAL THINKING

17. Explain how the traces on an ECG relate to what is occurring in the heart.
18. Explain hepatic portal circulation. How is it different from normal circulation, and what advantages are gained from this type of circulation?
19. Explain the differences between normal postnatal circulation and fetal circulation. Based on the environment of the fetus, explain how these differences make fetal circulation more efficient.
20. Explain why a pressure difference must exist between the aorta and the right atrium.

CHAPTER TEST

1. Ventricles are the thicker chambers of the heart, which are sometimes called the discharging chambers.
2. The atria are the thinner chambers of the heart, which are sometimes called the receiving chambers of the heart.
3. Cardiac muscle tissue is called myocardium
4. The ventricles of the heart are separated into right and left sides by the interventricular septum
5. The thin layer of tissue lining the interior of the heart chambers is called the ~~epicardium~~ endocardium
6. Another term for the visceral pericardium is the epicardium
7. Contraction of the heart is called systole.
8. Relaxation of the heart is called distole.
9. The heart valve located between the right atrium and right ventricle is called the tricuspid valve.
10. The term stroke volume refers to the volume of blood ejected from the ventricle during each beat.
11. The sinoatrial node is the pacemaker of the heart and causes the contraction of the atria.
12. The __________ are extensions of the atrioventricular fibers and cause the contraction of the ventricles.
13. The ECG tracing that occurs when the ventricles depolarize is called the __________.
14. The ECG tracing that occurs when the atria depolarize is called the __________.
15. The __________ are the blood vessels that carry blood back to the heart.
16. The __________ are the blood vessels that carry blood away from the heart.
17. The __________ are the microscopic blood vessels where substances are exchanged between the blood and tissues.
18. The innermost layer of tissue in an artery is called the __________.
19. The outermost layer of tissue in an artery is called the __________.
20. Systemic circulation involves the moving of blood throughout the body; __________ involves moving blood from the heart to the lungs and back.
21. The two structures in the developing fetus that allow most of the blood to bypass the lungs are the __________ and the __________.
22. The strength of the heart contraction and blood volume are two factors that influence blood pressure. Two other factors that influence blood pressure are __________ and __________.
23. Place the following structures in their proper order in blood flow through the heart by putting a 1 in front of the first structure the blood would pass through and a 10 in front of the last structure the blood would pass through.
    - **a.** ____ left atrium
    - **b.** ____ tricuspid valve (right atrioventricular valve)
    - **c.** ____ right ventricle
    - **d.** ____ pulmonary vein
    - **e.** ____ aortic semilunar valve
    - **f.** ____ mitral valve (left atrioventricular valve)
    - **g.** ____ left ventricle
    - **h.** ____ pulmonary artery
    - **i.** ____ right atrium
    - **j.** ____ pulmonary semilunar valve

STUDY TIPS

Before studying Chapter 12, review the synopsis of the circulatory system in Chapter 4. Chapter 12 deals with the heart, the pump that moves the blood; and the vessels, the tubing that carries the blood. The term *cardio-* refers to the heart, in Chapter 7 you learned that *myo-* means muscle. *Myocardium* is the heart muscle. The structures of the heart can be learned with flash cards. The location of the semilunar valves should be easy to remember because their names tell you where they are. It is harder to remember where the tricuspid and mitral valves are because the names don't help. An easier way to remember them is to use their other names, the right and left atrioventricular valves, respectively. This name tells you exactly where they are: between the atria and ventricles on the right or left side. Blood moves through the cardiovascular system in one direction, from the right heart, to the lungs, to the left heart, to the rest of the body and back to the right heart. If you are asked to learn the sequence of blood flow through the heart, don't forget the valves. Heart conduction may make more sense if you remember that atria contract from the top down, but ventricles must contract from the bottom up. The letters that are used in an ECG trace don't stand for anything; the P, Q, R, S, and T are arbitrary.

The arteries and veins are composed of three layers of tissue. There is a difference in thickness in these vessels because the arteries carry blood under higher pressure. Arteries and veins carry blood in opposite directions—arteries away from the heart, veins toward the heart. Capillaries need to be thin-walled because this is where the exchange of material between the blood and the tissues takes place. If you are asked to learn the names and locations of specific blood vessels, use flash cards and the figures. Fetal circulation makes sense if you remember the environment in which the fetus is living. The blood is oxygenated and full of digested food, so it doesn't have to go to the lungs or the liver. A liquid moves from high to low pressure, so it is logical that the pressure in the cardiovascular system is highest in the aorta and lowest in the vena cava.

In your study groups, bring photocopies of the figures of the heart and of the blood vessels if you need to learn them. Blacken out the labels and quiz each other on the name of each structure and its function. Discuss the sequence of heart circulation, the parts of an ECG, the heart conduction system, the structure and function of the blood vessels, and the structures in fetal circulation. Go over the questions at the end of the chapter and discuss possible test questions.

13 The Lymphatic System and Immunity

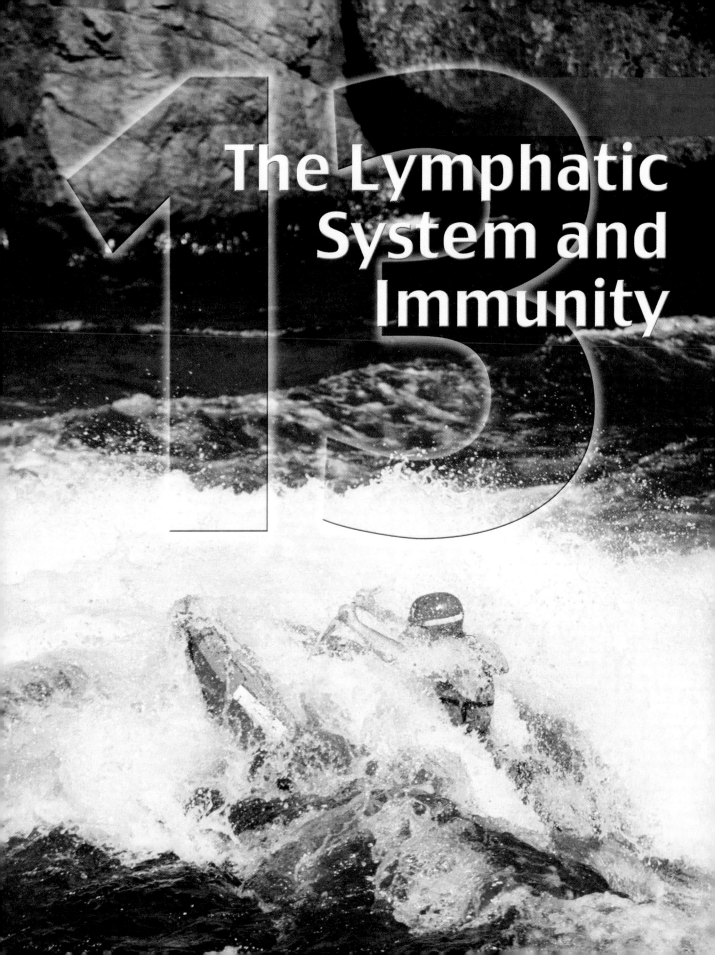

Outline

Objectives

AFTER YOU HAVE COMPLETED THIS CHAPTER, YOU SHOULD BE ABLE TO:

1. Describe the generalized functions of the lymphatic system and list the primary lymphatic structures.
2. Discuss and compare nonspecific and specific immunity, inherited and acquired immunity, and active and passive immunity.
3. Discuss the major types of immune system molecules and indicate how antibodies and complements function.
4. Discuss and contrast the development and functions of B and T cells.
5. Compare and contrast humoral and cell-mediated immunity.

All of us live in a hostile and dangerous environment. Each day we are faced with potentially harmful toxins, disease-causing bacteria, viruses, and even cells from our own bodies that have been transformed into cancerous invaders. Fortunately, we are protected from this staggering variety of differing biological enemies by a remarkable set of defense mechanisms. We refer to this protective "safety net" as the **immune system.**

This chapter deals with the lymphatic system and immunity. This system is characterized by structural components, many of them lymphatic organs, and by a functional group of specialized cells and molecules that protect us from infection and disease. This chapter begins with an overview of the lymphatic system, discussing vessels that help maintain fluid balance and lymphoid tissues that help protect the internal environment. We will then discuss the concept of immunity and the ways that highly specialized cells and molecules provide us with effective and very specific resistance to disease.

THE LYMPHATIC SYSTEM

Lymph and Lymph Vessels

Maintaining the constancy of the fluid around each body cell is possible only if numerous homeostatic mechanisms function effectively together in a controlled and integrated response to changing conditions. We know from Chapter 12 that the circulatory system plays a key role in bringing many needed substances to cells and then removing the waste products that accumulate as a result of metabolism. This exchange of substances between blood and tissue fluid occurs in capillary beds. Many additional substances that cannot enter or return through the capillary walls, including excess fluid and protein molecules, are returned to the blood as **lymph.** Lymph is a specialized fluid formed in the tissue spaces that is transported by way of specialized **lymphatic vessels** to eventually reenter the circulatory system. In addition to lymph and the lymphatic vessels, the lymphatic system includes lymph nodes and specialized lymphatic organs such as the thymus and spleen (Figure 13-1).

Lymph forms in this way: blood plasma filters out of the capillaries into the microscopic spaces between tissue cells because of the pressure generated by the pumping action of the heart. There, the liquid is called **interstitial fluid** or tissue fluid. Much of the interstitial fluid goes back into the blood by the same route it came out (that is, through the capillary membrane). The remainder of the interstitial fluid enters the lymphatic system before it returns to the blood. The fluid, now called *lymph*, enters a network of tiny blind-ended tubes distributed in the tissue spaces. These tiny vessels, called *lymphatic capillaries*, permit excess tissue fluid and some other substances such as dissolved protein molecules to leave the tissue spaces. Figure 13-2 shows the role of the lymphatic system in fluid homeostasis.

Lymphatic and blood capillaries are similar in many ways. Both types of vessels are microscopic and both are formed from sheets consisting of a cell layer of simple squamous epithelium called *endothelium* (en-doe-THEE-lee-um). The flattened endothelial cells that form blood capillaries, however, fit tightly together so that large molecules cannot enter or exit from the vessel. The "fit" between endothelial cells forming the lymphatic capillaries is not as tight. As a result, they are more porous and allow larger molecules, including proteins and other substances, as well as the fluid itself, to enter the vessel and eventually return to the general circulation. The movement of lymph in the lymphatic vessels is one way. Unlike blood, lymph does not flow over and over again through vessels that form a circular route.

Lymph flowing through the lymphatic capillaries next moves into successively larger and larger vessels called *lymphatic venules* and *veins* and eventually empties into two terminal vessels called the **right lymphatic duct** and the **thoracic duct,** which empty their lymph into the blood in veins in the neck region. Lymph from about three fourths of the body eventually drains into the thoracic duct, which is the largest lymphatic vessel in the body. Lymph from the right upper extremity and from the right side of the head, neck, and upper torso flows into the right lymphatic duct (Figure 13-1). The lymphatic vessels have a "beaded" appearance caused by the presence of valves that assist in maintaining a one-way flow of lymph. Note in Figure 13-1 that the thoracic duct in the abdomen has an enlarged pouchlike structure called the **cisterna chyli** (sis-TER-nah KI-li) that serves as a storage area for lymph moving toward its point of entry into the venous system.

Lymphatic capillaries in the wall of the small intestine are given the special name of **lacteals** (LAK-tee-als). They transport fats obtained from food to the bloodstream and are discussed in Chapter 15.

Lymph Nodes

As lymph moves from its origin in the tissue spaces toward the thoracic or right lymphatic ducts and then into the venous blood, it is filtered by moving through **lymph nodes,** which are located in clusters along the pathway of lymphatic vessels. Some of these nodes may be as small as a pinhead, and others may be as large as a lima bean. With the exception of a comparatively few single nodes, most lymph nodes occur in groups or clusters in certain

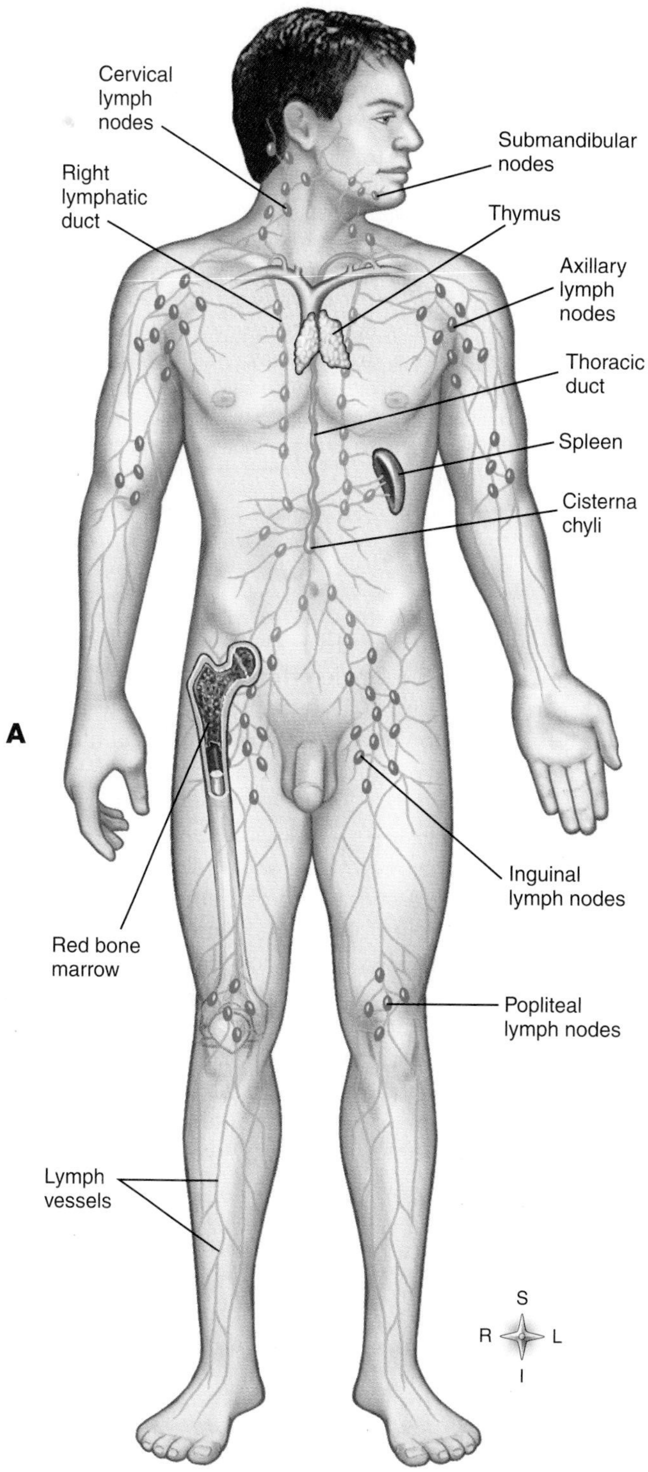

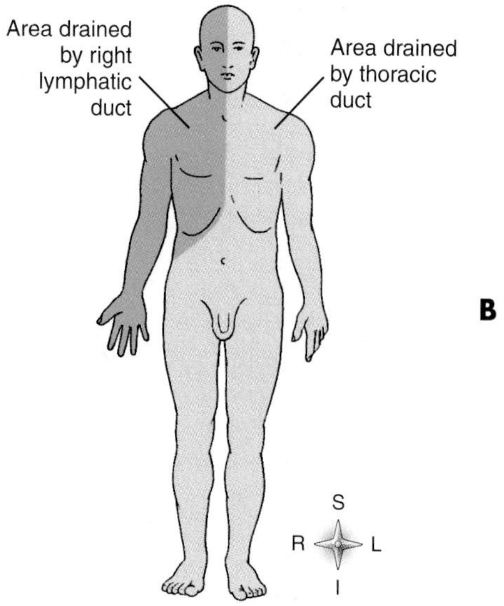

FIGURE 13-1

The lymphatic system. A, Principal organs of the lymphatic system. **B,** The inset shows the areas drained by the right lymphatic duct (green) and the thoracic duct (blue).

FIGURE 13-2

Role of lymphatic system in fluid homeostasis.
Fluid from blood plasma that is not reabsorbed by blood vessels drains into lymphatic vessels. Lymphatic drainage prevents accumulation of too much tissue fluid.

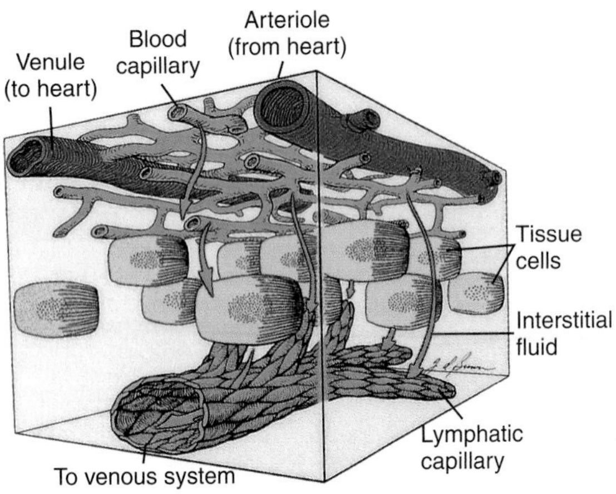

Health & Well-Being

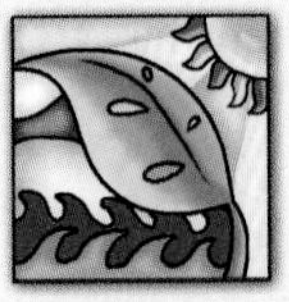

Effects of Exercise on Immunity

Exercise physiologists have found that moderate exercise increases the number of WBCs, specifically granular leukocytes and lymphocytes. Not only is the number of circulating immune cells higher after exercise, but the activity of sensitized T cells is also increased. But at the same time, research also shows that strenuous exercise may actually inhibit immune function. Nevertheless, immediate moderate exercise such as walking after a trauma such as surgery is often encouraged because of its immunity-strengthening effects.

areas (Figures 13-1 and 13-4). Figure 13-1 shows the locations of the clusters of greatest clinical importance. The structure of the lymph nodes makes it possible for them to perform two important functions: defense and white blood cell formation.

Defense Function: Biological Filtration

Figure 13-3 shows the structure of a typical lymph node. In this example, a small node located next to an infected hair follicle is shown filtering bacteria from lymph. Lymph nodes perform biological filtration, a process in which cells (phagocytic cells in this case) alter the contents of the filtered fluid. Biological filtration of bacteria and other abnormal cells by phagocytosis prevents local infections from spreading. Note in Figure 13-3 that lymph enters the node through four **afferent** (from the Latin "to carry toward") **lymph vessels.** These vessels deliver lymph to the node. Once lymph enters the node, it "percolates' slowly through spaces called *sinuses* that surround *nodules* found in the outer (cortex) and inner (medullary) areas of the node (Figure 13-3). In passing through the node, lymph is filtered so that injurious particles such as bacteria and cancer cells are removed and prevented from entering the blood and circulating all over the body. Lymph exits from the node through a single **efferent** (from the Latin "to carry away from") **lymph vessel.** Clusters of lymph nodes allow a very effective biological filtration of lymph flowing from specific body areas. Figure 13-4 shows an x-ray called a *lymphangiogram* (lym-FAN-go-o-gram). Dye material was injected into the soft tissues below the area visualized in the x-ray. Note the presence of lymph in the vessels and nodes of the inguinal and pelvic regions. A knowledge of lymph node location and function is important in clinical medicine. A surgeon uses knowledge of lymph node function when removing lymph nodes under the arms (axillary nodes) and in other areas during an operation for breast cancer. These nodes may contain cancer cells filtered out of the lymph drained from the breast. Cancer of the breast is one of the most common forms of this disease in women. Unfortunately, cancer cells from a single tumorous growth in the breast often spread to other areas of the body through the lymphatic system. Figure 13-5 shows how lymph from the breast drains into many different and widely placed nodes.

Thymus

The **thymus** (THYE-mus) (see Figure 13-1) is a small lymphoid tissue organ located in the mediastinum, extending upward in the midline of the

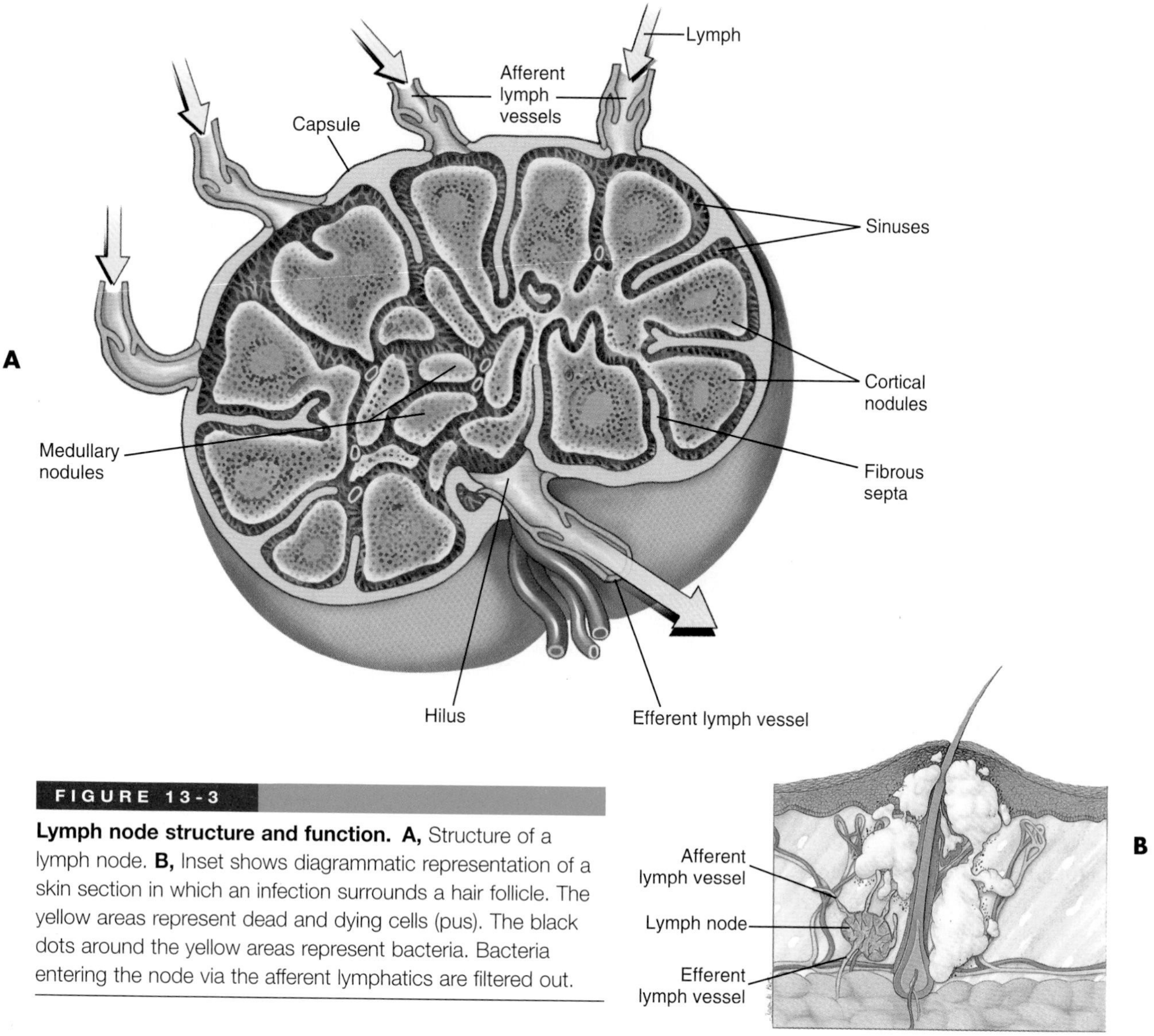

FIGURE 13-3

Lymph node structure and function. A, Structure of a lymph node. **B,** Inset shows diagrammatic representation of a skin section in which an infection surrounds a hair follicle. The yellow areas represent dead and dying cells (pus). The black dots around the yellow areas represent bacteria. Bacteria entering the node via the afferent lymphatics are filtered out.

neck. It is composed of lymphocytes in a unique epithelial tissue framework. The thymus is largest at puberty and even then weighs only about 35 or 40 g—a little more than an ounce. Although small in size, the thymus plays a central and critical role in the body's vital immunity mechanism. First, it is a source of lymphocytes before birth and is then especially important in the "maturation" or development of specialized lymphocytes that then leave the thymus and circulate to the spleen, tonsils, lymph nodes, and other lymphatic tissues. These **T-lymphocytes** or T cells are critical to the functioning of the immune system and are discussed later. They develop under the influence of hormones secreted by the thymus, **thymosins** (THYE-mo-sinz). The thymus completes most of its work early in childhood and is then replaced largely by fat and connective tissue, a process called *involution*. A tiny bit of functional thymus tissue remains, however.

FIGURE 13-4

Lymphangiogram. Dye material was injected into the soft tissues below the area visualized in the x-ray.

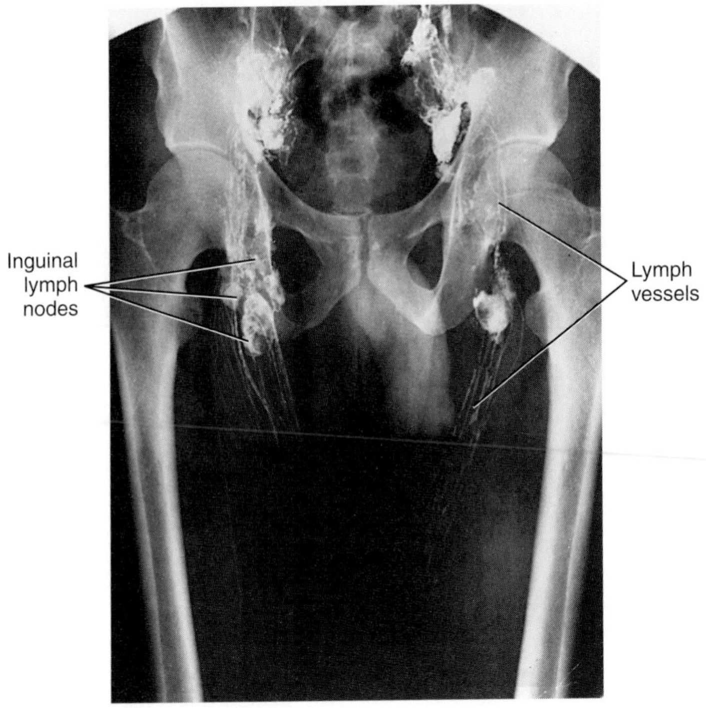

FIGURE 13-5

Lymphatic drainage of the breast. Note the extensive network of nodes that receive lymph from the breast.

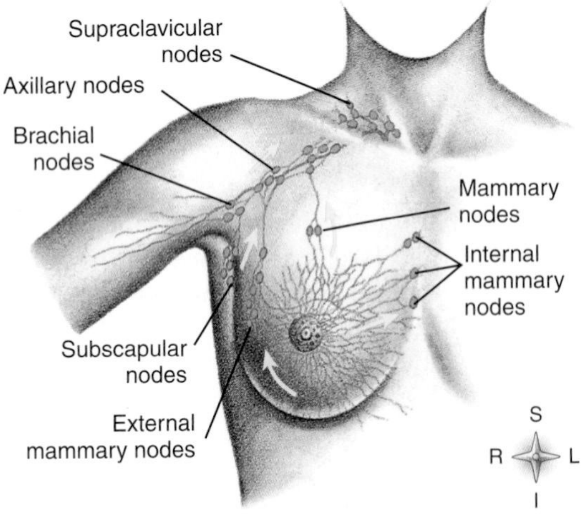

Tonsils

Masses of lymphoid tissue called tonsils are located in a protective ring under the mucous membranes in the mouth and back of the throat (Figure 13-6). They help protect against bacteria that may invade tissues in the area around the openings between the nasal and oral cavities. The **palatine tonsils** are located on each side of the throat. The **pharyngeal tonsils,** known as **adenoids** (AD-e-noyds) when they become swollen, are near the posterior opening of the nasal cavity. A third type of tonsil, the **lingual tonsils,** is near the base of the tongue. The tonsils serve as the first line of defense from the exterior and as such are subject to chronic infection. In rare cases, they may be removed surgically if antibiotic therapy is not successful or if swelling impairs breathing.

FIGURE 13-6

Location of the tonsils. Small segments of the roof and floor of the mouth have been removed to show the protective ring of tonsils (lymphoid tissue) around the internal opening of the nose and throat.

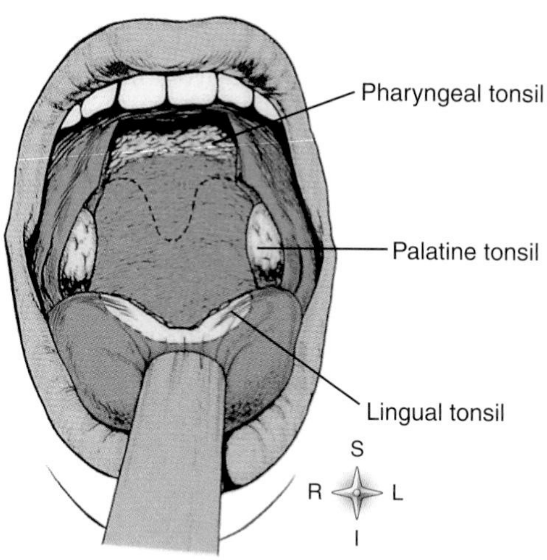

Clinical Application

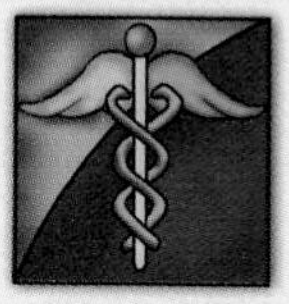

Allergy

The term **allergy** is used to describe hypersensitivity of the immune system to relatively harmless environmental antigens. One in six Americans has a genetic predisposition to an allergy. Immediate allergic responses involve antigen-antibody reactions that trigger the release of histamine, kinins, and other inflammatory substances. These responses usually cause symptoms such as a runny nose, conjunctivitis, and hives. In some cases, these substances may cause constriction of airways, relaxation of blood vessels, and irregular heart rhythms that can lead to a life-threatening condition called *anaphylactic shock*. Delayed allergic responses, on the other hand, involve cell-mediated immunity. In contact dermatitis, for example, T-lymphocytes trigger events that lead to local skin inflammation a few hours or days after initial exposure.

Spleen

The spleen is the largest lymphoid organ in the body. It is located high in the upper left quadrant of the abdomen lateral to the stomach (see Figures 13-1 and 1-7). Although the spleen is protected by the lower ribs, it can be injured by abdominal trauma. The spleen has a very rich blood supply and may contain more than 500 ml (about 1 pint) of blood. If the spleen is damaged and bleeding, surgical removal, called a **splenectomy** (splen-NEK-toe-mee), may be required to stop the loss of blood.

After entering the spleen, blood flows through dense, pulplike accumulations of lymphocytes. As blood flows through the pulp, the spleen removes by filtration and phagocytosis many bacteria and other foreign substances, destroys worn out RBCs and salvages the iron found in hemoglobin for future use, and serves as a reservoir for blood that can be returned to the circulatory system when needed.

Quick

1. How does the lymphatic system return fluid to the blood?
2. What is the role of lymph nodes in the body?
3. Why is the thymus important for immunity?

THE IMMUNE SYSTEM

Function of the Immune System

The body's defense mechanisms protect us from disease-causing microorganisms that invade our bodies, foreign tissue cells that may have been transplanted into our bodies, and our own cells that have turned malignant or cancerous. The body's specific defense system is called the **immune system.** The immune system makes us immune (that is, able to resist these enemies). Unlike other systems of the body, which are made up of groups of organs, the immune sys-

FIGURE 13-7

Inflammatory response. In this example, bacterial infection triggers a set of responses that tend to inhibit or destroy the bacteria.

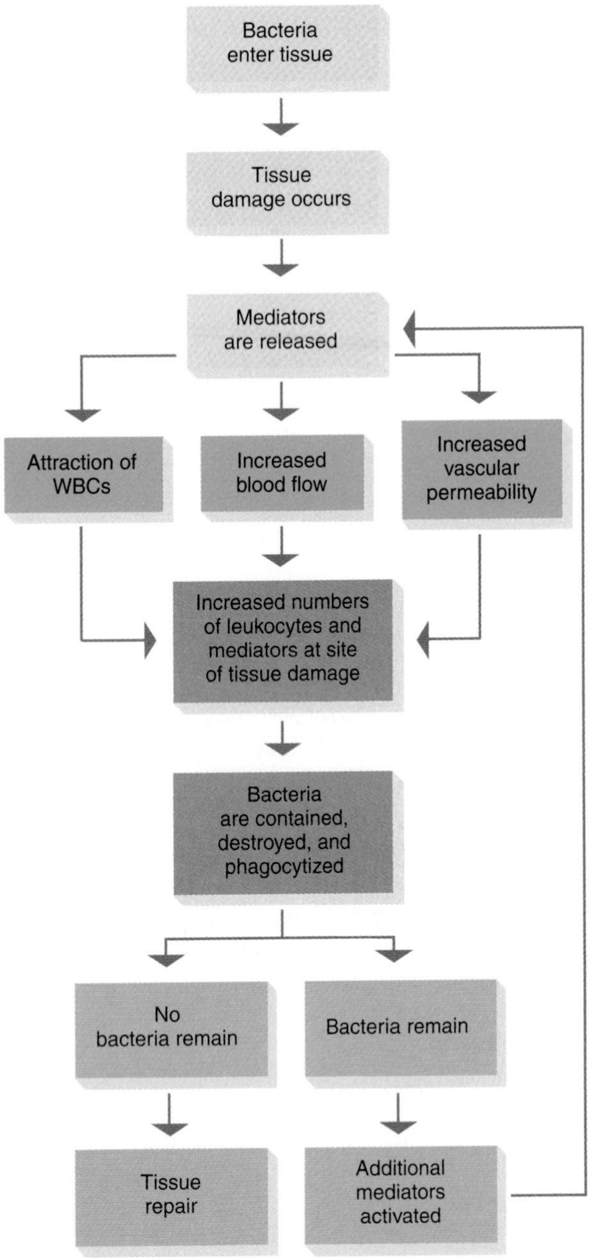

tem is made up of billions of cells and trillions of molecules.

Nonspecific Immunity

Nonspecific immunity is maintained by mechanisms that attack any irritant or abnormal substance that threatens the internal environment. In other words, nonspecific immunity confers general protection rather than protection from certain kinds of invading cells or chemicals. The skin and mucous membranes, for example, are mechanical barriers to prevent entry into the body by bacteria and many other substances such as toxins and harmful chemicals. Tears and mucus also contribute to nonspecific immunity. Tears wash harmful substances from the eyes, and mucus traps foreign material that may enter the respiratory tract. Phagocytosis of bacteria by WBCs is a nonspecific form of immunity.

The **inflammatory response** is a set of nonspecific responses that often occurs in the body. In the example shown in Figure 13-7, bacteria cause tissue damage that, in turn, triggers the release of mediators from any of a variety of immune cells. Some of the mediators attract WBCs to the area. Many of these factors produce the characteristic signs of inflammation: heat, redness, pain, and swelling. These signs are caused by increased blood flow (resulting in heat and redness) and vascular permeability (resulting in tissue swelling and the pain it causes) in the affected region. Such changes help phagocytic WBCs reach the general area and enter the affected tissue.

Specific Immunity

Specific immunity includes protective mechanisms that confer very specific protection against certain types of invading bacteria or other toxic materials. Specific immunity involves memory and the ability to recognize and respond to certain particular harmful substances or bacteria. For example, when the body is first attacked by particular bacteria or viruses, disease symptoms may occur as the body fights to destroy the invading

TABLE 13-1

Specific Immunity

TYPE	EXAMPLE
Inborn immunity	Immunity to certain diseases (for example, canine distemper) is inherited.
Acquired immunity	
Natural immunity	Exposure to the causative agent is not deliberate.
Active (exposure)	A child develops measles and acquires an immunity to a subsequent infection.
Passive (exposure)	A fetus receives protection from the mother through the placenta, or an infant receives protection via the mother's milk.
Artificial immunity	Exposure to the causative agent is deliberate
Active (exposure)	Injection of the causative agent, such as a vaccination against polio, confers immunity
Passive (exposure)	Injection of protective material (antibodies) that was developed by another individual's immune system is given

organism. However, if the body is exposed a second time, no symptoms occur because the organism is destroyed quickly—the person is said to be **immune.** Immunity to one type of disease-causing bacteria or virus does not protect the body against others. Immunity can be very selective.

Immunity to disease is classified as **inherited** or acquired. If inherited, it is described as **inborn immunity** (Table 13-1). Humans are immune from birth to certain diseases that affect other animals. Distemper, for example, is an often fatal viral disease in dogs. The virus does not produce symptoms in humans; we have an inborn or inherited immunity to the disease.

Acquired immunity may be further classified as "natural" or "artificial" depending on how the body is exposed to the harmful agent. Natural exposure is not deliberate and occurs in the course of everyday living. We are naturally exposed to many disease-causing agents on a regular basis. Artificial exposure is called *immunization* and is the deliberate exposure of the body to a potentially harmful agent.

Natural and artificial immunity may be "active" or "passive." Active immunity occurs when an individual's own immune system responds to a harmful agent, regardless of whether that agent was naturally or artificially encountered. Passive immunity results when immunity to a disease that has developed in another individual or animal is transferred to an individual who was not previously immune. For example, antibodies in a mother's milk confer passive immunity to her nursing infant. Active immunity generally lasts longer than passive immunity. Passive immunity, although temporary, provides immediate protection. Table 13-1 lists the various forms of specific immunity and gives examples of each.

Quick

1. What is the difference between *specific immunity* and *nonspecific immunity*?
2. Can you outline the changes that occur in the body's inflammatory response?

IMMUNE SYSTEM MOLECULES

The immune system functions because of adequate amounts of highly specialized protein molecules and unique cells. The protein molecules critical to immune system functioning are called **antibodies** (AN-ti-bod-ees) and **complements** (KOM-ple-ments).

Antibodies

Definition

Antibodies are protein compounds that are normally present in the body. A defining characteristic of an antibody molecule is the uniquely shaped concave regions called *combining sites* on its surface. Another defining characteristic is the ability of an antibody molecule to combine with a specific compound called an **antigen** (AN-ti-jen). All antigens are compounds whose molecules have small regions on their surfaces that are uniquely shaped to fit into the combining sites of a specific antibody molecule as precisely as a key fits into a specific lock. Antigens may be foreign proteins, most often the molecules in the surface membranes of invading or diseased cells such as microorganisms or cancer cells.

Functions

In general, antibodies produce **humoral** or **antibody-mediated immunity** by changing the antigens so that they cannot harm the body (Figure 13-8). To do this, an antibody must first bind to its specific antigen. This forms an antigen-antibody complex. The antigen-antibody complex then acts in one or more ways to make the antigen, or the cell on which it is present, harmless. For example, if the antigen is a toxin, a substance poisonous to body cells, the toxin is neutralized or made nonpoisonous by becoming part of an antigen-antibody complex. Or if antigens are molecules in the surface membranes of invading cells, when antibodies combine with them, the resulting antigen-antibody complexes may agglutinate the enemy cells (that is, make them stick together in clumps). Then macrophages or the other phagocytes can rapidly destroy them by ingesting and digesting large numbers of them at one time.

Another important function of antibodies is promotion and enhancement of phagocytosis. Certain antibody fractions help promote the attachment of phagocytic cells to the object they will engulf. As a result, the contact between the phagocytic cell and its victim is enhanced, and the object is more easily ingested. This process contributes to the efficiency of immune system phagocytic cells, which is described on p. 346.

Probably the most important way in which antibodies act is one we will consider last. It is a process called **complement fixation.** Often when antigens that are molecules on an antigenic or foreign cell's surface combine with antibody molecules, they change the shape of the antibody molecule slightly but just enough to expose two previously hidden regions. These are called **complement-binding sites.** Their exposure initiates a series of events that kill the cell on whose surface they take place. The next section describes these events.

Complement Proteins

Complement is the name used to describe a group of at least 14 proteins normally present in an inactive state in blood. These proteins are activated by exposure of complement-binding sites on antibodies. The result is formation of highly specialized antigen-antibody complexes that target foreign cells for destruction. The process is a rapid-fire cascade or sequence of events collectively called *complement fixation.* In this process a doughnut-shaped assemblage (complete with a hole in the middle) is formed when antibodies, antigens in the invading cell's plasma membrane, and complement molecules combine.

Complement fixation kills invading cells of various types. How? In effect, by drilling a hole in their plasma membranes! The tiny holes allow sodium to rapidly diffuse into the cell; then water follows through osmosis. The cell literally bursts as the internal osmotic pressure increases (Figure 13-9).

Quick Check

1. What are antibodies? How do they work?
2. What are complements? How do they work?

FIGURE 13-8

Antibody function. Antibodies produce humoral immunity by binding to specific antigens to form antigen-antibody complexes. These complexes produce a variety of changes that inactivate or kill invading cells.

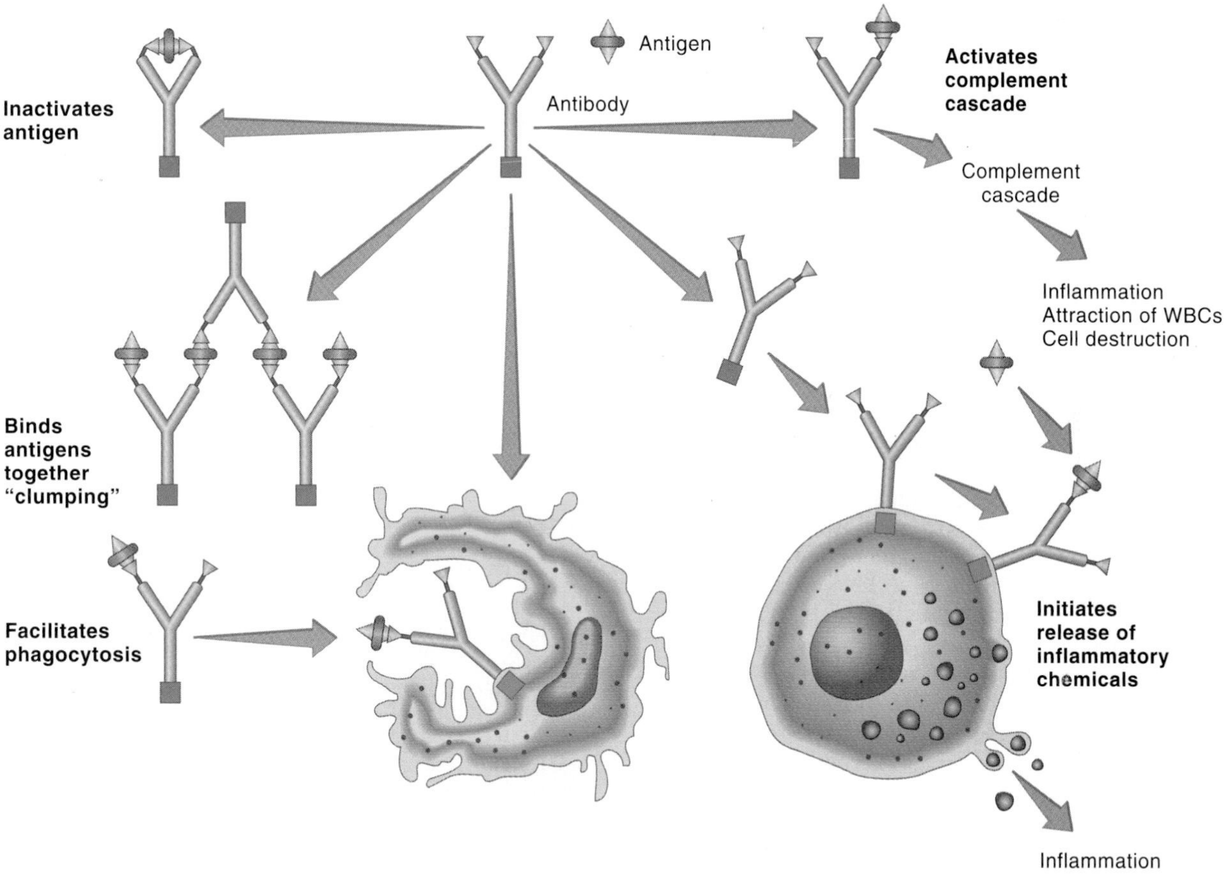

FIGURE 13-9

Complement fixation. A, Complement molecules activated by antibodies form doughnut-shaped complexes in a bacterium's plasma membrane. **B,** Holes in the complement complex allow sodium (Na^+) and then water (H_2O) to diffuse into the bacterium. **C,** After enough water has entered, the swollen bacterium bursts.

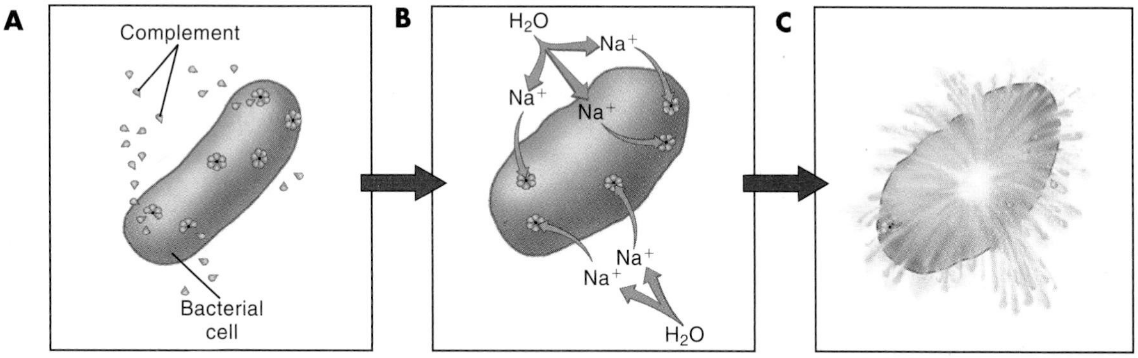

Research, Issues & Trends

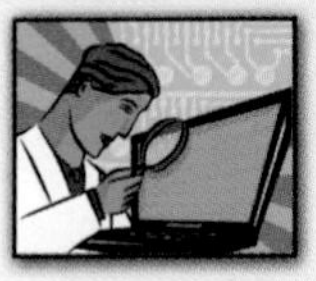

Monoclonal Antibodies

Techniques that have permitted biologists to produce large quantities of pure and very specific antibodies have resulted in dramatic advances in medicine. As a new medical technology, the development of **monoclonal antibodies** has been compared in importance with advances in recombinant DNA or genetic engineering.

Monoclonal antibodies are specific antibodies produced or derived from a population or culture of identical, or **monoclonal,** cells. In the past, antibodies produced by the immune system against a specific antigen had to be "harvested" from serum containing literally hundreds of other antibodies. The total amount of a specific antibody that could be recovered was very limited, so the cost of recovery was high. Monoclonal antibody techniques are based on the ability of immune system cells to produce individual antibodies that bind to and react with very specific antigens. We know, for example, that if the body is exposed to the varicella virus of chickenpox, WBCs will produce an antibody that will react very specifically with that virus and no other.

With monoclonal antibody techniques, lymphocytes that are produced by the body after the injection of a specific antigen are "harvested" and then "fused" with other cells that have been transformed to grow and divide indefinitely in a tissue culture medium. These fused or hybrid cells, called *hybridomas* (HYE-brid-o-mahs) continue to produce the same antibody produced by the original lymphocyte. The result is a rapidly growing population of identical or monoclonal cells that produce large quantities of a very specific antibody. Monoclonal antibodies have now been produced against a wide array of different antigens, including disease-producing organisms and various types of cancer cells.

The availability of very pure antibodies against specific disease-producing agents is the first step in the commercial preparation of diagnostic tests that can be used to identify viruses, bacteria, and even specific cancer cells in the blood or other body fluids. The use of monoclonal antibodies may serve as the basis for specific treatment of many human diseases.

Monoclonal antibodies are also used in over-the-counter early pregnancy test kits. The antibodies in such kits bind to the hormone *human chorionic gonadotropin* (hCG) found in the urine of women in the early stages of pregnancy. When the antibodies in the kit bind to hCG molecules, they trigger a chemical reaction that produces a color change.

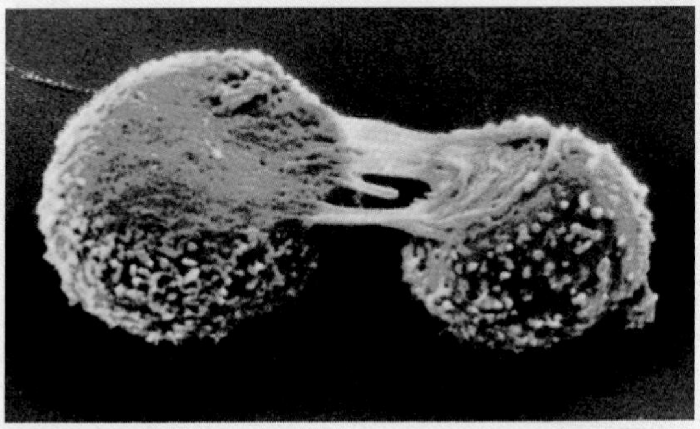

IMMUNE SYSTEM CELLS

The primary cells of the immune system include:

1. Phagocytes
   a. Neutrophils
   b. Monocytes
   c. Macrophages
2. Lymphocytes
   a. T-lymphocytes
   b. B-lymphocytes

Phagocytes

Phagocytic WBCs are an important part of the immune system. In Chapter 11, phagocytes were described as cells derived from the bone marrow that carry on phagocytosis or ingestion and digestion of foreign cells or particles. The most important phagocytes are neutrophils and monocytes (see Figure 11-4, p. 287). These blood phagocytes migrate out of the blood and into the tissues in response to an infection. The neutrophils are functional but short lived in the tissues. Once in the tissues, monocytes develop into phagocytic cells called **macrophages** (MAK-ro-fay-jes). Some macrophages "wander" through the tissues to engulf bacteria wherever they find them. Other macrophages become permanent residents of other organs. Macrophages found in spaces between liver cells, for example, are called *Kupffer's cells*, whereas those that ingest particulate matter in the small air sacs of the lungs are

FIGURE 13-10

Phagocytosis. This series of scanning electron micrographs shows the progressive steps in phagocytosis of damaged RBCs by a macrophage. **A,** RBCs *(R)* attach to the macrophage *(M)*. **B,** Plasma membrane of the macrophage begins to enclose the RBC. **C,** The RBCs are almost totally ingested by the macrophage.

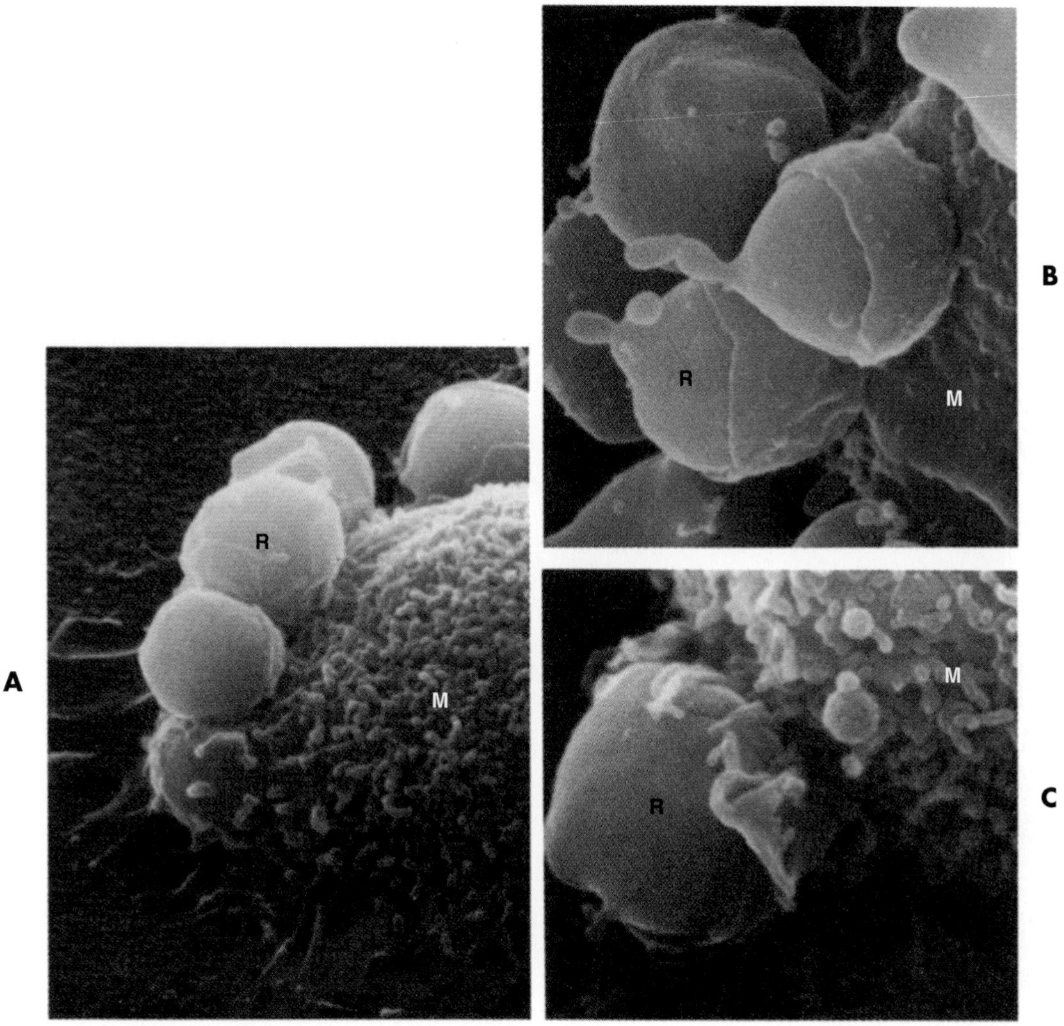

called *dust cells*. Macrophages can also be found in the spleen and lymph nodes and on the lining membranes of the abdominal and thoracic cavities. Specialized antibodies that bind to and coat certain foreign particles help macrophages function effectively. They serve as "flags" that alert the macrophage to the presence of foreign material, infectious bacteria, or cellular debris. They also help bind the phagocyte to the foreign material so that it can be engulfed more effectively (Figure 13-10).

Lymphocytes

The most numerous cells of the immune system are the lymphocytes; they are ultimately responsible for antibody production. Several million strong, lymphocytes continually patrol the body, searching out any enemy cells that may have entered. Lymphocytes circulate in the body's fluids. Huge numbers of them wander vigilantly through most of its tissues. Lymphocytes densely populate the body's widely scattered lymph nodes and its other lymphatic tissues, especially the thymus gland in the chest and the spleen and liver in the abdomen. There are two major types of lymphocytes, designated as *B-* and *T-lymphocytes* but usually called *B cells* and *T cells*.

Development of B Cells

All lymphocytes that circulate in the tissues arise from primitive cells in the bone marrow called *stem cells* and go through two stages of development. The first stage of B-cell development—transformation of stem cells into immature B cells—occurs in the liver and bone marrow before birth but only in the bone marrow in adults. Because this process was first discovered in a bird organ called the *bursa*, these cells were named B cells.

Immature B cells are small lymphocytes that have synthesized and inserted into their cytoplasmic membranes numerous molecules of one specific kind of antibody (Figure 13-11). These antibody-bearing immature B cells leave the tissue where they were formed, enter the blood, and are transported to their new place of residence, chiefly the lymph nodes. There they act as seed cells. Each immature B cell undergoes repeated mitosis (cell division) and forms a clone of immature B cells. A **clone** is a family of many identical cells all descended from one cell. Because all the cells in a clone of immature B cells have descended from one immature B cell, all of them bear the same surface antibody molecules as their single ancestor cell.

The second stage of B-cell development changes an immature B cell into an activated B cell. Not all immature B cells undergo this change. They do so only if an immature B cell comes in contact with certain protein molecules—antigens—whose shape fits the shape of the immature B cell's surface antibody molecules. If this happens, the antigens lock onto the antibodies and by so doing change the immature B cell into an activated B cell. Then the activated B cell, by dividing rapidly and repeatedly, develops into clones of two kinds of cells: **plasma cells** and **memory cells** (see Figure 13-11). Plasma cells secrete copious amounts of antibody into the blood—reportedly, 2000 antibody molecules per second by each plasma cell for every second of the few days that it lives. Antibodies circulating in the blood constitute an enormous, mobile, ever-on-duty army.

Memory cells can secrete antibodies but do not immediately do so. They remain in reserve in the lymph nodes until they are contracted by the same antigen that led to their formation. Then, very quickly, the memory cells develop into plasma cells and secrete large amounts of antibody. Memory cells, in effect, seem to remember their ancestor-activated B cell's encounter with its appropriate antigen. They stand ready, at a moment's notice, to produce antibody that will combine with this antigen.

Function of B Cells

B cells function indirectly to produce humoral immunity. Recall that humoral immunity is resistance to disease organisms produced by the

Clinical Application

Interferon

Interferon (in-ter-FEER-on) is a small protein compound that plays a very significant role in producing immunity from viral infections. It is produced by T cells within hours after they have been infected by a virus. The interferon released from the T cells protects other cells by interfering with the ability of the virus to reproduce as it moves from cell to cell. In the past, thousands of pints of blood had to be processed to harvest tiny quantities of leukocyte (T cell) interferon for study. Synthetic human interferon is now being "manufactured" in bacteria as a result of gene-splicing techniques and is available in quantities sufficient for clinical use. Synthetic interferon decreases the severity of many virus-related diseases including chickenpox, measles, and hepatitis C. Interferon also shows promise as an anticancer agent. It has been shown to be effective in treating breast, skin, and other forms of cancer.

FIGURE 13-11

B-cell development. B-cell development takes place in two stages. First stage: Shortly before and after birth, stem cells develop into immature B cells. Second stage (occurs only if the immature B-cell contacts its specific antigen): Immature B cell develops into activated B cell, which divides rapidly and repeatedly to form a clone of plasma cells and a clone of memory cells. Plasma cells secrete antibodies capable of combining with specific antigen that caused immature B cell to develop into active B cell. Stem cells maintain a constant population of newly differentiating cells.

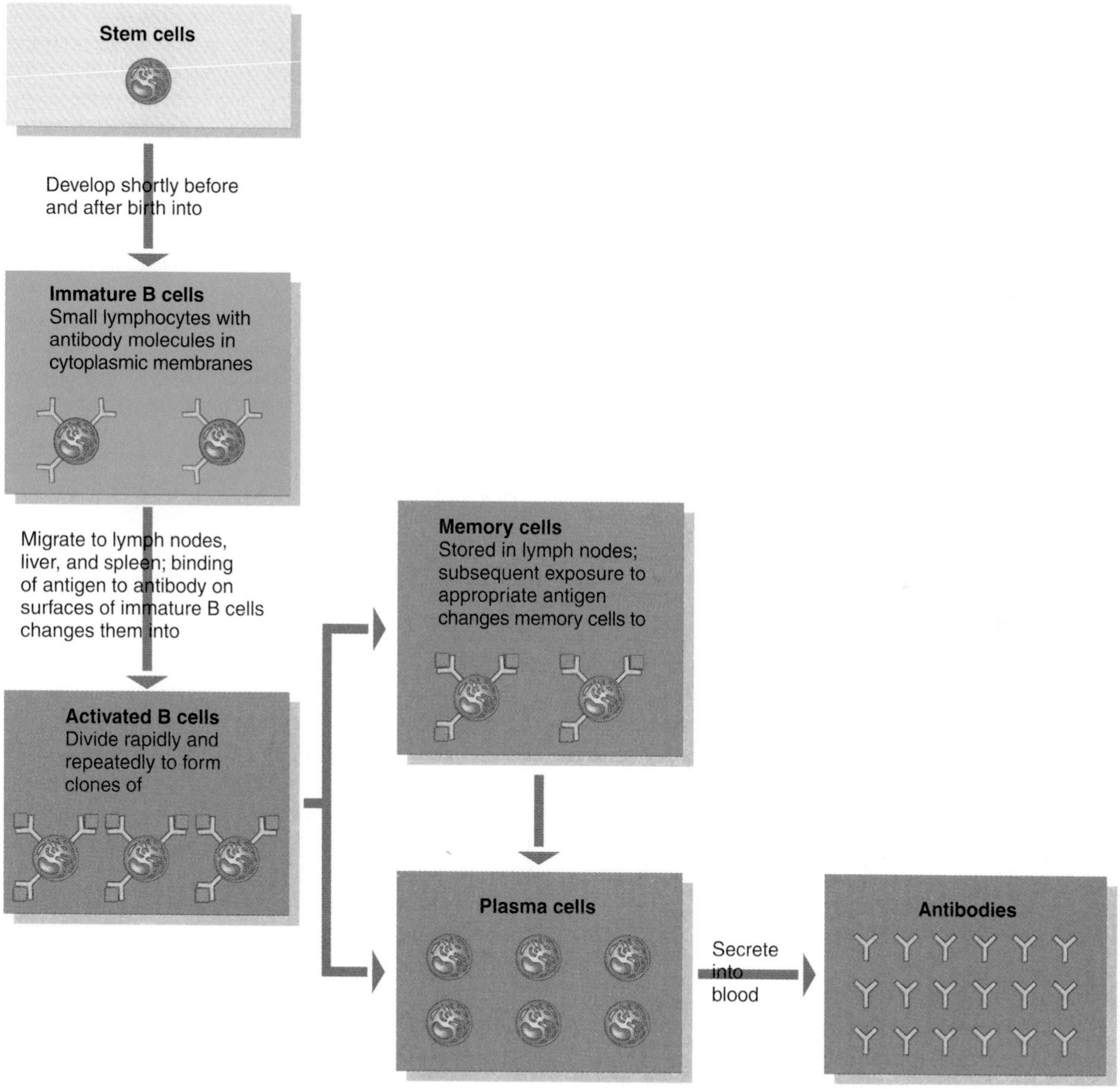

Clinical Application

AIDS

AIDS, or **acquired immunodeficiency syndrome** was first recognized as a new disease by the Centers for Disease Control and Prevention (CDC) in 1981. This syndrome (collection of symptoms) is caused by the human immunodeficiency virus, or HIV. HIV, a retrovirus, contains RNA that undergoes reverse transcription inside infected cells to form its own DNA. The viral DNA often becomes part of the cell's DNA. When the viral DNA is activated, it directs the synthesis of its own RNA and protein coat, thus "stealing" raw materials from the cell. When this occurs in certain T cells, the cell is destroyed, and immunity is impaired. As the T cell dies, it releases new retroviruses that can spread the HIV infection.

Although HIV can invade several types of cells, it has its most obvious effects in a certain type of T cell called a $CD4^+$ T cell. When T cell function is impaired, infectious organisms and cancer cells can grow and spread much more easily than normal. Unusual conditions, such as pneumocystosis (a protozoan infection) and Kaposi sarcoma (a type of skin cancer), may also appear. Because their immune systems are deficient, AIDS patients usually die from one of these infections or cancers.

After infection with HIV, a person may not show signs of AIDS for months or years. This is because the immune system can hold the infection at bay for a long time before finally succumbing to it.

There are several strategies for controlling AIDS. Many agencies are trying to slow the spread of AIDS by educating people about how to avoid contact with the HIV retrovirus. HIV is spread by means of direct contact of body fluids, so preventing such contact reduces HIV transmission. Sexual relations, contaminated blood transfusions, and intravenous use of contaminated needles are the usual modes of HIV transmission. Several teams of researchers are working on HIV vaccines. Like many viruses, such as those that cause the common cold, HIV changes rapidly enough to make development of a vaccine difficult at best.

Another way to inhibit the disease is by means of chemicals such as azidothymidine (AZT) and ritonavir (Norvir) that block HIV's ability to reproduce within infected cells. A breakthrough in the treatment of HIV came a few years ago when it was discovered that a "cocktail" of several antiviral drugs working together greatly reduce the number of virus particles in a patient's blood. More than 100 such compounds in various combinations are being evaluated for use in halting the progress of HIV infections.

actions of antibodies binding to specific antigens while circulating in body fluids. Activated B cells develop into plasma cells. Plasma cells secrete antibodies into the blood; they are the "antibody factories" of the body. These antibodies, like other proteins manufactured for extracellular use, are formed on the endoplasmic reticulum of the cell.

Development of T Cells

T cells are lymphocytes that have undergone their first stage of development in the thymus gland. Stem cells from the bone marrow seed the thymus, and shortly before and after birth, they develop into T cells. The newly formed T cells stream out of the thymus into the blood and migrate chiefly to the lymph nodes, where they take up residence. Embedded in each T cell's cytoplasmic membrane are protein molecules shaped so that they can fit only one specific kind of antigen molecule. The second stage of T-cell development takes place when and if a T cell comes into contact with its specific antigen. If this happens, the antigen binds to the protein on the T cell's surface, thereby changing the T cell into a sensitized T cell (Figure 13-12).

Functions of T Cells

Sensitized T cells produce cell-mediated immunity. As the name suggests, **cell-mediated immunity** is resistance to disease organisms resulting from the actions of cells—chiefly sensitized T cells. Some sensitized T cells kill invading cells directly (Figure 13-13). When bound to antigens on an in-

FIGURE 13-12

T cell development. The first stage takes place in the thymus gland shortly before and after birth. Stem cells maintain a constant population of newly differentiating cells as they are needed. The second stage occurs only if a T cell contacts antigen, which combines with certain proteins on the T cell's surface.

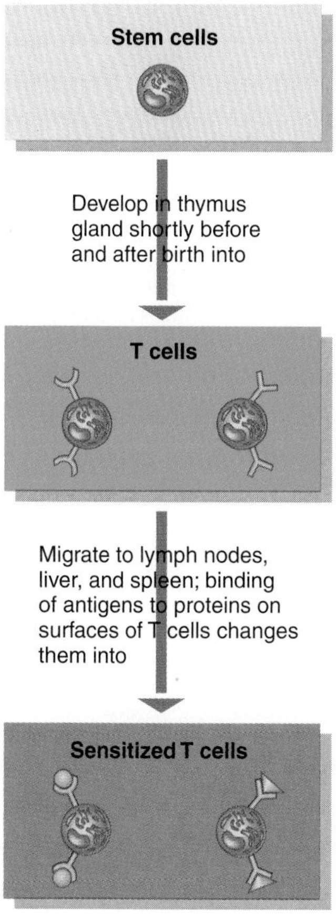
Stem cells
Develop in thymus gland shortly before and after birth into
T cells
Migrate to lymph nodes, liver, and spleen; binding of antigens to proteins on surfaces of T cells changes them into
Sensitized T cells

FIGURE 13-13

T cells. The blue spheres seen in this scanning electron microscope view are T cells attacking a much larger cancer cell. The cells are a significant part of our defense against cancer and other types of foreign cells.

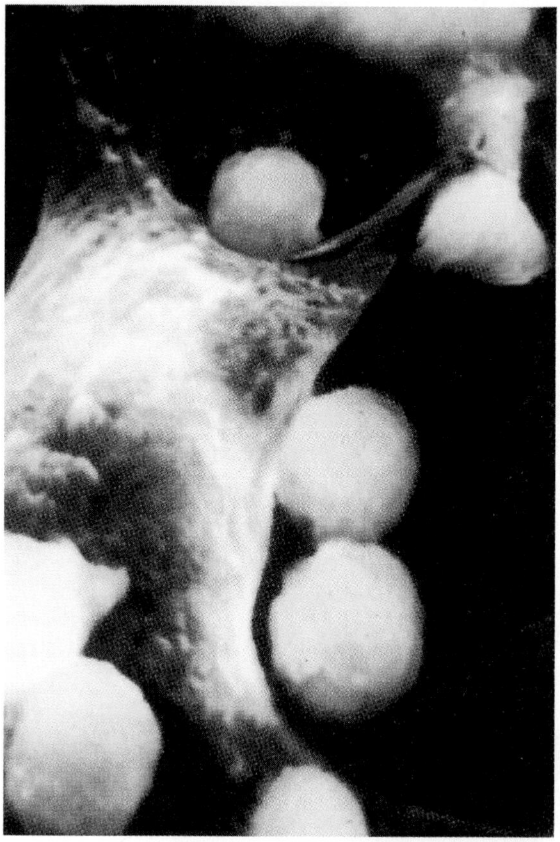

vading cell's surface, they release a substance that acts as a specific and lethal poison against the bound cell. Many sensitized cells produce their deadly effects indirectly by means of compounds that they release into the area around enemy cells. Among these is a substance that attracts macrophages into the neighborhood of the enemy cells. The assembled macrophages then destroy the cells by phagocytosing (ingesting and digesting) them (Figure 13-14).

Quick Check

1. What are phagocytes? How do they work?
2. What is the role of B cells in immunity?
3. What is the role of T cells in immunity?
4. What are memory cells?

FIGURE 13-14

T-cell function. Sensitized T cells produce cell-mediated immunity by releasing various compounds in the vicinity of invading cells. Some act directly, and some act indirectly to kill invading cells.

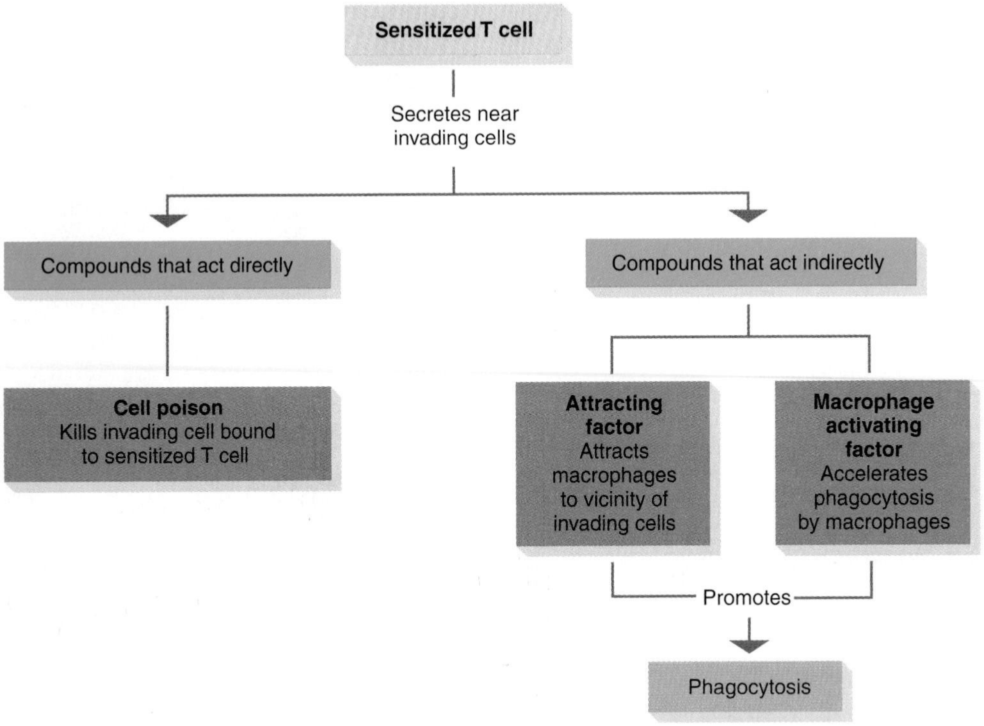

Science Applications

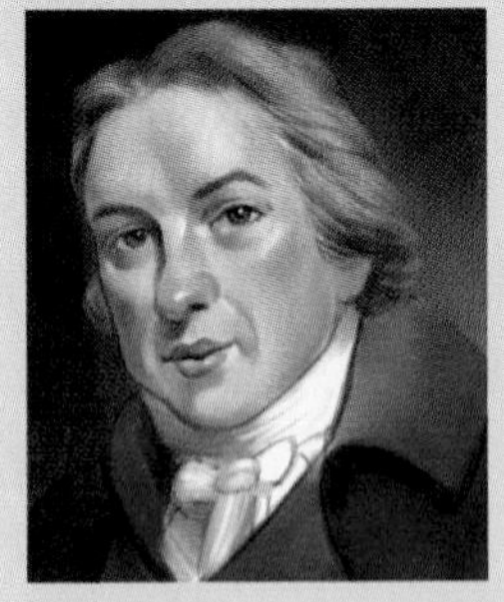

Edward Jenner (1749-1823).

English surgeon Edward Jenner changed the world forever in 1789 when he inoculated his young son and two others against the terrible viral disease, smallpox. Using material from the blisters of a patient with the milder disease swinepox, he was able to trigger immunity to smallpox—the world's first vaccination. Later, in 1796, he found that vaccination with material from cowpox blisters worked even better in protecting people from smallpox. A disease that had formerly killed millions upon millions of people worldwide eventually disappeared from the human population in the 20th century because of Jenner's pioneering efforts.

In this century, interest in smallpox vaccinations has resurfaced because of the threat of smallpox as a weapon. As immunologists work on improving this important vaccine to protect against such weapons, they continue to work on vaccines for other infectious diseases such as AIDS and even disorders such as heart disease and cancer. Many health care professionals use vaccines in their practice, of course, to boost the immune systems of their clients. Many physicians also treat disorders of the immune system itself. For example, immune deficiencies such as AIDS, allergies such as "hay fever" and autoimmune disorders such as lupus and rheumatoid arthritis, are treated every day by physicians and other health professionals.

OUTLINE SUMMARY

THE LYMPHATIC SYSTEM (FIGURE 13-1)

A. Lymph—fluid in the tissue spaces that carries protein molecules and other substances back to the blood
B. Lymphatic vessels—permit only one-way movement of lymph
   1. Lymphatic capillaries—tiny blind-ended tubes distributed in tissue spaces (Figure 13-2)
      a. Microscopic in size
      b. Sheets consisting of one cell layer of simple squamous epithelium
      c. Poor "fit" between adjacent cells results in porous walls
      d. Called *lacteals* in the intestinal wall (for fat transportation)
   2. Right lymphatic duct
      a. Drains lymph from the right upper extremity and right side of head, neck, and upper torso
   3. Thoracic duct
      a. Largest lymphatic vessel
      b. Has an enlarged pouch along its course, called *cisterna chyli*
      c. Drains lymph from about three fourths of the body (Figure 13-3)
C. Lymph nodes
   1. Filter lymph (Figure 13-3)
   2. Located in clusters along the pathway of lymphatic vessels (Figures 13-1, 13-4, and 13-5)
   3. Functions include defense and WBC formation
   4. Flow of lymph: to node via several afferent lymph vessels and drained from node by a single efferent lymph vessel
D. Thymus
   1. Lymphoid tissue organ located in mediastinum
   2. Total weight of 35 to 40 g—a little more than an ounce
   3. Plays a vital and central role in immunity
   4. Produces T-lymphocytes or T cells
   5. Secretes hormones called *thymosins*
   6. Lymphoid tissue is largely replaced by fat in the process called *involution*
E. Tonsils (Figure 13-6)
   1. Composed of three masses of lymphoid tissue around the openings of the mouth and throat
      a. Palatine tonsils ("the tonsils")
      b. Pharyngeal tonsils (adenoids)
      c. Lingual tonsils
   2. Subject to chronic infection
   3. Enlargement of pharyngeal tonsils may impair breathing
F. Spleen
   1. Largest lymphoid organ in body
   2. Located in upper left quadrant of abdomen
   3. Often injured by trauma to abdomen
   4. Surgical removal called *splenectomy*
   5. Functions include phagocytosis of bacteria and old RBCs; acts as a blood reservoir

THE IMMUNE SYSTEM (TABLE 13-1)

A. Protects body from pathological bacteria, foreign tissue cells, and cancerous cells
B. Made up of specialized cells and molecules
C. Nonspecific immunity
   1. Skin—mechanical barrier to bacteria and other harmful agents
   2. Tears and mucus—wash eyes and trap and kill bacteria
   3. Inflammation—attracts immune cells to site of injury, increases local blood flow, increases vascular permeability; promotes movement of WBCs to site of injury or infection (Figure 13-7)
D. Specific immunity—ability of body to recognize, respond to, and remember harmful substances or bacteria
E. Inherited or inborn immunity—inherited immunity to certain diseases from birth

Continued

OUTLINE SUMMARY—*cont'd*

F. Acquired immunity
  1. Natural immunity—exposure to causative agent is not deliberate
     a. Active—active disease produces immunity
     b. Passive—immunity passes from mother to fetus through placenta or from mother to child through mother's milk
  2. Artificial immunity—exposure to causative agent is deliberate
     a. Active—vaccination results in immunity
     b. Passive—protective material developed in another individual's immune system and given to previously nonimmune individual

IMMUNE SYSTEM MOLECULES

A. Antibodies
  1. Protein compounds with specific combining sites
  2. Combining sites attach antibodies to specific antigens (foreign proteins), forming an antigen-antibody complex—called *humoral* or *antibody-mediated immunity* (Figure 13-8)
  3. Antigen-antibody complexes may:
     a. Neutralize toxins
     b. Clump or agglutinate enemy cells
     c. Promote phagocytosis

B. Complement proteins
  1. Group of at least 14 proteins normally present in blood in inactive state
  2. Complement fixation
     a. Important mechanism of action for antibodies
     b. Causes cell lysis by permitting entry of water through a defect created in the plasma membrane (Figure 13-9)

IMMUNE SYSTEM CELLS

A. Phagocytes—ingest and destroy foreign cells or other harmful substances via phagocytosis (Figure 13-10)
  1. Types
     a. Neutrophils
     b. Monocytes
     c. Macrophages (Figure 13-10)
        (1) Kupffer cells (liver)
        (2) Dust cells (lung)

B. Lymphocytes
  1. Most numerous of immune system cells
  2. Development of B cells—primitive stem cells migrate from bone marrow and go through two stages of development (Figure 13-11)
     a. First stage—stem cells develop into immature B cells; takes place in the liver and bone marrow before birth and in the bone marrow only in adults; immature B cells are small lymphocytes with antibody molecules (which they have synthesized) in their plasma membranes; migrate chiefly to lymph nodes
     b. Second stage—immature B cell develops into activated B cell; initiated by immature B cell's contact with antigens, which bind to its surface antibodies; activated B cell, by dividing repeatedly, forms two clones of cells—plasma cells and memory cells—plasma cells secrete antibodies into blood; memory cells stored in lymph nodes; if subsequent exposure to antigen that activated B cell occurs, memory cells become plasma cells and secrete antibodies

OUTLINE SUMMARY—*cont'd*

3. Function of B cells—indirectly, B cells produce humoral immunity; activated B cells develop into plasma cells; plasma cells secrete antibodies into the blood; circulating antibodies produce humoral immunity (Figure 13-11)
4. Development of T cells—stem cells from bone marrow migrate to thymus gland (Figure 13-12)
   a. Stage 1—stem cells develop into T cells; occurs in thymus during few months before and after birth; T cells migrate chiefly to lymph nodes
   b. Stage 2—T cells develop into sensitized T cells; occurs when, and if, antigen binds to T cell's surface proteins
5. Functions of T cells—produce cell-mediated immunity; kill invading cells by releasing a substance that poisons cells and also by releasing chemicals that attract and activate macrophages to kill cells by phagocytosis (Figures 13-13 and 13-14)

NEW WORDS

afferent
AIDS
antibodies
antigen
B cells (lymphocytes)
cell-mediated immunity
clone
combining sites
complement
complement fixation
efferent
humoral immunity
inflammatory response
interferon
lymph
macrophage
memory cells
monoclonal antibodies
plasma cells
T cells (lymphocytes)

REVIEW QUESTIONS

1. Define *lymph* and explain its function.
2. Name the two lymphatic ducts and the areas of the body each of them drain.
3. Describe the structure of the lymph node.
4. Explain the defense function of the lymph node.
5. Where is the thymus gland? What are its functions?
6. Name the three pairs of tonsils and give the location of each.
7. Give the location and function of the spleen.
8. Explain the types of nonspecific immunity.
9. Name and differentiate between the four types of acquired immunity.
10. What are antibodies? What are antigens?

Continued

REVIEW QUESTIONS—*cont'd*

11. Explain the role of complement in the immune system.
12. Explain the role of macrophages in the immune system.
13. Explain the development and functioning of B cells.
14. Explain the development and functioning of T cells.

CRITICAL THINKING

15. Differentiate between lymphatic capillaries and blood capillaries. Explain how the differences in structure relate to their function.
16. Explain the role of lymph nodes in the possible spread of cancer.

CHAPTER TEST

1. Lymph is the fluid that leaves the blood capillaries and is not returned to the blood.
2. Lymph from about three fourths of the body drains into the Thoracic Duct.
3. Lymph from the right upper extremity and the right side of the head drains into the Right lymph duct
4. The enlarged, pouchlike structure in the abdomen that serves as a storage area for lymph is called the cisterna chyli
5. The function of the lymph nodes is to filter and clean the lymph.
6. The many lymph vessels that enter the lymph node are called the afferent vessels. The single vessel leaving the lymph node is called the efferent vessel.
7. The thymus gland is the site of maturation for these WBCs: T-cells. It also produces the hormone thymosis
8. The three pairs of tonsils are the palatine tonsils, the pharyngeal tonsils and the lingual tonsils.
9. The largest lymphoid organ is the spleen.
10. The signs inflammation of are heat, redness, pain, and swelling.
11. Complement fixation kills invading cells by drilling holes in their plasma membrane, which disrupts the sodium and water balance.
12. Macrophages were originally Monocytes that migrated into the tissues.
13. The immunity that develops against polio after receiving a polio vaccination is an example of:
    a. active natural immunity
    b. passive natural immunity
    c. active artificial immunity
    d. passive artificial immunity
14. The immunity that is given to the fetus or newborn by the immune system of the mother is an example of:
    a. active natural immunity
    b. passive natural immunity
    c. active artificial immunity
    d. passive artificial immunity
15. The immunity that comes from the injection of antibodies made by another individual's immune system is an example of:
    a. active natural immunity
    b. passive natural immunity
    c. active artificial immunity
    d. passive artificial immunity
16. The immunity that develops after a person has had a disease is an example of:
    a. active natural immunity
    b. passive natural immunity
    c. active artificial immunity
    d. passive natural immunity

CHAPTER TEST—*cont'd*

If the following statement describes the development or functioning of a B-cell, write a B in front of it. If it describes the development or functioning of a T-cell, write a T in front of it.

17. __B__ produces antibodies
18. __B__ some develop into plasma cells
19. __T__ the main cell involved in cell-mediated immunity
20. __B__ the main cell involved in humoral immunity
21. __T__ develops in the thymus gland
22. __T__ moves to the site of the antigen and releases cell poison
23. __B__ once this cell is activated, it divides rapidly into clones
24. __T__ releases a substance which attracts macrophages
25. __B__ some of these cells develop into memory cells

25/25

STUDY TIPS

Before starting Chapter 13, review the synopsis of the lymphatic system in Chapter 4.

The lymphatic system is the "sewer" system of the body. Plasma is pushed out of the capillaries and washes over the tissue cells. The fluid carries bacteria and cellular debris into the open-ended capillaries in the lymphatic system. The fluid is now called *lymph*. It is carried to the lymph node, where it is filtered, cleaned, and carried in the ducts back to the blood. Keep this process in mind when you study the structures of the lymphatic system. There are several specific organs in the lymphatic system. Flash cards with their names, locations, and functions will help you learn them.

The immune system is divided into nonspecific and specific immunity. Most of the nonspecific immunity is fairly simple; the most complex part is the inflammatory response, so study that well. Specific immunity can be classified as natural or artificial depending on how the body was exposed to the antigen, and active or passive depending on how much work the body had to do to develop the response. The natural, active immune response is divided into two parts also: humoral immunity and cell-mediated immunity. Humoral immunity is mediated by B-lymphocytes or B cells. They stay in the lymph node and secrete antibodies into the blood, a body humor. They also form memory cells for lifelong immunity. T-lymphocytes or T cells provide the cell-mediated immunity. They leave the lymph node and actively engage the antigen.

In your study groups, use flash cards to quiz each other on the terms and structures of the lymphatic and immune systems. Discuss the process of how lymph is formed, filtered, and returned to the blood. Discuss nonspecific immunity, especially the inflammatory response. Discuss what type of immunity getting a vaccination or coming down with the disease would be. Discuss the steps in humoral and cell-mediated immunity. Go over the questions in the back of the chapter and discuss possible test questions.

14 The Respiratory System

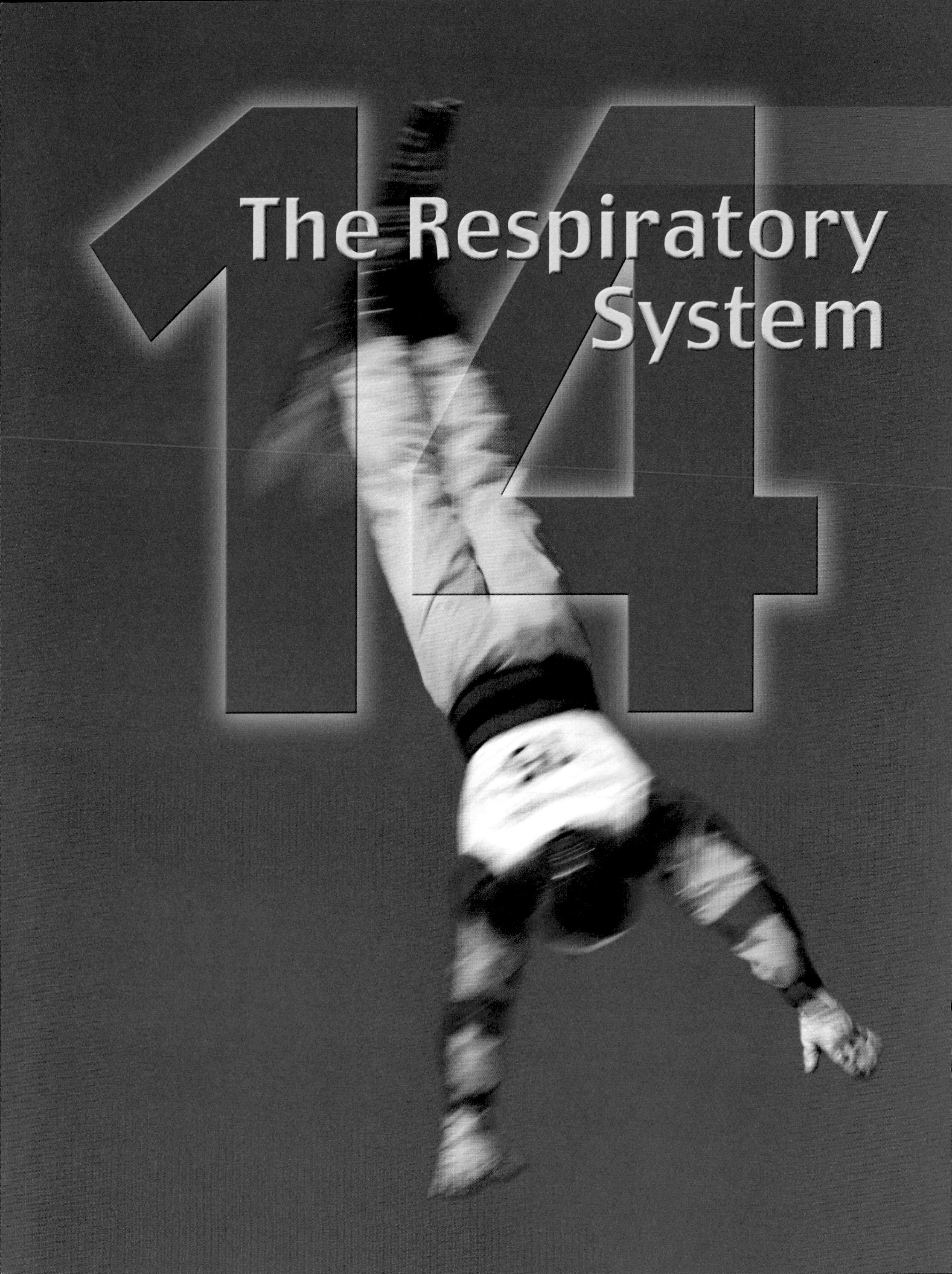

Outline

Objectives

AFTER YOU HAVE COMPLETED THIS CHAPTER, YOU SHOULD BE ABLE TO:

1. Discuss the generalized functions of the respiratory system.
2. List the major organs of the respiratory system and describe the function of each.
3. Compare, contrast, and explain the mechanism responsible for the exchange of gases that occurs during internal and external respiration.
4. List and discuss the volumes of air exchanged during pulmonary ventilation.
5. Identify and discuss the mechanisms that regulate respiration.

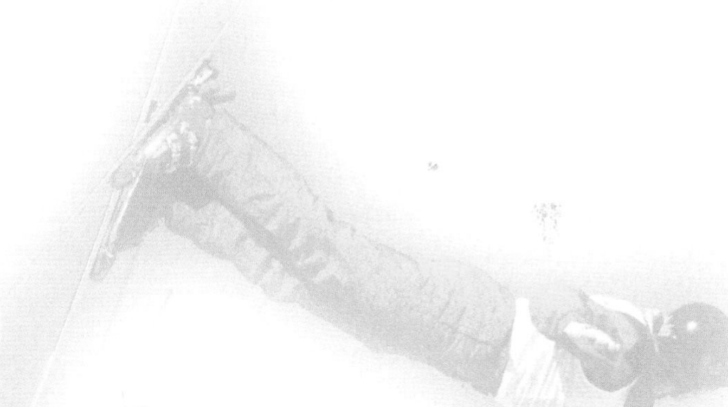

No one needs to be told how important the **respiratory system** is. The respiratory system serves the body much as a lifeline to an oxygen tank serves a deep-sea diver. Think how panicked you would feel if suddenly your lifeline became blocked—if you could not breathe for a few seconds! Of all the substances that cells and therefore the body as a whole must have to survive, oxygen is by far the most crucial. A person can live a few weeks without food, a few days without water, but only a few minutes without oxygen. Constant removal of carbon dioxide from the body is just as important for survival as a constant supply of oxygen.

The organs of the respiratory system are designed to perform two basic functions: they serve as an **air distributor** and as a **gas exchanger** for the body. The respiratory system ensures that oxygen is supplied to and carbon dioxide is removed from the body's cells. The process of respiration therefore is an important **homeostatic mechanism.** By constantly supplying adequate oxygen and by removing carbon dioxide as it forms, the respiratory system helps maintain a constant environment that enables our body cells to function effectively.

In addition to air distribution and gas exchange, the respiratory system effectively **filters, warms,** and **humidifies** the air we breathe. Respiratory

Clinical Application

Oxygen Therapy

Oxygen therapy is the administration of oxygen to individuals suffering from **hypoxia** (hi-POX-see-ah)—an insufficient oxygen supply to the tissues. Individuals with certain respiratory problems, such as emphysema, may require supplemental oxygen in order to maintain a normal lifestyle. Many of these patients respond well to home treatment with oxygen therapy—often under the supervision of a registered *respiratory therapist* or other health care provider.

Oxygen (O_2) in the form of compressed gas or in liquid form is commonly stored in and dispensed from small, green, metal cylinders or tanks that can be kept in the home or transported in small carts or backpacks for ambulatory use. Because the oxygen dispensed from such tanks is often cold and dry, it may need to be warmed and moistened, generally by bubbling the released gas through water, to prevent damage to the respiratory tract. Home treatment using *oxygen concentrators*, which are rather large and nonportable electrical devices that can both concentrate oxygen and eliminate other gases from room air, are also used in some situations. Regardless of source, supplemental oxygen is delivered to the patient through a mask or tubes that lead into the nasal passage (nasal prongs).

Supplemental (and generally very expensive) oxygen is now being dispensed for recreational purposes at trendy "oxygen bars." Delivery is at low flow levels and, although considered safe for healthy individuals, has more psychological than measurable physiological effects. Breathing supplemental oxygen after strenuous exercise is another nonmedical application of oxygen therapy. Although it may shorten recovery times for some athletes, it seldom provides more than transitory benefits.

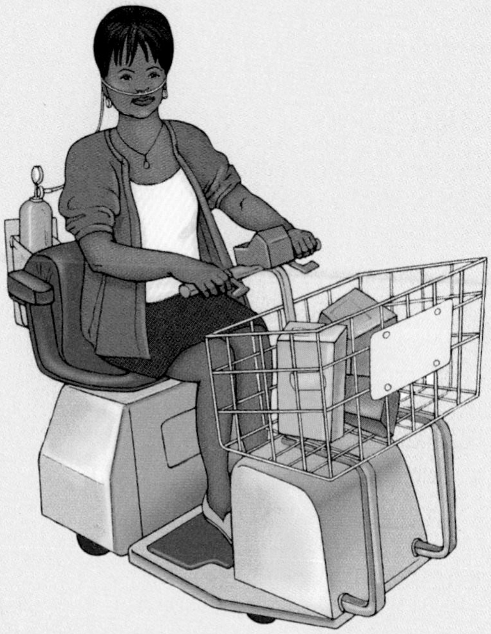

organs or organs closely associated with the respiratory system, such as the **sinuses,** also influence speech or sound production and make possible the sense of smell or **olfaction** (ol-FAK-shun). In this chapter, the structural plan of the respiratory system will be considered first, then the respiratory organs will be discussed individually, and finally some facts about gas exchange and the nervous system's control of respiration will be discussed.

STRUCTURAL PLAN

Respiratory organs include the **nose, pharynx** (FAIR-inks), **larynx** (LAIR-inks), **trachea** (TRAY-kee-ah), **bronchi** (BRONG-ki), and **lungs.** The basic structural design of this organ system is that of a tube with many branches ending in millions of extremely tiny, very thin-walled sacs called **alveoli** (al-VEE-o-li). Figure 14-1 shows the extensive branching of the "respiratory tree" in both lungs. Think of this air distribution system as an "upside-down tree." The trachea or windpipe then becomes the trunk and the bronchial tubes the branches. This idea will be developed when the types of bronchi and the alveoli are studied in more detail later in the chapter. A network of capillaries fits like a hairnet around each microscopic alveolus. Incidentally, this is a good place for us to think again about a principle already mentioned several times—namely, that structure and function are intimately related. The function of alveoli—in

FIGURE 14-1

Structural plan of the respiratory organs showing the pharynx, trachea, bronchi, and lungs. The inset shows the alveolar sacs where the interchange of oxygen and carbon dioxide takes place through the walls of the grapelike alveoli. Capillaries surround the alveoli.

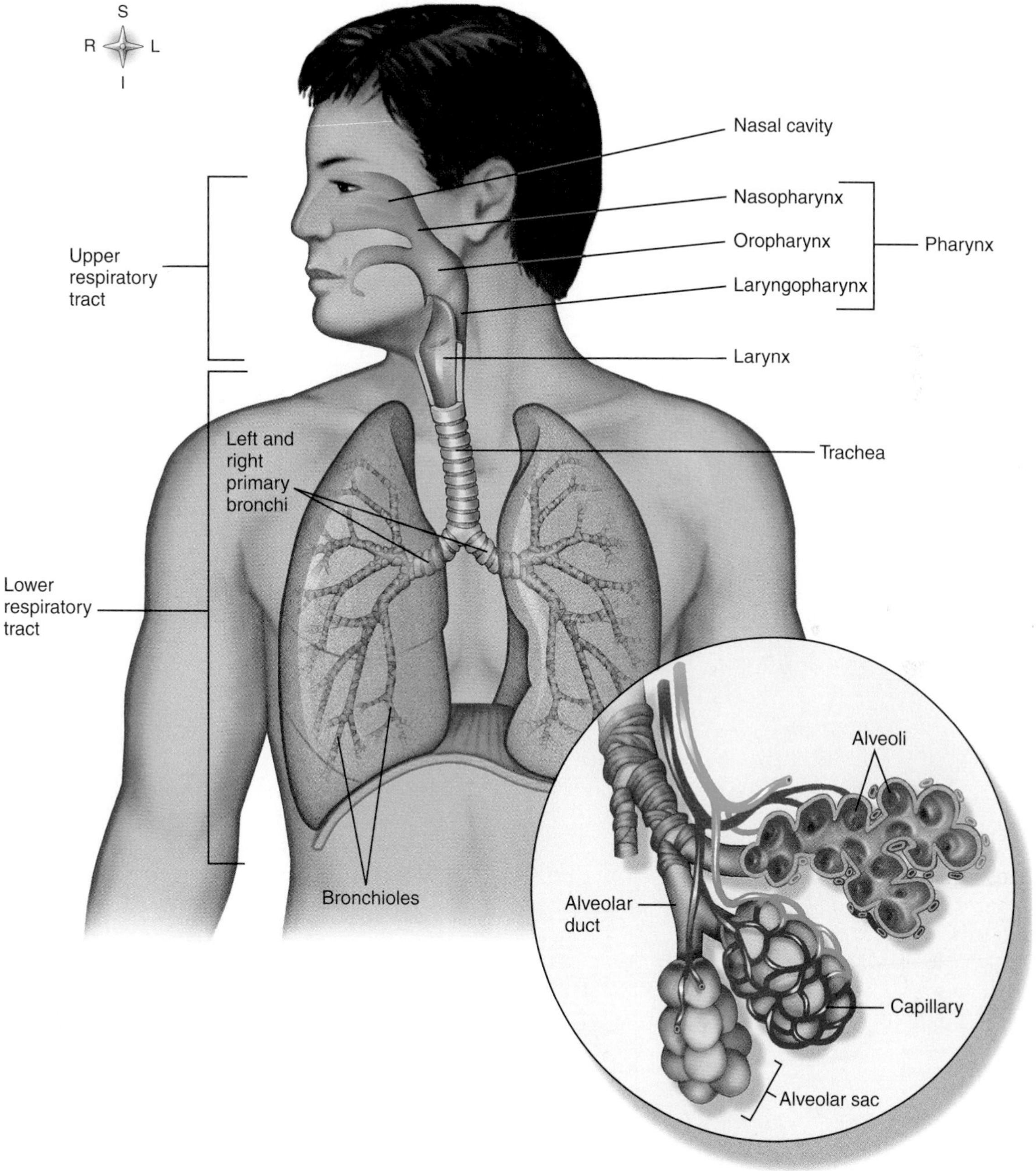

fact, the function of the entire respiratory system—is to distribute air close enough to blood for a gas exchange to take place between air and blood. The passive transport process of **diffusion,** which was described in Chapter 3, is responsible for the exchange of gases that occurs in the respiratory system. You may want to review the discussion of diffusion on p. 50 before you study the mechanism of gas exchange that occurs in the lungs and body tissues.

Two characteristics about the structure of alveoli assist in diffusion and make them able to perform this function admirably. First, the wall of each alveolus is made up of a single layer of cells and so are the walls of the capillaries around it. This means that, between the blood in the capillaries and the air in the alveolus, there is a barrier probably less than 1 micron thick. This extremely thin barrier is called the **respiratory membrane** (Figure 14-2). Second, there are millions of alveoli.

FIGURE 14-2

The gas-exchange structures of the lung. Each alveolus is continually ventilated with fresh air. The inset shows a magnified view of the respiratory membrane composed of the alveolar wall (surfactant, epithelial cells, and basement membrane), interstitial fluid, and the wall of a pulmonary capillary (basement membrane and endothelial cells). The gases, CO_2 (carbon dioxide) and O_2 (oxygen), diffuse across the respiratory membrane.

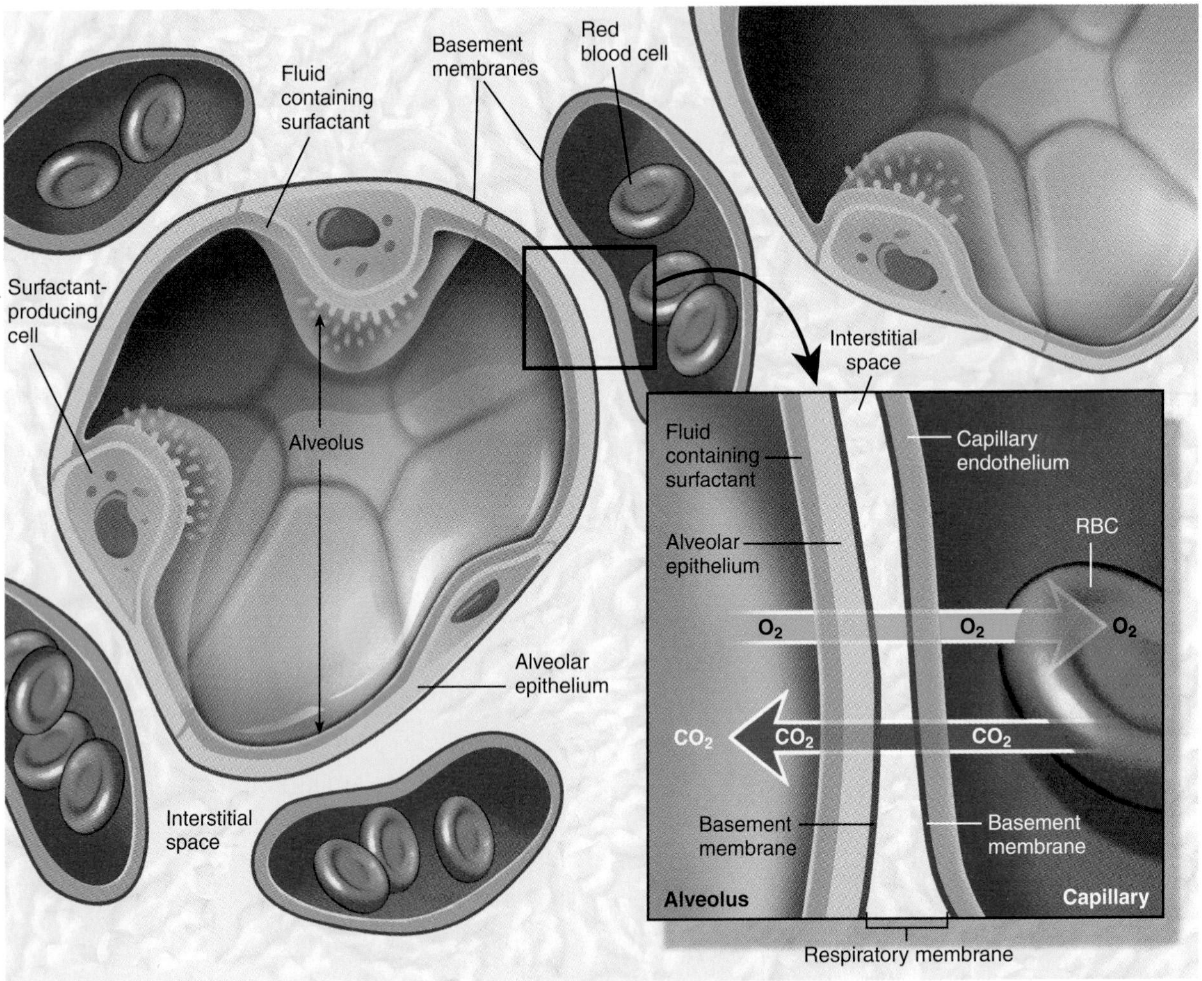

This means that together they make an enormous surface (approximately 100 square meters, an area many times larger than the surface of the entire body) where larger amounts of oxygen and carbon dioxide can rapidly be exchanged.

RESPIRATORY TRACTS

The respiratory system is often divided into upper and lower tracts or divisions to assist in the description of symptoms associated with common respiratory problems such as a cold. The organs of the upper respiratory tract are located outside of the thorax or chest cavity, whereas those in the lower tract or division are located almost entirely within it. The **upper respiratory tract** is composed of the nose, pharynx, and larynx. The **lower respiratory tract** or division consists of the trachea, all segments of the bronchial tree, and the lungs. The designation *upper respiratory infection* or URI is often used to describe what many patients call a "head cold." Typically the symptoms of an upper respiratory infection involve the sinuses, nasal cavity, pharynx, and larynx, whereas the symptoms of what is often referred to as a "chest cold" are similar to pneumonia and involve the organs of the lower respiratory tract.

RESPIRATORY MUCOSA

Before beginning the study of individual organs in the respiratory system, it is important to review the histology or microscopic anatomy of the **respiratory mucosa**—the membrane that lines most of the air distribution tubes in the system. Do not confuse the respiratory membrane with the respiratory mucosa! The **respiratory membrane** (Figure 14-2) separates the air in the alveoli from the blood in surrounding capillaries. The respiratory mucosa (Figure 14-3) is covered with mucus and lines the tubes of the respiratory tree.

Recall that in addition to serving as air distribution passageways or gas exchange surfaces, the anatomical components of the respiratory tract and lungs cleanse, warm, and humidify inspired air. Air entering the nose is generally contaminated with one or more common irritants; examples include insects, dust, pollen, and bacterial organisms. A remarkably effective air purification mechanism removes almost every form of contaminant before inspired air reaches the alveoli or terminal air sacs in the lungs.

The layer of protective mucus that covers a large portion of the membrane that lines the respiratory tree serves as the most important air purification

FIGURE 14-3

Respiratory mucosa lining the trachea. A layer of mucus covers the hairlike cilia.

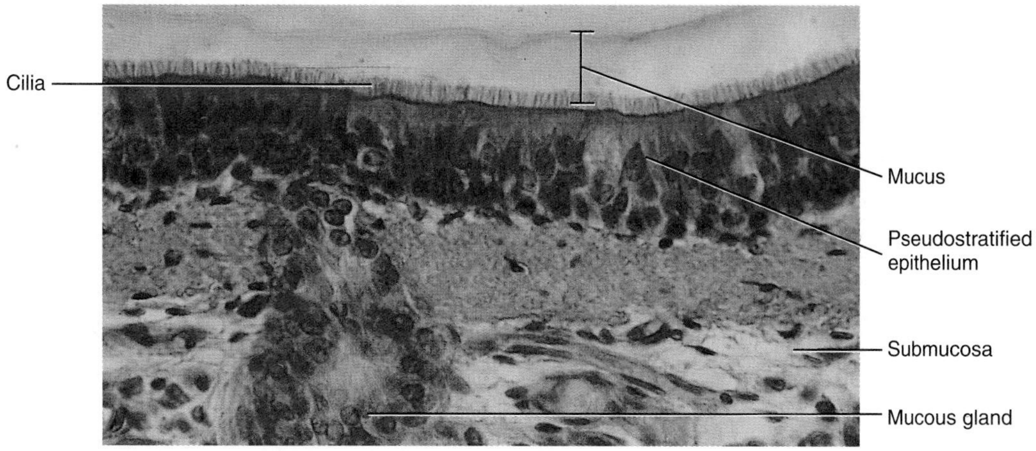

mechanism. More than 125 ml of respiratory mucus is produced daily. It forms a continuous sheet called a *mucous blanket* that covers the lining of the air distribution tubes in the respiratory tree. This layer of cleansing mucus moves upward to the pharynx from the lower portions of the bronchial tree on millions of hairlike cilia that cover the epithelial cells in the respiratory mucosa (see Figure 14-3). The microscopic cilia that cover epithelial cells in the respiratory mucosa beat or move only in one direction. The result is movement of mucus toward the pharynx. Cigarette smoke paralyzes these cilia and results in accumulations of mucus and the typical smoker's cough, which is an effort to clear the secretions.

Quick Check

1. What are the primary functions of the respiratory system?
2. Can you distinguish the upper respiratory tract from the lower respiratory tract?
3. What is the role of the respiratory membrane?

NOSE

Air enters the respiratory tract through the **external nares** (NA-rees) or nostrils. It then flows into the right and left **nasal cavities,** which are lined by respiratory mucosa. A partition called the *nasal septum* separates these two cavities.

The surface of the nasal cavities is moist from mucus and warm from blood flowing just under it. Nerve endings responsible for the sense of smell (olfactory receptors) are located in the nasal mucosa. Four **paranasal sinuses**—frontal, maxillary, sphenoidal, and ethmoidal—drain into the nasal cavities (Figure 14-4). Because the mucosa that lines the sinuses is continuous with the mucosa that lines the nose, sinus infections, called **sinusitis** (sye-nyoo-SYE-tis), often develop from colds in which the nasal mucosa is inflamed. The paranasal sinuses are lined with a mucous membrane that assists in the production of mucus for the respiratory tract. In addition, these hollow spaces help to lighten the skull bones and serve as resonant chambers for the production of sound.

Two ducts from the **lacrimal sacs** (LAK-rim-al saks) also drain into the nasal cavity, as Figure 14-4 shows. The lacrimal sacs collect tears from the corner of the each eyelid and drain them into the nasal cavity.

Note in Figure 14-5 that three shelflike structures called **conchae** (KONG-kee) protrude into the nasal cavity on each side. The mucosa-covered conchae greatly increase the surface over which air must flow as it passes through the naval cavity. As air moves over the conchae and through the nasal cavities, it is warmed and humidified. This helps explain why breathing through the nose is more effective in humidifying inspired air than is breathing through the mouth. If an individual who is ill requires supplemental oxygen, it is first bubbled through water to reduce the amount of moisture that would otherwise have to be removed from the lining of the respiratory tree to humidify it. Administration of "dry" oxygen pulls water from the mucosa and results in respiratory discomfort and irritation.

PHARYNX

The **pharynx** is the structure that many of us call the throat. It is about 12.5 cm (5 inches) long and can be divided into three portions (see Figure 14-5). The uppermost part of the tube just behind the nasal cavities is called the **nasopharynx** (nay-zo-FAIR-inks). The portion behind the mouth is called the **oropharynx** (o-ro-FAIR-inks). The last or lowest segment is called the **laryngopharynx** (lah-ring-go-FAIR-inks). The pharynx as a whole serves the same purpose for the respiratory and digestive tracts as a hallway serves for a house. Air and food pass through the pharynx on their way to the lungs and the stomach respectively. Air enters the pharynx from the two nasal cavities and leaves it by way of the larynx; food enters it from the mouth and leaves it by way of the esophagus. The right and left **auditory** or *eustachian* (yoo-STAY-she-an) **tubes** open into the nasopharynx; they connect the middle ears with the nasopharynx (see Figure 14-5). This connection permits equalization of air pressure between the middle and the exterior ear. The lining of the

FIGURE 14-4

The paranasal sinuses. The anterior view shows the anatomical relationship of the paranasal sinuses to each other and to the nasal cavity. The inset is a lateral view of the position of the sinuses.

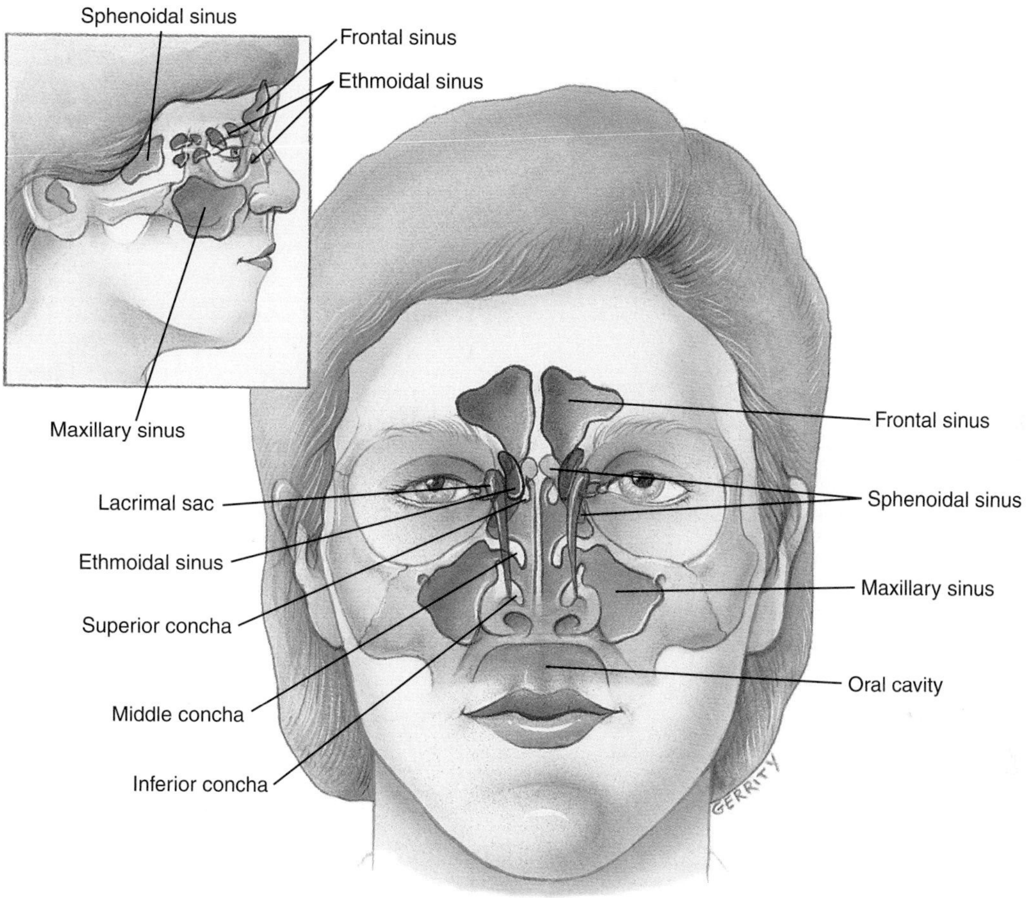

auditory tubes is continuous with the lining of the nasopharynx and middle ear. Thus just as sinus infections can develop from colds in which the nasal mucosa is inflamed, middle ear infections can develop from inflammation of the nasopharynx.

Masses of lymphatic tissue called **tonsils** are embedded in the mucous membrane of the pharynx (see p. 340). The **pharyngeal** (fa-RIN-jee-al) **tonsils** or **adenoids** (AD-e-noyds) are in the nasopharynx. The **palatine tonsils** are located in the oropharynx (see Figure 14-5). Both tonsils are generally removed in a **tonsillectomy** (ton-si-LEK-toe-mee). This procedure, with its potentially serious complications, is now performed only reluctantly, and the number of tonsillectomies reported each year continues to decrease. Physicians now recognize the value of lymphatic tissue in the body defense mechanism and delay removal of the tonsils—even in cases of inflammation or **tonsillitis**—unless antibiotic treatment is ineffective. When the pharyngeal tonsils become swollen, they are referred to as adenoids. Such swelling caused by infections may

FIGURE 14-5

Sagittal section of the head and neck. The nasal septum has been removed, exposing the right lateral wall of the nasal cavity so that the nasal conchae can be seen. Note also the divisions of the pharynx and the position of the tonsils.

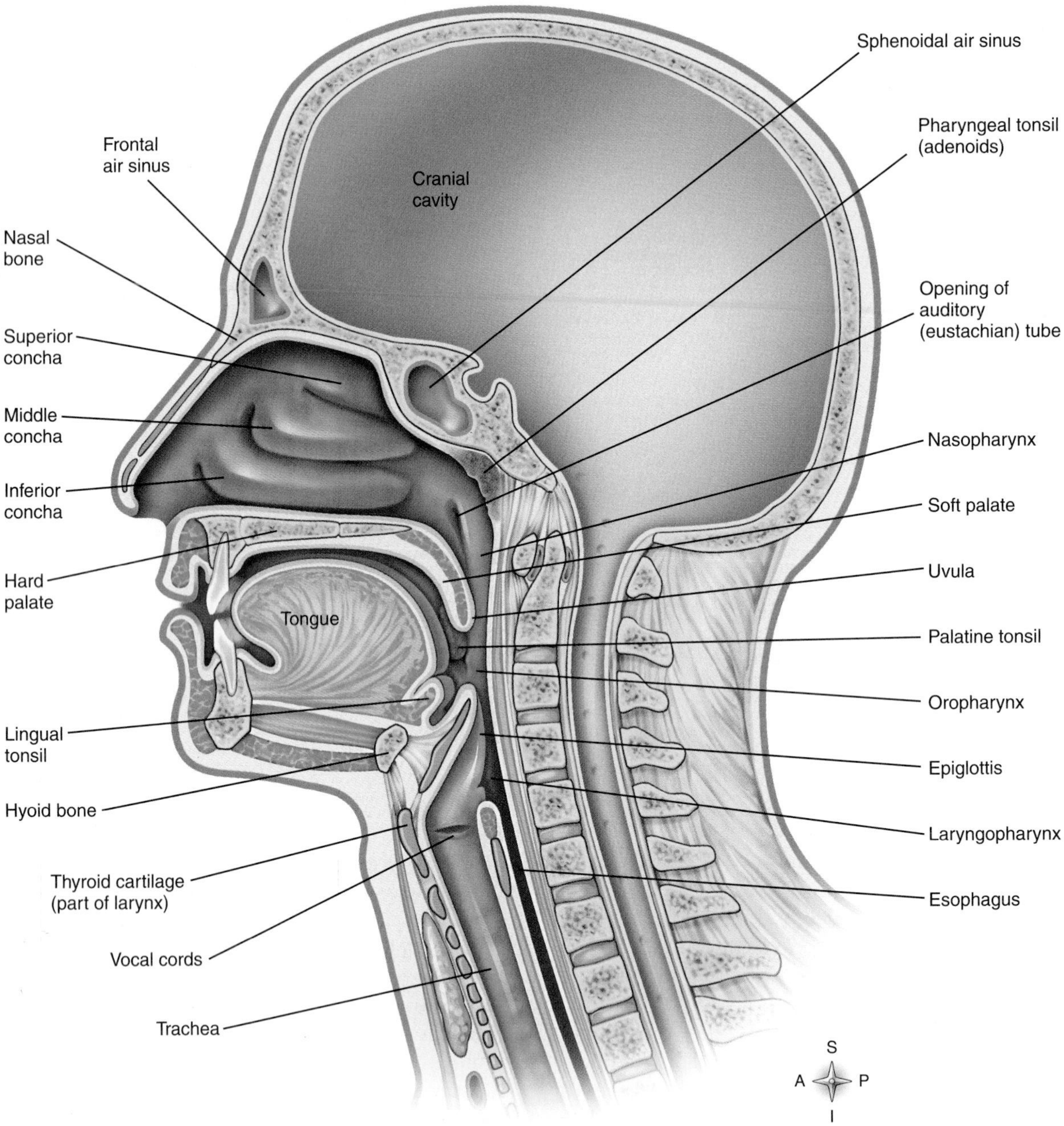

FIGURE 14-6

The larynx. A, Sagittal section of the larynx. **B,** Superior view of the larynx. **C,** Photograph of the larynx taken with an endoscope (optical device) inserted through the mouth and pharynx to the epiglottis.

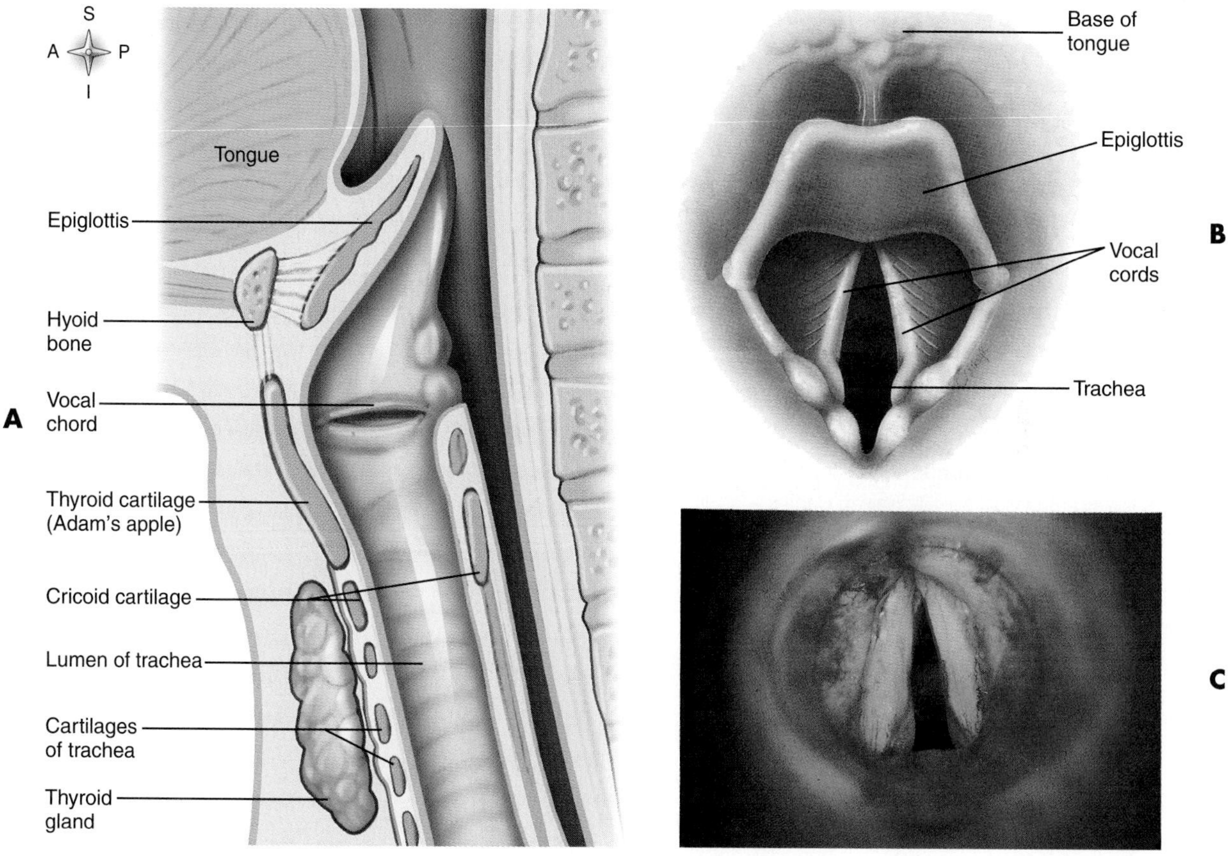

make it difficult or impossible for air to travel from the nose into the throat. In these cases the individual is forced to breathe through his or her mouth.

LARYNX

The **larynx** or voice box is located just below the pharynx. It is composed of several pieces of cartilage. You know the largest of these (the *thyroid cartilage*) as the "Adam's apple" (Figure 14-6).

Two short fibrous bands, the **vocal cords,** stretch across the interior of the larynx. Muscles that attach to the larynx cartilages can pull on these cords in such a way that they become tense or relaxed. When they are tense, the voice is high pitched; when they are relaxed, it is low pitched. The space between the vocal cords is the **glottis.** Another cartilage, the **epiglottis** (ep-i-GLOT-is) partially covers the opening of the larynx (Figure 14-6). The epiglottis acts like a trapdoor, closing off the larynx during swallowing and preventing food from entering the trachea.

TRACHEA

The **trachea** or windpipe is a tube about 11 cm (4.5 inches) long that extends from the larynx in the neck to the bronchi in the chest cavity (Figures 14-1 and 14-7). The trachea performs a simple but vital function: it furnishes part of the open passageway through which air can reach the lungs from the outside.

By pushing with your fingers against your throat about an inch above the sternum, you can feel the shape of the trachea or windpipe. Only if you use considerable force can you squeeze it closed. Nature has taken precautions to keep this lifeline open. Its framework is made of an almost noncollapsible material—15 or 20 C-shaped rings of cartilage placed one above the other with only a little soft tissue between them (Figure 14-7). The trachea is lined by the typical respiratory mucosa. Glands below the ciliated epithelium help produce the blanket of mucus that continually moves upward toward the pharynx.

Despite the structural safeguard of cartilage rings, closing of the trachea sometimes occurs. A tumor or an infection may enlarge the lymph nodes of the neck so much that they squeeze the trachea shut, or a person may aspirate (breathe in) a piece of food or something else that blocks the windpipe. Because air has no other way to get to the lungs, complete tracheal obstruction causes

FIGURE 14-7

Cross section of the trachea. Inset at top shows where the section was cut. The scanning electron micrograph shows the tip of one of the C-shaped cartilage rings.

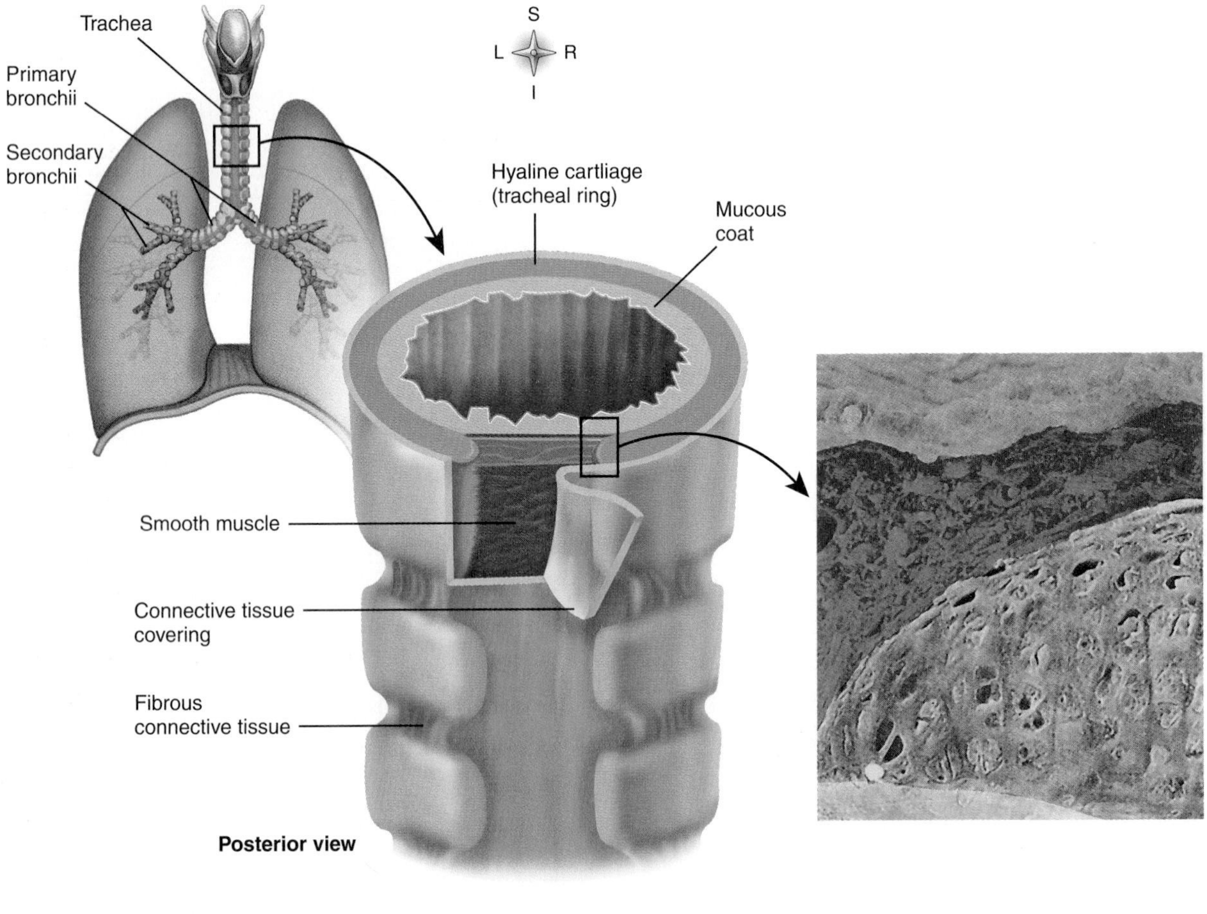

Clinical Application

Heimlich Maneuver

The **Heimlich maneuver** is an effective and often lifesaving technique that can be used to open a windpipe that is suddenly obstructed. The maneuver (see figures) uses air already present in the lungs to expel the object obstructing the trachea. Most accidental airway obstructions result from pieces of food aspirated (breathed in) during a meal; the condition is sometimes referred to as a *café coronary*. Other objects such as chewing gum or balloons are frequently the cause of obstructions in children.

Individuals trained in emergency procedures must be able to tell the difference between airway obstruction and other conditions such as heart attacks that produce similar symptoms. The key question they must ask the person who appears to be choking is, "Are you choking?" A person with an obstructed airway will not be able to speak, even while conscious. The Heimlich maneuver, if the victim is standing, consists of the rescuer's grasping the victim with both arms around the victim's waist just below the rib cage and above the navel. The rescuer makes a fist with one hand, grasps it with the other, and then delivers an upward thrust against the diaphragm just below the xiphoid process of the sternum. Air trapped in the lungs is compressed, forcing the object that is choking the victim out of the airway.

Technique if victim can be lifted (see *A*):

1. The rescuer stands behind the victim and wraps both arms around the victim's chest slightly below the rib cage and above the navel. The victim is allowed to fall forward with the head, arms, and chest over the rescuer's arms.
2. The rescuer makes a fist with one hand and grasps it with the other hand, pressing the thumb side of the fist against the victim's abdomen below the end of the xiphoid process and above the navel.
3. The hands only are used to deliver the upward subdiaphragmatic thrusts. It is performed with sharp flexion of the elbows, in an upward rather than inward direction. It is very important not to compress the rib cage or actually press on the sternum during the Heimlich maneuver. Thrusts are usually repeated four times or as many as needed to dislodge the obstruction. Thrusting should be stopped periodically to assess the victim but otherwise should continue as long as the victim is conscious and the airway is obstructed.

Technique if victim has collapsed or cannot be lifted (see *B*):

1. Rescuer places victim on floor face up.
2. Facing victim, rescuer straddles the victim's hips.
3. Rescuer places one hand on top of the other, with the bottom hand on the victim's abdomen slightly above the navel and below the rib cage.
4. Rescuer performs a forceful upward thrust with the heel of the bottom hand, repeating several times if necessary.

A

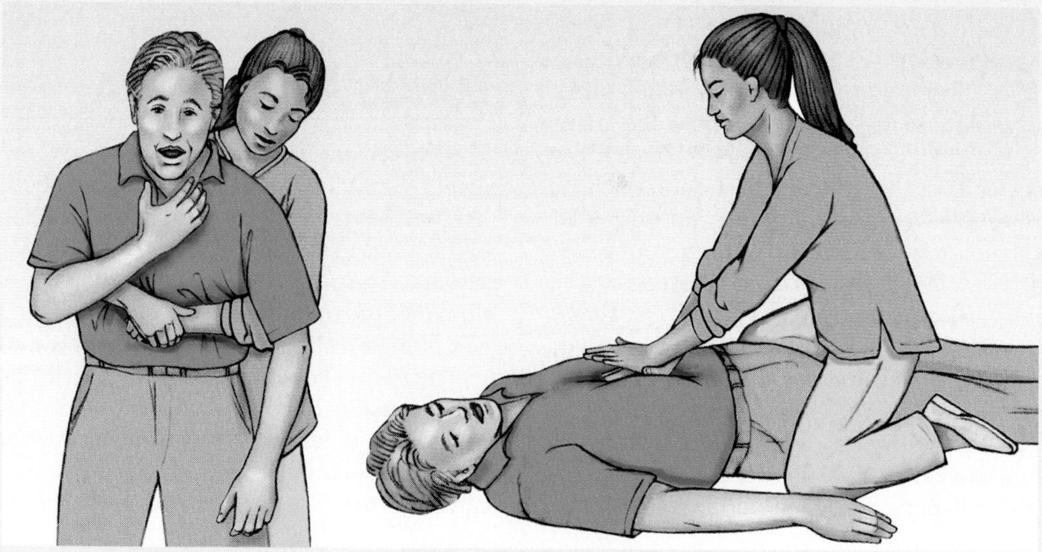

B

death in a matter of minutes. Choking on food and other substances caught in the trachea kills more than 4000 people each year and is the fifth major cause of accidental death in the United States. A lifesaving technique developed by Dr. Henry Heimlich (see the box on p. 381), is now widely used to free the trachea of ingested food or other foreign objects that would otherwise block the airway and cause death in choking victims.

Quick Check

1. What are the paranasal sinuses? What is their role?
2. What are the three divisions of the pharynx?
3. What is the scientific term for the voice box?
4. What keeps the trachea from collapsing?

FIGURE 14-8

Alveoli. Bronchioles subdivide to form tiny tubes called alveolar ducts, which end in clusters of alveoli called *alveolar sacs*.

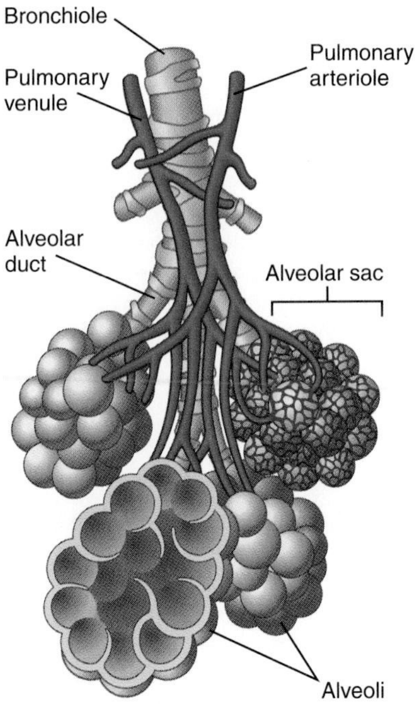

BRONCHI, BRONCHIOLES, AND ALVEOLI

Recall that one way to picture the thousands of air tubes that make up the lungs is to think of an upside-down tree. The trachea is the main trunk of this tree; the right bronchus (the tube leading into the right lung) and the left bronchus (the tube leading into the left lung) are the trachea's first branches or **primary bronchi.** In each lung, they branch into smaller or **secondary bronchi** whose walls, as with those of the trachea and bronchi, are kept open by rings of cartilage for air passage. These bronchi divide into smaller and smaller tubes, ultimately branching into tiny tubes whose walls contain only smooth muscle. These very small passageways are called **bronchioles.** The bronchioles subdivide into microscopic tubes called **alveolar ducts,** which resemble the main stem of a bunch of grapes (Figure 14-8). Each alveolar duct ends in several **alveolar sacs,** each of which resembles a cluster of grapes, and the wall of each alveolar sac is made up of numerous **alveoli,** each of which resembles a single grape.

Alveoli are very effective in gas exchange, mainly because they are extremely thin walled; each alveolus lies in contact with a blood capillary, and there are millions of alveoli in each lung. The surface of the respiratory membrane inside the alveolus is covered by a substance called **surfactant** (sur-FAK-tant). This important substance helps reduce surface tension in the alveoli and keeps them from collapsing as air moves in and out during respiration.

LUNGS AND PLEURA

The **lungs** are fairly large organs. Note in Figure 14-9 that the right lung has three lobes and the left lung has two. Figure 14-9 shows the relationship of the lungs to the rib cage at the end of a normal expiration. The narrow, superior position of each lung, up under the collarbone, is the apex; the broad, inferior portion resting on the diaphragm is the base.

The **pleura** covers the outer surface of the lungs and lines the inner surface of the rib cage. The pleura resembles other serous membranes in structure and function. As with the peritoneum or pericardium, the pleura is an extensive, thin, moist,

Clinical Application

Infant Respiratory Distress Syndrome

Infant respiratory distress syndrome or **IRDS** is a very serious, life-threatening condition that often affects prematurely born infants of less than 37 weeks' gestation or those who weigh less than 2.2 kg (5 lbs) at birth. IRDS is the leading cause of death among premature infants in the United States, claiming more than 5000 premature babies each year. The disease, characterized by a lack of **surfactant** in the alveolar air sacs, affects 50,000 babies annually.

Surfactant is manufactured by specialized cells in the walls of the alveoli. Surfactant reduces the surface tension of the fluid on the free surface of the alveolar walls and permits easy movement of air into and out of the lungs. The ability of the body to manufacture this important substance is not fully developed until shortly before birth—normally about 40 weeks after conception.

In newborn infants who are unable to manufacture surfactant, many air sacs collapse during expiration because of the increased surface tension. The effort required to reinflate these collapsed alveoli is much greater than that needed to reinflate normal alveoli with adequate surfactant. The baby soon develops labored breathing, and symptoms of respiratory distress appear shortly after birth.

In the past, treatment of IRDS was limited to keeping the alveoli open so that delivery and exchange of oxygen and carbon dioxide could occur. To accomplish this, a tube was inserted into the respiratory tract and oxygen-rich air was delivered under sufficient pressure to keep the alveoli from collapsing at the end of expiration. A newer treatment involves delivering air under pressure and applying prepared surfactant directly into the baby's airways by means of a tube.

slippery membrane. It lines a large, closed cavity of the body and covers the organs located within it. The parietal pleura lines the walls of the thoracic cavity; the visceral pleura covers the lungs, and the intrapleural space lies between the two pleural membranes (Figure 14-10). Pleurisy is an inflammation of the pleura that causes pain when the pleural membranes rub together.

Normally the intrapleural space contains just enough fluid to make both portions of the pleura moist and slippery and able to glide easily against each other as the lungs expand and deflate with each breath. **Pneumothorax** (noo-mo-THO-raks) is the presence of air in the intrapleural space on one side of the chest. The additional air increases the pressure on the lung on that side and causes it to collapse. While collapsed, the lung does not function in breathing.

Quick Check

1. What are bronchi? What is their role?
2. What is the function of the alveoli?
3. Can you describe the structure and function of the pleura?

RESPIRATION

Respiration means exchange of gases (oxygen and carbon dioxide) between a living organism and its environment. If the organism consists of only one cell, gases can move directly between it and the environment. If, however, the organism consists of billions of cells, as do our bodies, most of its cells are too far from the air for a direct exchange of gases. To overcome this difficulty, a pair of organs—the lungs—provides a place where air and a circulating fluid (blood) can come close enough to each other for oxygen to move out of the air into blood while carbon dioxide moves out of the blood into air. Breathing or **pulmonary ventilation** is the process that moves air into and out of the lungs. It makes possible the exchange of gases between air in the lungs and in the blood. This exchange is often called **external respiration.** In addition, exchange of gases occurs between the blood and the cells of the body—a process called **internal respiration.** *Cellular respiration* refers to the actual use of oxygen by cells in the process of metabolism, which is discussed in Chapter 16.

FIGURE 14-9

Lungs. The trachea is an airway that branches to form an inverted tree of bronchi and bronchioles. Note that the right lung has three lobes and that the left lung has two lobes.

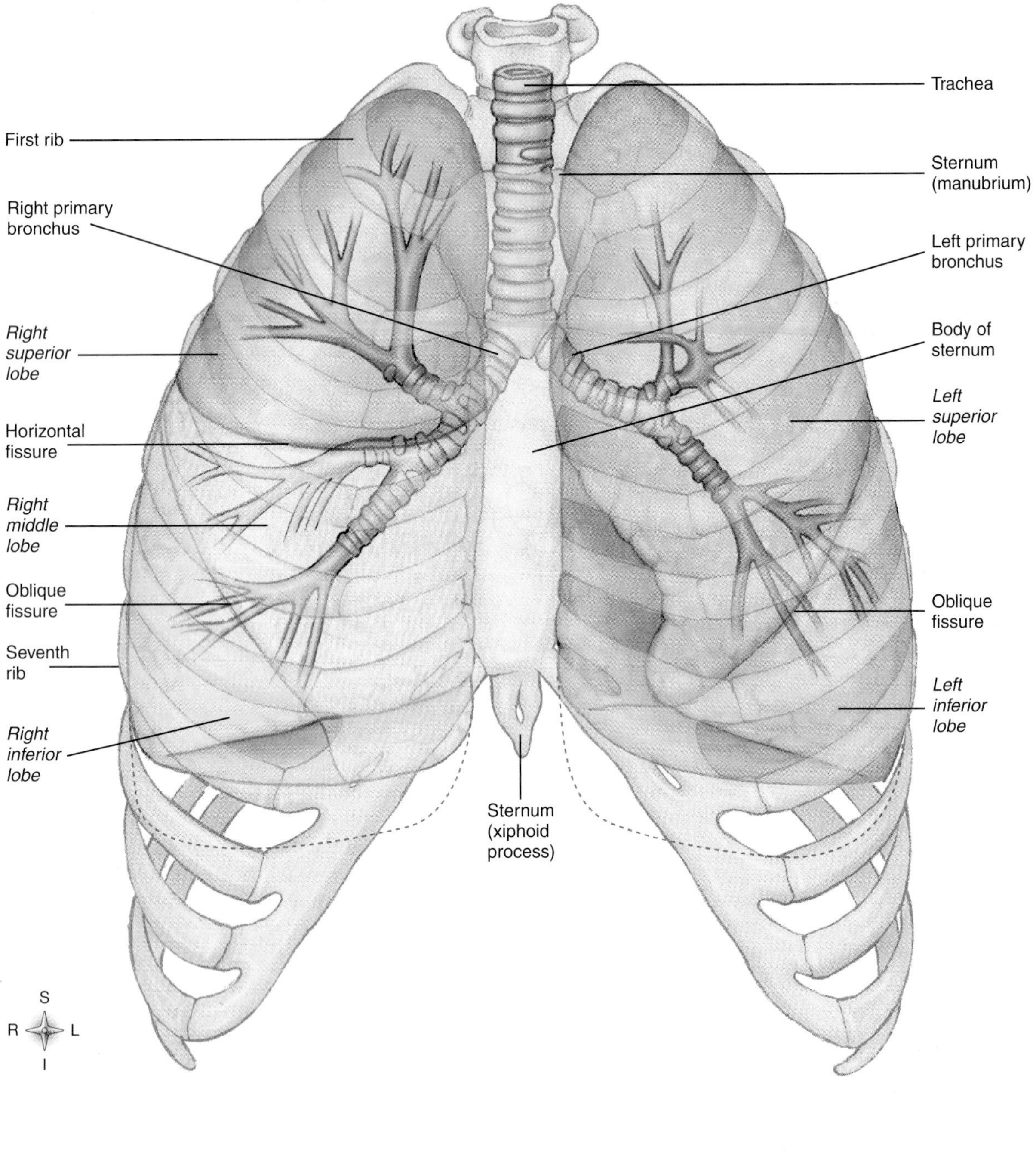

FIGURE 14-10

Lungs and pleura. The inset shows where the body was cut to show this transverse section of the thorax. A serous membrane lines the thoracic wall (parietal pleura) and then folds inward near the bronchi to cover the lung (visceral pleura). The intrapleural space contains a small amount of serous pleural fluid.

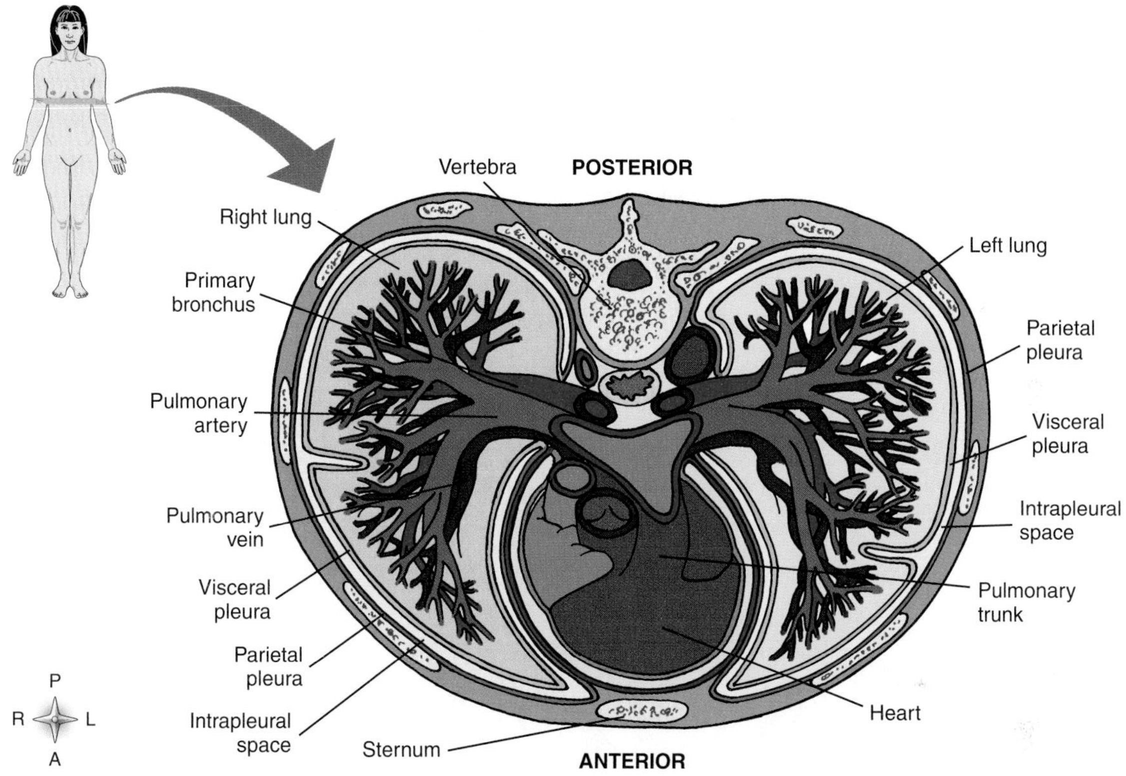

Mechanics of Breathing

Pulmonary ventilation or breathing has two phases. **Inspiration** or inhalation moves air into the lungs, and **expiration** or exhalation moves air out of the lungs. The lungs are enclosed within the thoracic cavity. Thus changes in the shape and size of the thoracic cavity result in changes in the air pressure within that cavity and in the lungs. This difference in air pressure causes the movement of air into and out of the lungs. Air moves from an area where pressure is high to an area where pressure is lower. Respiratory muscles are responsible for the changes in the shape of the thoracic cavity that cause the air movements involved in breathing.

Inspiration

Inspiration occurs when the chest cavity enlarges. As the thorax enlarges, the lungs expand along with it, and air rushes into them and down into the alveoli. Muscles of respiration that are classified as **inspiratory muscles** include the **diaphragm** (DYE-a-fram) and the external intercostals. The diaphragm is the dome-shaped muscle separating the abdominal cavity from the thoracic cavity. The diaphragm flattens out when it contracts during inspiration.

Research, Issues & Trends

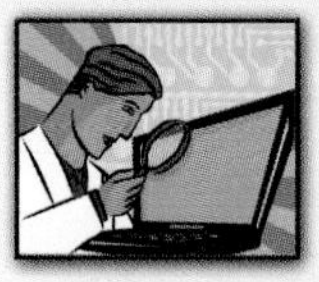

Lung Volume Reduction Surgery (LVRS)

Clinical trials to study the effects of lung volume reduction surgery (LVRS) have been under way for several years. LVRS was developed as a treatment option for patients in the last stages of emphysema and involves removal of 20% to 30% of each lung. Current data now show that LVRS treatment benefits emphysema patients beyond what could be expected with traditional medical therapy and rehabilitation.

More than 2 million Americans, most older than age 50 and current or former smokers, have emphysema—a major cause of disability and death in the United States. In the end stages of this chronic disease, breathing becomes labored as the lungs fill with large irregular spaces resulting from the enlargement and rupture of many alveoli (see illustration). The LVRS procedure removes part of the diseased open space and is intended to help improve the efficiency of air movement into and out of the remaining lung tissue. We now know that LVRS reduces the need for lung transplantation procedures and augments the effectiveness of such supporting medical treatments as nutritional supplementation and physical (exercise) rehabilitation in the treatment of many late-stage emphysema patients.

Emphysema. The effects of emphysema can be seen in these scanning electron micrographs of lung tissue. **A,** Normal lung with many small alveoli. **B,** Lung tissue affected by emphysema. Notice that the alveoli have merged into larger air spaces, reducing the surface area for gas exchange.

A

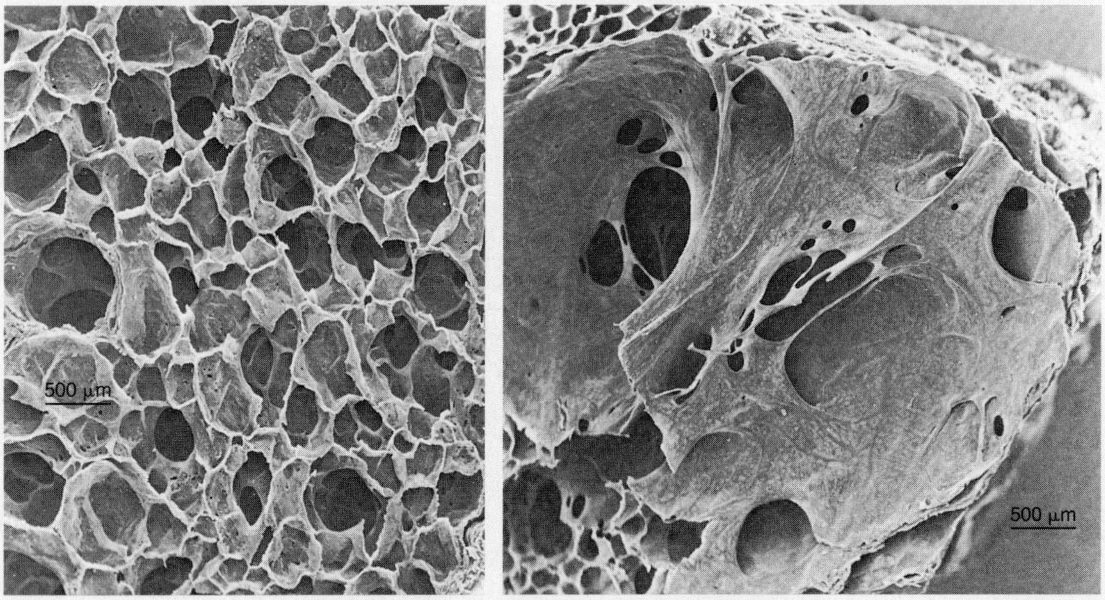

B

Instead of protruding up into the chest cavity, it moves down toward the abdominal cavity. Thus the contraction or flattening of the diaphragm makes the chest cavity longer from top to bottom. The diaphragm is the most important muscle of inspiration. Nerve impulses passing through the *phrenic nerve* stimulate the diaphragm to contract. The external intercostal muscles are located between the ribs. When they contract, they enlarge the thorax by increasing the size of the cavity from front to back and from side to side. Contraction of the inspiratory muscles increases the volume of the thoracic cavity and reduces the air pressure within it, drawing air into the lungs (Figure 14-11).

FIGURE 14-11

Mechanics of breathing. During *inspiration*, the diaphragm contracts, increasing the volume of the thoracic cavity. This increase in volume results in a decrease in pressure, which causes air to rush into the lungs. During *expiration*, the diaphragm returns to an upward position, reducing the volume in the thoracic cavity. Air pressure increases then, forcing air out of the lungs. The insets show the classic model in which a jar represents the rib cage, a rubber sheet represents the diaphragm, and a balloon represents the lungs.

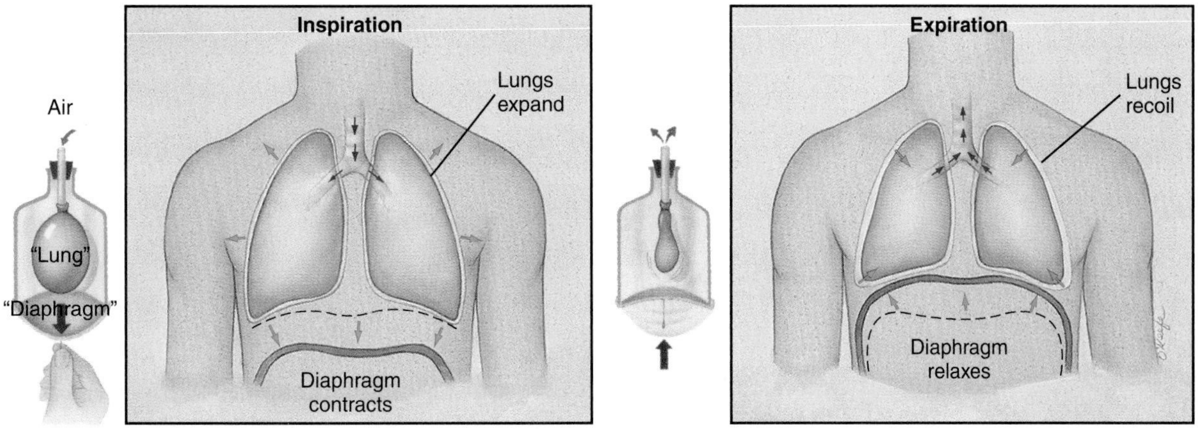

Expiration

Quiet expiration is ordinarily a passive process that begins when the inspiratory muscles relax. The thoracic cavity then returns to its smaller size. The elastic nature of lung tissue also causes these organs to "recoil" and decrease in size as air leaves the alveoli and flows outward through the respiratory passageways. When we speak, sing, or do heavy work, we may need more forceful expiration to increase the rate and depth of ventilation. During more forceful expiration, the **expiratory muscles** (internal intercostals and abdominal muscles) contract. When contracted, the internal intercostal muscles depress the rib cage and decrease the front-to-back size of the thorax. Contraction of the abdominal muscles pushes the abdominal organs against the underside of the diaphragm, thus elevating it and making it more "dome shaped." The result is to further shorten or decrease the top-to-bottom size of the thoracic cavity. As the thoracic cavity decreases in size, the air pressure within it increases and air flows out of the lungs (see Figure 14-11).

Exchange of Gases in Lungs

Blood pumped from the right ventricle of the heart enters the pulmonary artery and eventually enters the lungs. It then flows through the thousands of tiny lung capillaries that are in close proximity to the air-filled alveoli (see Figure 14-1). External respiration or the exchange of gases between the blood and alveolar air occurs by diffusion.

Diffusion is a passive process that results in movement down a concentration gradient; that is, substances move from an area of high concentration to an area of low concentration of the diffusing substance. Oxygen is continually removed from the blood and used by the cells of the body. By the time blood flows into the lung capillaries, it is low in oxygen content. Because alveolar air is rich in oxygen, diffusion causes movement of oxygen from the area of high concentration (alveolar air) to the area of low concentration (capillary blood). Note in Figure 14-12 that most of the oxygen (O_2) entering the blood combines with hemoglobin (Hb) in the red blood cells (RBCs) to form **oxyhemoglobin** (ok-see-

FIGURE 14-12

Exchange of gases in lung and tissue capillaries. The right insets show O_2 diffusing out of alveolar air into blood and associating with hemoglobin (Hb) in lung capillaries to form oxyhemoglobin. In tissue capillaries, oxyhemoglobin dissociates, releasing O_2, which diffuses from the red blood cells (RBCs) and then crosses the capillary wall to reach the tissue cells. As the left insets show, CO_2 diffuses in the opposite direction (into RBCs) and some of it associates with Hb to form carbaminohemoglobin. However, most CO_2 combines with water to form carbonic acid (H_2CO_3), which dissociates to form H^+ and HCO_3^- (bicarbonate) ions. Back in the lung capillaries, CO_2 dissociates from the bicarbonate and carbaminohemoglobin molecules and diffuses out of blood into alveolar air.

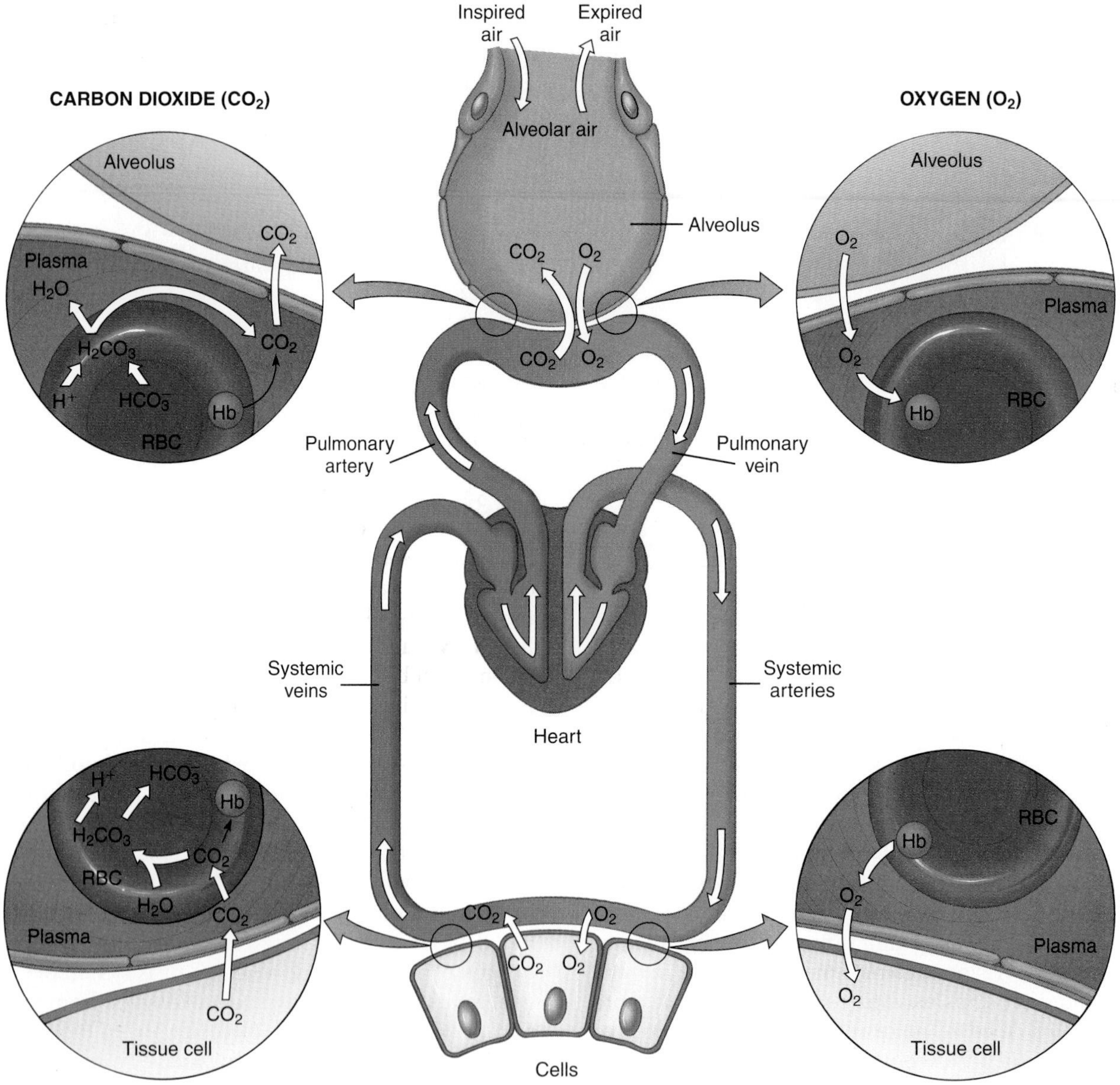

HEE-mo-glo-bin) (HbO_2) so that it can be carried to the tissues and used by the body cells.

Diffusion of carbon dioxide (CO_2) also occurs between blood in lung capillaries and alveolar air. Blood flowing through the lung capillaries is high in carbon dioxide. Most carbon dioxide is carried as bicarbonate ion (HCO_3^-) in the blood. Some, as in Figure 14-12, combines with the hemoglobin in RBCs to form **carbaminohemoglobin** (kar-bam-i-no-HEE-mo-glo-bin) (HbNHCOOH). As cells remove oxygen from circulating blood, they add the waste product carbon dioxide to it. As a result, the blood in pulmonary capillaries eventually becomes low in oxygen and high in carbon dioxide. Diffusion of carbon dioxide results in its movement from an area of high concentration in the pulmonary capillaries to an area of low concentration in alveolar air. Then from the alveoli, carbon dioxide leaves the body in expired air.

Exchange of Gases in Tissues

The exchange of gases that occurs between blood in tissue capillaries and the body cells is called *internal respiration*. As you would expect, the direction of movement of oxygen and carbon dioxide during internal respiration is just the opposite of that noted in the exchange that occurs during external respiration when gases are exchanged between the blood in the lung capillaries and the air in alveoli. As shown in Figure 14-12, oxyhemoglobin breaks down into oxygen and hemoglobin in the tissue capillaries. Oxygen molecules move rapidly out of the blood through the tissue capillary membrane into the interstitial fluid and on into the cells that make up the tissues. The oxygen is used by the cells in their metabolic activities. Diffusion results in the movement of oxygen from an area of high concentration to an area of low concentration in the cells where it is needed. While this is happening, carbon dioxide molecules leave the cells, entering the tissue capillaries where bicarbonate ions are formed and where hemoglobin molecules unite with carbon dioxide to form carbaminohemoglobin. Once again, diffusion is responsible for the movement of carbon dioxide from an area of high concentration in the cells to an area of lower concentration in the capillary blood. In other words, oxygenated blood enters tissue capillaries and is changed into deoxygenated blood as it flows through them. In the process of losing oxygen, the waste product carbon dioxide is picked up and transported to the lungs for removal from the body.

Volumes of Air Exchanged in Pulmonary Ventilation

A special device called a **spirometer** is used to measure the amount of air exchanged in breathing. Figure 14-13 illustrates the various pulmonary volumes, which can be measured as a subject breathes into a spirometer. We take 500 ml (about a pint) of air into our lungs with each normal inspiration and expel it with each normal expiration. Because this amount comes and goes regularly like the tides of the sea, it is referred to as the **tidal volume (TV).** The largest amount of air that we can breathe out in one expiration is known as the **vital capacity (VC).** In normal young men, this is about 4800 ml. Tidal volume and vital capacity are frequently measured in patients with lung disease such as emphysema or heart problems, conditions that often lead to abnormal volumes of air being moved in and out of the lungs.

Observe the area in Figure 14-13 that represents the **expiratory reserve volume (ERV).** This is the amount of air that can be forcibly exhaled after expiring the tidal volume. Compare this with the area in Figure 14-13 that represents the **inspiratory reserve volume (IRV).** The IRV is the amount of air that can be forcibly inspired over and above a normal inspiration. As the tidal volume increases, the ERV and IRV decrease. Note in Figure 14-13 that vital capacity (VC) is the total of tidal volume, inspiratory reserve volume, and expiratory reserve volume—or expressed in another way: VC = TV + IRV + ERV. **Residual volume (RV)** is simply the air that remains in the lungs after the most forceful expiration.

Quick Check

1. How does the diaphragm operate during inspiration? During expiration?
2. In what form does oxygen travel in the blood? Carbon dioxide?
3. What is the vital capacity? How is it measured?

FIGURE 14-13

Pulmonary ventilation volumes. The chart in **A** shows a tracing like that produced with a spirometer. The diagram in **B** shows the pulmonary volumes as relative proportions of an inflated balloon (see Figure 14-11). During normal, quiet breathing, about 500 ml of air is moved into and out of the respiratory tract, an amount called the *tidal volume*. During forceful breathing (like that during and after heavy exercise), an extra 3300 ml can be inspired (the inspiratory reserve volume), and an extra 1000 ml or so can be expired (the expiratory reserve volume). The largest volume of air that can be moved in and out during ventilation is called the *vital capacity*. Air that remains in the respiratory tract after a forceful expiration is called the *residual volume*.

A

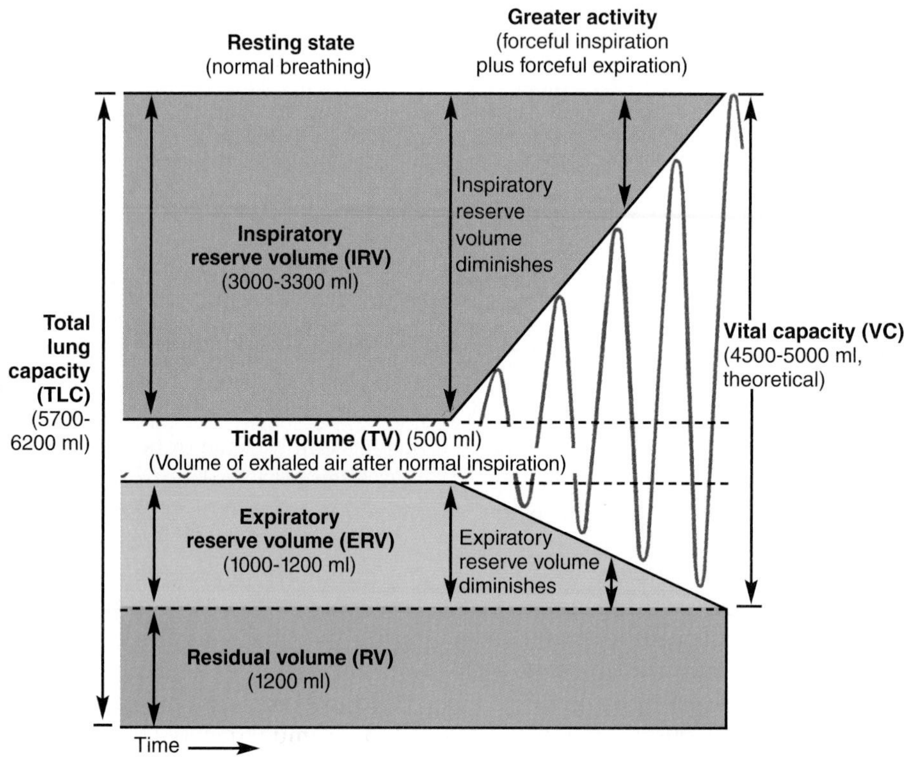

B

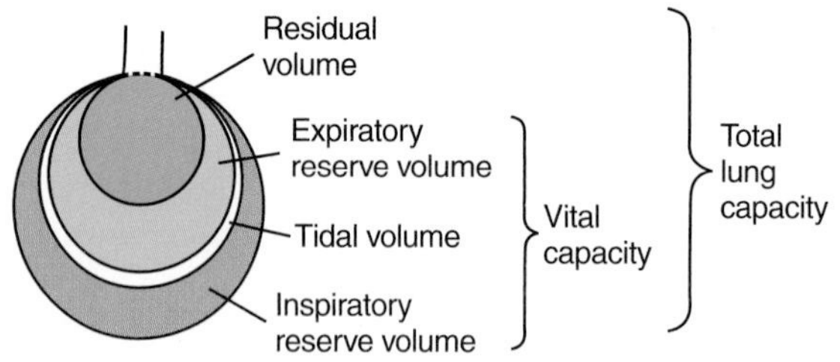

Health & Well-Being

Maximum Oxygen Consumption

Exercise physiologists use **maximum oxygen consumption** ($VO_{2\ max}$) as a predictor of a person's capacity to do aerobic exercise. An individual's $VO_{2\ max}$ represents the amount of oxygen taken up by the lungs, transported to the tissues, and used to do work. $VO_{2\ max}$ is determined largely by hereditary factors, but aerobic (endurance) training can increase it by as much as 35%. Many endurance athletes are now using $VO_{2\ max}$ measurements to help them determine and then maintain their peak condition.

Clinical Application

Sudden Infant Death Syndrome (SIDS)

Sudden infant death syndrome (SIDS) is the third-ranking cause of infant death and accounts for about 1 in 9 of the nearly 30,000 infant deaths reported each year in the United States. Sometimes called "crib-death," SIDS occurs most frequently in babies with no obvious medical problems who are younger than 3 months of age. The exact cause of death can seldom be determined even after extensive testing and autopsy.

SIDS occurs at a higher rate in African-American and Native American babies than in white, Hispanic, or Asian infants, although the reasons remain a mystery. Regardless of infant ethnicity, recent data suggest that certain precautions, such as having babies sleep only on their backs and keeping cribs free of pillows or plush toys that might partially cover the nose or mouth, may reduce the incidence of SIDS. Also important is the elimination of smoking during pregnancy and protecting infants from exposure to "second-hand" cigarette smoke after birth. Although the exact cause of SIDS remains unknown, genetic defects involving the structure and function of the respiratory system or unusual physiological responses to common flu or cold viruses may also play a role in this tragic problem.

REGULATION OF RESPIRATION

We know that the body uses oxygen to obtain energy for the work it has to do. The more work the body does, the more oxygen that must be delivered to its millions of cells. One way this is accomplished is by increasing the rate and depth of respirations. Although we may take only 12 to 18 breaths a minute when we are not moving about, we take considerably more than this when we are exercising. Not only do we take more breaths, but our tidal volume also increases.

To help supply cells with more oxygen when they are doing more work, automatic adjustments occur not only in respirations but also in circulation. Most notably, the heart beats faster and harder and therefore pumps more blood through the body each minute. This means that the millions of RBCs make more round trips between the lungs and tissues each minute and so deliver more oxygen per minute to tissue cells.

Working cells not only require more oxygen, they also produce more waste products such as carbon dioxide and certain metabolic acids. The increase in respirations during exercise shows us how the body automatically regulates its vital functions. By increasing the rate and depth of respiration, we can adjust to the varying demands for increased oxygen while increasing the elimination of metabolic waste products in expired air to maintain homeostasis.

Normal respiration depends on proper functioning of the muscles of respiration. These muscles are stimulated by nervous impulses that originate in **respiratory control centers** located in the medulla and pons of the brain. These centers are in turn regulated by a number of inputs from receptors located in varying areas of the body. These receptors can sense the need for changing the rate or depth of respirations to maintain homeostasis. Certain receptors sense carbon dioxide or oxygen levels, whereas others sense blood acid levels or the amount of stretch in lung tissues. The two most important control centers are in the medulla and are called the **inspiratory center** and the **expiratory center.** Centers in the pons have a modifying function. Under rest conditions, neurons in the inspiratory and expiratory centers "fire" at a rate that will produce a normal breathing rate of about 12 to 18 breaths a minute.

The depth and rate of respiration can be influenced by many "inputs" to the respiratory control centers from other areas of the brain or from specialized receptors located outside of the central nervous system (Figure 14-14).

Cerebral Cortex

The cerebral cortex can influence respiration by modifying the rate at which neurons "fire" in the inspiratory and expiratory centers of the medulla. In other words, an individual may voluntarily speed up or slow down the breathing rate or greatly change the pattern of respiration during activities. This ability permits us to change respiratory patterns and even to hold our breath for short periods to accommodate activities such as speaking, eating, or underwater swimming. This voluntary control of respiration, however, has limits. As indicated in a later section, other factors such as blood carbon dioxide levels are much more powerful in controlling respiration than conscious control. Regardless of cerebral intent to the contrary, we resume breathing when our bodies sense the need for more oxygen or if carbon dioxide levels increase to certain levels.

FIGURE 14-14

Regulation of respiration. Respiratory control centers in the brainstem control the basic rate and depth of breathing. The brainstem also receives input from other parts of the body; information from chemoreceptors and stretch receptors can alter the basic breathing pattern, as can emotional and sensory input. Despite these controls, the cerebral cortex can override the "automatic" control of breathing to some extent to accomplish activities such as singing or blowing up a balloon. Green arrows show how regulatory information flows into the respiratory control centers. The purple arrow shows the flow of regulatory information from the control centers to the respiratory muscles that drive breathing.

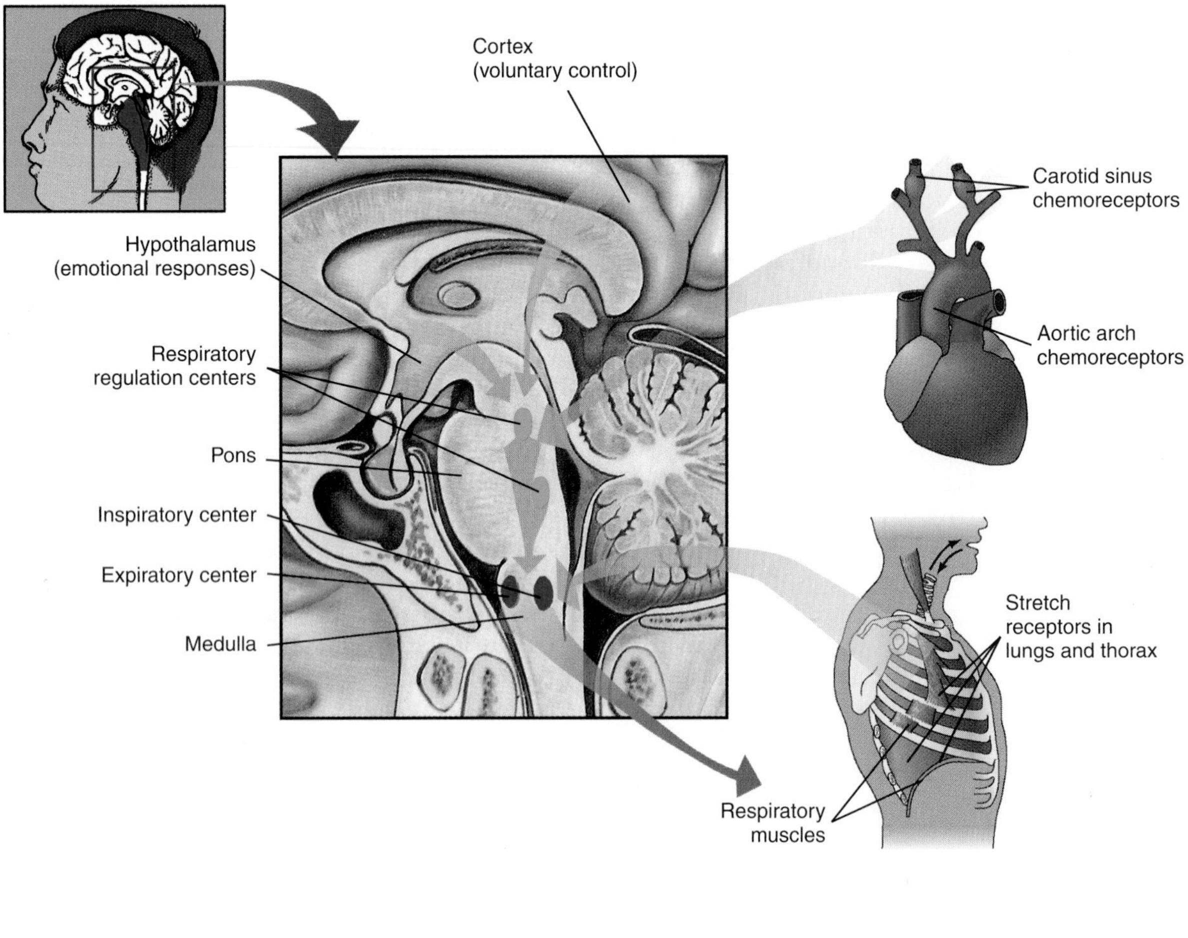

Receptors Influencing Respiration

Chemoreceptors

Chemoreceptors (KEE-mo-ree-SEP-tors) located in the **carotid** and **aortic bodies** are specialized receptors that are sensitive to increases in blood carbon dioxide level and decreases in blood oxygen level. They also can sense and respond to increasing blood acid levels. The carotid body receptors are found at the point where the common carotid arteries divide, and the aortic bodies are small clusters of chemosensitive cells that lie adjacent to the aortic arch near the heart (see Figure 14-14). When stimulated by increasing levels of blood carbon dioxide, decreasing oxygen levels, or increasing blood acidity, these receptors send nerve impulses to the respiratory regulatory centers that in turn modify respiratory rates.

Pulmonary Stretch Receptors

Specialized stretch receptors in the lungs are located throughout the pulmonary airways and in the alveoli (see Figure 14-14). Nervous impulses generated by these receptors influence the normal pattern of breathing and protect the respiratory system from excess stretching caused by harmful overinflation. When the tidal volume of air has been inspired, the lungs are expanded enough to stimulate stretch receptors that then send inhibitory impulses to the inspiratory center. Relaxation of inspiratory muscles occurs, and expiration follows. After expiration, the lungs are sufficiently deflated to inhibit the stretch receptors, and inspiration is then allowed to start again.

TYPES OF BREATHING

Several terms are used to describe breathing patterns. **Eupnea** (YOOP-nee-ah), for example, refers to a normal respiratory rate. During eupnea, the need for oxygen and carbon dioxide exchange is being met, and the individual is usually not aware of the breathing pattern. The terms **hyperventilation** and **hypoventilation** describe very rapid and deep or slow and shallow respirations, respectively. Hyperventilation sometimes results from a conscious voluntary effort preceding exertion or from psychological factors—"hysterical hyperventilation." **Dyspnea** (DISP-nee-ah) refers to labored or difficult breathing and is often associated with hypoventilation. If breathing stops completely for a brief period, regardless of cause, it is called **apnea** (ap-nee-ah). *Sleep apnea* is a condition that results in brief but often frequent stops in breathing during sleep. It is often caused by enlarged tonsil tissue and may necessitate tonsillectomy. Failure to resume breathing after a prolonged period of apnea is called **respiratory arrest.**

Quick Check

1. Where are the respiratory control centers located?
2. What is a chemoreceptor? How does it influence breathing?
3. What is hyperventilation? Hypoventilation?

Science Applications

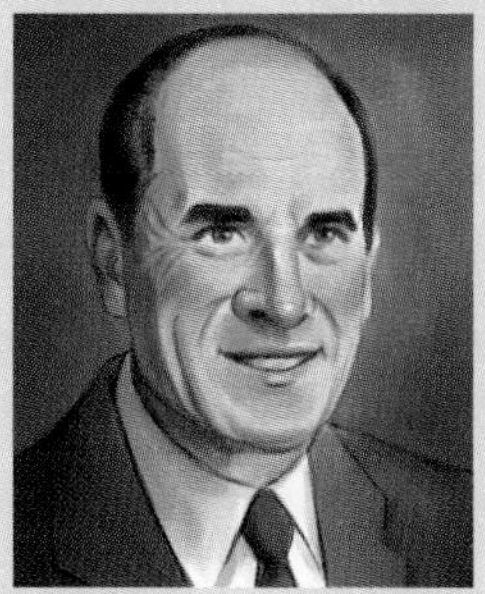

Respiratory Medicine

Henry Heimlich (b. 1920).

The name of American physician Henry Heimlich is known to many people around the world because of the Heimlich maneuver that he developed in 1974 to save the lives of people who are choking (see box on p. 369). What many do not know is that Heimlich has made important breakthroughs throughout his life. For example, after witnessing a soldier die after being shot in the chest in 1945 he went on to develop the Heimlich Chest Drain Valve that drains blood and air out of the chest. In 1980, he developed a tiny tube called the Heimlich MicroTrach that can be inserted into the trachea under local anesthesia and used in oxygen therapy (see box on p. 360). Later, he developed a method for teaching stroke victims who were fed through a tube to swallow again.

Today, Heimlich's first aid techniques are being used by countless emergency medical technicians, paramedics, police and firefighters trained in first aid, and even ordinary citizens who have been trained in these lifesaving procedures. Physicians, respiratory therapists, and many other health professionals continue to use Heimlich's medical procedures along with many other respiratory treatments to save the lives of their patients.

OUTLINE SUMMARY

STRUCTURAL PLAN

Basic plan of respiratory system would be similar to an inverted tree if it were hollow; leaves of the tree would be comparable to alveoli, with the microscopic sacs enclosed by networks of capillaries (Figure 14-1)

RESPIRATORY TRACTS

A. Upper respiratory tract—nose, pharynx, and larynx
B. Lower respiratory tract—trachea, bronchial tree, and lungs

RESPIRATORY MUCOSA

A. Specialized membrane that lines the air distribution tubes in the respiratory tree (Figure 14-3)
B. More than 125 ml of mucus produced each day forms a "mucous blanket" over much of the respiratory mucosa
C. Mucus serves as an air purification mechanism by trapping inspired irritants such as dust and pollen
D. Cilia on mucosal cells beat in only one direction, moving mucus upward to pharynx for removal

NOSE

A. Structure
  1. Nasal septum separates interior of nose into two cavities
  2. Mucous membrane lines nose
  3. Frontal, maxillary, sphenoidal, and ethmoidal sinuses drain into nose (Figure 14-4)
B. Functions
  1. Warms and moistens inhaled air
  2. Contains sense organs of smell

PHARYNX

A. Structure (Figure 14-5)
  1. Pharynx (throat) about 12.5 cm (5 inches) long
  2. Divided into nasopharynx, oropharynx, and laryngopharynx
  3. Two nasal cavities, mouth, esophagus, larynx, and auditory tubes all have openings into pharynx
  4. Pharyngeal tonsils and openings of auditory tubes open into nasopharynx; tonsils found in oropharynx
  5. Mucous membrane lines pharynx
B. Functions
  1. Passageway for food and liquids
  2. Air distribution; passageway for air

LARYNX

A. Structure (Figure 14-6)
  1. Several pieces of cartilage form framework
    a. Thyroid cartilage (Adam's apple) is largest
    b. Epiglottis partially covers opening into larynx
  2. Mucous lining
  3. Vocal cords stretch across interior of larynx
B. Functions
  1. Air distribution; passageway for air to move to and from lungs
  2. Voice production

TRACHEA

A. Structure (Figure 14-7)
  1. Tube about 11 cm (4.5 inches) long that extends from larynx into the thoracic cavity
  2. Mucous lining
  3. C-shaped rings of cartilage hold trachea open
B. Function—passageway for air to move to and from lungs
C. Obstruction
  1. Blockage of trachea occludes the airway and if complete causes death in minutes
  2. Tracheal obstruction causes more than 4000 deaths annually in the United States
  3. Heimlich maneuver (p. 369) is a lifesaving technique used to free the trachea of obstructions

OUTLINE SUMMARY—*cont'd*

BRONCHI, BRONCHIOLES, AND ALVEOLI

A. Structure
  1. Trachea branches into right and left bronchi
  2. Each bronchus branches into smaller and smaller tubes eventually leading to bronchioles
  3. Bronchioles end in clusters of microscopic alveolar sacs, the walls of which are made up of alveoli (Figure 14-8)

B. Function
  1. Bronchi and bronchioles—air distribution; passageway for air to move to and from alveoli
  2. Alveoli—exchange of gases between air and blood

LUNGS AND PLEURA

A. Structure (Figure 14-9)
  1. Size—large enough to fill the chest cavity, except for middle space occupied by heart and large blood vessels
  2. Apex—narrow upper part of each lung, under collarbone
  3. Base—broad lower part of each lung; rests on diaphragm
  4. Pleura—moist, smooth, slippery membrane that lines chest cavity and covers outer surface of lungs; reduces friction between the lungs and chest wall during breathing (Figure 14-10)

B. Function—breathing (pulmonary ventilation)

RESPIRATION

A. Mechanics of breathing (Figure 14-11)
  1. Pulmonary ventilation includes two phases called *inspiration* (movement of air into lungs) and *expiration* (movement of air out of lungs)
  2. Changes in size and shape of thorax cause changes in air pressure within that cavity and in the lungs
  3. Air pressure differences actually cause air to move into and out of the lungs

B. Inspiration
  1. Active process—air moves into lungs
  2. Inspiratory muscles include diaphragm and external intercostals
     a. Diaphragm flattens during inspiration—increases top-to-bottom length of thorax
     b. External intercostals contraction elevates the ribs and increases the size of the thorax from the front to the back and from side to side
  3. The increase in the size of the chest cavity reduces pressure within it, and air enters the lungs

C. Expiration
  1. Quiet expiration is ordinarily a passive process
  2. During expiration, thorax returns to its resting size and shape
  3. Elastic recoil of lung tissues aids in expiration
  4. Expiratory muscles used in forceful expiration are internal intercostals and abdominal muscles
     a. Internal intercostals—contraction depresses the rib cage and decreases the size of the thorax from the front to back
     b. Contraction of abdominal muscles elevates the diaphragm, thus decreasing size of the thoracic cavity from the top to bottom
  5. Reduction in the size of the thoracic cavity increases its pressure and air leaves the lungs

D. Exchange of gases in lungs (Figure 14-12)
  1. Carbaminohemoglobin breaks down into carbon dioxide and hemoglobin
  2. Carbon dioxide moves out of lung capillary blood into alveolar air and out of body in expired air

Continued

OUTLINE SUMMARY—*cont'd*

3. Oxygen moves from alveoli into lung capillaries
4. Hemoglobin combines with oxygen, producing oxyhemoglobin

E. Exchange of gases in tissues
1. Oxyhemoglobin breaks down into oxygen and hemoglobin
2. Oxygen moves out of tissue capillary blood into tissue cells
3. Carbon dioxide moves from tissue cells into tissue capillary blood
4. Hemoglobin combines with carbon dioxide, forming carbaminohemoglobin

F. Volumes of air exchanged in pulmonary ventilation (Figure 14-13)
1. Volumes of air exchanged in breathing can be measured with a spirometer
2. Tidal volume (TV)—amount normally breathed in or out with each breath
3. Vital capacity (VC)—greatest amount of air that one can breathe out in one expiration
4. Expiratory reserve volume (ERV)—amount of air that can be forcibly exhaled after expiring the tidal volume
5. Inspiratory reserve volume (IRV)—amount of air that can be forcibly inhaled after a normal inspiration
6. Residual volume (RV)—air that remains in the lungs after the most forceful expiration
7. Rate—usually about 12 to 18 breaths a minute; much faster during exercise

G. Regulation of respiration (Figure 14-14)
1. Regulation of respiration permits the body to adjust to varying demands for oxygen supply and carbon dioxide removal
2. Most important central regulatory centers in medulla are called *respiratory control centers* (inspiratory and expiratory centers)
   a. Under resting conditions, nervous activity in the respiratory control centers produces a normal rate and depth of respirations (12 to 18 per minute)
3. Respiratory control centers in the medulla are influenced by "inputs" from receptors located in other body areas:
   a. Cerebral cortex—voluntary (but limited) control of respiratory activity
   b. Chemoreceptors respond to changes in carbon dioxide, oxygen, and blood acid levels—located in carotid and aortic bodies
   c. Pulmonary stretch receptors—respond to the stretch in lungs, thus protecting respiratory organs from overinflation

TYPES OF BREATHING

A. Eupnea—normal breathing
B. Hyperventilation—rapid and deep respirations
C. Hypoventilation—slow and shallow respirations
D. Dyspnea—labored or difficult respirations
E. Apnea—stopped respiration
F. Respiratory arrest—failure to resume breathing after a period of apnea

NEW WORDS

alveoli	expiratory reserve volume (ERV)	paranasal sinuses	spirometer
aortic body	Heimlich maneuver	pharynx	surfactant
apnea	hyperventilation	pleurisy	tidal volume (TV)
bronchi	hypoventilation	pulmonary ventilation	tonsillectomy
carbaminohemoglobin	inspiratory reserve volume (IRV)	residual volume (RV)	trachea
carotid body	larynx	respiration	vital capacity (VC)
conchae	oxyhemoglobin	respiratory arrest	
dyspnea		respiratory membrane	
eupnea			

REVIEW QUESTIONS

1. Differentiate between the respiratory membrane and the respiratory mucosa.
2. List the functions of the paranasal sinuses.
3. What is the function of the auditory tube?
4. What is the function of the epiglottis?
5. Describe, in decreasing order of size, the structures that make up the air tubes of the lung.
6. Describe the pleura. What is the function of pleural fluid?
7. Differentiate between external respiration, internal respiration, and cellular respiration.
8. Explain the mechanical process of inspiration.
9. Explain the mechanical process of expiration.
10. Explain how gas is exchanged between the lung and the blood, and between the blood and the tissues.
11. How is oxygen carried in the blood? How is carbon dioxide carried in the blood?
12. Name and explain the volumes that make up vital capacity.
13. Explain the function of chemoreceptors in regulating respiration.
14. Explain the function of stretch receptors in the lung.

CRITICAL THINKING

15. Explain the effect smoking has on the body's ability to remove trapped material in the respiratory mucosa.
16. The developing fetus does not produce lung surfactant until late in its development. Explain what problem a premature infant would have if it were born before it had produced surfactant.
17. Explain the role of other systems in the regulation of respiration.

CHAPTER TEST

1. The organs of the respiratory system are designed to perform two basic functions: *air distribution* and *gas exchange*

2. The upper respiratory tract consists of the *nose*, the *pharynx* and the *larynx*

3. The lower respiratory tract consists of the *trachea* the *bronchial tree* and the *lungs*.

4. The membrane that separates the air in the alveoli from the blood in the surrounding capillaries is called the *respiratory membrane*

5. The membrane that lines most of the air distribution tubes in the respiratory system is called the *respiratory mucosa*

6. The frontal, maxillary, sphenoidal, and ethmoidal cavities make up the *paranasal sinus*

7. The *lacrimal* sacs drain tears into the nasal cavity.

8. The *conchae* protrude into the nasal cavities and function to warm and humidify the air.

9. The *pharynx* is the structure that can also be called the throat.

10. The *larynx* is also called the voice box.

11. The *trachea* is the large air tube in the neck.

12. The four progressively smaller air tubes that connect the trachea and the alveolar sacs are the *primary bronchi, 2ndary bronchi, bronchioles* and the *alveolar ducts*

13. A *surfactant* is a substance made by the lungs to help reduce the surface tension of water in the alveoli.

14. The right lung is made up of ___3___ lobes, while the left lung is made up of ___2___ lobes.

15. The exchange of gases between the blood and the tissues is called *internal respiratory*

16. The exchange of gases between the blood and the air in the lungs is called *external respiratory*

17. The *Diaphragm* is the most important muscle in respiration.

18. Oxygen is carried in the blood as *oxyhemoglobin*

19. Carbon dioxide can be carried in the blood as the *bicarbonat* ion or combined with hemoglobin as *carbaminohemoglobin*

20. The inspiratory and expiratory centers are located in this part of the brain: *Medulla*.

21. *Stretch receptors* are the receptors that inhibit the inspiratory center that keep the lungs from overexpanding.

22. *Chemoreceptors* are the receptors that modify respiratory rates by responding to the amount of carbon dioxide, oxygen, or acid levels in the blood.

23. The amount of air that is moved in and out of the lung during normal breathing is called *Tidal* volume.

24. The three volumes that make up vital capacity are *tidal* *expiratory reserve*, and *inspiratory reserve*.

25. The volume included in total lung capacity but not vital capacity is *residual* volume.

STUDY TIPS

Before starting Chapter 14, review the synopsis of the respiratory system in Chapter 4. The structure of the respiratory system can be described as tubes and bags. All the structures except the alveoli are tubes. Their job is to get air to and from the alveoli where oxygen and carbon dioxide are exchanged within the blood. Flash cards can be used to learn the names, locations, and functions of the structures. Lungs are passive organs. To move air in or out of the lungs, the pressure of the chest cavity must be raised or lowered. To lower the pressure, the volume must increase (Boyle's law). This is done by contracting the diaphragm, which causes air to enter the lung. When the diaphragm relaxes, the volume of the chest cavity decreases, the pressure goes up, and air is pushed out of the lung. The function of the respiratory system is to supply the cells with oxygen and remove carbon dioxide. All it really does is to supply the blood with oxygen and remove carbon dioxide from the blood. Oxygen moves into the blood, forming a weak bond with the hemoglobin. When the blood gets to the tissue, it gives up the oxygen and takes on carbon dioxide. It carries carbon dioxide as the bicarbonate ion or by combining it with hemoglobin. The *carbon* dioxide joins with an *amino* acid in the *hemoglobin* forming the compound *carbaminohemoglobin* (see how easy that will be to remember?). When the blood gets to the lung, the carbon dioxide dissociates and is exhaled. Figure 14-2 shows this very well. The volumes are fairly easy and can be learned using flash cards.

In your study group you should go over the flash cards of the structures of the respiratory system and pulmonary volumes. Discuss the processes of inspiration, expiration, and regulation of respiration. Use a photocopy of Figure 14-2 with the information blackened out to explain both internal (in the tissues) and external (in the lung) respiration. Go over the questions at the end of the chapter and discuss possible test questions.

15
The Digestive System

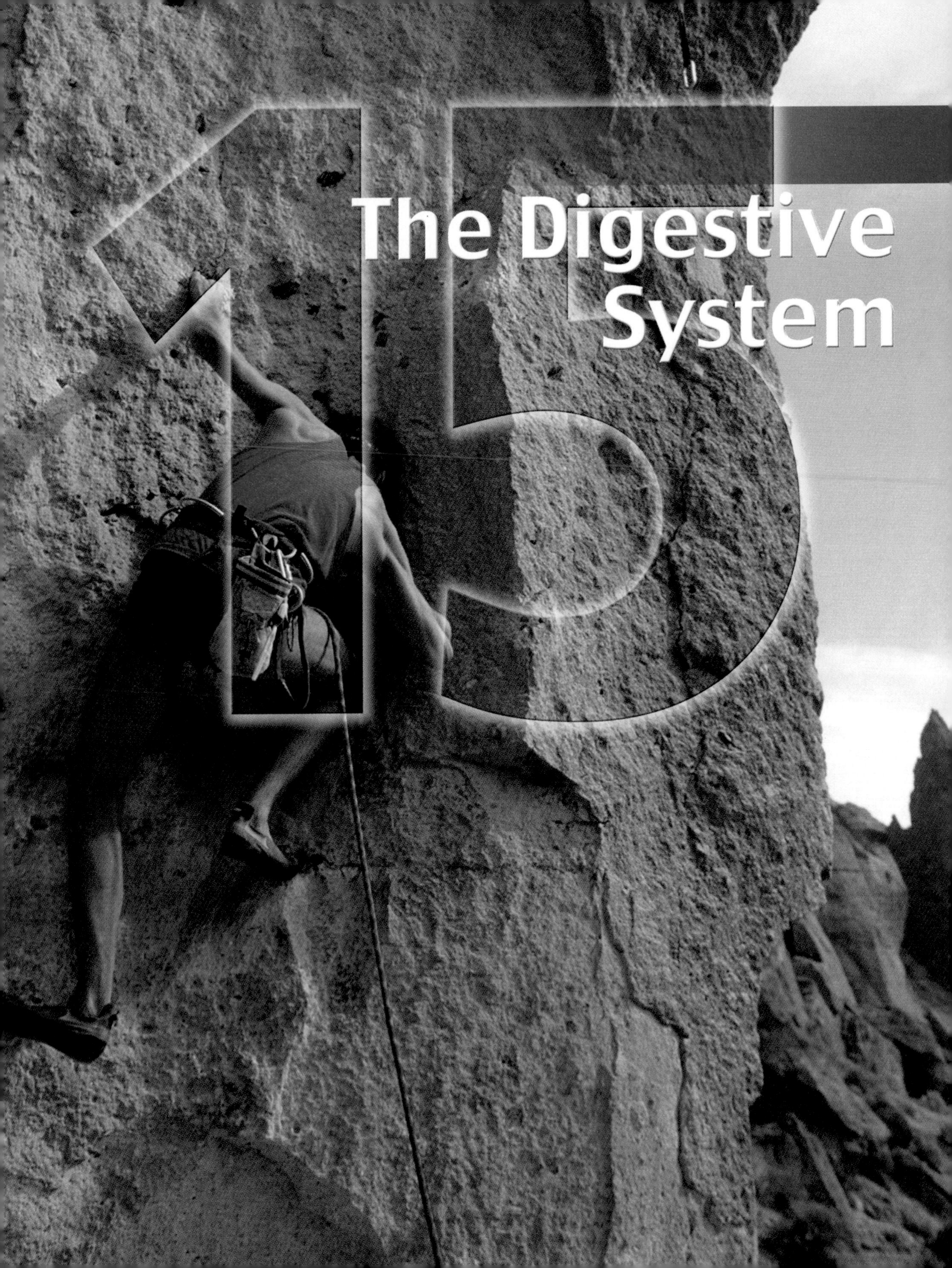

Outline

Objectives

AFTER YOU HAVE COMPLETED THIS CHAPTER, YOU SHOULD BE ABLE TO:

1. List in sequence each of the component parts or segments of the alimentary canal from the mouth to the anus and identify the accessory organs of digestion.
2. List and describe the four layers of the wall of the alimentary canal. Compare the lining layer in the esophagus, stomach, small intestine, and large intestine.
3. Discuss the basics of protein, fat, and carbohydrate digestion and give the end products of each process.
4. Define and contrast mechanical and chemical digestion.
5. Define *peristalsis, bolus, chyme, jaundice, ulcer,* and *diarrhea.*

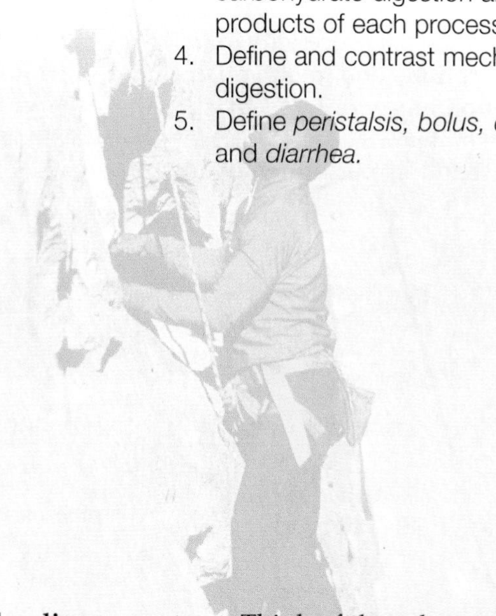

T*he principal structure* of the **digestive system** is an irregular tube, open at both ends, called the **alimentary** (al-i-MEN-tar-ee) **canal** or the **gastrointestinal** (gas-tro-in-TES-ti-nal) **(GI) tract.** In the adult, this hollow tube is about 9 m (29 feet) long. Although this may seem strange, food or other material that enters the digestive tube is not really inside the body. Most parents of young children quickly learn that a button or pebble swallowed by their child will almost always pass unchanged and with little difficulty through the tract. Think of the tube as a passageway that extends through the body like a hallway through a building. Food must be broken down or **digested** and then absorbed through the walls of the digestive tube before it can actually enter the body and be used by cells. The breakdown or digestion of food material is both mechanical and chemical in nature. The teeth are used to physically break down food material before it is swallowed. The churning of food in the stomach then continues the mechanical breakdown process. Chemical breakdown results from the action of digestive enzymes and other chemicals acting on food as it passes through the GI tract. In chemical digestion, large food molecules are reduced to smaller molecules that can be absorbed through the lining of the intestinal wall and then distributed to body cells for use. This process of altering the chemical and physical composition of food so that it can be absorbed and used by body cells is known as *digestion*, and it is the function of the digestive system. Part of the digestive system, the large intestine, serves also as an organ of elimination, ridding the body of the waste material or **feces** resulting from the digestive process. Table 15-1 names both main and accessory digestive organs. Note that the accessory organs include the teeth, tongue, gallbladder, and appendix, as well as a number of glands that secrete their products into the digestive tube.

Foods undergo three kinds of processing in the body: **digestion, absorption,** and **metabolism.** Digestion and absorption are performed by the organs of the digestive system (Figure 15-1). Metabolism, on the other hand, is performed by all body cells. In this chapter, we shall begin by describing digestive organs and then discuss digestion and absorption. Later, in Chapter 16, we will discuss the metabolism of food after it has been absorbed.

WALL OF THE DIGESTIVE TRACT

The digestive tract has been described as a tube that extends from the mouth to the anus. The wall of this digestive tube is fashioned of four layers of tissue (Figure 15-2). The inside or hollow space within the tube is called the **lumen.** The four layers, named from the inside coat to the outside of the tube, follow:

1. Mucosa or mucous membrane
2. Submucosa
3. Muscularis
4. Serosa

Although the same four tissue coats form the organs of the alimentary tract, their structures

TABLE 15-1

Organs of the Digestive System

MAIN ORGAN	ACCESSORY ORGAN	MAIN ORGAN	ACCESSORY ORGAN
Mouth	Teeth and tongue	Large intestine	Vermiform appendix
	Salivary glands	Cecum	
	Parotid	Colon	
	Submandibular	Ascending colon	
	Sublingual	Transverse colon	
Pharynx (throat)		Descending colon	
Esophagus		Sigmoid colon	
Stomach		Rectum	
Small intestine	Liver	Anal canal	
Duodenum	Gallbladder		
Jejunum	Pancreas		
Ileum			

FIGURE 15-1

Location of digestive organs.

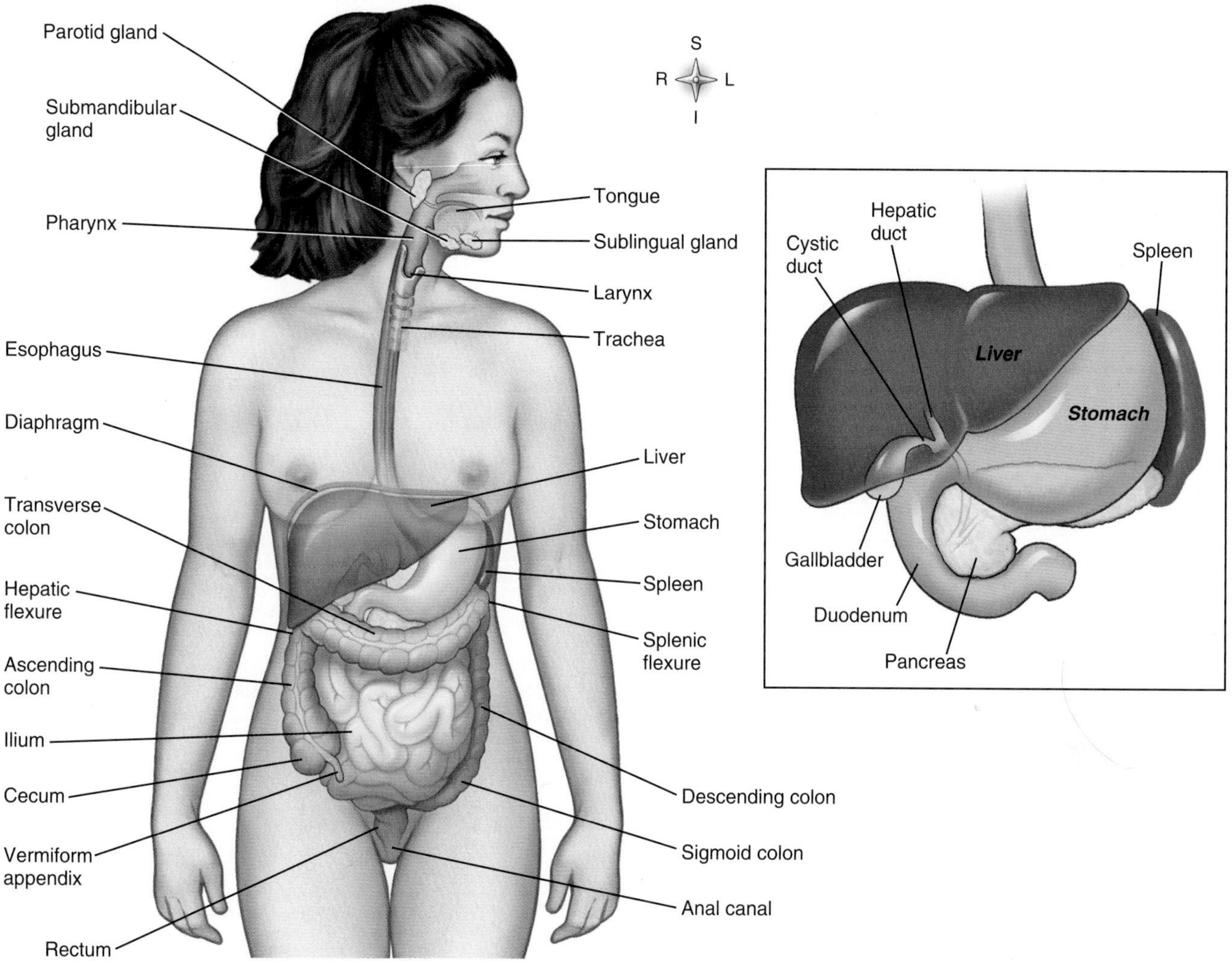

vary in different organs. The **mucosa** of the esophagus, for example, is composed of tough and stratified abrasion-resistant epithelium. The mucosa of the remainder of the tract is a delicate layer of simple columnar epithelium designed for absorption and secretion. The mucus produced by either type of epithelium coats the lining of the alimentary canal.

The **submucosa,** as the name implies, is a connective tissue layer that lies just below the mucosa. It contains many blood vessels and nerves. The two layers of muscle tissue called the **muscularis** have an important function in the digestive process. By a wavelike, rhythmic contraction of the muscular coat, called **peristalsis** (pair-i-STAL-sis), food material is moved through the digestive

FIGURE 15-2

Section of the small intestine. The four layers typical of walls of the gastrointestinal tract are shown. Circular folds of mucous membrane called plicae increase the surface area of the lining coat.

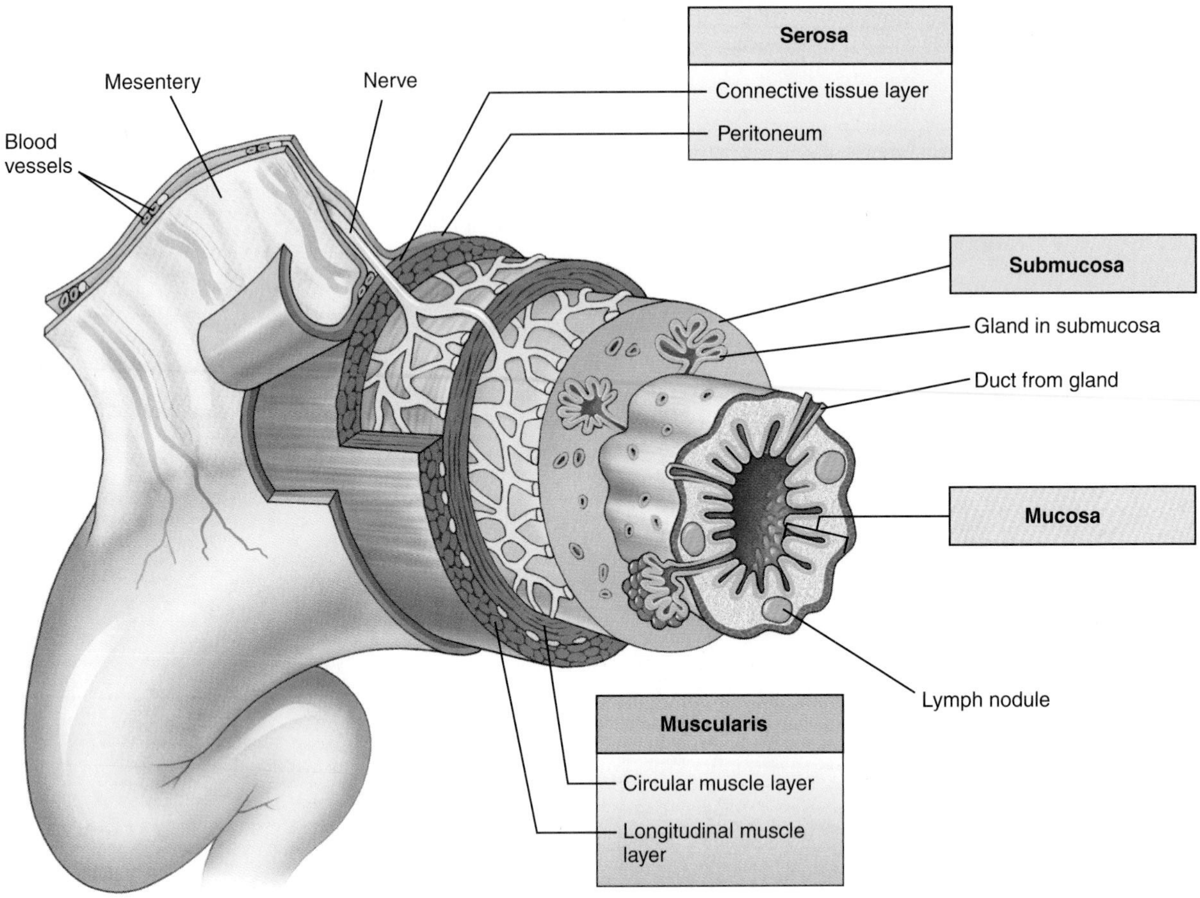

tube (Figure 15-3). In addition, the contraction of the muscularis also assists in the mixing of food with digestive juice and in the further mechanical breakdown of larger food particles.

The **serosa** is the outermost covering or coat of the digestive tube. In the abdominal cavity it is composed of the visceral peritoneum. The loops of the digestive tract are anchored to the posterior wall of the abdominal cavity by a large double fold of peritoneal tissue called the **mesentery** (MEZ-en-tair-ee).

MOUTH

The **mouth** or **oral cavity** is a hollow chamber with a roof, a floor, and walls. Food enters or is ingested into the digestive tract through the mouth, and the process of digestion begins immediately. As with the remainder of the digestive tract, the mouth is lined with mucous membrane. It may be helpful if you review the structure and function of mucous membranes in Chapter 5. Typically, mucous membranes line hollow organs, such as the digestive

FIGURE 15-3

Peristalsis. Peristalsis moves a *bolus* (chunk) of food by a wavelike contraction of muscle in the wall of the digestive tract that pushes material in front of it as moves along.

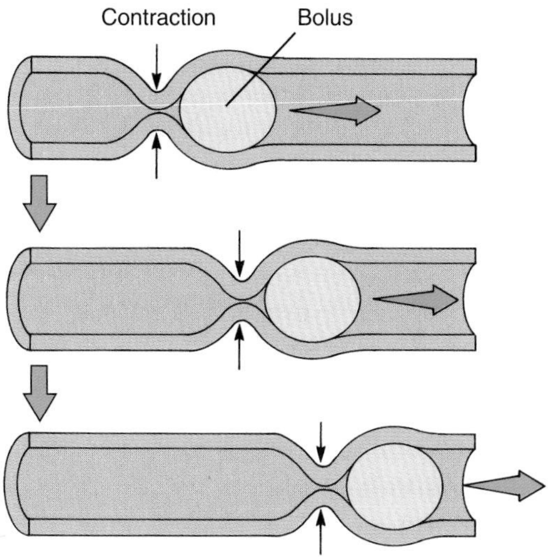

FIGURE 15-4

The mouth cavity.

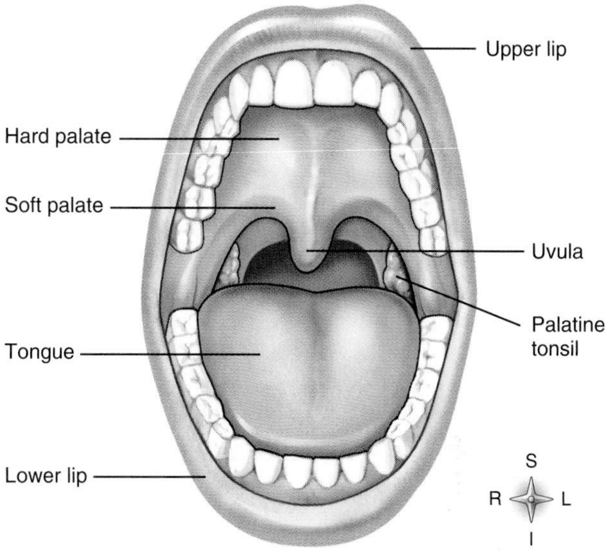

tube, that open to the exterior of the body. Mucus produced by the lining of the GI tract protects the epithelium from digestive juices and lubricates food passing through the lumen.

The roof of the mouth is formed by the **hard** and **soft palates** (Figure 15-4). The hard palate is a bony structure in the anterior or front portion of the mouth formed by parts of the palatine and maxillary bones. The soft palate is located above the posterior or rear portion of the mouth. It is soft because it consists chiefly of muscle. Hanging down from the center of the soft palate is a cone-shaped structure, the **uvula** (YOO-vyoo-lah). If you look in the mirror, open your mouth wide, and say "Ah," you can see your uvula. The uvula and the soft palate prevent any food and liquid from entering the nasal cavities above the mouth.

The floor of the mouth consists of the tongue and its muscles. The tongue is made of skeletal muscle covered with mucous membrane. It is anchored to bones in the skull and to the hyoid bone in the neck. A thin membrane called the **frenulum** (FREN-yoo-lum) attaches the tongue to the floor of the mouth. Occasionally the frenulum is too short to allow free movements of the tongue. Individuals with this condition cannot enunciate words normally and are said to be tongue-tied. Note in Figure 15-5 that the tongue can be divided into a blunt rear portion called the *root*, a pointed *tip*, and a central *body*.

Have you ever noticed the many small elevations on the surface of your tongue? They are **papillae.** The largest are the **vallate** type; as you can see in Figure 15-5, they form an inverted V-shaped row of about 10 to 12 mushroomlike elevations. The taste buds, which contain sensory receptors for salty, sour, sweet, and bitter compounds, are located on the papillae (see Chapter 9).

Quick Check

1. What is the alimentary canal?
2. What three kinds of processing does food undergo in the body?
3. Can you describe the layers of the digestive tract's wall?
4. What is the uvula? What does it do?

FIGURE 15-5

The tongue. A, Surface. **B,** Mouth cavity showing the undersurface of the tongue.

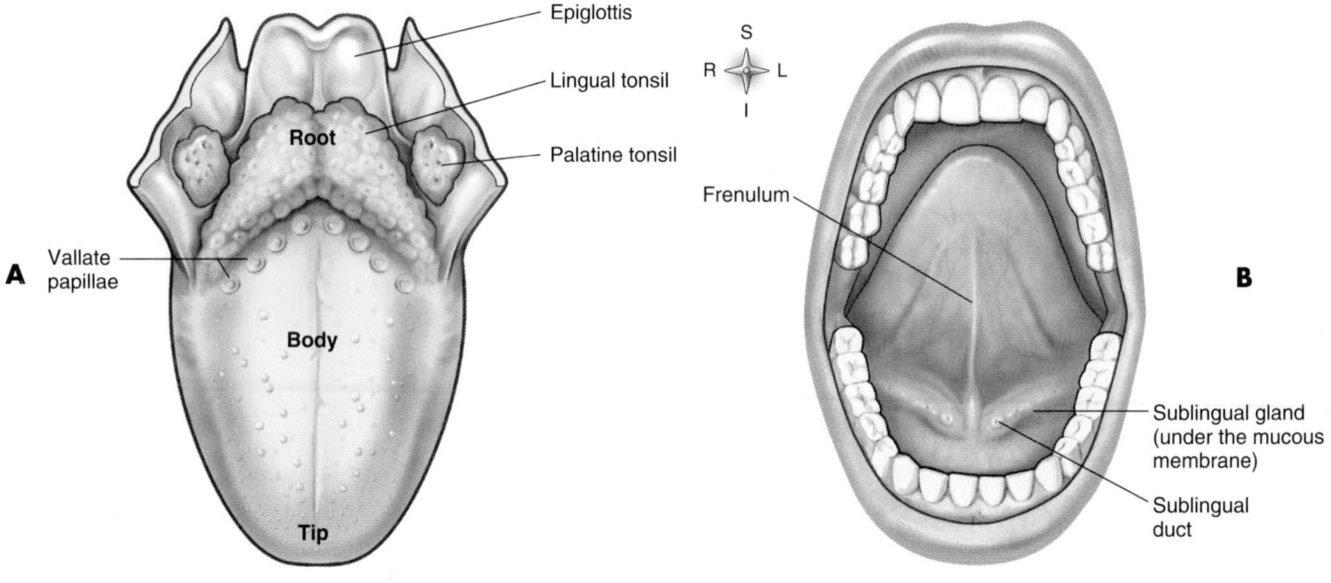

TEETH

The shape and placement of the teeth assist in their functions. The four major types of teeth follow:

1. Incisors
2. Canines
3. Premolars
4. Molars

Note in Figure 15-6 that the incisors have a sharp cutting edge. They have a cutting function during **mastication** (mas-ti-KAY-shun) or chewing of food. The canine teeth are sometimes called **cuspids.** They pierce or tear the food that is being eaten. This tooth type is particularly apparent in meat-eating mammals such as dogs. Premolars or **bicuspids** and molars or **tricuspids** have rather large, flat surfaces with two or three grinding or crushing "cusps" on their surface. They provide extensive breakdown of food in the mouth. After food has been chewed, it is formed into a small rounded mass called a **bolus** (BO-lus) so that it can be swallowed.

By the time a baby is 2 years old, the child probably has a full set of 20 baby teeth. When a young adult is somewhere between 17 and 24 years old, a full set of 32 permanent teeth is generally present. The average age for cutting the first tooth is about 6 months, and the average age for losing the first baby tooth and starting to cut the permanent teeth is about 6 years. Figure 15-6 gives the names of the teeth and shows which ones are lacking in the deciduous or baby set.

Typical Tooth

A typical tooth can be divided into three main parts: crown, neck, and root. The **crown** is the portion that is exposed and visible in the mouth. It is covered by enamel—the hardest tissue in the body. Enamel is ideally suited to withstand the grinding that occurs during the chewing of hard and brittle foods. In addition to enamel, the outer shell of each tooth is covered by two other dental

FIGURE 15-6

The deciduous (baby) teeth and adult teeth. In the deciduous set, there are no premolars and only two pairs of molars in each jaw. Generally the lower teeth erupt before the corresponding upper teeth.

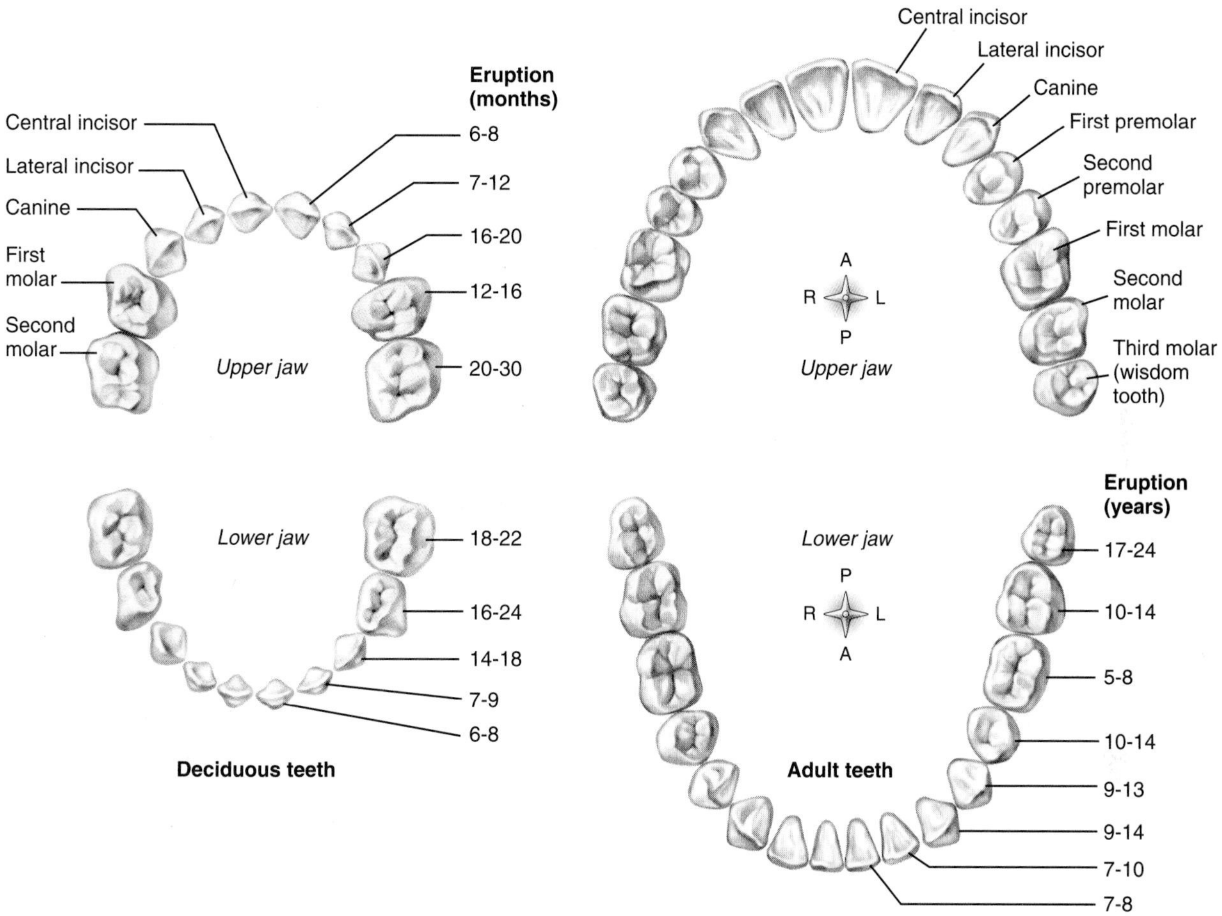

tissues—dentin and cementum (Figure 15-7). Dentin makes up the greatest proportion of the tooth shell. It is covered by enamel in the crown and by cementum in the neck and root areas. The center of the tooth contains a pulp cavity consisting of connective tissue, blood and lymphatic vessels, and sensory nerves.

The **neck** of a tooth is the narrow portion, shown in Figure 15-7, surrounded by the pink gingiva or gum tissue. It joins the crown of the tooth to the root. The **root** fits into the socket of the upper or lower jaw. A fibrous **periodontal membrane** lines each tooth socket.

Tooth decay or *dental caries* is a disease of the enamel, dentin, and cementum of teeth that results in the formation of a permanent defect called a **cavity.** Decay occurs on tooth surfaces where food debris, acid-secreting bacteria, and plaque accumulate. Regular and thorough brushing of the teeth and the introduction of fluoride to water supplies have proven to be the most effective and practical methods of reducing the rate of tooth decay.

FIGURE 15-7

Longitudinal section of a tooth. A molar is sectioned to show its bony socket and details of its three main parts: crown, neck, and root. Enamel (over the crown) and cementum (over the neck and root) surround the dentin layer. The pulp contains nerves and blood vessels.

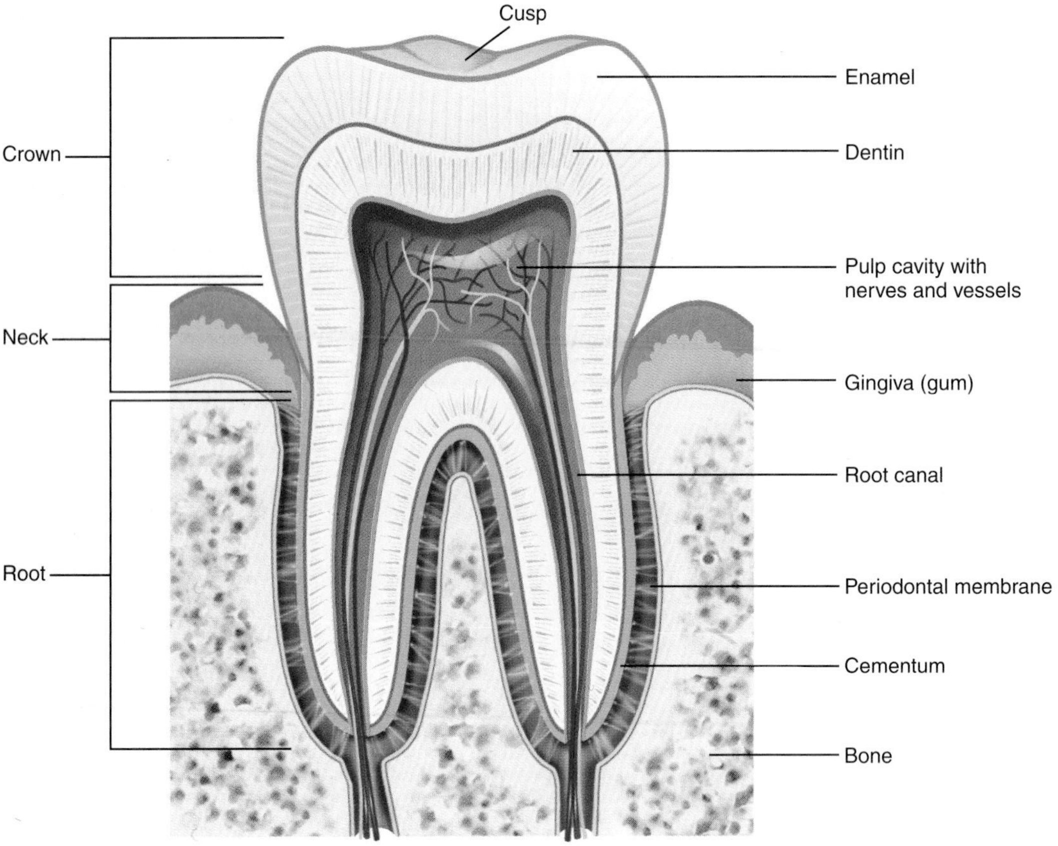

SALIVARY GLANDS

Three pairs of salivary glands—the parotids, submandibulars, and sublinguals—secrete most (about 1 L) of the saliva produced each day in the adult. The salivary glands (Figure 15-8) are typical of the accessory glands associated with the digestive system. They are located outside of the digestive tube itself and must convey their secretions by way of ducts into the tract.

The **parotid glands,** largest of the salivary glands, lie just below and in front of each ear at the angle of the jaw—an interesting anatomical position because it explains why people who have mumps (an infection of the parotid gland) often complain that it hurts when they open their mouths or chew; these movements squeeze the tender, inflamed gland. To see the openings of the parotid ducts, look in a mirror at the insides of your cheeks opposite the second molar tooth on either side of the upper jaw.

The ducts of the **submandibular glands** open into the mouth on either side of the lingual frenulum (see Figure 15-5). The ducts of the **sublingual glands** open into the floor of the mouth.

Saliva contains mucus and a digestive enzyme that is called **salivary amylase** (AM-i-lase). Mucus moistens the food and allows it to pass with less friction through the esophagus and into the stomach. Salivary amylase begins the chemical digestion of carbohydrates.

PHARYNX

The **pharynx** is a tubelike structure made of muscle and lined with mucous membrane. Observe its location in Figure 15-1. Because of its location behind the nasal cavities and mouth, it functions as part of the respiratory and digestive systems. Air must pass through the pharynx on its way to the lungs, and food must pass through it on its way to the stomach. The pharynx as a whole is subdivided into three anatomical components, as described in Chapter 14.

ESOPHAGUS

The **esophagus** (e-SOF-ah-gus) is the muscular, mucus-lined tube that connects the pharynx with the stomach. It is about 25 centimeters (10 inches) long. The esophagus serves as a dynamic passageway for food, pushing the food toward the stomach. The production of mucus by glands in the mucosal lining lubricates the tube to permit easier passage of food moving toward the stomach.

Quick Check

1. What are the four major types of teeth?
2. What digestive enzyme is found in saliva?
3. How do the pharynx and esophagus play roles in the digestive tract?

STOMACH

The **stomach** (Figure 15-9) lies in the upper part of the abdominal cavity just under the diaphragm. It serves as a pouch that food enters after it has been chewed, swallowed, and passed through the esophagus. The stomach looks small after it is emptied, not much bigger than a large sausage, but it expands considerably after a large meal. Have you ever felt so uncomfortably full after eating that you could not take a deep breath? If so, it probably meant that your stomach was so full of food that it occupied more space than usual and pushed up against the diaphragm. This made it hard for the diaphragm to contract and move downward as much as necessary for a deep breath.

After food has entered the stomach by passing through the muscular **gastroesophageal** (GAS-tro-e-SOF-ah-JEE-al) or **cardiac sphincter** (SFINGK-ter) at the end of the esophagus, the digestive process continues. Sphincters are rings of muscle tissue. The cardiac sphincter keeps food from reentering the esophagus when the stomach contracts. Occasionally, the opening in the diaphragm that permits the passage of the esophagus into the abdomen is enlarged. This may permit a bulging of the end of the esophagus and part or even all of the stomach upward through the diaphragm and into the chest.

FIGURE 15-8

Location of the salivary glands.

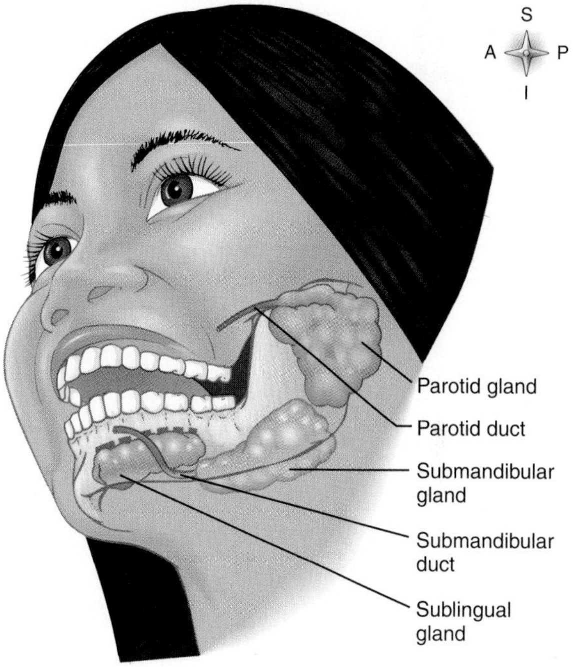

Clinical Application

Malocclusion

Malocclusion of the teeth occurs when missing teeth create wide spaces in the dentition, when teeth overlap, or when malposition of one or more teeth prevents correct alignment of the maxillary and mandibular dental arches (Figures *A* and *B*). Malocclusion that results in protrusion of the upper front teeth causing them to hang over the lower front teeth is called *overbite* (Figure *A*), whereas the positioning of the lower front teeth outside the upper front teeth is called *underbite* (Figure *B*).

Dental malocclusion may cause significant problems and chronic pain in the functioning of the temporomandibular joint, contribute to the generation of headaches, or complicate routine mastication of food. Fortunately, even severe malocclusion problems can be corrected by the use of braces and other dental appliances. Orthodontics (or-tho-DON-tiks) is that branch of dentistry that deals with the prevention and correction of positioning irregularities of the teeth and malocclusion.

A

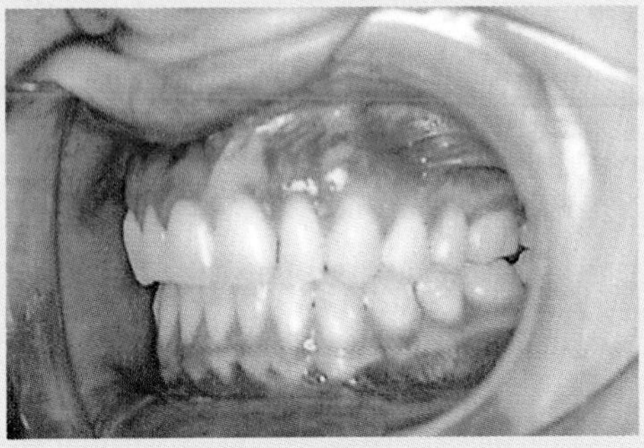

Overbite

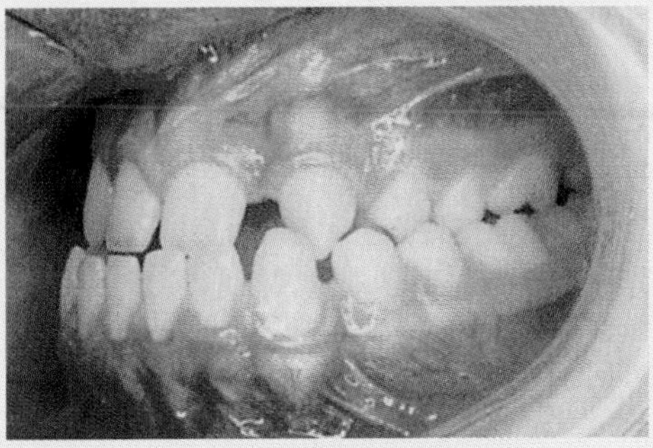

B

Underbite

The condition, called a **hiatal** (hi-AY-tal) **hernia,** may result in backward movement or reflux of stomach contents into the lower portion of the esophagus. The resulting symptoms are referred to as **gastroesophageal reflux disease** (see box).

Contraction of the stomach's muscular walls mixes the food thoroughly with the gastric juice and breaks it down into a semisolid mixture called **chyme** (KIME). Gastric juice contains hydrochloric acid and enzymes that function in the digestive process. Chyme formation is a continuation of the mechanical digestive process that begins in the mouth.

Note in Figure 15-9 that there are three layers of smooth muscle in the stomach wall. The muscle fibers that run lengthwise, around, and obliquely make the stomach one of the strongest internal organs—well able to break up food into tiny particles and to mix them thoroughly with gastric juice to form chyme. Stomach muscle contractions result in **peristalsis,** which propels food down the digestive tract. Mucous membrane lines the stomach; it contains thousands of microscopic **gastric glands** that secrete gastric juice and hydrochloric acid into the stomach. When the stomach is empty, its lining lies in folds called **rugae.**

The three divisions of the stomach shown in Figure 15-9 are the **fundus, body,** and **pylorus** (pye-LOR-us). The fundus is the enlarged portion to the left of and above the opening of the esophagus into the stomach. The body is the central part of the stomach, and the pylorus is its lower narrow section, which joins the first part of the small intestine. Partial digestion occurs after food is held in the stomach by the **pyloric** (pi-LOR-ik) **sphincter** muscle. The smooth muscle fibers of the sphincter stay contracted most of the time and thereby close off the opening of the pylorus into the small intestine.

FIGURE 15-9

Stomach. A portion of the anterior wall has been cut away to reveal the muscle layers of the stomach wall. Notice that the mucosa lining the stomach forms folds called *rugae*.

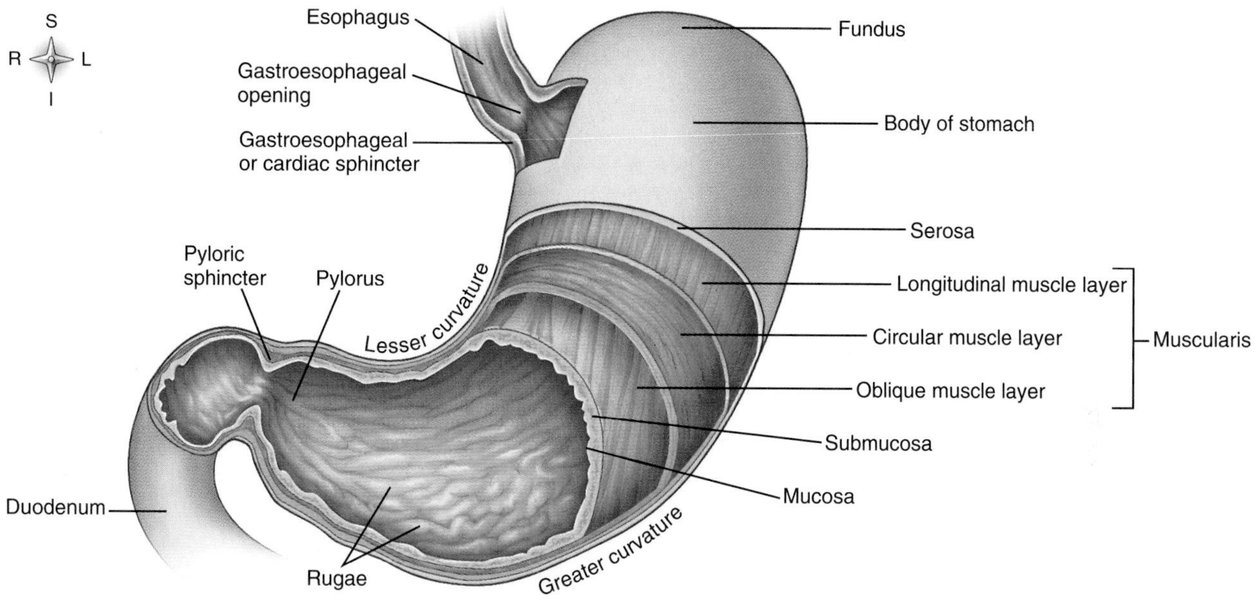

Clinical Application

Gastroesophageal Reflux Disease (GERD)

The terms *heartburn* or *acid indigestion* are often used to describe a number of unpleasant symptoms experienced by more than 60 million Americans each month. Backward flow of stomach acid up into the esophagus causes these symptoms, which typically include burning and pressure behind the breastbone. The term **gastroesophageal reflux disease (GERD)** is now used to better describe this very common and sometimes serious medical condition.

In its simplest form, GERD produces mild symptoms that occur only infrequently (twice a week or less). In these cases, avoiding problem foods or beverages, stopping smoking, or losing weight if needed may solve the problem. Additional treatment with over-the-counter antacids or nonprescription-strength acid-blocking medications called H2-receptor antagonists such as Tagamet, Zantac, or Pepcid may also be used. More severe and frequent episodes of GERD can trigger asthma attacks, cause severe chest pain, result in bleeding, or promote a narrowing (stricture) or chronic irritation of the esophagus. In these cases, more powerful inhibitors of stomach acid production called proton pump inhibitors, such as Prilosec and Prevacid, may be added to the treatment prescribed. As a last resort, a surgical procedure called *fundoplication* is performed to strengthen the sphincter. The procedure involves wrapping a layer of the upper stomach wall around the sphincter and terminal esophagus to lessen the possibility of acid reflux. If GERD is left untreated, serious pathological (precancerous) changes in the esophageal lining may develop—a condition called *Barrett's esophagus*.

Note also in Figure 15-9 that the upper right border of the stomach is known as the **lesser curvature,** and the lower left border is called the **greater curvature.** After food has been mixed in the stomach, chyme begins its passage through the pyloric sphincter into the first part of the small intestine.

Quick Check

1. What is chyme?
2. How does a sphincter muscle help the stomach perform its function?
3. What are the main divisions of the stomach?

SMALL INTESTINE

The **small intestine** seems to be misnamed if you look at its length—it is roughly 7 meters (20 feet) long. However, it is noticeably smaller in diameter than the large intestine, so in this respect its name is appropriate. Different names identify different sections of the small intestine. In the order in which food passes through them, they are the **duodenum** (doo-o-DEE-num), **jejunum** (je-JOO-num), and **ileum** (IL-ee-um).

The mucous lining of the small intestine, as with that of the stomach, contains thousands of microscopic glands. These **intestinal glands** secrete the intestinal digestive juice. Another structural feature of the lining of the small intestine makes it especially well suited to absorption of food and water; it is not perfectly smooth, as it appears to the naked eye. Instead, the intestinal lining is arranged into multiple circular folds called **plicae** (PLYE-kee) (Figures 15-2 and 15-10). These folds are themselves covered with thousands of tiny "fingers" called **villi** (VILL-eye). Under the microscope, the villi can be seen projecting into the hollow interior of the intestine. Inside each villus lies a rich network of blood capillaries that absorb the products of carbohydrate and protein digestion (sugars and amino acids). Millions and millions of villi jut inward from the mucous lining. Imagine the lining as perfectly smooth without any villi; think how much less surface area there would be for contact between capillaries and intestinal lining. Consider what an advantage a large contact area offers for faster absorption of food from the intestine into the blood and lymph—one more illustration that structure and function are intimately related.

Note also in Figure 15-10 that each villus in the intestine contains a lymphatic vessel or **lacteal** that absorbs lipid or fat materials from the chyme passing through the small intestine. In addition to the thousands of villi that increase surface area in the small intestine, each villus is itself covered by

Clinical Application

Treatment of Ulcers

Current statistics show that about 1 in 10 individuals in the United States will suffer from either a gastric (stomach) or duodenal ulcer in their lifetime. These craterlike lesions, which destroy areas of stomach or intestinal lining, cause gnawing or burning pain and may ultimately result in hemorrhage, perforation, scarring, and other very serious medical complications. Long-term use of certain pain medications such as aspirin and ibuprofen, called *nonsteroidal antiinflammatory agents* (NSAIDs), can cause ulcers. However, we now know that most gastric and duodenal ulcers result from infection with the *Helicobacter pylori* (*H. pylori*) bacterium. This is especially so if the infected individual has a genetic predisposition to ulcer development. *H. pylori* infection is diagnosed by biopsy, breath, or blood antibody tests.

Knowing that most ulcers are caused by a bacterial organism led to development of a number of treatment programs that were designed to eradicate the bacteria by use of antibiotics while simultaneously blocking or reducing stomach acid secretion. Currently, the standard antibiotic-based treatment used most frequently to both heal ulcers and prevent recurrences is called **triple therapy.** It is successful in 80% to 95% of cases and requires three medications be taken concurrently for 2 weeks. Triple therapy combines bismuth subsalicylate (Pepto-Bismol) with tetracycline and metronidazole (Flagyl) or clarithromycin (Biaxin). Recently, triple therapy has also been shown to be effective in treatment of Crohn's disease, a chronic bowel disorder. The same types of antisecretory drugs used to reduce stomach acid in GERD, including H2-receptor antagonists (e.g., Tagamet) and proton (H^+) pump inhibitors (e.g., Prilosec), are also used in ulcer therapy and treatment of irritable bowel syndrome.

FIGURE 15-10

The small intestine. Note that the folds of mucosa are covered with villi and that each villus is covered with epithelium, which increases the surface area for absorption of food.

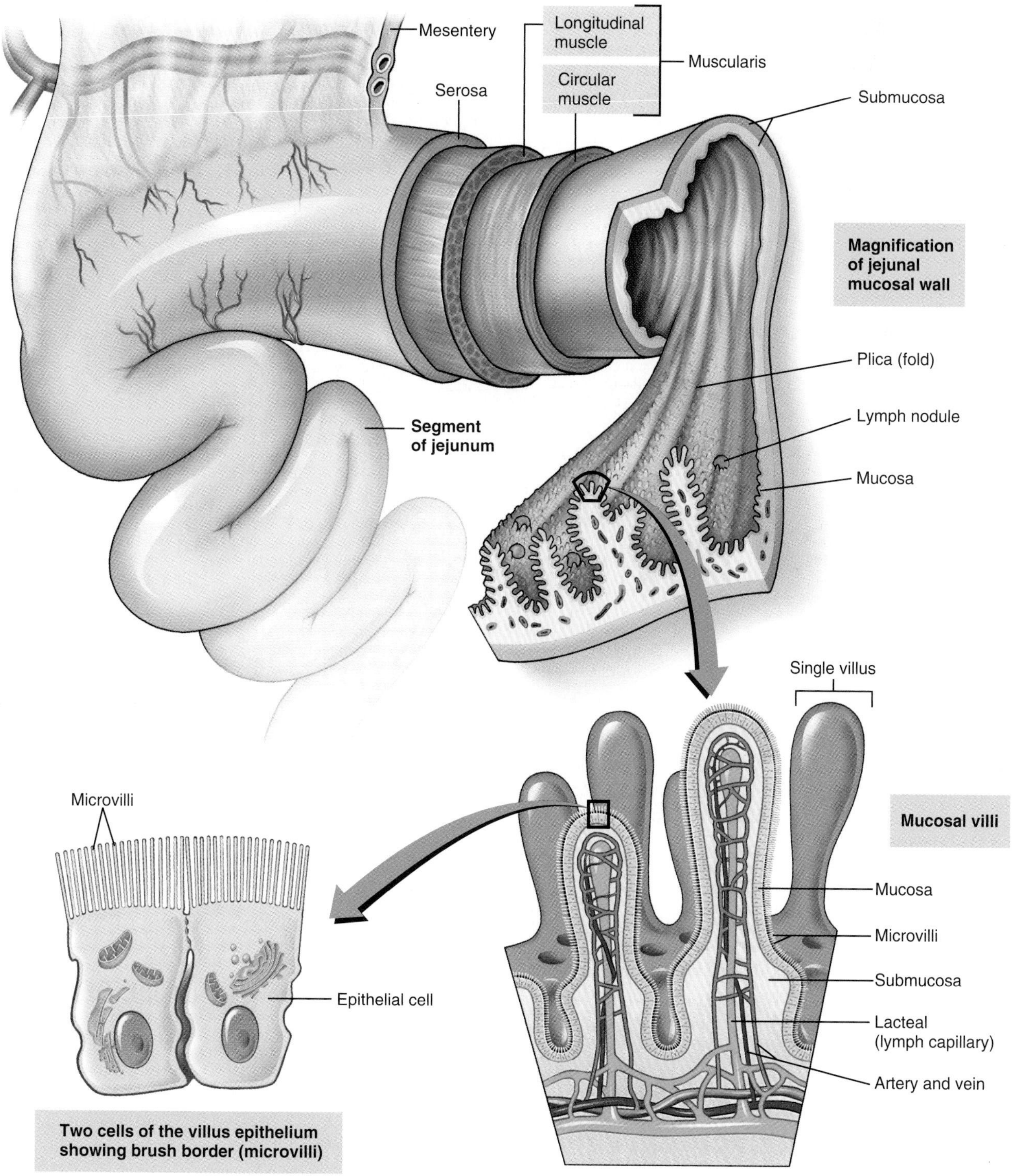

FIGURE 15-11

The gallbladder and bile ducts. Obstruction of the hepatic or common bile duct by stone or spasm blocks the exit of bile from the liver, where it is formed, and prevents bile from being ejected into the duodenum.

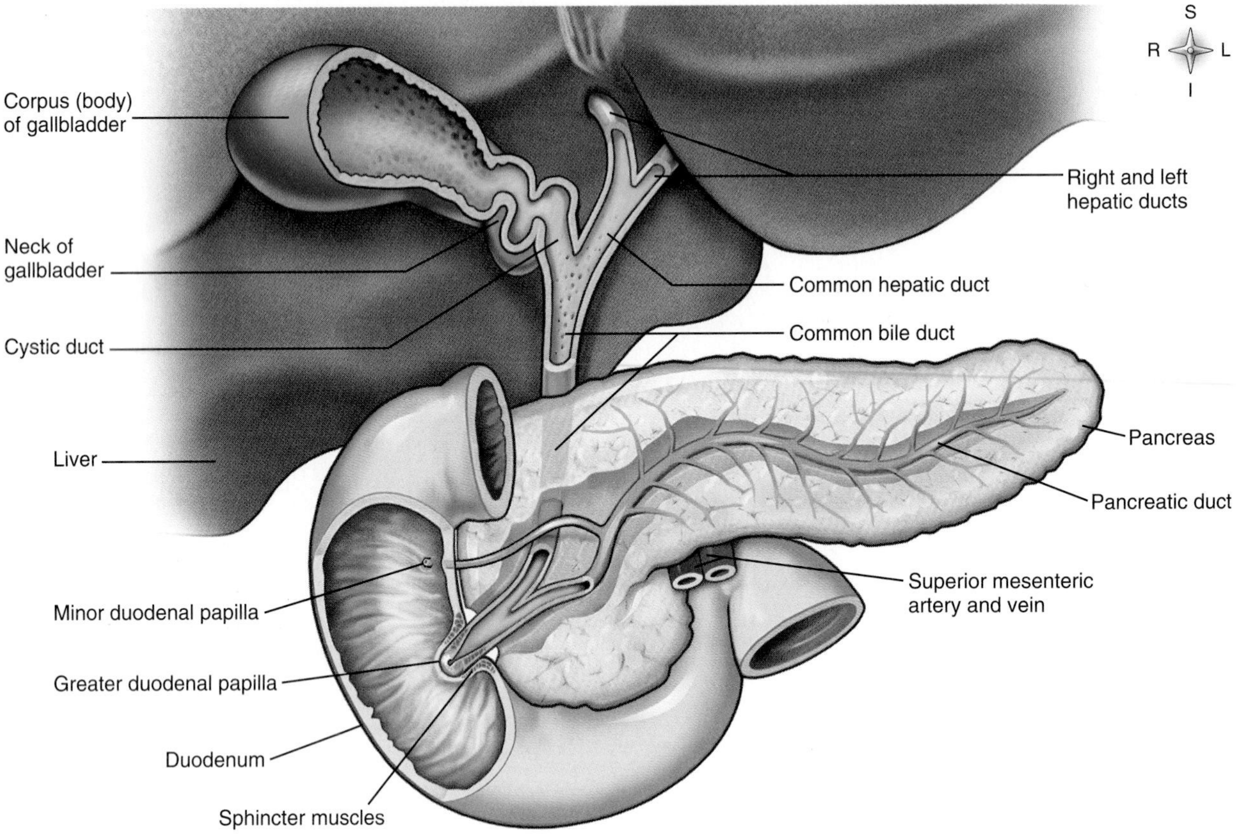

epithelial cells, which have a brushlike border composed of **microvilli.** The microvilli further increase the surface area of each villus for absorption of nutrients.

Most of the chemical digestion occurs in the first subdivision of the small intestine or duodenum. The duodenum is C-shaped (Figure 15-11) and curves around the head of the pancreas. The acid chyme enters the duodenum from the stomach. This area is the site of frequent ulceration (duodenal ulcers). The middle third of the duodenum contains the openings of ducts that empty pancreatic digestive juice and bile from the liver into the small intestine. As you can see in Figure 15-11, the two openings are called the **minor** and **major duodenal papillae.** Occasionally a gallstone blocks the major duodenal papilla, causing symptoms such as severe pain, jaundice, and digestive problems. Smooth muscle in the wall of the small intestine contracts to produce peristalsis, the wavelike contraction that moves food through the tract.

LIVER AND GALLBLADDER

The liver is so large that it fills the entire upper right section of the abdominal cavity and even extends part way into the left side. Because its cells

Clinical Application

Gallstones and Weight Loss

Gallstones are solid clumps of material (mostly cholesterol) that form in the gallbladder of 1 in 10 Americans (Figure *A*). Some gallstones never cause problems and are called *silent gallstones*, whereas others produce painful symptoms or other medical complications and are called *symptomatic gallstones*. Gallstones often form when the cholesterol concentration in bile becomes excessive, causing crystallization or precipitation to occur. Stone formation is much more likely to occur if the gallbladder does not empty regularly and chemically imbalanced or cholesterol-laden bile remains in the gallbladder for long periods.

The relationship of dieting and weight loss to gallstone formation is currently under intense scrutiny. Physicians have known for years that, in severely obese individuals (BMI or body mass index greater than 40), the liver produces higher levels of cholesterol and the risk of developing gallstones is increased. However, only recently have scientists established with certainty that significant and rapid weight loss greatly increases the risk of symptomatic gallstone formation that may require surgery—a procedure called *cholecystectomy* (KO-le-cys-TEK-toe-me).

Surgical procedures used for producing weight loss, such as restrictive gastric banding (vertical-banded gastroplasty) or more extensive bypass operations (RGB or Roux-en-Y gastric bypass), almost always result in rapid postsurgical weight loss, but more than one third of these patients develop gallstones. Unfortunately, individuals who choose nonsurgical approaches to achieve significant and rapid weight loss, such as very–low-calorie or ultra–low-fat diets, also experience higher rates of gallstone formation. In these cases, stone formation is related to imbalances in bile chemistry and delayed emptying or incomplete gallbladder contractions.

If surgery is required for removal of symptomatic gallstones, laparoscopic techniques have now made the need for open abdominal surgical procedures less common. Laparoscopic surgery means using instruments to gain access to internal body content through "punched holes" rather than through the traditional incision. To punch the holes, a trocar (a sharp pointed rod inside a tube) is inserted through the skin. Once inside the body cavity, the rod is removed but the tube remains in place. Then, instruments, lights, and gases may be inserted into the cavity as needed to conduct the surgery. In the case of laparoscopic cholecystectomy surgery, sometimes up to five holes are created. Figure *B* shows the most common locations for abdominal cavity access. Gallstones can sometimes be treated (dissolved) over time or prevented from developing in individuals experiencing rapid weight loss by oral administration of a naturally occurring bile constituent called *ursodeoxycholic acid* (Actigall).

A

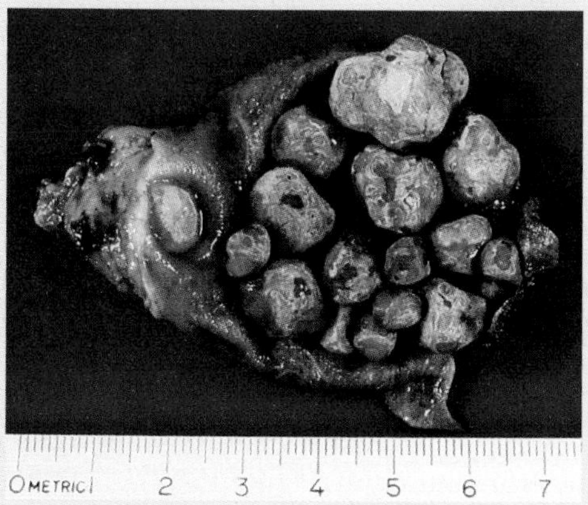

B

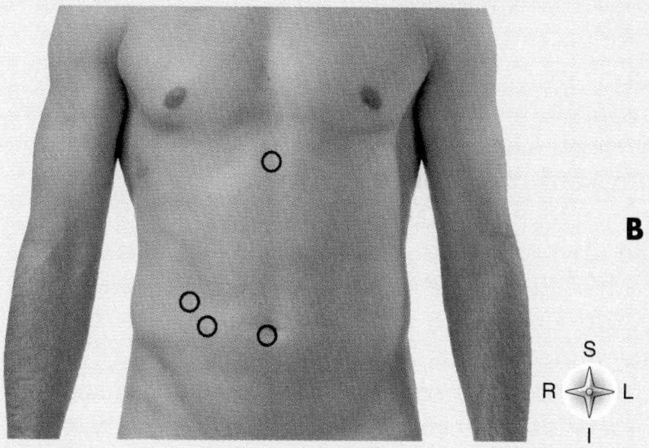

secrete a substance called **bile** into ducts, the liver is classified as an exocrine gland; in fact, it is the largest gland in the body.

Look again at Figure 15-11. First, identify the hepatic ducts. They drain bile out of the liver, a fact suggested by the name "hepatic," which comes from the Greek word for liver (*hepar*). Next, notice the duct that drains bile into the small intestine (duodenum), the common bile duct. It is formed by the union of the common hepatic duct with the cystic duct.

Chemically, bile contains significant quantities of cholesterol and substances *(bile salts)* that act as detergents to mechanically break up or **emulsify** (e-MUL-se-fye) fats. Because fats form large globules, they must be broken down or emulsified to form smaller particles to increase the surface area for digestion. In addition to emulsification of fats, loss of bile in the feces also serves as a mechanism to excrete cholesterol from the body. Both emulsification of fats and elimination of cholesterol from the body are primary functions of bile.

When chyme containing lipid or fat enters the duodenum, it initiates a mechanism that contracts the gallbladder and forces bile into the small intestine. Fats in chyme stimulate or "trigger" the secretion of the hormone **cholecystokinin** (ko-le-sis-toe-KYE-nin) or **CCK** from the intestinal mucosa of the duodenum. This hormone then stimulates the contraction of the gallbladder, and bile flows into the duodenum. Between meals, a lot of bile moves up the cystic duct into the gallbladder on the undersurface of the liver. The gallbladder thus concentrates and stores bile produced in the liver.

Visualize a gallstone blocking the common bile duct shown in Figure 15-11. Bile could not then drain into the duodenum. Feces would then appear gray-white because the pigments from bile give feces its characteristic color. Furthermore, excessive amounts of bile would be absorbed into the blood. A yellowish skin discoloration called **jaundice** (JAWN-dis) would result. Obstruction of the common hepatic duct also leads to jaundice. Because bile cannot then drain out of the liver, excessive amounts of it are absorbed. Because bile is not resorbed from the gallbladder, no jaundice occurs if the cystic duct is blocked.

PANCREAS

The pancreas lies behind the stomach in the concavity produced by the C shape of the duodenum. It is an exocrine gland that secretes pancreatic juice into ducts and an endocrine gland that secretes hormones into the blood. Pancreatic juice is the most important digestive juice. It contains enzymes that digest all three major kinds of foods. It also contains sodium bicarbonate, an alkaline substance that neutralizes the hydrochloric acid in the gastric juice that enters the intestines. Pancreatic juice enters the duodenum of the small intestine at the same place that bile enters. As you can see in Figure 15-11, the common bile and pancreatic ducts open into the duodenum at the major duodenal papilla.

Between the cells that secrete pancreatic juice into ducts lie clusters of cells that have no contact with any ducts. These are the pancreatic islets (of Langerhans), which secrete the hormones of the pancreas described in Chapter 10. Locate the pancreas and nearby structures in Figure 15-12, which shows a transverse section of the abdomen of a human cadaver.

Quick Check

1. What are the main divisions of the small intestine?
2. What is bile and where does it come from?
3. What is the role of the gallbladder?
4. Is the pancreas an exocrine gland or an endocrine gland?

LARGE INTESTINE

The **large intestine** is only about 1.5 meters (5 feet) in length. As the name implies, however, it has a much larger diameter than the small intestine. It forms the lower or terminal portion of the digestive tract. Undigested and unabsorbed food material enters the large intestine after passing through a sphincterlike structure (Figure 15-13) called the **ileocecal** (il-ee-o-SEE-kal) **valve.** The word *chyme* is no longer appropriate in describing the contents of the large intestine. Chyme, which has the consistency of soup and is found in the small intestine, changes to the consistency of fecal matter as water and salts are reabsorbed during its passage through the small intestine. During its movement through the large in-

FIGURE 15-12

Horizontal (transverse) section of the abdomen. The photograph of a cadaver section shows the relative position of some of the major digestive organs of the abdomen. Such a view is typical in imaging methods such as computed tomography (CT) scanning and magnetic resonance imaging (MRI).

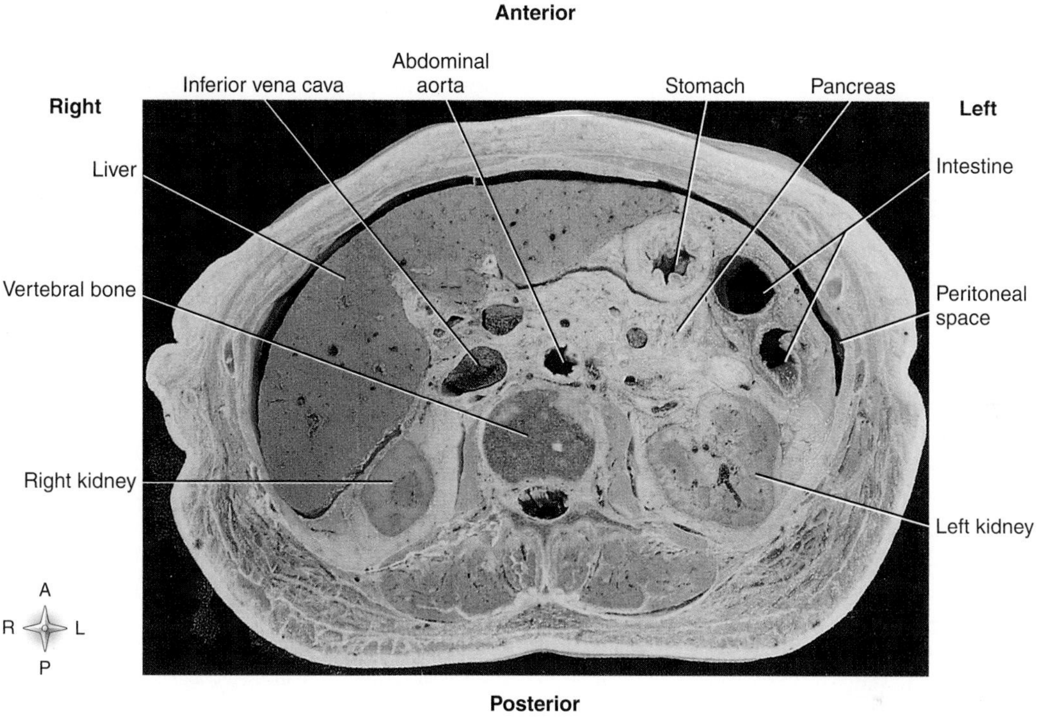

testine, material that escaped digestion in the small intestine is acted on by bacteria. As a result of this bacterial action, additional nutrients may be released from cellulose and other fibers and absorbed. In addition to their digestive role, bacteria in the large intestine have other important functions. They are responsible for the synthesis of vitamin K needed for normal blood clotting and for the production of some of the B-complex vitamins. After they are formed, these vitamins are absorbed from the large intestine and enter the blood.

Although some absorption of water, salts, and vitamins occurs in the large intestine, this segment of the digestive tube is not as well suited for absorption as is the small intestine. Salts, especially sodium, are absorbed by active transport, and water is moved into the blood by osmosis. No villi are present in the mucosa of the large intestine. As a result, much less surface area is available for absorption, and the efficiency and speed of movement of substances through the wall of the large intestine is lower than in the small intestine. Normal passage of material through the large intestine takes about 3 to 5 days. If the rate of passage of material quickens, the consistency of the stools or fecal material becomes more and more fluid, and **diarrhea** (dye-ah-REE-ah) results. If the time of passage through the large intestine is prolonged beyond 5 days, the feces lose volume and becomes more solid because of excessive water absorption. This reduces stimulation of the bowel emptying reflex, resulting in retention of feces, a condition called **constipation.**

The subdivisions of the large intestine are listed below in the order in which food material or feces passes through them.

1. Cecum
2. Ascending colon
3. Transverse colon
4. Descending colon
5. Sigmoid colon
6. Rectum
7. Anal canal

FIGURE 15-13

Divisions of the large intestine.

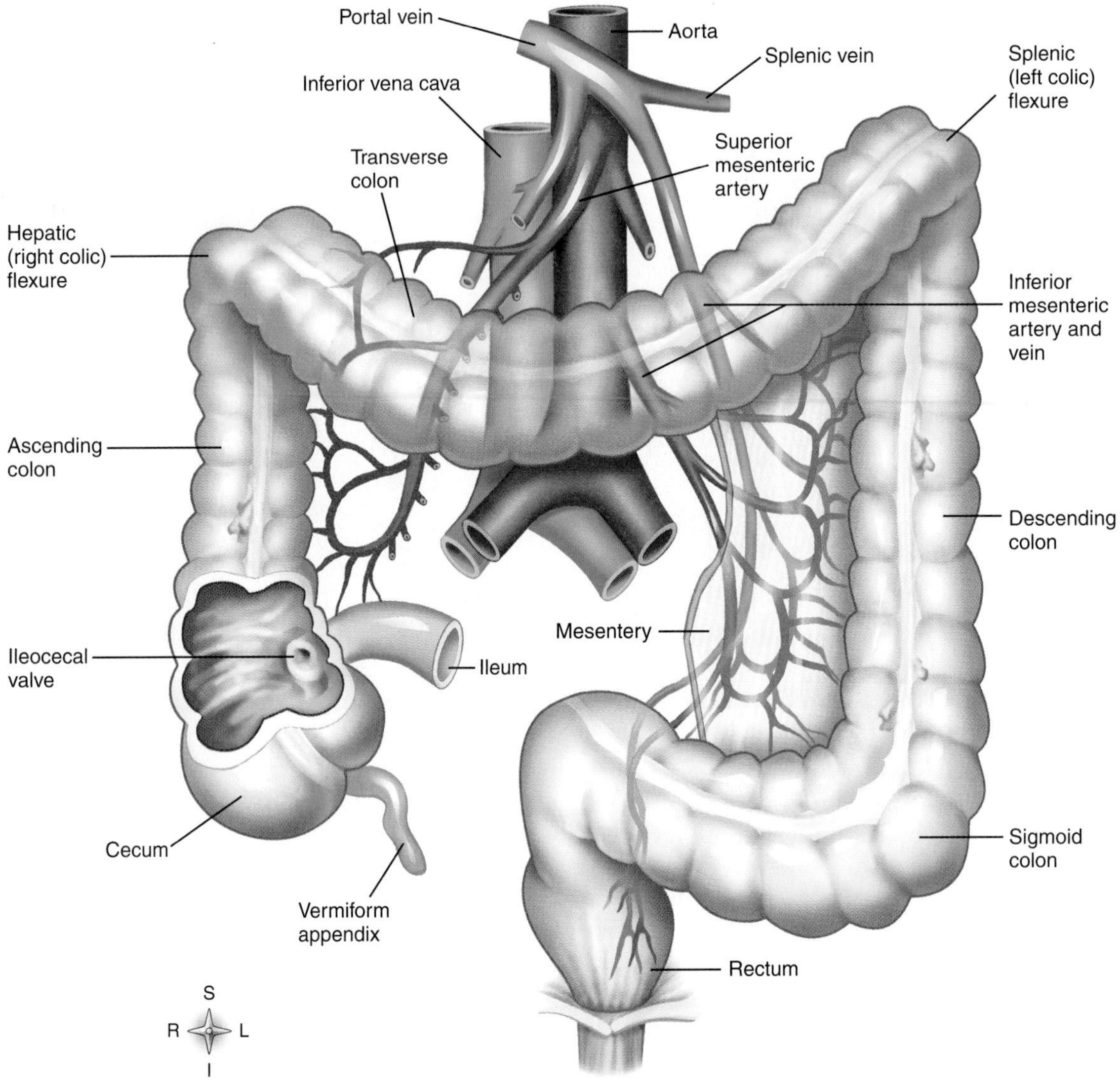

These areas can be studied and identified by tracing the passage of material from its point of entry into the large intestine at the ileocecal valve to its elimination from the body through the external opening called the **anus.**

Note in Figure 15-13 that the ileocecal valve opens into a pouchlike area called the **cecum** (SEE-kum). The opening itself is about 5 or 6 cm (2 inches) above the beginning of the large intestine. Food residue in the cecum flows upward on the right side of the body in the **ascending colon.** The **hepatic** or **right colic flexure** is the bend between the ascending colon and the **transverse colon,** which extends across the front of the abdomen from right to left. The **splenic** or **left colic flexure** marks the point where the **descending colon** turns downward on the left side of the abdomen. The **sigmoid colon** is the S-shaped segment that terminates in the **rectum.** The terminal portion of the rectum is called the **anal canal,** which ends at the external opening or anus.

Two sphincter muscles stay contracted to keep the anus closed except during defecation. Smooth or involuntary muscle composes the **inner anal sphincter,** but striated, or voluntary, muscle composes the outer one. This anatomical fact sometimes becomes highly important from a practical standpoint. For example, often after a person has had a stroke, the voluntary anal sphincter at first becomes paralyzed. This means, of course, that the individual has no control at this time over bowel movements.

FIGURE 15-14

The large intestine. A special x-ray technique produces a clear image of the large intestine and its position relative to the skeleton.

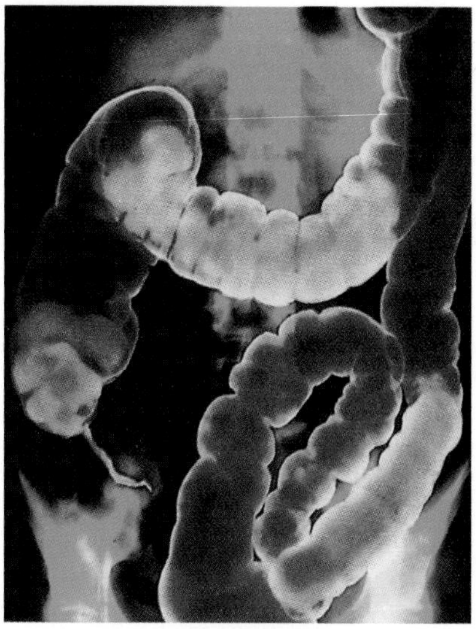

APPENDIX

The **vermiform appendix** (Latin *vermiformis* from *vermis* "worm" and *forma* "shape") is, as the name implies, a wormlike, tubular structure. Although it serves no important digestive function in humans, it contains lymphatic tissue and may play a minor role in the immunologic defense mechanisms of the body described in Chapter 13. Note in Figure 15-13 that the appendix is directly attached to the cecum. The appendix contains a blind, tubelike interior lumen that communicates with the lumen of the large intestine 3 cm (1 inch) below the opening of the ileocecal valve into the cecum. If the mucous lining of the appendix becomes inflamed, the resulting condition is the well-known affliction, **appendicitis.** As you can see in Figures 15-13 and 15-14, the appendix is very close to the rectal wall. For patients with suspected appendicitis, a physician often evaluates the appendix by a digital rectal examination.

PERITONEUM

The **peritoneum** is a large, moist, slippery sheet of serous membrane that lines the abdominal cavity and covers the organs located in it, including most of the digestive organs. The parietal layer of the peritoneum lines the abdominal cavity. The visceral layer of the peritoneum forms the outer or covering layer of each abdominal organ. The small space between the parietal and visceral layers is called the *peritoneal space.* It contains just enough peritoneal fluid to keep both layers of the peritoneum moist and able to slide freely against each other during breathing and digestive movements (Figure 15-15). Organs outside of the peritoneum are said to be retroperitoneal.

Extensions

The two most prominent extensions of the peritoneum are the mesentery and the greater omentum. The **mesentery,** an extension between the parietal and visceral layers of the peritoneum, is shaped like a giant, pleated fan. Its smaller edge attaches to the lumbar region of the posterior abdominal wall, and its long, loose outer edge encloses most of the small intestine, anchoring it to the posterior abdominal wall. The **greater omentum** is a pouchlike extension of the visceral peritoneum from the lower edge of the stomach, part of the duodenum, and the transverse colon.

Shaped like a large apron, it hangs down over the intestines, and because spotty deposits of fat give it a lacy appearance, it has been nicknamed the *lace apron*. It usually envelops a badly inflamed appendix, walling it off from the rest of the abdominal organs.

Quick

1. What is the role of the large intestine?
2. Can you name the divisions of the large intestine?
3. Where is the appendix?
4. What are mesenteries? What is their function?

DIGESTION

Digestion, a complex process that occurs in the alimentary canal, consists of physical and chemical changes that prepare food for absorption. **Mechanical digestion** breaks food into tiny particles, mixes them with digestive juices, moves them along the alimentary canal, and finally eliminates the digestive wastes from the body. Chewing or mastication, swallowing or **deglutition** (deg-loo-TISH-un), peristalsis (Figure 15-3), and defecation are the main processes of mechanical digestion. **Chemical diges-**

FIGURE 15-15

The peritoneum. The parietal layer of the peritoneum lines the abdominopelvic cavity and then extends as a series of mesenteries to form the visceral layer that covers abdominal organs.

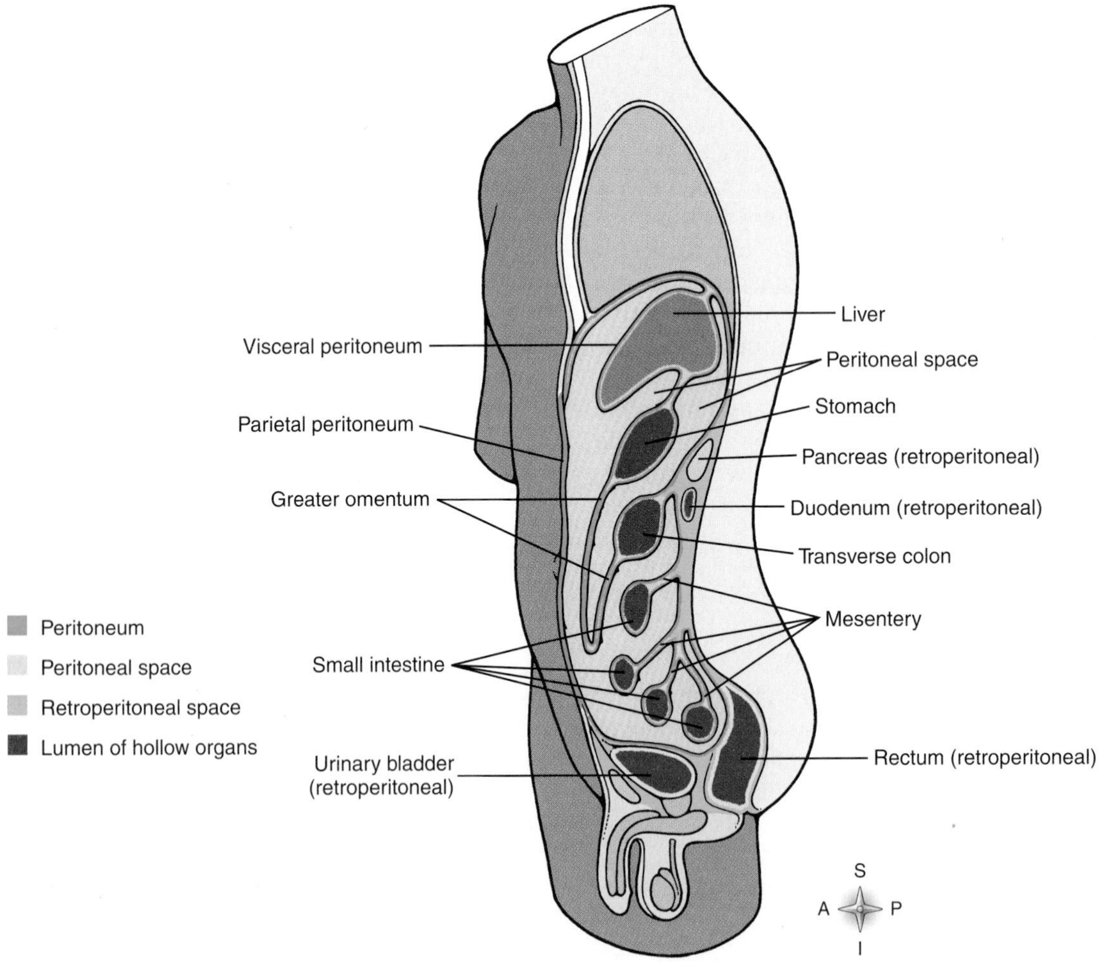

tion breaks down large, nonabsorbable food molecules into smaller, absorbable molecules—molecules that are able to pass through the intestinal mucosa into blood and lymph (Figure 15-16). Chemical digestion consists of numerous chemical reactions catalyzed by enzymes in saliva, gastric juice, pancreatic juice, and intestinal juice.

Carbohydrate Digestion

Very little digestion of carbohydrates (starches and sugars) occurs before food reaches the small intestine. Salivary amylase usually has little time to do its work because so many of us swallow our food so fast. Gastric juice contains no carbohydrate-digesting enzymes. But after the food reaches the small intestine, pancreatic and intestinal juice enzymes digest the starches and sugars. A pancreatic enzyme (amylase) starts the process by breaking down polysaccharides such as starches into disaccharides (double sugars). Three intestinal enzymes—maltase, sucrase, and lactase—digest disaccharides by changing them into monosaccharides (simple sugars). Maltase digests maltose (malt sugar), sucrase digests sucrose (ordinary cane sugar), and lactase digests lactose (milk sugar). The end products of carbohydrate digestion are the monosaccharides; the most abundant is glucose.

Protein Digestion

Protein digestion starts in the stomach. Pepsin, an enzyme in the gastric juice, causes the giant protein molecules to break up into somewhat simpler com-

FIGURE 15-16

Digestion and absorption of nutrients, minerals, and water.

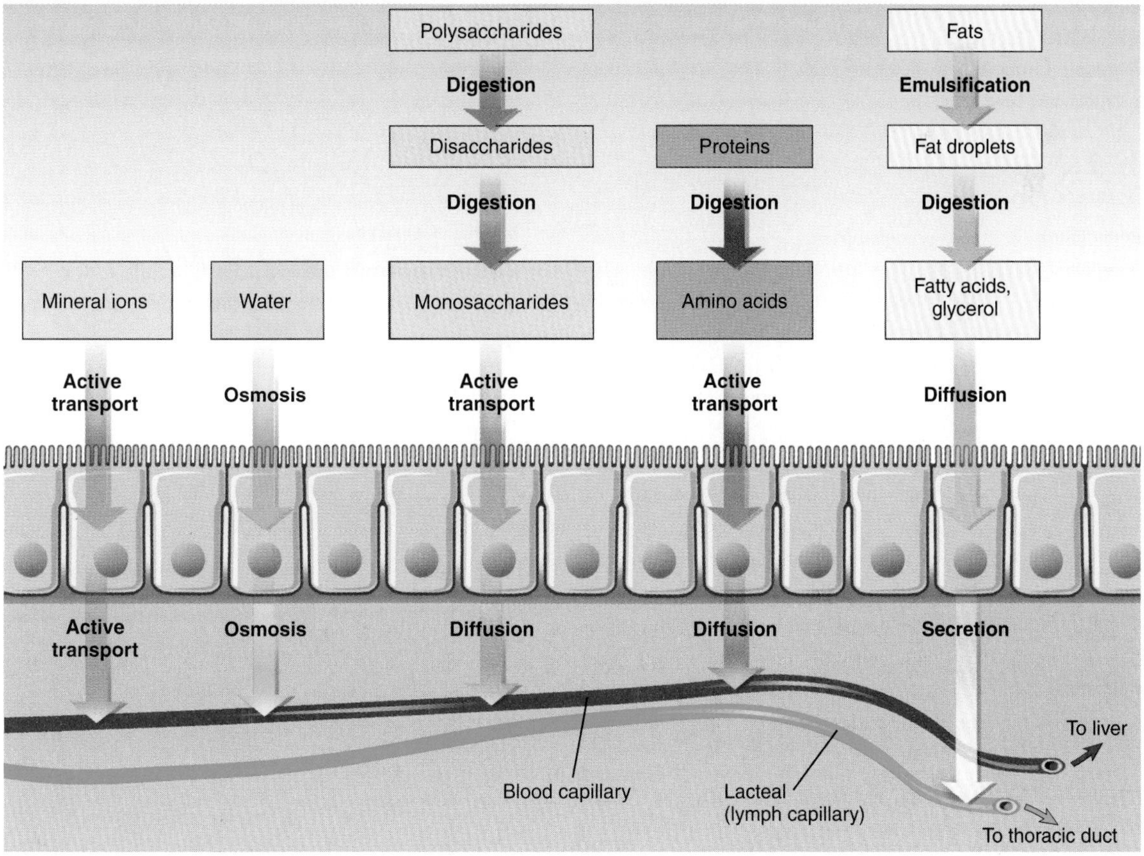

pounds. Pepsinogen, a component of gastric juice, is converted into active pepsin enzyme by hydrochloric acid (also in gastric juice). In the intestine, other enzymes (trypsin in the pancreatic juice and peptidases in the intestinal juice) finish the job of protein digestion. Every protein molecule is made up of many amino acids joined together. When enzymes have split up the large protein molecule into its separate amino acids, protein digestion is completed. Hence the end product of protein digestion is amino acids. For obvious reasons, the amino acids are also referred to as *protein building blocks*.

Fat Digestion

Very little carbohydrate and fat digestion occurs before food reaches the small intestine. Most fats are undigested until after emulsification by bile in the duodenum (that is, fat droplets are broken into very small droplets). After this takes place, pan-

TABLE 15-2

Chemical Digestion

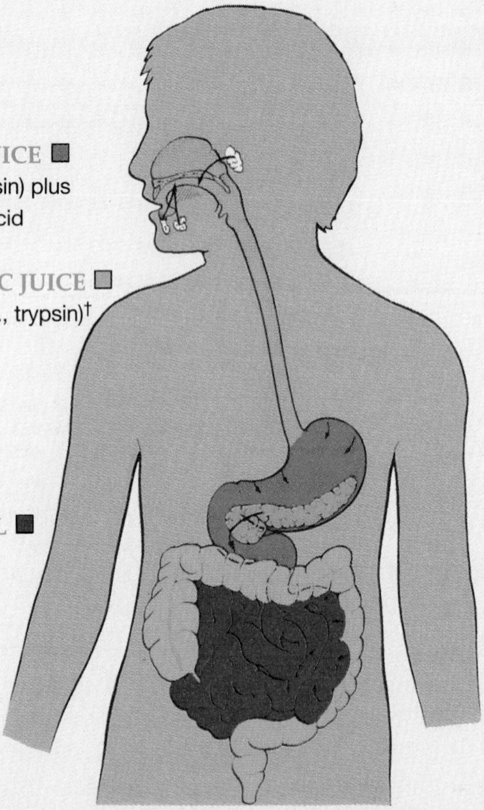

DIGESTIVE JUICES AND ENZYMES	SUBSTANCE DIGESTED (OR HYDROLYZED)	RESULTING PRODUCT*
SALIVA □		
Amylase	Starch (polysaccharide)	Maltose (a double sugar, or disaccharide)
GASTRIC JUICE ■		
Protease (pepsin) plus hydrochloric acid	Proteins	Partially digested proteins
PANCREATIC JUICE ■		
Proteases (e.g., trypsin)[†]	Proteins (intact or partially digested)	Peptides and **amino acids**
Lipases	Fats emulsified by bile	**Fatty acids, monoglycerides,** and **glycerol**
Amylase	Starch	Maltose
INTESTINAL ENZYMES[‡] ■		
Peptidases	Peptides	**Amino acids**
Sucrase	Sucrose (cane sugar)	**Glucose and fructose**[§] (simple sugars, or monosaccharides)
Lactase	Lactose (milk sugar)	**Glucose and galactose** (simple sugars)
Maltase	Maltose (malt sugar)	**Glucose**

*Substances in boldface type are end products of digestion (that is, completely digested nutrients ready for absorption).
[†]Secreted in inactive form (trypsinogen); activated by enterokinase, an enzyme in the intestinal brush border.
[‡]Brush-border enzymes.
[§]Glucose is also called dextrose; fructose is also called *levulose*.

creatic lipase splits up the fat molecules into fatty acids and glycerol (glycerin). The end products of fat digestion, then, are fatty acids and glycerol.

Table 15-2 summarizes the main facts about chemical digestion. Enzyme names indicate the type of food digested by the enzyme. For example, the name *amylase* indicates that the enzyme digests carbohydrates (starches and sugars), *protease* indicates a protein-digesting enzyme, and *lipase* means a fat-digesting enzyme. When carbohydrate digestion has been completed, starches (polysaccharides) and double sugars (disaccharides) have been changed mainly to glucose, a simple sugar (monosaccharide). The end products of protein digestion, on the other hand, are amino acids. Fatty acid and glycerol are the end products of fat digestion.

ABSORPTION

After food is digested, it is absorbed; that is, it moves through the mucous membrane lining of the small intestine into the blood and lymph (Figure 15-16). In other words, food absorption is the process by which molecules of amino acids, glucose, fatty acids, and glycerol go from the inside of the intestines into the circulating fluids of the body. Absorption of foods is just as essential as digestion of foods. The reason is fairly obvious. As long as food stays in the intestines, it cannot nourish the millions of cells that compose all other parts of the body. Their lives depend on the absorption of digested food and its transportation to them by the circulating blood.

Structural adaptations of the digestive tube, including folds in the lining mucosa, villi, and microvilli, increase the absorptive surface and the efficiency and speed of transfer of materials from the intestinal lumen to body fluids. Many salts such as sodium are actively transported through the intestinal mucosa. Water follows by osmosis. Other nutrients such as monosaccharides and amino acids are also actively transported through the intestinal mucosa and diffuse into the blood of capillaries in the intestinal villi. Fatty acids and glycerol diffuse into the absorptive cells of the GI tract and then are secreted into the lymphatic vessels or lacteals found in intestinal villi.

Quick

1. What is the difference between mechanical and chemical digestion?
2. In what form are carbohydrates absorbed into the bloodstream?
3. What must happen to fat before it can be chemically digested?

Science Applications

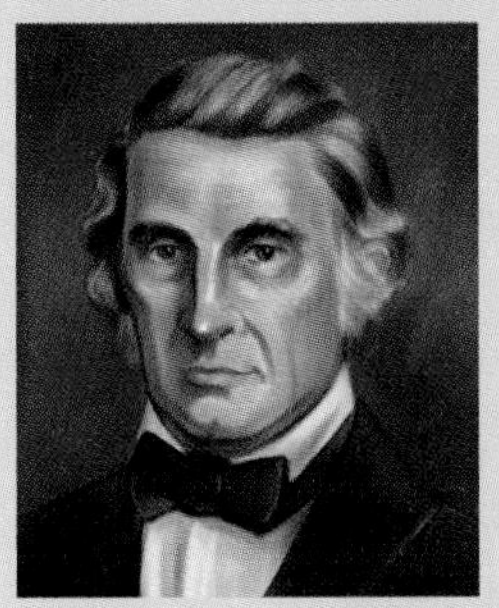

Gastroenterology

William Beaumont (1785-1853).

Analyzing the word gastroenterology tells you it is the study *(-ology)* and treatment of the stomach *(gastro-)* and the intestines *(-entero-)*. One of the pioneering gastroenterologists was the American physician William Beaumont. In 1822, the young Québécois trapper Alexis St. Martin was shot with a musket near the Army hospital in Michigan where Beaumont was working. Beaumont treated his wound—expecting St. Martin to die. St. Martin recovered and lived a long life even though the wound did not heal properly. For his entire life, there remained an open hole in his abdomen leading directly into the stomach. St. Martin allowed Beaumont to study gastric secretion through the opening. Over many years, Beaumont made careful observations about how the stomach works. Many of his conclusions are still valid today and serve as the foundation for modern gastroenterology.

Of course, many physicians and nurses specialize in gastroenterology today. However, many health care providers such as health care technicians and nursing assistants need a basic knowledge of digestive structure and function in order to care for patients effectively. In addition, even those in dietetics, nutrition, and food service benefit by knowledge of the principles of digestion.

OUTLINE SUMMARY

DIGESTIVE SYSTEM (FIGURE 15-1)

A. Irregular tube called alimentary canal or gastrointestinal (GI) tract
B. Food must first be digested, then absorbed, and later metabolized

WALL OF THE DIGESTIVE TRACT (FIGURE 15-2)

The wall of the digestive tube is formed by four layers of tissue:
A. Mucosa—mucous epithelium
B. Submucosa—connective tissue
C. Muscularis—two or three layers of smooth muscle
D. Serosa—serous membrane that covers the outside of abdominal organs; it attaches the digestive tract to the wall of the abdominopelvic cavity by forming folds called *mesenteries*

MOUTH

A. Roof—formed by hard palate (parts of maxillary and palatine bones) and soft palate, an arch-shaped muscle separating mouth from pharynx; uvula, a downward projection of soft palate (Figure 15-4)
B. Floor—formed by tongue and its muscles; papillae, small elevations on mucosa of tongue; taste buds, found in many papillae; lingual frenulum, fold of mucous membrane that helps anchor tongue to floor of mouth (Figure 15-5)

TEETH

A. Names of teeth—incisors, cuspids, bicuspids, and tricuspids
B. Twenty teeth in temporary set; average age for cutting first tooth about 6 months; set complete at about 2 years of age
C. Thirty-two teeth in permanent set; 6 years about average age for starting to cut first permanent tooth; set complete usually between ages of 17 and 24 years (Figure 15-6)
D. Structures of a typical tooth—crown, neck, and root (Figure 15-7)

SALIVARY GLANDS (FIGURE 15-8)

A. Parotid glands
B. Submandibular glands
C. Sublingual glands

PHARYNX

ESOPHAGUS

STOMACH (Figure 15-9)

A. Size—expands after large meal; about size of large sausage when empty
B. Pylorus—lower part of stomach; pyloric sphincter muscle closes opening of pylorus into duodenum
C. Wall—many smooth muscle fibers; contractions produce churning movements (peristalsis)
D. Lining—mucous membrane; many microscopic glands that secrete gastric juice and hydrochloric acid into stomach; mucous membrane lies in folds (rugae) when stomach is empty

SMALL INTESTINE (FIGURE 15-10)

A. Size—about 7 meters (20 feet) long but only 2 cm or so in diameter
B. Divisions
  1. Duodenum
  2. Jejunum
  3. Ileum
C. Wall—contains smooth muscle fibers that contract to produce peristalsis

OUTLINE SUMMARY—*cont'd*

D. Lining—mucous membrane; many microscopic glands (intestinal glands) secrete intestinal juice; villi (microscopic finger-shaped projections from surface of mucosa into intestinal cavity) contain blood and lymph capillaries

LIVER AND GALLBLADDER

A. Size and location—liver is largest gland; fills upper right section of abdominal cavity and extends over into left side
B. Liver secretes bile
C. Ducts (Figure 15-11)
   1. Hepatic—drains bile from liver
   2. Cystic—duct by which bile enters and leaves gallbladder
   3. Common bile—formed by union of hepatic and cystic ducts; drains bile from hepatic or cystic ducts into duodenum
D. Gallbladder
   1. Location—undersurface of the liver
   2. Function—concentrates and stores bile produced in the liver

PANCREAS

A. Location—behind stomach
B. Functions
   1. Pancreatic cells secrete pancreatic juice into pancreatic ducts; main duct empties into duodenum
   2. Pancreatic islets (of Langerhans)—cells not connected with pancreatic ducts; secrete hormones glucagon and insulin into the blood

LARGE INTESTINE (FIGURE 15-13)

A. Divisions
   1. Cecum
   2. Colon—ascending, transverse, descending, and sigmoid
   3. Rectum
B. Opening to exterior—anus
C. Wall—contains smooth muscle fibers that contract to produce churning, peristalsis, and defecation
D. Lining—mucous membrane

APPENDIX

Blind tube off cecum; no important digestive functions in humans

PERITONEUM (FIGURE 15-15)

A. Definitions—peritoneum, serous membrane lining abdominal cavity and covering abdominal organs; parietal layer of peritoneum lines abdominal cavity; visceral layer of peritoneum covers abdominal organs; peritoneal space lies between parietal and visceral layers
B. Extensions—largest ones are the mesentery and greater omentum; mesentery is extension of parietal peritoneum, which attaches most of small intestine to posterior abdominal wall; greater omentum, or "lace apron," hangs down from lower edge of stomach and transverse colon over intestines

DIGESTION (TABLE 15-2)

Meaning—changing foods so that they can be absorbed and used by cells
A. Mechanical digestion—chewing, swallowing, and peristalsis break food into tiny particles, mix them well with digestive juices, and move them along the digestive tract
B. Chemical digestion—breaks up large food molecules into compounds having smaller molecules; brought about by digestive enzymes (Figure 15-16)
C. Carbohydrate digestion—mainly in small intestine
   1. Pancreatic amylase—breaks polysaccharides down to disaccharides

Continued

OUTLINE SUMMARY—*cont'd*

2. Intestinal juice enzymes
   a. Maltase—changes maltose to glucose
   b. Sucrase—changes sucrose to glucose
   c. Lactase—changes lactose to glucose

D. Protein digestion—starts in stomach; completed in small intestine
   1. Gastric juice enzyme pepsin partially digests proteins
   2. Pancreatic enzyme, trypsin, continues digestion of proteins
   3. Intestinal enzymes, peptidases, complete digestion of partially digested proteins to amino acids

E. Fat digestion
   1. Bile contains no enzymes but emulsifies fats (breaks fat droplets into very small droplets)
   2. Pancreatic lipase changes emulsified fats to fatty acids and glycerol in small intestine

ABSORPTION

A. Meaning—digested food moves from intestine into blood or lymph

B. Where absorption occurs—foods and most water from small intestine; some water also absorbed from large intestine

NEW WORDS

absorption	digestion	hiatal hernia	plica
alimentary canal	emesis	jaundice	rugae
appendicitis	emulsify	lumen	ulcer
bolus	feces	mastication	uvula
cavity	frenulum	mesentery	villus
cholecystectomy	gastroesophageal reflux disease (GERD)	papilla	
chyme		peristalsis	
diarrhea		peritoneum	

REVIEW QUESTIONS

1. Name and describe the four layers of the wall of the gastrointestinal tract.
2. What is the function of the uvula and soft palate?
3. Explain the function of the different types of teeth.
4. Describe the three main parts of a tooth.
5. Name the three pairs of salivary glands and describe where the duct from each enters the mouth.
6. What are the functions of the cardiac and pyloric sphincter muscles?
7. Define *peristalsis*.
8. Explain how bile from the liver and gallbladder reaches the small intestine. What is the function of cholecystokinin?
9. What is contained in pancreatic juice?
10. What do the bacteria in the large intestine contribute to the body?
11. List the seven subdivisions of the large intestine.
12. Describe the mesentery and the greater omentum.
13. Differentiate between mechanical digestion and chemical digestion.
14. Briefly describe the process of carbohydrate digestion.

REVIEW QUESTIONS—*cont'd*

15. Briefly describe the process of fat digestion.
16. Briefly describe the process of protein digestion.
17. Explain the process of absorption. What function do the lacteals have in absorption?

CRITICAL THINKING

18. What structures in the small intestine increase the internal surface area? What advantage is gained by this increase in surface area?
19. Bile does not cause a chemical change; what is the effect of bile on fat and why does this make fat digestion more efficient?
20. Some people are lactose intolerant. This means they are unable to digest lactose sugar. What enzyme is probably not functioning properly and what types of food should these people try to avoid?

30/30

CHAPTER TEST

1. Food undergoes three kinds of processing in the body. All cells perform metabolism, but digestion and absorption are performed by the digestive system.
2. The muscularis layer of the wall of the gastrointestinal tract produces peristalsis.
3. The submucosa layer of the wall of the gastrointestinal tract contains blood vessels and nerves.
4. mucosa is the innermost layer of the wall of the gastrointestinal tract.
5. serosa is the outermost layer of the wall of the gastrointestinal tract.
6. The uvula and soft palate prevent food and liquid from entering the nasal cavity above the mouth when food is swallowed.
7. The three main parts of a tooth are crown, neck, and root.
8. The names of the three pairs of salivary glands are the parotid, the submandibular, and the sublingual
9. The tube connecting the pharynx and the stomach is the esophagus
10. The three divisions of the stomach are the fundus the body and the pylorus
11. The three divisions of the small intestine are the duodenum the jejunum, and the ileum.
12. The tiny fingerlike projections covering the plicae of the small intestine are called villi.
13. The lymphatic vessel in the villi is called the lacteal.
14. The common bile duct is formed by the union of the common hepatic duct from the liver and the cystic duct from the gallbladder.
15. The part of the large intestine between the ascending and descending colon is the transverse colon.
16. The part of the large intestine between the descending colon and the rectum is called the sigmoid colon
17. The two most prominent extensions of the peritoneum are the mesentery and the greater omentum
18. The process by which digested food is moved from the digestive system to the circulating fluids is called absorption

Continued

CHAPTER TEST—*cont'd*

Match the statement in Column B with the correct term in Column A.

COLUMN A	COLUMN B
19. __e__ Emulsification	**a.** this enzyme is made in the pancreas and digests fat
20. __i__ Amylase	**b.** this enzyme is made in the small intestine and digests protein
21. __j__ Pepsin	**c.** this gland produces bile
22. __k__ Cholecystokinin	**d.** this is the final end product of protein digestion
23. __b__ Peptidase	**e.** bile has this effect on fat droplets
24. __l__ Cystic	**f.** this enzyme is made in an inactive form in the pancreas and digests protein
25. __f__ Trypsin	**g.** this is the final end product of carbohydrate digestion
26. __g__ Simple sugars	**h.** this is one of the final end products of fat digestion
27. __d__ Amino acids	**i.** this enzyme is made in both the salivary gland and the pancreas and digests starch
28. __c__ Liver	**j.** this enzyme is made in the stomach in an inactive form and digests protein
29. __a__ Lipase	**k.** this hormone stimulates the contraction of the gallbladder
30. __h__ Glycerol	**l.** this duct connects the gallbladder to the common bile duct

STUDY TIPS

Before studying Chapter 15, review the synopsis of the digestive system in Chapter 4. The structure of the digestive system can be divided into two parts: a tube called the gastrointestinal tract, and accessory organs—organs that are not in the tube. In most cases, the accessory organs produce substances that are released into the tube. The tube is composed of four layers of tissue, and the actual process of digestion occurs in this tube. The names, locations, and functions of both the organs making up the gastrointestinal tract and the accessory organs can be learned using flash cards. The two processes of the digestive system are digestion and absorption. Digestion is what happens physically and chemically to the food. Absorption is moving the digested food into the blood. The process of digestion is explained in terms of what type of food is being digested: carbohydrates, fats, or proteins. The chemical process of digestion uses some suffixes that can make the processes easier to learn. The suffix *–ose* indicates the substance is a carbohydrate. The suffix *–ase* indicates the substance is an enzyme. In many cases, the first part of an enzyme's name tells you what substance is being digested: mal*tose* is digested by the enzyme malt*ase*. If you know this general rule, remembering what digests what becomes easier. Fats are lipids, so they are digested by lipase. Large carbohydrates are held together by amyl bonds, so they are digested by amylase. Remember that bile is not an enzyme; it causes a physical, not a chemical change. The protein enzymes pepsin and trypsin do not fit this rule. Also, they need to be made in an inactive form. The suffix for an inactive form is *–ogen*. Pepsin is made as pepsinogen and trypsin is made as trypsinogen. Absorption usually occurs by diffusion of nutrients into the cells of the small intestine and then into the blood. The structure of the interior of the small intestine greatly increases its internal surface area by forming villi. This makes the process of absorption much more efficient.

In your study group, you should go through the flash cards of the structures of the digestive system. The table with the list of enzymes, substances that they digest, and the end products they produce should be used to quiz each other. Discuss the process of absorption, go over the questions in the back of the chapter, and discuss possible test questions.

16 Nutrition and Metabolism

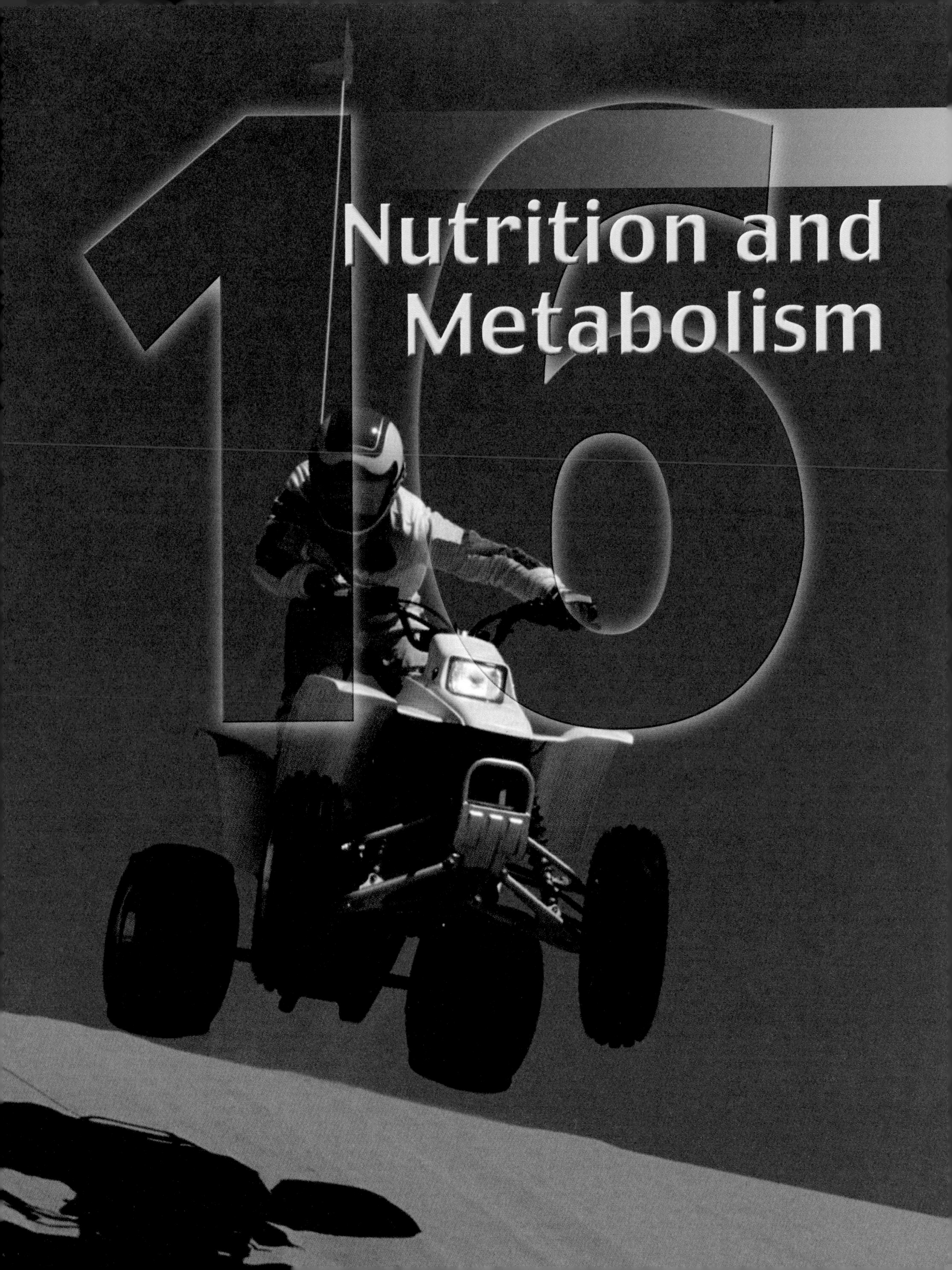

Outline

Objectives

AFTER YOU HAVE COMPLETED THIS CHAPTER, YOU SHOULD BE ABLE TO:

1. Define and contrast catabolism and anabolism.
2. Describe the metabolic roles of carbohydrates, fats, proteins, vitamins, and minerals.
3. Define basal metabolic rate and list some factors that affect it.
4. Discuss the physiological mechanisms that regulate body temperature.

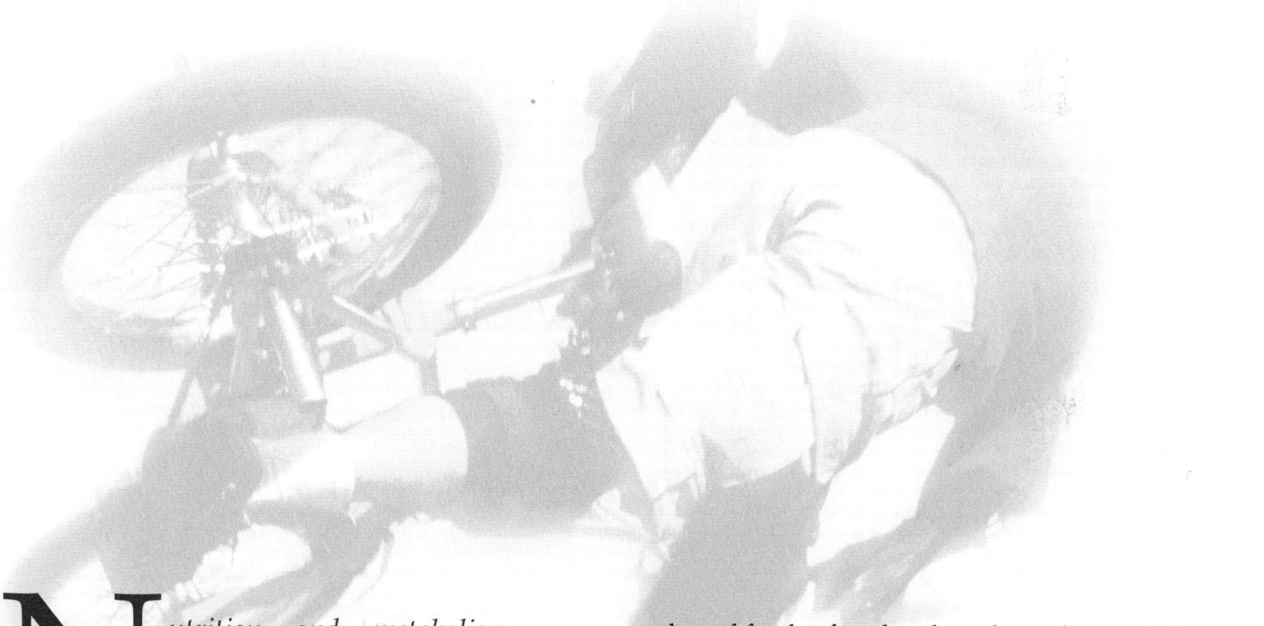

Nutrition and metabolism are words that are often used together—but what do they mean? *Nutrition* is a term that refers to the food (nutrients) that we eat. Proper nutrition requires a balance of the three basic food types: *carbohydrates*, *fats*, and *proteins*, plus essential *vitamins* and *minerals*. Malnutrition is a deficiency or imbalance in the consumption of food, vitamins, and minerals.

A good phrase to remember in connection with the word *metabolism* is "use of foods" because basically this is what metabolism is—the use the body makes of foods after they have been digested, absorbed, and circulated to cells. It uses them in two ways: as an energy source and as building blocks for making complex chemical compounds. Before they can be used in these two ways, foods have to be *assimilated*. Assimilation occurs when food molecules enter cells and undergo many chemical changes there. All the chemical reactions that release energy from food molecules make up the process of catabolism, a vital process because it is the only way that the body has of supplying itself with energy for doing any work. The many chemical reactions that build food molecules into more complex chemical compounds constitute the process of anabolism. Catabolism and anabolism make up the process of metabolism.

This chapter explores many of the basic ideas about why certain nutrients are necessary for survival and how they are used by the body.

ROLE OF THE LIVER

As we discussed in Chapter 15, the liver plays an important role in the mechanical digestion of lipids because it secretes *bile*. As you recall, bile breaks large fat globules into smaller droplets of fat that are more easily broken down. In addition, liver cells perform other functions necessary for healthy survival. They play a major role in the metabolism of all three kinds of foods. They help maintain a normal blood glucose concentration by carrying on complex and essential chemical reactions. Liver cells also carry on the first steps of protein and fat metabolism and synthesize several kinds of protein compounds. They release them into the blood, where they are called the *blood proteins or plasma proteins*. Prothrombin and fibrinogen, two of the plasma proteins formed by liver cells, play essential parts in blood clotting (see pp. 287-290). Another protein made by liver cells, albumin, helps maintain normal blood volume. Liver cells detoxify various poisonous substances such as bacterial products and certain drugs. Liver cells store several substances, notably iron and vitamins A and D.

The liver is assisted by an interesting structural feature of the blood vessels that supply it. As you may recall from Chapter 12, the hepatic portal vein delivers blood directly from the gastrointestinal tract to the liver (see Figure 12-12). This arrangement allows blood that has just absorbed nutrients and other substances to be processed by the liver before being distributed throughout the body. Thus excess nutrients and vitamins can be stored and toxins can be removed from the bloodstream.

Quick Check

1. What are the three basic food types?
2. What is metabolism?
3. How many of the liver's functions can you describe?

NUTRIENT METABOLISM

Carbohydrate Metabolism

Carbohydrates are the preferred energy food of the body. The larger carbohydrate molecules are composed of smaller "building blocks," primarily *glucose* (see Chapter 2). Human cells catabolize (break down) glucose rather than other substances as long as enough glucose enters them to supply their energy needs. Three series of chemical reactions, occurring in a precise sequence, make up the process of glucose catabolism. **Glycolysis** (glye-KOL-i-sis) is the name given the first series of reactions, **citric acid cycle** is the name of the second series, and **electron transfer system** is the third. Glycolysis, as Figure 16-1 shows, changes glucose to pyruvic acid. The citric acid cycle changes the pyruvic acid to carbon dioxide. Glycolysis takes place in the cytoplasm of a cell, whereas the citric acid cycle goes on in the mitochondria, the cell's miniature power plants. Glycolysis uses no oxygen; it is an **anaerobic** (an-er-O-bik) process. The citric acid cycle, in contrast, is an oxygen-using or **aerobic** (aer-O-bik) process.

While the chemical reactions of glycolysis and the citric acid cycle occur, energy stored in the glucose molecule is being released. More than half of the released energy is in the form of high-energy electrons. The electron transport system, located in the mitochondria, almost immediately transfers the energy to molecules of adenosine triphosphate (ATP). The rest of the energy originally stored in the glucose molecule is released as heat. ATP serves as the direct source of energy for doing cellular work in all kinds of living organisms from one-cell plants to billion-cell animals, including man. Among biological compounds, therefore, ATP ranks as one of the most important. The energy transferred to ATP molecules differs in two ways from the energy stored in food molecules: the energy in ATP molecules is not stored but is released almost instantaneously, and it can be used directly to do cellular work. Release of energy from food molecules occurs much more slowly because it accompanies the long series of chemical reactions that make up the process of catabolism. Energy released from food molecules cannot be used directly for doing cellular work. It must first

FIGURE 16-1

Catabolism of glucose. Glycolysis splits one molecule of glucose (six carbon atoms) into two molecules of pyruvic acid (three carbon atoms each). The citric acid cycle converts each pyruvic acid molecule into three carbon dioxide molecules (one carbon atom each).

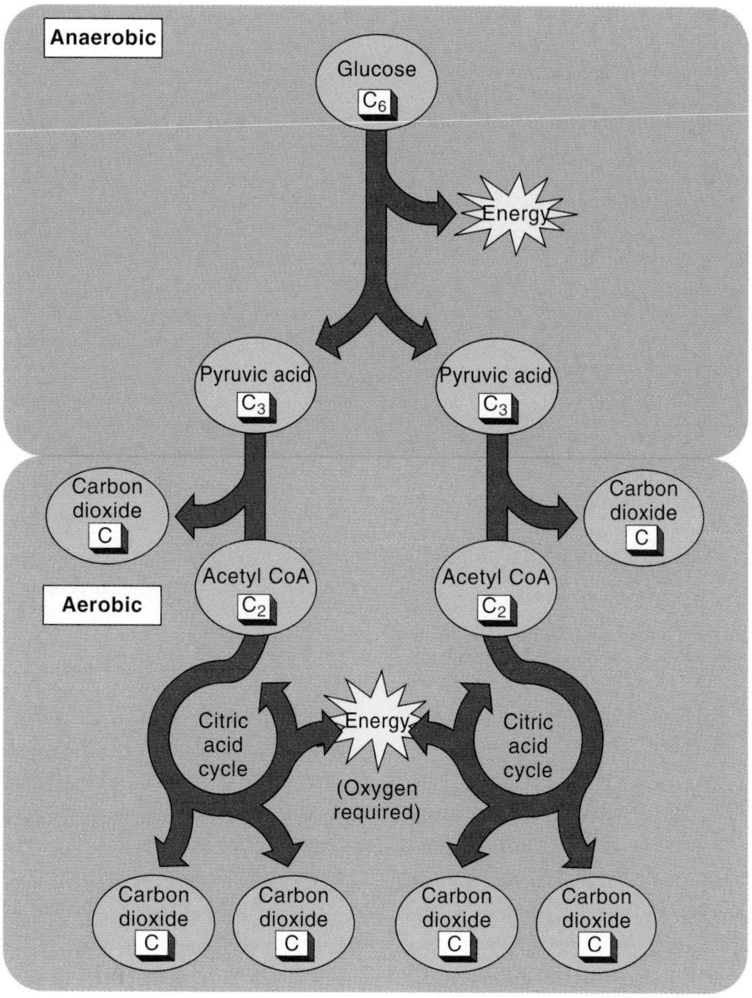

be transferred to ATP molecules and then be explosively released from them.

As Figure 16-2 shows, ATP is made up of an adenosine group and three phosphate groups. The capacity of ATP to store large amounts of energy is found in the high-energy bonds that hold the phosphate groups together, illustrated as curvy lines. When a phosphate group breaks off of the molecule, an adenosine diphosphate (ADP) molecule and free phosphate group result. Energy that had been holding the phosphate bond together is freed to do cellular work (muscle fiber contractions, for example). As you can see in Figure 16-2, the ADP and phosphate are reunited by the energy produced by carbohydrate catabolism, making ATP a reusable energy-storage molecule. Only enough ATP for immediate cellular requirements is made at any one time. Glucose that is not

FIGURE 16-2

ATP. A, The structure of ATP. A single adenosine group (*A*) has three attached phosphate groups (*P*). The high-energy bonds between the phosphate groups can release chemical energy to do cellular work. **B,** ATP energy cycle. ATP stores energy in its last high-energy phosphate bond. When that bond is later broken, energy is released to do cellular work. The ADP and phosphate groups that result can be resynthesized into ATP capturing additional energy from nutrient catabolism.

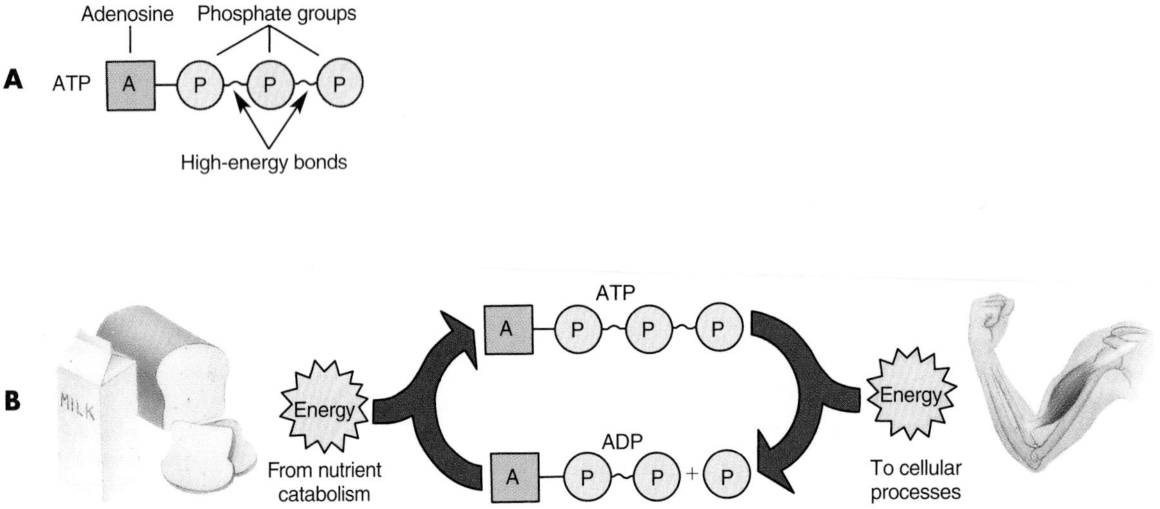

needed is anabolized into larger molecules that are stored for later use.

Glucose anabolism is called **glycogenesis** (glye-ko-JEN-e-sis). Carried on chiefly by liver and muscle cells, glycogenesis consists of a series of reactions that join glucose molecules together, like many beads in a necklace, to form *glycogen*, a compound sometimes called *animal starch*.

Something worth noting is that the amount of nutrients in the blood normally does not change very much, not even when we go without food for many hours, when we exercise and use a lot of food for energy, or when we sleep and use little food for energy. The amount of glucose in our blood, for example, usually stays at about 70 to 110 mg in 100 ml of blood.

Several hormones help regulate carbohydrate metabolism to keep blood glucose normal. **Insulin** is one of the most important of these. It acts in some way not yet definitely known to make glucose leave the blood and enter the cells at a more rapid rate. As insulin secretion increases, more glucose leaves the blood and enters the cells. The amount of glucose in the blood therefore decreases as the rate of glucose metabolism in cells increases (see p. 268). Too little insulin secretion, such as occurs with diabetes mellitus, produces the opposite effects. Less glucose leaves the blood and enters the cells; more glucose therefore remains in the blood, and less glucose is metabolized by cells. In other words, high blood glucose (hyperglycemia) and a low rate of glucose metabolism characterize insulin deficiency. Insulin is the only hormone that lowers the blood glucose level. Several other hormones, on the other hand, increase it. Growth hormone secreted by the anterior pituitary gland, hydrocortisone secreted by the adrenal cortex, epinephrine secreted by the adrenal medulla, and glucagon secreted by the pancreatic islets are four of the most important hormones that increase blood glucose. More information about these hormones appears in Chapter 10.

Health & Well-Being

Carbohydrate Loading

A number of athletes and others who must occasionally sustain endurance exercise for a significant period practice **carbohydrate loading** or **glycogen loading.** As with liver cells, some skeletal muscle fibers can take up and store glucose in the form of glycogen. By ceasing intense exercise and switching to a diet high in carbohydrates 2 or 3 days before an endurance event, an athlete can cause the skeletal muscles to store almost twice as much glycogen as usual. This allows the muscles to sustain aerobic exercise for up to 50% longer than usual. The concept of carbohydrate loading has been used to promote the use of "energy bar" sport snacks.

FIGURE 16-3

Catabolism of nutrients. Fats, carbohydrates, and proteins can be converted to products that enter the citric acid cycle to yield energy.

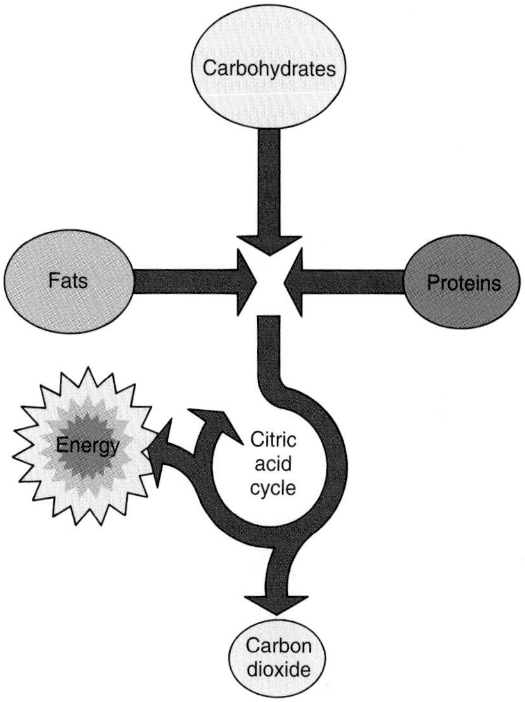

Fat Metabolism

Fats, like carbohydrates, are primarily energy foods. If cells have inadequate amounts of glucose to catabolize, they immediately shift to the catabolism of fats for energy. Fats are simply converted into a form of glucose that can enter the citric acid cycle. This happens normally when a person goes without carbohydrates for many hours. It happens abnormally in untreated diabetic individuals. Because of an insulin deficiency, too little glucose enters the cells of a diabetic person to supply all energy needs. The result is that the cells catabolize fats to make up the difference (Figure 16-3). In all persons, fats not needed for catabolism are anabolized to form triglycerides and stored in adipose tissue.

Protein Metabolism

In a healthy person, proteins are catabolized to release energy to a very small extent. When fat reserves are low, as they are in the starvation that accompanies certain eating disorders such as anorexia nervosa, the body can start to use its protein molecules as an energy source. Specifically, the amino acids that make up proteins are each broken apart to yield an amine group that is converted to a form of glucose that can enter the citric acid cycle. After a shift to reliance on protein catabolism as a major energy source occurs, death may quickly follow because vital proteins in the muscles and nerves are catabolized (see Figure 16-3).

A more common situation in normal bodies is protein anabolism, the process by which the body builds amino acids into complex protein compounds (for example, enzymes and proteins that form the structure of the cell). Proteins are assembled from a pool of 20 different kinds of amino acids. If any one type of amino acid is deficient, vital proteins cannot be synthesized—a serious health threat. One way your body maintains a constant supply of amino acids is by making them from other compounds already present in the body. Only about half of the required 20 types of amino acids can be made by the body, however. The remaining types of amino acids must be supplied in the diet. **Essential amino acids** are those

TABLE 16-1
Amino Acids

ESSENTIAL (INDISPENSABLE)	NONESSENTIAL (DISPENSABLE)
Histidine*	Alanine
Isoleucine	Arginine
Leucine	Asparagine
Lysine	Aspartic acid
Methionine	Cysteine
Phenylalanine	Glutamic acid
Threonine	Glutamine
Tryptophan	Glycine
Valine	Proline
	Serine
	Tyrosine†

*Essential in infants and, perhaps, adult males.
†Can be synthesized from phenylalanine, therefore is nonessential as long as phenylalanine is in the diet.

that must be in the diet. **Nonessential amino acids** can be missing from the diet because they can be made by the body. See Table 16-1.

Quick Check

1. How are aerobic and anaerobic respiration different? How are they alike?
2. How is energy transferred from glucose to ATP?
3. How are proteins used once they are absorbed into the body?
4. What are essential amino acids?

VITAMINS AND MINERALS

One glance at the label of any packaged food product reveals the importance we place on vitamins and minerals. We know that carbohydrates, fats, and proteins are used by our bodies to build important molecules and to provide energy. So why do we need vitamins and minerals?

First, let's discuss the importance of vitamins. Vitamins are organic molecules needed in small quantities for normal metabolism throughout the body. Vitamin molecules attach to enzymes and help them work properly. Many enzymes are totally useless without the appropriate vitamins to activate them. Most vitamins cannot be made by the body, so we must eat them in our food. The body can store fat-soluble vitamins—A, D, E, and K—in the liver for later use. Because the body cannot store water-soluble vitamins such as B vitamins and vitamin C, they must be continually supplied in the diet. Vitamin deficiencies can lead to severe metabolic problems. Table 16-2 lists some of the more well-known vitamins, their sources, functions, and symptoms of deficiency.

Minerals are just as important as vitamins. Minerals are inorganic elements or salts found naturally in the earth. As with vitamins, mineral ions can attach to enzymes and help them work. Minerals also function in a variety of other vital chemical reactions. For example, sodium, calcium, and other minerals are required for nerve conduction and for contraction in muscle fibers. Without these minerals, the brain, heart, and respiratory tract would cease to function. Information about some of the more important minerals is summarized in Table 16-3.

METABOLIC RATES

The **basal metabolic rate (BMR)** is the rate at which food is catabolized under basal conditions (that is, when the individual is resting but awake, is not digesting food, and is not adjusting to a cold external temperature). Or, stated differently, the BMR is the number of calories of heat that must be produced per hour by catabolism just to keep the body alive, awake, and comfortably warm. To provide energy for muscular work and digestion and absorption of food, an additional amount of food must be catabolized. The amount of additional food depends mainly on how much work

TABLE 16-2

Major Vitamins

VITAMIN	DIETARY SOURCE	FUNCTIONS	SYMPTOMS OF DEFICIENCY
Vitamin A	Green and yellow vegetables, dairy products, and liver	Maintains epithelial tissue and produces visual pigments	Night blindness and flaking skin
B-complex vitamins			
B_1 (thiamine)	Grains, meat, and legumes	Helps enzymes in the citric acid cycle	Nerve problems (beriberi), heart muscle weakness, and edema
B_2 (riboflavin)	Green vegetables, organ meats, eggs, and dairy products	Aids enzymes in the citric acid cycle	Inflammation of skin and eyes
B_3 (niacin)	Meat and grains	Helps enzymes in the citric acid cycle	Pellagra (scaly dermatitis and mental disturbances) and nervous disorders
B_5 (pantothenic acid)	Organ meat, eggs, and liver	Aids enzymes that connect fat and carbohydrate metabolism	Loss of coordination (rare)
B_6 (pyridoxine)	Vegetables, meats, and grains	Helps enzymes that catabolize amino acids	Convulsions, irritability, and anemia
B_{12} (cyanocobalamin)	Meat and dairy products	Involved in blood production and other processes	Pernicious anemia
Biotin	Vegetables, meat, and eggs	Helps enzymes in amino acid catabolism and fat and glycogen synthesis	Mental and muscle problems (rare)
Folic acid	Vegetables	Aids enzymes in amino acid catabolism and blood production	Digestive disorders and anemia
Vitamin C (ascorbic acid)	Fruits and green vegetables	Helps in manufacture of collagen fibers	Scurvy and degeneration of skin, bone, and blood vessels
Vitamin D (calciferol)	Dairy products and fish liver oil	Aids in calcium absorption	Rickets and skeletal deformity
Vitamin E (tocopherol)	Green vegetables and seeds	Protects cell membranes from being catabolized	Muscle and reproductive disorders (rare)

TABLE 16-3

Major Minerals

MINERAL	DIETARY SOURCE	FUNCTIONS	SYMPTOMS OF DEFICIENCY
Calcium (Ca)	Dairy products, legumes, and vegetables	Helps blood clotting, bone formation, and nerve and muscle function	Bone degeneration and nerve and muscle malfunction
Chlorine (Cl)	Salty foods	Aids in stomach acid production and acid-base balance	Acid-base imbalance
Cobalt (Co)	Meat	Helps vitamin B_{12} in blood cell production	Pernicious anemia
Copper (Cu)	Seafood, organ meats, and legumes	Involved in extracting energy from the citric acid cycle and in blood production	Fatigue and anemia
Iodine (I)	Seafood and iodized salt	Aids in thyroid hormone synthesis	Goiter (thyroid enlargement) and decrease of metabolic rate
Iron (Fe)	Meat, eggs, vegetables, and legumes	Involved in extracting energy from the citric acid cycle and in blood production	Fatigue and anemia
Magnesium (Mg)	Vegetables and grains	Helps many enzymes	Nerve disorders, blood vessel dilation, and heart rhythm problems
Manganese (Mn)	Vegetables, legumes, and grains	Helps many enzymes	Muscle and nerve disorders
Phosphorus (P)	Dairy products and meat	Aids in bone formation and is used to make ATP, DNA, RNA, and phospholipids	Bone degeneration and metabolic problems
Potassium (K)	Seafood, milk, fruit, and meats	Helps muscle and nerve function	Muscle weakness, heart problems, and nerve problems
Sodium (Na)	Salty foods	Aids in muscle and nerve function and fluid balance	Weakness and digestive upset
Zinc (Zn)	Many foods	Helps many enzymes	Metabolic problems

FIGURE 16-4

Factors that determine the basal and total metabolic rates.

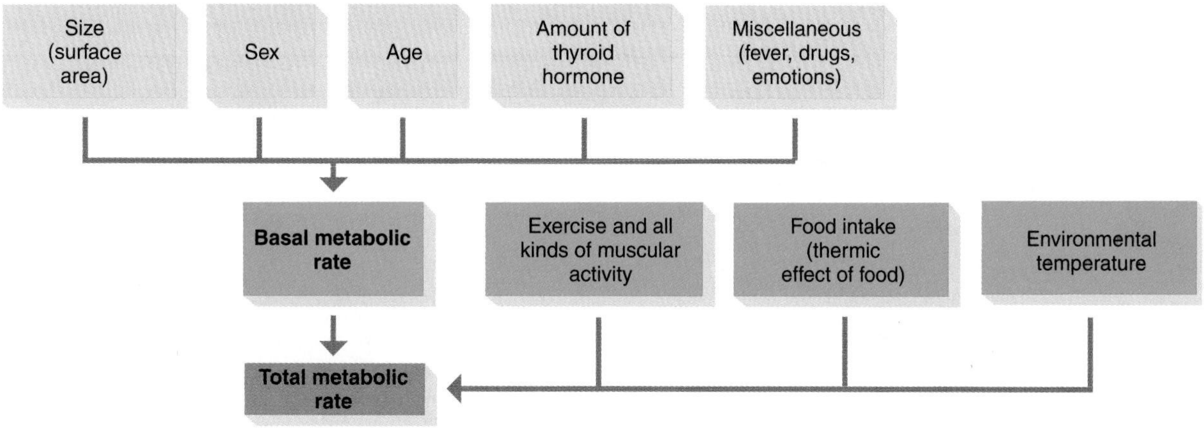

Health & Well-Being

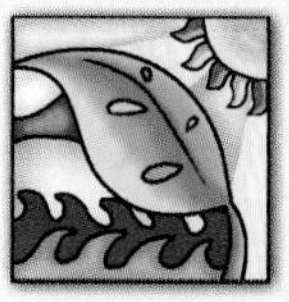

Vitamin Supplements for Athletes

Because a deficiency of vitamins **(avitaminosis)** can cause poor athletic performance, many athletes regularly consume vitamin supplements. However, research suggests that vitamin supplementation has little or no effect on athletic performance. A reasonably well-balanced diet supplies more than enough vitamins for even the elite athlete. The use of vitamin supplements therefore has fueled some controversy among exercise experts. Opponents of vitamin supplements cite the cost and the possibility of liver damage associated with some forms of **hypervitaminosis,** whereas supporters cite the benefit of protecting against vitamin deficiency.

Research, Issues & Trends

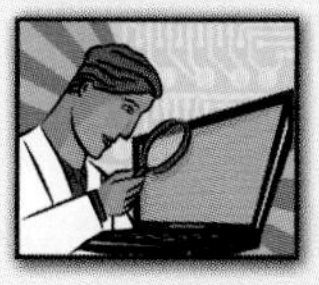

Measuring Energy

Physiologists studying metabolism must be able to express a quantity of energy in mathematical terms. The unit of energy measurement most often used is the calorie (cal). A calorie is the amount of energy needed to raise the temperature of 1 g of water 1° C. Because physiologists often deal with very large amounts of energy, the larger unit, *kilocalorie* (kcal) or *Calorie* (notice the upper-case C), is used. There are 1000 cal in 1 kcal or Calorie. Nutritionists prefer to use *Calorie* when they express the amount of energy stored in a food.

the individual does. The more active he or she is, the more food the body must catabolize and the higher the total metabolic rate will be. The **total metabolic rate (TMR)** is the total amount of energy used by the body per day (Figure 16-4).

When the number of calories in your food intake equals your TMR, your weight remains constant (except for possible variations resulting from water retention or water loss). When your food intake provides more calories than your TMR, you gain weight; when your food intake provides fewer calories than your TMR, you lose weight. These weight control principles rarely fail

FIGURE 16-5

The skin as a thermoregulatory organ. When homeostasis requires that the body conserve heat, blood flow in the warm organs of the body's core increases *(left).* When heat must be lost to maintain the stability of the internal environment, flow of warm blood to the skin increases *(right).* Heat can be lost from the blood and skin by means of radiation, conduction, convection, and evaporation.

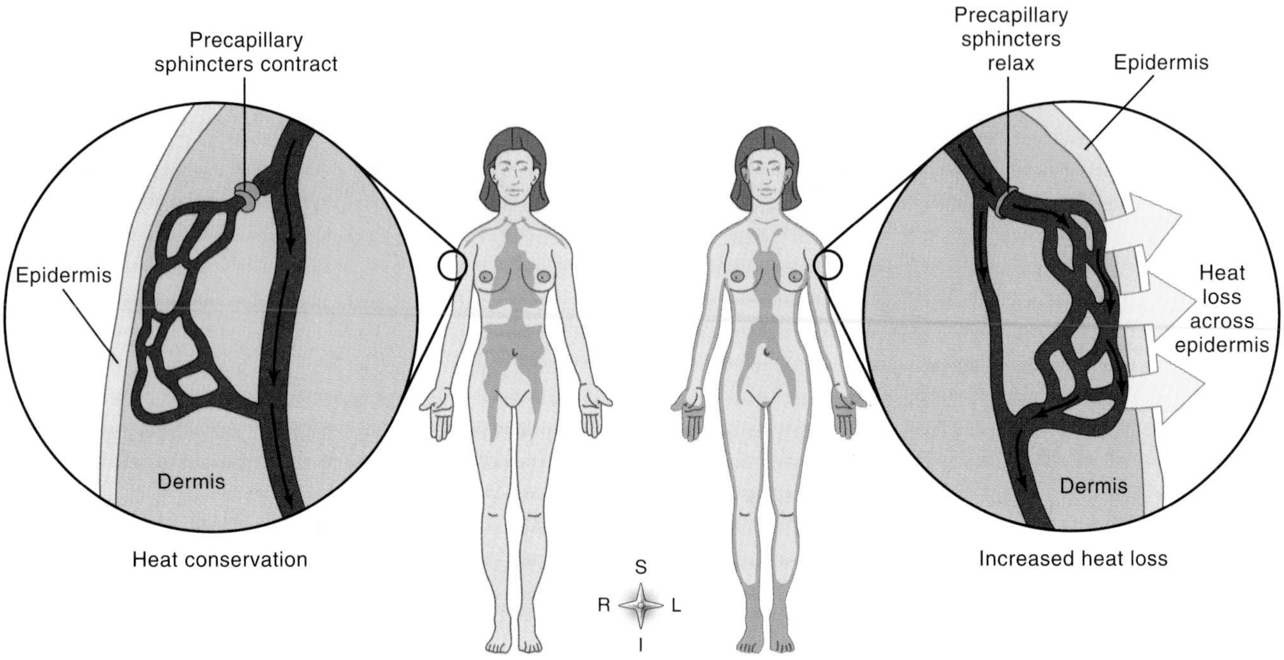

to operate. Nature does not forget to count calories. Reducing diets make use of this knowledge. They contain fewer calories than the TMR of the individual eating the diet. See Appendix A for information on the *body mass index (BMI)* and its relationship to body weight.

BODY TEMPERATURE

Considering the fact that more than 60% of the energy released from food molecules during catabolism is converted to heat rather than being transferred to ATP, it is no wonder that maintaining a constant body temperature is a challenge. Maintaining homeostasis of body temperature or thermoregulation is the function of the hypothalamus. The hypothalamus operates a variety of negative-feedback mechanisms that keep body temperature in its normal range (36.2° to 37.6° C or 97° to 100° F).

The skin is often involved in negative-feedback loops that maintain body temperature. When the body is overheated, blood flow to the skin increases (Figure 16-5). Warm blood from the body's core can then be cooled by the skin, which acts as a radiator. At the skin, heat can be lost from blood by the following mechanisms:

1. Radiation—flow of heat waves away from the blood
2. Conduction—transfer of heat energy to the skin and then the external environment
3. Convection—transfer of heat energy to air that is continually flowing away from the skin
4. Evaporation—absorption of heat by water (sweat) vaporization

When necessary, heat can be conserved by reducing blood flow in the skin (see Figure 16-5).

A number of other mechanisms can be called on to help maintain the homeostasis of body temperature. Heat-generating muscle activity such as shivering and secretion of metabolism-regulating hormones are two of the body's processes that can be altered to adjust the body's temperature. The concept of using feedback control loops in homeostatic mechanisms was introduced in Chapter 1.

Quick

1. What is the overall job of vitamins in the body?
2. What is another name for the rate at which food is catabolized under resting conditions?
3. How does calories consumed relate to a person's body weight?
4. Can you describe the four main ways that heat leaves the body?

Science Applications

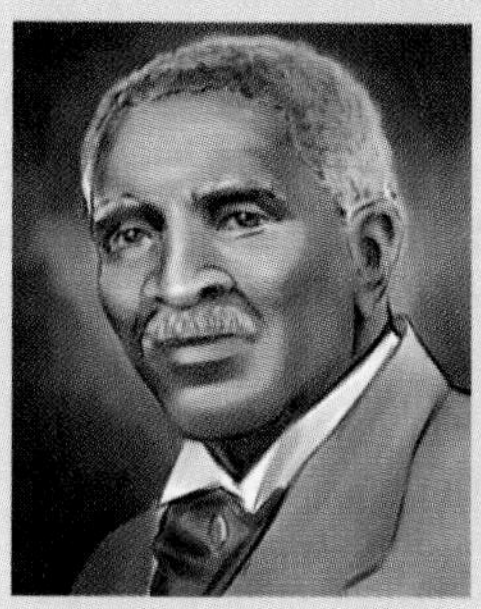

Food Science

George Washington Carver (1864-1943).

At the dawn of the twentieth century, one figure loomed large in the world of food science—George Washington Carver. Born a slave on a Missouri plantation during the Civil War, Carver overcame great obstacles to become one of the most admired American scientists in history. Although talented in music and art, it was his knack for agriculture that led him to a long and successful career as a professor, researcher, and inventor in the agriculture department of Alabama's Tuskegee Institute. There, his work resulted in the creation of 325 products from peanuts, nearly 200 products from yams (sweet potatoes), and hundreds more from other plants native to the Southern United States. Development of these new products helped poor farmers survive by allowing them to make money from a variety of crops that thrived on their land.

Today, breakthroughs continue in the world of agriculture and food science. Farmers and ranchers work closely with agricultural scientists and technicians to improve food crops and livestock—and ways of raising them. As did Carver, they strive to work in ways that benefit the land as well as the people. Of course, nutritionists, dieticians, chefs, and food preparers all play a role in getting these crops to our table in a healthy and appetizing way. Food scientists and other industrial scientists work to develop technologies and methods for preparing, preserving, storing, and packaging foods.

OUTLINE SUMMARY

DEFINITIONS

A. Nutrition—food, vitamins, and minerals that are ingested and assimilated into the body
B. Metabolism—process of using food molecules as energy sources and as building blocks for our own molecules
C. Catabolism—breaks food molecules down, releasing their stored energy; oxygen used in catabolism
D. Anabolism—builds food molecules into complex substances

ROLE OF THE LIVER

A. Processes blood immediately after it leaves the gastrointestinal tract
   1. Helps maintain normal blood glucose level
   2. Site of protein and fat metabolism
   3. Removes toxins from the blood

NUTRIENT METABOLISM

A. Carbohydrates are primarily catabolized for energy (Figure 16-1), but small amounts are anabolized by glycogenesis (a series of chemical reactions that changes glucose to glycogen—occurs mainly in liver cells where glycogen is stored)
B. Blood glucose (imprecisely, blood sugar)—normally stays between about 80 and 120 mg per 100 ml of blood; insulin accelerates the movement of glucose out of the blood into cells, therefore decreases blood glucose and increases glucose catabolism
C. Adenosine triphosphate (ATP)—molecule in which energy obtained from breakdown of foods is stored; serves as a direct source of energy for cellular work (Figure 16-2)
D. Fats catabolized to yield energy and anabolized to form adipose tissue (Figure 16-3)
E. Proteins primarily anabolized and secondarily catabolized

VITAMINS AND MINERALS

A. Vitamins—organic molecules that are needed in small amounts for normal metabolism (Table 16-2)
B. Minerals—inorganic molecules required by the body for normal function (Table 16-3)

METABOLIC RATES

A. Basal metabolic rate (BMR)—rate of metabolism when a person is lying down but awake and not digesting food and when the environment is comfortably warm
B. Total metabolic rate (TMR)—the total amounts of energy, expressed in calories, used by the body per day (Figure 16-4)

BODY TEMPERATURE

A. Hypothalamus—regulates the homeostasis of body temperature through a variety of processes
B. Skin—can cool the body by losing heat from the blood through four processes: radiation, conduction, convection, evaporation (Figure 16-5)

NEW WORDS

anabolism	catabolism	glycogenesis	total metabolic rate (TMR)
basal metabolic rate (BMR)	citric acid cycle	glycolysis	vitamin
calorie	electron transport system	kilocalorie	
		thermoregulation	

REVIEW QUESTIONS

1. Define *anabolism* and *catabolism.*
2. Explain the function of the liver.
3. Briefly explain the process of glycolysis.
4. Briefly explain the citric acid cycle.
5. What is the function of the electron transfer system?
6. Explain the ways in which energy stored in ATP is different than the energy stored in food molecules.
7. List the hormones that tend to increase the amount of sugar in the blood.
8. When does fat catabolism usually occur?
9. When does protein catabolism usually occur?
10. Explain what is meant by a nonessential amino acid.
11. Name three water-soluble and three fat-soluble vitamins.
12. Name three minerals needed by the body.
13. What is the function of vitamins and minerals in the body?
14. Differentiate between basal and total metabolic rate.
15. Name and explain three ways heat can be lost by the skin.

CRITICAL THINKING

16. Differentiate between absorption and assimilation.
17. Explain the advantage the body gains by having the blood go to the liver through the hepatic portal system.
18. Diagram the ATP-ADP cycle. Include where the energy is added and where it is released.
19. A man went on a 10-day vacation. His total metabolic rate was 2600 calories a day. His calorie intake was 3300 calories a day. He began his trip weighing 178 pounds, what did he weigh by the end of his vacation? (3500 excess calories = 1 pound)

CHAPTER TEST

1. The process of __________ occurs when food molecules enter the cells and undergo chemical changes.
2. __________ is the term used to describe all the chemical processes that release energy from food.
3. __________ is the term used to describe all the chemical processes that build food molecules into larger compounds.
4. The plasma proteins __________ and __________ are made by the liver and are important in blood clot formation.
5. The vitamins __________ and __________ can be stored in the liver.
6. The B vitamins are __________ soluble, whereas vitamins K and E are __________ soluble.
7. __________ is the total amount of energy used by the body per day.
8. __________ is the number of calories that must be used just to keep the body alive, awake, and comfortably warm.
9. To lose weight, your total caloric intake must be less than your __________.
10. One way heat can be lost by the skin is __________, which is the transfer of heat to the air that is continually flowing away from the skin.
11. One way heat can be lost by the skin is __________, which is the absorption of heat by water (sweat) vaporization.
12. __________ is the process used by the body as its second choice of energy metabolism. People with diabetes frequently must use this process.
13. In a healthy body, __________ is used almost exclusively for anabolism rather than catabolism.
14. __________ are amino acids needed by the body, but they can be made from other amino acids if they are not supplied by the diet.

Match the statement in Column B with the correct term in Column A.

COLUMN A

15. _____ Glycolysis
16. _____ Citric acid cycle
17. _____ Electron transfer system
18. _____ Mitochondriacycle
19. _____ Cytoplasm
20. _____ ATP
21. _____ Glycogenesis
22. _____ ADP

COLUMN B

a. glycolysis occurs in this part of the cell
b. this part of carbohydrate metabolism does not require oxygen
c. this process converts high-energy molecules from the citric acid to ATP
d. this part of carbohydrate metabolism requires oxygen
e. this is the body's direct source of energy
f. when adenosine triphosphate loses a phosphate group it becomes this molecule
g. the citric acid cycle takes place in this part of the cell
h. this is glucose anabolism

STUDY TIPS

This chapter begins with an explanation of the functions of the liver and the importance of the portal system, both of which were discussed previously. The process of metabolism refers to the body's use of food. Fats and carbohydrates are used primarily for energy. Carbohydrate metabolism begins with glycolysis. *Glyco-* refers to carbohydrates, and *-lysis* means "to destroy or break down," and the process does exactly that. Glycolysis occurs in the cytoplasm, requires no oxygen, and releases very little energy. The end products of glycolysis enter the citric acid (or Krebs) cycle, which occurs in the mitochondria, requires oxygen, and produces high-energy molecules. The electron transfer system converts these high-energy molecules into ATP. ATP is the only energy source your body can use directly. The energy is stored between the phosphates in the molecule, and these phosphates can be broken off to release energy and replaced to store energy. Fat and protein molecules can be modified so they can enter the citric acid cycle. The term *nonessential amino acids* does not mean your body doesn't need these amino acids; nonessential amino acids are necessary for you to live, but your body has the ability to make the nonessential amino from other amino acids. Vitamins and minerals assist in enzyme function. You can learn the names and functions of the vitamins and minerals from flash cards. Metabolic rates describe how quickly the food is used. Basal metabolic rate is the amount of food you use just to stay alive and awake. The total metabolic rate depends on how active you are.

In your study group, go over the flash cards for vitamins and minerals. Discuss the processes of carbohydrate, protein, and fat metabolism. Discuss what constitutes basal and total metabolic rates and the ways heat can be lost from the body. Go over the questions in the back of the chapter and discuss possible test questions.

17 The Urinary System

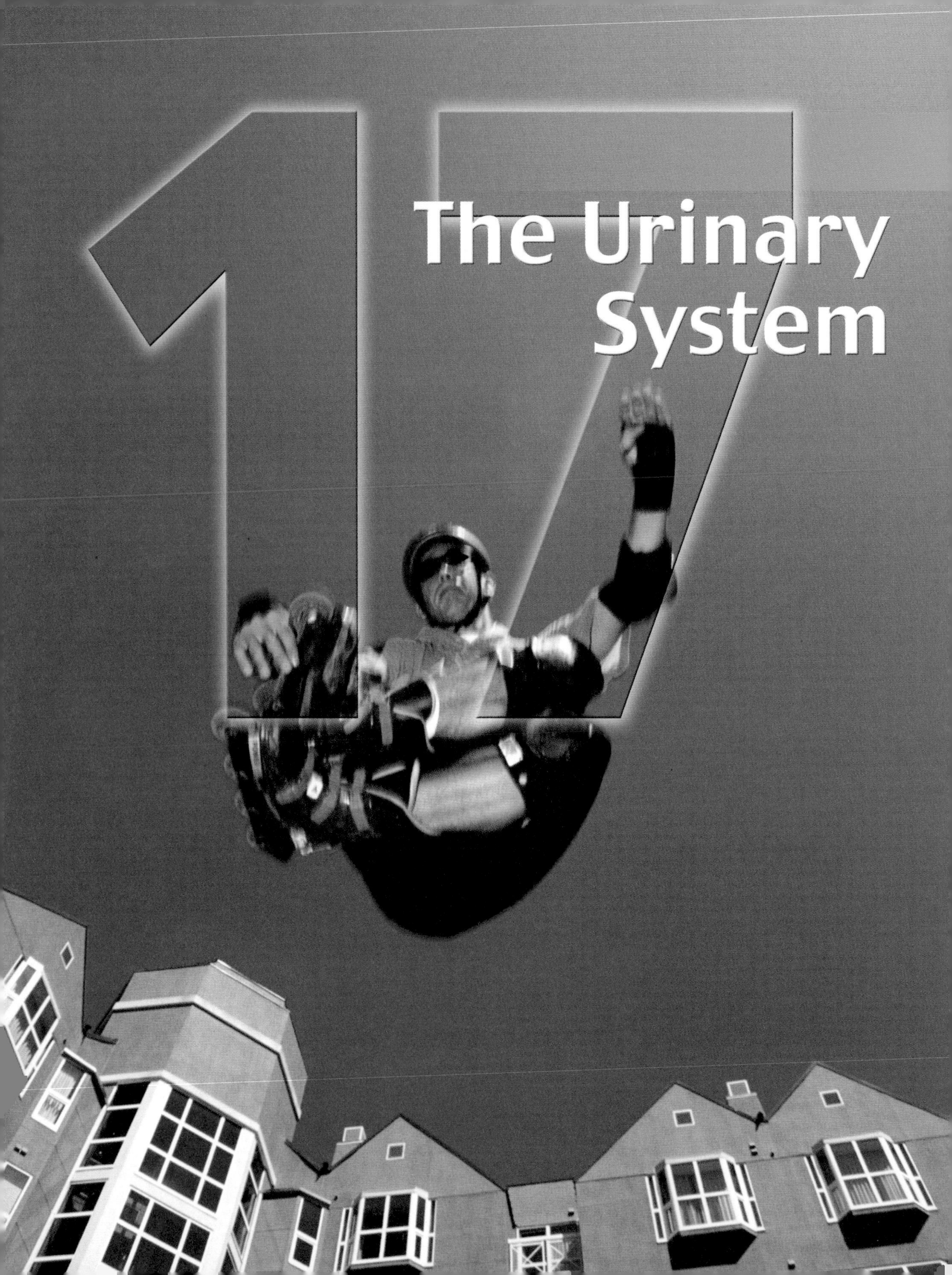

Outline

Objectives

AFTER YOU HAVE COMPLETED THIS CHAPTER, YOU SHOULD BE ABLE TO:

1. Identify the major organs of the urinary system and give the generalized function of each.
2. Name the parts of a nephron and describe the role each component plays in the formation of urine.
3. Explain the importance of filtration, tubular reabsorption, and tubular secretion in urine formation.
4. Discuss the mechanisms that control urine volume.
5. Explain how the kidneys act as vital organs in maintaining homeostasis.

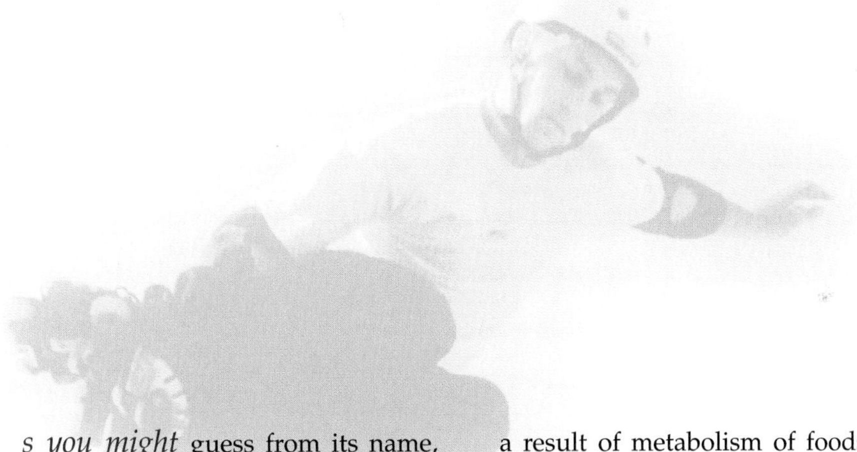

A*s you might* guess from its name, the urinary system performs the functions of producing and excreting urine from the body. What you might not guess so easily is how essential these functions are for the maintenance of homeostasis and healthy survival. The constancy of body fluid volumes and the levels of many important chemicals depend on normal urinary system function. Unless the urinary system operates normally, the normal composition of blood cannot be maintained for long, and serious consequences soon follow. The kidneys "clear" or clean the blood of the many waste products continually produced as a result of metabolism of foodstuffs in the body cells. As nutrients are burned for energy, the waste products produced must be removed from the blood, or they quickly accumulate to toxic levels—a condition called **uremia** (yoo-REE-mee-ah) or **uremic poisoning.** The kidneys also play a vital role in maintaining electrolyte, water, and acid-base balances in the body. In this chapter, we will discuss the structure and function of each organ of the urinary system. There are two kidneys, two ureters, one bladder, and one urethra (Figure 17-1). We will also briefly mention disease conditions produced by abnormal functioning of the urinary system.

FIGURE 17-1

Urinary system. A, Anterior view of urinary organs. **B,** Surface markings of the kidneys, 11th and 12th ribs, spinous processes of L1 to L4, and lower edge of pleura viewed from behind. **C,** X-ray film of the urinary organs.

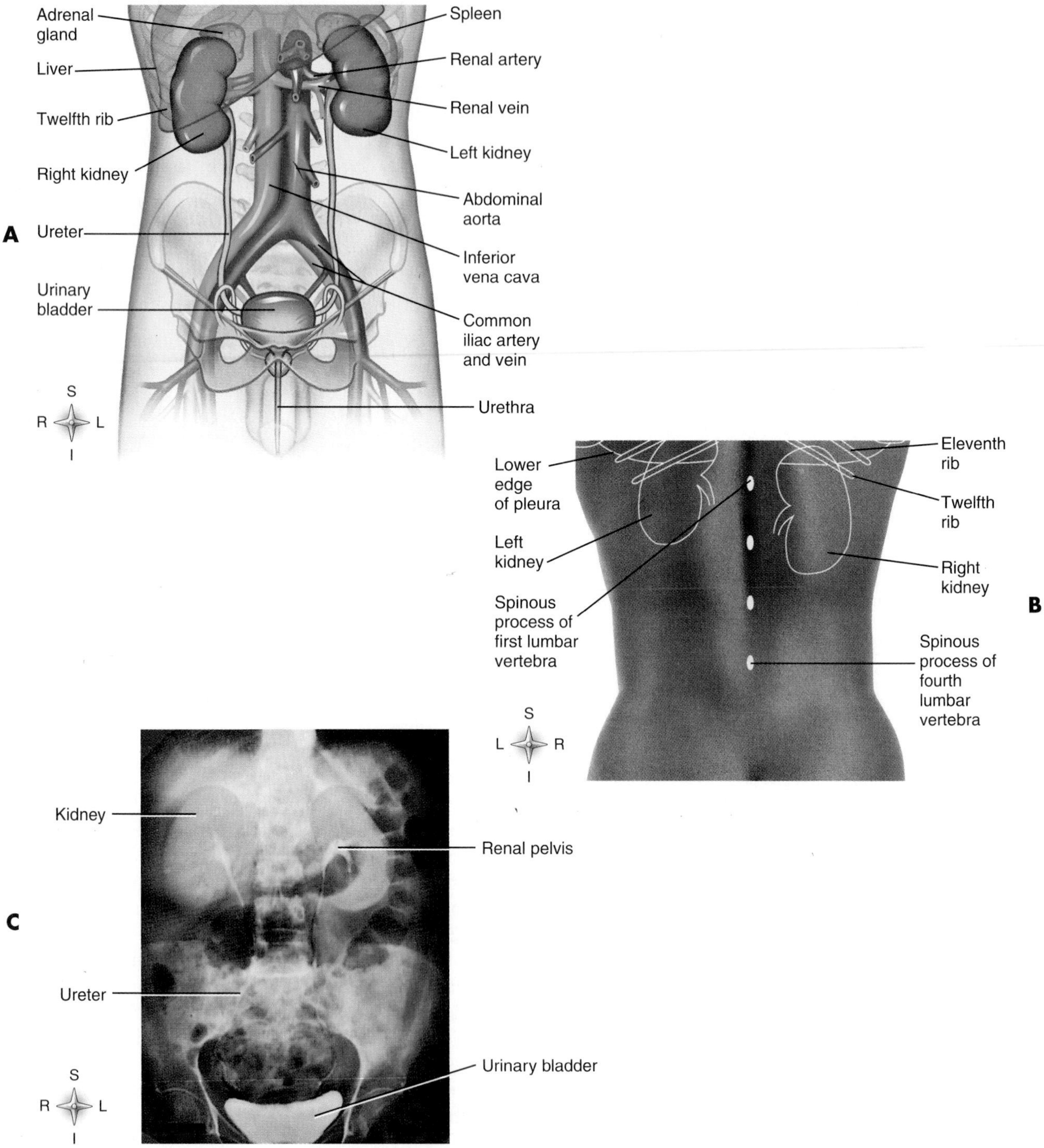

FIGURE 17-2

Internal structure of the kidney. A, Coronal section of the kidney in an artist's rendering. **B,** Photo of coronal section of a preserved human kidney.

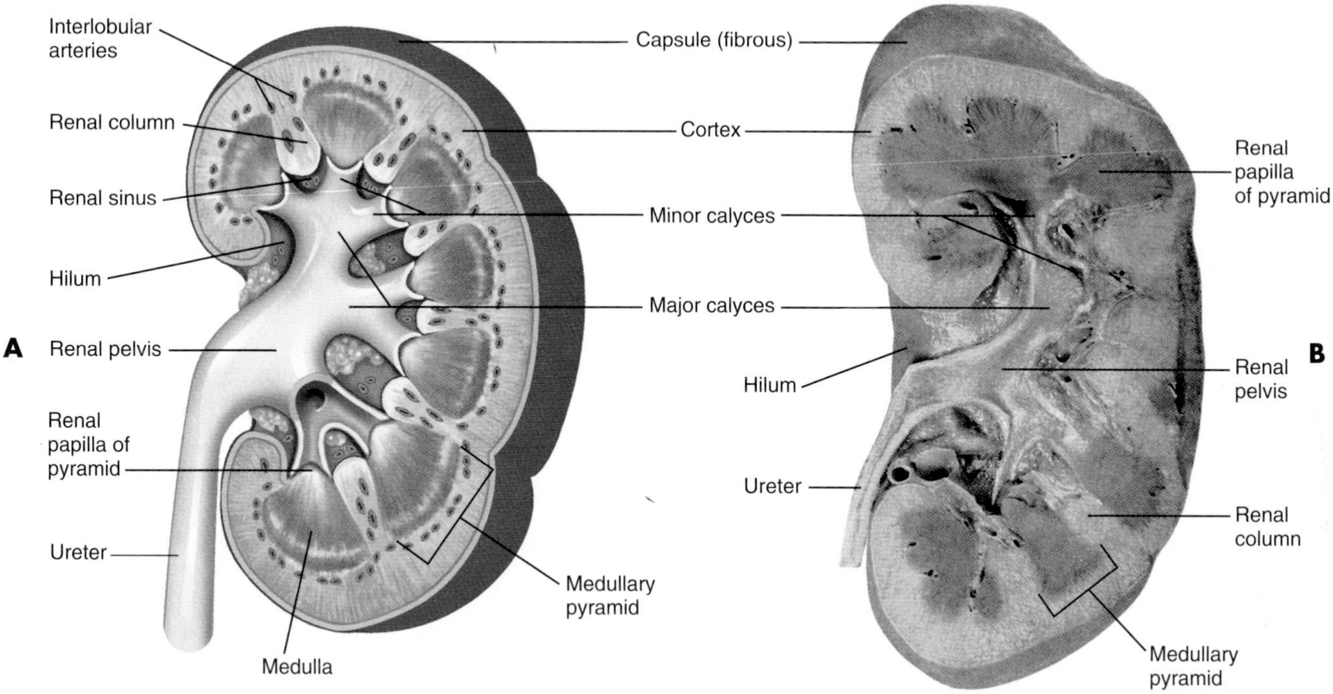

KIDNEYS

Location

To locate the kidneys on your own body, stand erect and put your hands on your hips with your thumbs meeting over your backbone. When you are in this position, your kidneys lie above your thumbs on either side of your spinal column, but their placement is higher than you might think. Note in Figure 17-1 that the right kidney, which touches the liver, is lower than the left. Both are protected a bit by the lower rib cage and are located under the muscles of the back and behind the parietal peritoneum (the membrane that lines the abdominal cavity). Because of this retroperitoneal location, a surgeon can operate on a kidney without cutting through the peritoneum. A heavy cushion of fat normally encases each kidney and helps hold it in place.

Note the relatively large diameter of the renal arteries in Figure 17-1. Normally a little more than 20% of the total blood pumped by the heart each minute enters the kidneys. The rate of blood flow through this organ is among the highest in the body. This is understandable because one of the main functions of the kidney is to remove waste products from the blood. Maintenance of a high rate of blood flow and normal blood pressure in the kidneys is essential for the formation of urine.

Internal Structure

If you were to slice through a kidney from side to side and open it like the pages of a book (called a coronal section), you would see the structures shown in Figure 17-2. Identify each of the following parts:

1. **Renal cortex** (KOR-teks)—the outer part of the kidney (the word *cortex* comes from the Latin

word for "bark," so the cortex of an organ is its outer layer).

2. **Renal medulla** (me-DUL-ah)—the inner portion of the kidney.
3. **Renal pyramids** (PIR-ah-mids)—the triangular divisions of the medulla of the kidney. Extensions of cortical tissue that dip down into the medulla between the renal pyramids are called *renal columns*.
4. **Renal papilla** (pah-PIL-ah) (pl. *papillae*)—narrow, innermost end of a pyramid.
5. **Renal pelvis**—(the kidney or renal pelvis) an expansion of the upper end of a ureter (the tube that drains urine into the bladder).
6. **Calyx** (KAY-liks) (pl. *calyces*)—a division of the renal pelvis (the papilla of a pyramid opens into each calyx).

Microscopic Structure

More than a million microscopic units called **nephrons** (NEF-rons) make up each kidney's interior. The shape of a nephron is unique, unmistakable, and admirably suited to its function of producing urine. It looks a little like a tiny funnel with a very long stem, but it is an unusual stem in that it is highly convoluted (that is, it has many bends in it). The nephron is composed of two principle components: the **renal corpuscle** and the **renal tubule.** The renal corpuscle can be subdivided still further into two parts and the renal tubule into four regions or segments. Identify each part of the renal corpuscle and renal tubule described below in Figures 17-3 and 17-4.

1. **Renal corpuscle**
   a. **Bowman's capsule**—the cup-shaped top of a nephron (the saclike Bowman's capsule surrounds the glomerulus).
   b. **Glomerulus** (glo-MAIR-yoo-lus) (pl. *glomeruli*)—a network of blood capillaries tucked into Bowman's capsule (note in Figure 17-3 that the small artery that delivers blood to the glomerulus, **[afferent arteriole]** is larger in diameter than the blood vessel that drains blood from it **[efferent arteriole]** and that it is relatively short. This explains the high blood pressure that exists in the glomerular capillaries. This high pressure is required to filter wastes from the blood).
2. **Renal tubule**
   a. **Proximal convoluted tubule**—the first segment of a renal tubule (it is called *proximal* because it lies nearest the tubule's origin from Bowman's capsule, and it is called *convoluted* because it has several bends).
   b. **Loop of Henle** (HEN-lee)—the extension of the proximal tubule (observe that the loop of Henle consists of a straight descending limb, a hairpin loop, and a straight ascending limb).
   c. **Distal convoluted tubule**—the part of the tubule distal to the ascending limb of the loop of Henle (it is the extension of the ascending limb).
   d. **Collecting tubule**—a straight (that is, not convoluted) part of a renal tubule (distal tubules of several nephrons join to form a single collecting tubule or duct).

Look again at Figure 17-3. Note that the renal corpuscles (glomeruli surrounded by Bowman's capsule) and both proximal and distal convoluted tubules are located in the cortex of the kidney. The medulla contains the loop of Henle and collecting tubules. Urine from the collecting tubules exits from the pyramid through the papilla and enters the calyx and renal pelvis before flowing into the ureter.

Function

The kidneys are vital organs. The function they perform, that of forming urine, is essential for homeostasis and maintenance of life. Early in the process of urine formation, fluid, electrolytes, and wastes from metabolism are *filtered* from the blood and enter the nephron. Additional wastes may be *secreted* into the tubules of the nephron as substances useful to the body are reabsorbed into the blood. Table 17-1 lists the components of normal versus abnormal urine. Normally the kidneys balance the amount of many substances entering and leaving the blood over time so that normal concentrations can be maintained. In short, the kidneys adjust their output to equal the intake of the body. By eliminating wastes and adjusting fluid balance, the kidneys play an essential part in maintaining homeostasis. Homeostasis cannot be maintained—nor can life itself—if the kidneys fail and the condition is not soon

FIGURE 17-3

Location and components of the nephron. A, Magnified wedge cut from a renal pyramid. **B,** Schematic showing relationship of glomerulus to Bowman's capsule and adjacent structures. **C,** Scanning electron micrograph showing several glomeruli and their associated blood vessels.

A

B

C

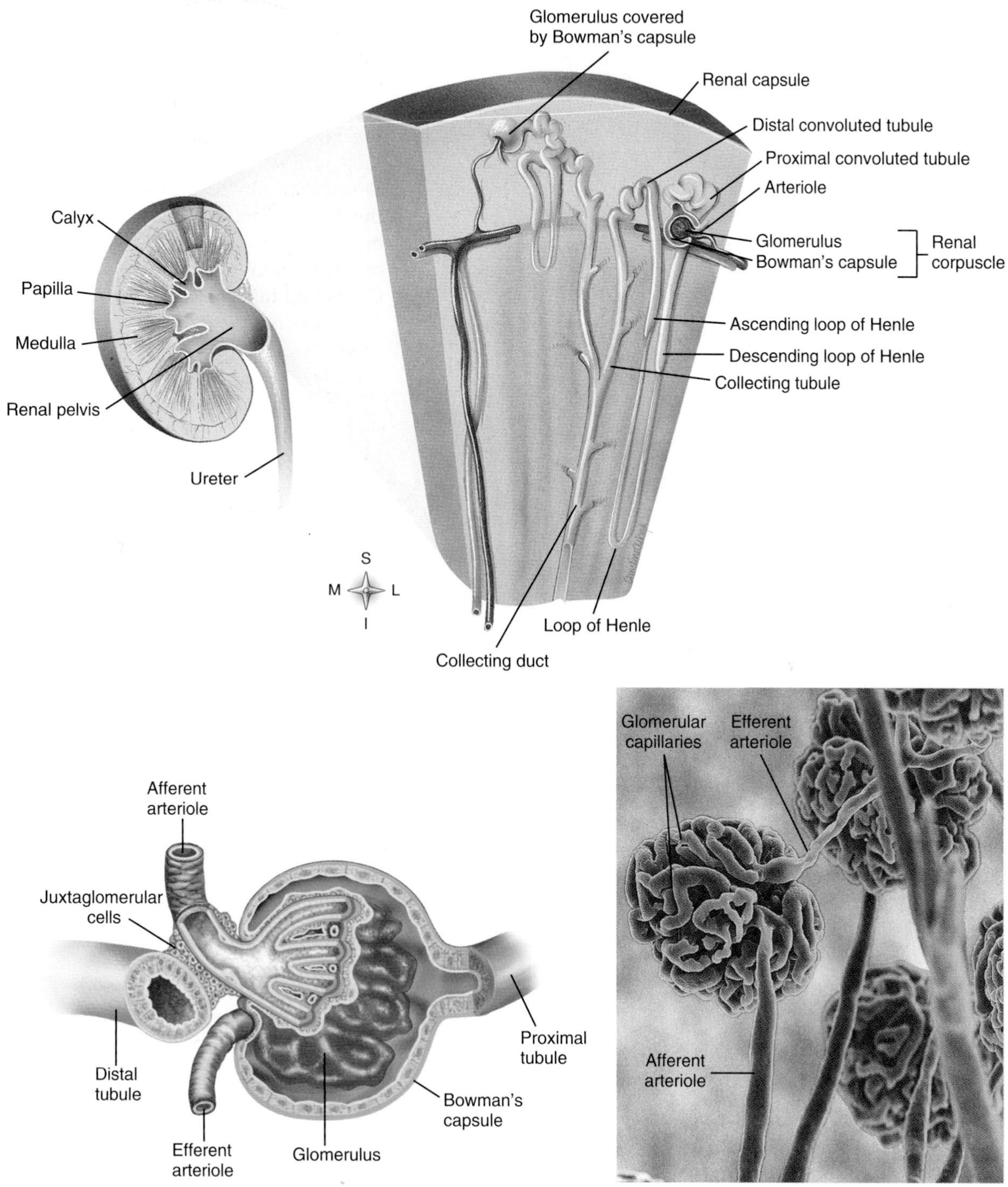

FIGURE 17-4

The nephron unit. Cross sections from the four segments of the renal tubule are shown. The differences in appearance in tubular cells seen in a cross section reflect the differing functions of each nephron segment.

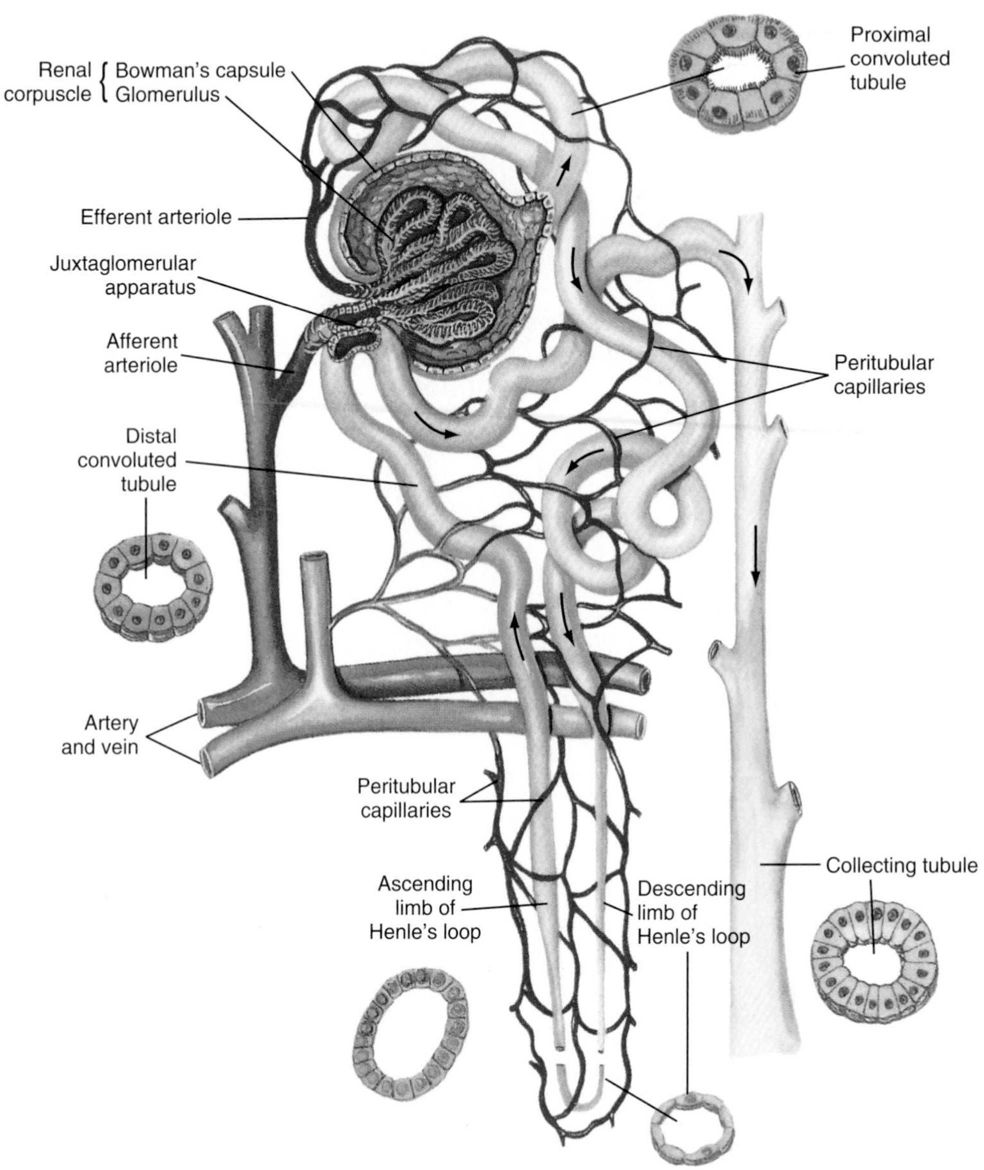

corrected. Nitrogenous waste products accumulate as a result of protein breakdown and quickly reach toxic levels if not excreted. If kidney function ceases because of injury or disease, life can be maintained by using an artificial kidney to cleanse the blood of wastes (see Clinical Application: Artificial Kidney on p. 446).

Excretion of toxins and of waste products containing nitrogen such as urea and ammonia represents only one of the important responsibilities of the kidney. The kidney also plays a key role in regulating the levels of many chemical substances in the blood such as chloride, sodium, potassium, and bicarbonate. The kidneys also regulate the proper balance between body water content and salt by selectively retaining or excreting both substances as requirements demand. In addition, the cells of the *juxtaglomerular apparatus* (see Figure 17-4) function in blood pressure regulation. When blood pressure is low, these cells secrete a hormone that initiates constriction of blood vessels and thus raises blood pressure. It is easy to understand why the kidneys are often considered to be the most important homeostatic organs in the body.

Quick Check

1. What are the two main regions of the kidney?
2. Can you describe the structure of a nephron?
3. What is the role of filtration in the kidney?

FORMATION OF URINE

The kidney's 2 million or more nephrons form urine by a series of three processes: (1) filtration, (2) reabsorption, and (3) secretion (Figure 17-5). Urine formation begins with the process of **filtration,** which goes on continually in the renal corpuscles (Bowman's capsules plus their encased glomeruli). Blood flowing through the glomeruli exerts pressure, and this glomerular blood pressure is high enough to push water and dissolved substances out of the glomeruli into the Bowman's capsule. Briefly, glomerular blood pressure causes filtration through the glomerular-capsular membrane. If the glomerular blood pressure drops below a certain level, filtration and urine formation cease. Hemorrhage, for example, may cause a precipitous drop in blood pressure followed by kidney failure.

Glomerular filtration normally occurs at the rate of 125 ml per minute. As a result, about 180 L (almost 190 quarts) of **glomerular filtrate** is produced by the kidneys every day.

Obviously no one ever excretes anywhere near 180 L of urine per day. Why? Because most of the fluid that leaves the blood by glomerular filtration, the first process in urine formation, returns to the blood by the second process—reabsorption.

TABLE 17-1

Characteristics of Urine

NORMAL CHARACTERISTICS	ABNORMAL CHARACTERISTICS
Transparent yellow, amber, or straw colored	Abnormal colors or cloudiness, which may indicate presence of blood, bile, bacteria, drugs, food pigments, or high-solute concentration
COMPOUNDS	
Mineral ions (for example, Na^+, Cl^-, K^+)	Acetone
Nitrogenous wastes: ammonia, creatinine, urea, uric acid	Albumin
Suspended solids, (sediment)*: bacteria, blood cells, casts (solid matter)	Bile
Urine pigments	Glucose
ODOR	
Slight odor	Acetone odor, which is common in diabetes mellitus
PH	
4.6-8.0	High in alkalosis; low in acidosis
SPECIFIC GRAVITY	
1.001-1.035	High specific gravity can cause precipitation of solutes and formation of kidney stones

*Occasional trace amounts.

Reabsorption is the movement of substances out of the renal tubules into the blood capillaries located around the tubules (peritubular capillaries). Water, glucose and other nutrients, and sodium

FIGURE 17-5

Formation of urine. Diagram shows the steps in urine formation in successive parts of a nephron: filtration, reabsorption, and secretion.

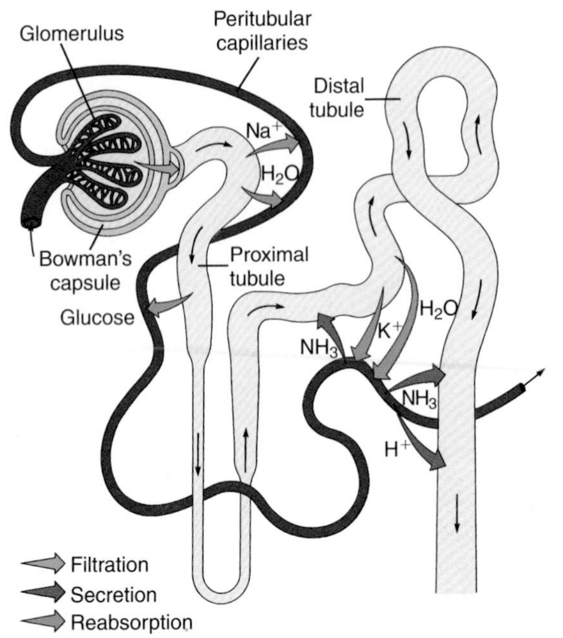

FIGURE 17-6

Glycosuria. Using a reagent strip to check the level of glucose in the urine of a diabetic patient.

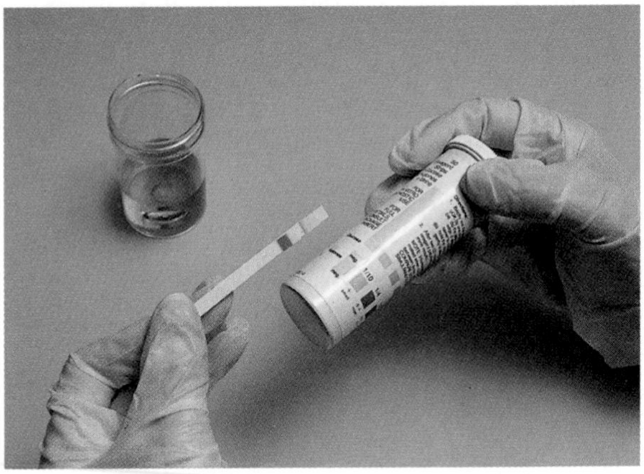

and other ions are substances that are reabsorbed. Reabsorption begins in the proximal convoluted tubules and continues in the loop of Henle, distal convoluted tubules, and collecting tubules.

Large amounts of water—approximately 178 L per day—are reabsorbed by osmosis from the proximal tubules. In other words, nearly 99% of the 180 L of water that leaves the blood each day by glomerular filtration returns to the blood by proximal tubule reabsorption.

The nutrient glucose is reabsorbed from the proximal tubules into peritubular capillary blood. None of this valuable nutrient is wasted by being lost in the urine. However, exceptions occur. For example, in *diabetes mellitus,* if blood glucose concentration increases above a certain level, the tubular filtrate then contains more glucose than kidney tubule cells can reabsorb. Some of the glucose therefore remains behind in the urine. Glucose in the urine—**glycosuria** (glye-ko-SOO-ree-ah)—is a well-known sign of diabetes mellitus (Figure 17-6).

Sodium ions and other ions are only partially reabsorbed from renal tubules. For the most part, sodium ions are actively transported back into blood from the tubular urine. The amount of sodium reabsorbed varies from time to time; it depends largely on salt intake. In general the greater the amount of salt intake, the less the amount of salt reabsorption and therefore the greater the amount of salt excreted in the urine. Also, the less the salt intake, the greater the salt reabsorption and the less salt excreted in the urine. By varying the amount of salt reabsorbed, the body usually can maintain homeostasis of the blood's salt concentration. This is an extremely important matter because cells are damaged by either too much or too little salt in the fluid around them.

Secretion is the process by which substances move into urine in the distal and collecting tubules from blood in the capillaries around these tubules. In this respect, secretion is reabsorption in reverse. Whereas reabsorption moves substances out of the urine into the blood, secretion moves substances out of the blood into the urine. Substances secreted are hydrogen ions, potassium ions, ammonia, and certain drugs. Hydrogen ions, potassium ions, and some drugs are secreted by being actively trans-

TABLE 17-2

Functions of Parts of Nephron in Urine Formation

PART OF NEPHRON	PROCESS IN URINE FORMATION	SUBSTANCES MOVED
Glomerulus	Filtration	Water and solutes (for example, sodium and other ions, glucose and other nutrients filtering out of glomeruli into Bowman's capsules)
Proximal tubule	Reabsorption	Water and solutes
Loop of Henle	Reabsorption	Sodium and chloride ions
Distal and collecting tubules	Reabsorption	Water, sodium, and chloride ions
	Secretion	Ammonia, potassium ions, hydrogen ions, and some drugs

ported out of the blood into tubular urine. Ammonia is secreted by diffusion. Kidney tubule secretion plays a crucial role in maintaining the body's acid-base balance (see Chapter 19).

In summary, the following processes occurring in successive portions of the nephron accomplish the function of urine formation (Table 17-2):

1. **Filtration**—of water and dissolved substances out of the blood in the glomeruli into Bowman's capsule
2. **Reabsorption**—of water and dissolved substances out of kidney tubules back into blood (this prevents substances needed by the body from being lost in urine. Usually, 97% to 99% of water filtered out of glomerular blood is retrieved from tubules).
3. **Secretion**—of hydrogen ions, potassium ions, and certain drugs

Control of Urine Volume

The body has ways to control the amount and composition of the urine that it excretes. It does this mainly by controlling the amount of water and dissolved substances that are reabsorbed by the convoluted tubules. For example, a hormone (antidiuretic hormone or ADH) from the posterior pituitary gland decreases the amount of urine by making collecting tubules permeable to water. If no ADH is present, the tubules are practically impermeable to water, so little or no water is reabsorbed from them. When ADH is present in the blood, collecting tubules are permeable to water and water is reabsorbed from them. As a result, less water is lost from the body as urine, or more water is retained from the tubules—whichever way you wish to say it. At any rate, for this reason ADH is accurately described as the "water-retaining hormone." You might also think of it as the "urine-decreasing hormone."

The hormone aldosterone, secreted by the adrenal cortex, plays an important part in controlling the kidney tubules' reabsorption of salt. Primarily it stimulates the tubules to reabsorb sodium salts at a faster rate. Secondarily, aldosterone also increases tubular water reabsorption. The term *salt- and water-retaining hormone* therefore is a descriptive nickname for aldosterone. This mechanism is discussed in chapter 18.

Another hormone, atrial natriuretic hormone (ANH), secreted from the heart's atrial wall, has the opposite effect of aldosterone. ANH stimulates kidney tubules to secrete more sodium and thus lose more water. Thus ANH is a *salt- and water-losing hormone*. The body secretes ADH, aldosterone, and ANH in different amounts, depending on the homeostatic balance of body fluids at any particular moment.

Health & Well-Being

Proteinuria after Exercise

Proteinuria is the presence of abnormally large amounts of plasma proteins in the urine. Proteinuria usually indicates kidney disease **(nephropathy)** because only damaged nephrons consistently allow many plasma protein molecules to leave the blood. However, intense exercise causes temporary proteinuria in many individuals. Some exercise physiologists believed that intense athletic activities cause kidney damage, but subsequent research has ruled out that explanation. One current hypothesis is that hormonal changes during strenuous exercise increase the permeability of the nephron's filtration membrane, allowing more plasma proteins to enter the filtrate. Some postexercise proteinuria is usually considered normal.

Sometimes the kidneys do not excrete normal amounts of urine as a result of kidney disease, cardiovascular disease, or stress. Here are some terms associated with abnormal amounts of urine:

1. **Anuria** (ah-NOO-ree-ah)—absence of urine
2. **Oliguria** (ol-i-GYOO-ree-ah)—scanty amounts of urine
3. **Polyuria** (pol-e-YOO-ree-ah)—an unusually large amount of urine

Quick

1. What are the three basic processes that occur in the nephron?
2. How do ADH and aldosterone affect urine output?
3. What is anuria? Polyuria?

URETERS

Urine drains out of the collecting tubules of each kidney into the renal pelvis and down the ureter into the urinary bladder (see Figures 17-1 and 17-8). The **renal pelvis** is the basinlike upper end of the ureter located inside the kidney. Ureters are narrow tubes less than 6 mm (¼ inch) wide and 25 to 30 cm (10 to 12 inches) long. Mucous membranes line both ureters and each renal pelvis. Note in Figure 17-7 that the ureter has a thick, muscular wall. Contraction of the muscular coat produces peristaltic-type movements that assist in moving urine down the ureters into the bladder. The lining membrane of the ureters is richly supplied with sensory nerve endings.

FIGURE 17-7

Ureter cross section. Note the thick layer of muscle around the tube.

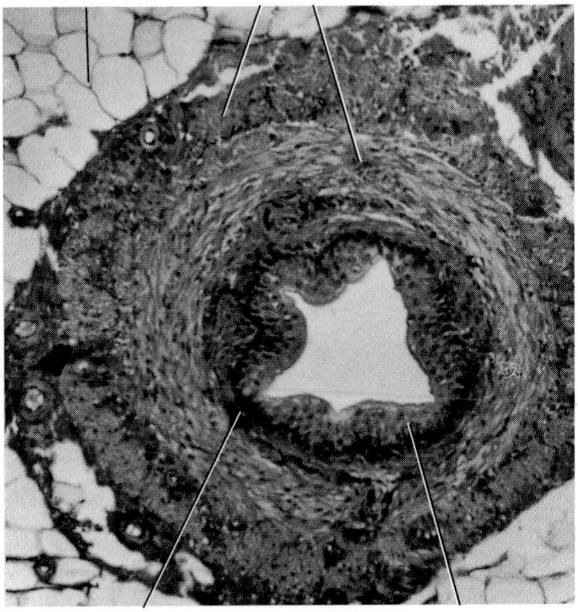

URINARY BLADDER

The empty urinary bladder lies in the pelvis just behind the pubic symphysis. When full of urine, it projects upward into the lower portion of the abdominal cavity. In women it sits in front of the uterus, whereas in men, it rests on the prostate (Figure 17-8).

Elastic fibers and involuntary muscle fibers in the wall of the urinary bladder make it well

FIGURE 17-8

The male urinary bladder. This view (with bladder cut to show the interior) shows how the prostate gland surrounds the urethra as it exits from the bladder. The glands associated with the male reproductive system are further discussed in Chapter 20.

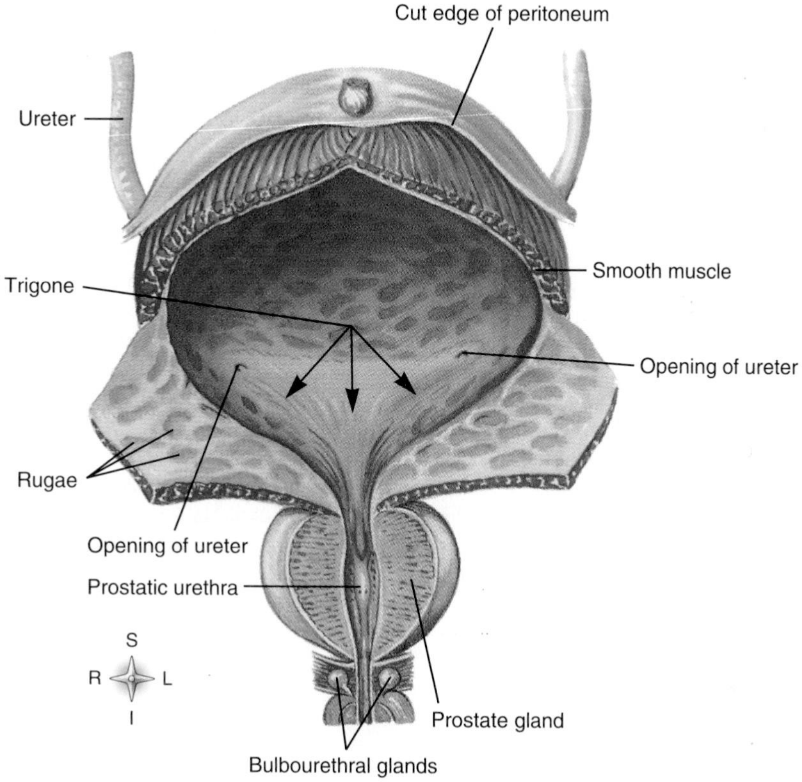

suited for expanding to hold variable amounts of urine and then contracting to empty itself. A specialized type of epithelial membrane lines the urinary bladder. The lining is loosely attached to the deeper muscular layer so that the bladder is very wrinkled and lies in folds called *rugae* when it is empty. When the bladder is filled, its inner surface is smooth. Note in Figure 17-8 that one triangular area on the back or posterior surface of the bladder is free of rugae. This area, called the *trigone*, is always smooth. There, the lining membrane is tightly fixed to the deeper muscle coat. The trigone extends between the openings of the two ureters above and the point of exit of the urethra below.

Attacks of *renal colic*—pain caused by the passage of a kidney stone—have been described in medical writings since antiquity. Kidney stones cause intense pain if they have sharp edges or are large enough to distend the walls or cut the lining of the ureters or urethra as they pass from the kidneys to the exterior of the body.

URETHRA

To leave the body, urine passes from the bladder, down the urethra, and out of its external opening, the **urinary meatus.** In other words, the urethra is the lowest part of the urinary tract. The same sheet

Clinical Application

Artificial Kidney

The artificial kidney is a mechanical device that uses the principle of dialysis to remove or separate waste products from the blood. In the event of kidney failure, the process, appropriately called **hemodialysis** (Greek *haima* "blood" and *lysis* "separate"), is a reprieve from death for the patient. During a hemodialysis treatment, a semipermeable membrane is used to separate large (nondiffusible) particles such as blood cells from small (diffusible) ones such as urea and other wastes. Figure A shows blood from the radial artery passing through a porous (semipermeable) cellophane tube that is housed in a tanklike container. The tube is surrounded by a bath or dialyzing solution containing varying concentrations of electrolytes and other chemicals. The pores in the membrane are small and allow only very small molecules, such as urea, to escape into the surrounding fluid. Larger molecules and blood cells cannot escape and are returned through the tube to reenter the patient via a wrist vein. By constantly replacing the bath solution in the dialysis tank with freshly mixed solution, levels of waste materials can be kept at low levels. As a result, wastes such as urea in the blood rapidly pass into the surrounding wash solution. For a patient with complete kidney failure, two or three hemodialysis treatments a week are required.

Dialysis treatments are now being monitored and controlled by sophisticated computer components and software integrated into modern hemodialysis equipment. New and dramatic advances in both treatment techniques and equipment are expected to continue. Although most hemodialysis treatments occur in hospital or clinical settings, equipment designed for use in the home is now available and appropriate for some individuals. Patients and their families using this equipment are initially instructed in its use and then monitored and supported on an ongoing basis by home health care professionals.

Another technique used in the treatment of renal failure is called **continuous ambulatory peritoneal dialysis (CAPD).** In this procedure, 1 to 3 L of sterile dialysis fluid is introduced directly into the peritoneal cavity through an opening in the abdominal wall (Figure B). Peritoneal membranes in the abdominal cavity transfer waste products from the blood into the dialysis fluid, which is then drained back into a plastic container after about 2 hours. This technique is less expensive than hemodialysis and does not require the use of complex equipment. CAPD is the more frequently used home-based dialysis treatment for patients with chronic renal failure. Successful long-term treatment is greatly enhanced by support from professionals trained in home health care services.

A

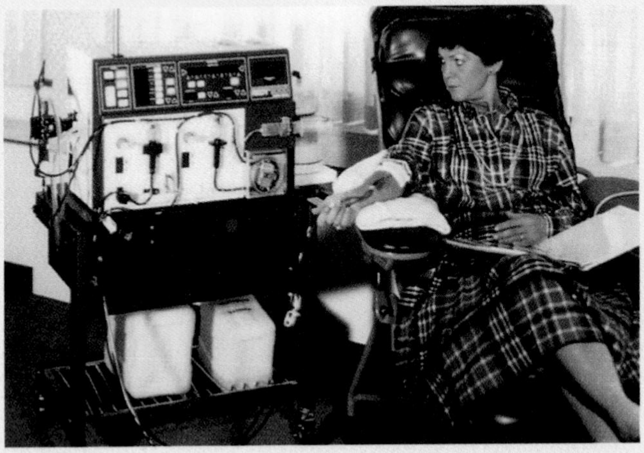

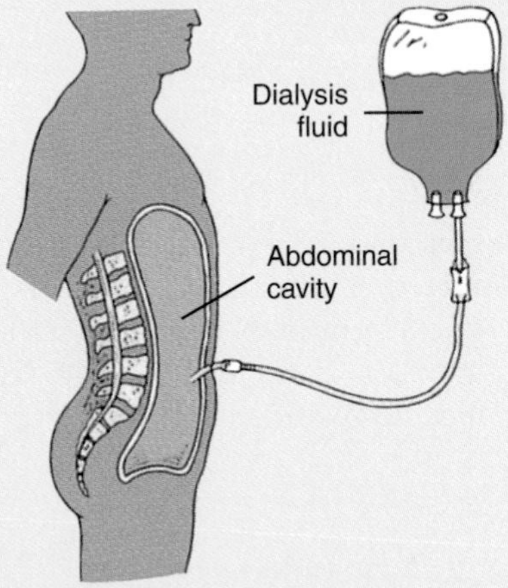

B

of mucous membrane that lines each renal pelvis, the ureters, and the bladder extends down into the urethra, too; this is a structural feature worth noting because it accounts for the fact that an infection of the urethra may spread upward through the urinary tract. The urethra is a narrow tube; it is only about 4 cm (1 ½ inches) long in a woman, but it is about 20 cm (8 inches) long in a man. In a man, the urethra has two functions: (1) it is the terminal portion of the urinary tract, and (2) it is the passageway for movement of the reproductive fluid (semen) from the body. In a woman, the urethra is a part of only the urinary tract.

MICTURITION

The terms **micturition** (mik-too-RISH-un), **urination** (yoor-i-NAY-shun), and **voiding** refer to the passage of urine from the body or the emptying of the bladder. This is a reflex action in infants or very young children. Although there is considerable variation between individuals, most children between 2 and 3 years of age learn to urinate voluntarily and also to inhibit voiding if the urge comes at an inconvenient time.

Two **sphincters** (SFINGK-ters) or rings of muscle tissue guard the pathway leading from the bladder. The **internal urethral sphincter** is located at the bladder exit, and the **external urethral sphincter** circles the urethra just below the neck of the bladder. When contracted, both sphincters seal off the bladder and allow urine to accumulate without leaking to the exterior. The internal urethral sphincter is involuntary, and the external urethral sphincter is composed of striated muscle and is under voluntary control.

The muscular wall of the bladder permits this organ to accommodate a considerable volume of urine with very little increase in pressure until a volume of 300 to 400 ml is reached. As the volume of urine increases, the need to void may be noticed at volumes of 150 ml, but micturition in adults does not normally occur much below volumes of 350 ml. As the bladder wall stretches, nervous impulses are transmitted to the second, third, and fourth sacral segments of the spinal cord, and an **emptying reflex** is initiated. The reflex causes contraction of the muscle of the bladder wall and relaxation of the internal sphincter. Urine then enters the urethra. If the external sphincter, which is under voluntary control, is relaxed, micturition occurs. Voluntary contraction of the external sphincter suppresses the emptying reflex until the bladder is filled to capacity with urine and loss of control occurs. Contraction of this powerful sphincter also abruptly terminates urination voluntarily.

Higher centers in the brain also function in micturition by integrating bladder contraction and internal and external sphincter relaxation, with the cooperative contraction of pelvic and abdominal muscles. Urinary **retention** is a condition in which no urine is voided. The kidneys produce urine, but the bladder for one reason or another cannot empty itself. In urinary **suppression** the opposite is true. The kidneys do not produce any urine, but the bladder retains the ability to empty itself.

Clinical Application

The Aging Kidney

As with other body organs, the kidneys undergo both age-related structural changes and decreasing functional capacity. Adults older than 35 years of age gradually lose functional nephron units and kidney weight actually decreases. By approximately 80 to 85 years of age, most individuals will have experienced a 30% reduction in total kidney mass. In spite of a numerical reduction in actual kidney nephron units and a decrease in the metabolic activity of remaining tubular cells, most of these individuals continue to exhibit normal kidney function. This is possible because older persons generally have a lower overall lean body mass and therefore a reduced production of waste products that must be excreted from the body. However, the "margin of safety" is reduced, and any stress on the remaining functional nephrons, such as a systemic infection or a reduction in kidney blood flow, can produce almost immediate symptoms of kidney failure. Marginal kidney function in old age may make it difficult to excrete drugs that are easily cleared from the blood of younger persons and dosages of many medications have to be adjusted accordingly for older patients.

Clinical Application

Removal of Kidney Stones Using Ultrasound

Statistics suggest that approximately 1 in every 1000 adults in the United States suffers from kidney stones or **renal calculi** (KAL-kyoo-lye) at some point in their life. Although symptoms of excruciating pain are common, many kidney stones are small enough to pass out of the urinary system spontaneously. If this is possible, no therapy is required other than treatment for pain and antibiotics if the calculi are associated with infection. Larger stones, however, may obstruct the flow of urine and are much more serious and difficult to treat.

Until recently, only traditional surgical procedures were effective in removing relatively large stones that formed in the calyces and renal pelvis of the kidney. In addition to the risks that always accompany major medical procedures, surgical removal of stones from the kidneys frequently requires rather extensive hospital and home recovery periods, lasting 6 weeks or more.

A technique that uses ultrasound to pulverize the stones so that they can be flushed out of the urinary tract without surgery is used in hospitals across the United States. The specially designed ultrasound generator required for the procedure is called a **lithotriptor** (li-tho-TRIP-ter). Using a lithotriptor, physicians break up the stones with ultrasound waves, in a process called *lithotripsy*, without making an incision. Recovery time is minimal, and patient risk and costs are reduced.

Incontinence (in-KON-ti-nens) is a condition in which the patient voids urine involuntarily. It frequently occurs in patients who have suffered a stroke or spinal cord injury. If the sacral segments of the spinal cord are injured, some loss of bladder function always occurs. Although the voiding reflex may be reestablished to some degree, the bladder does not empty completely. In these individuals the residual urine is often the cause of repeated bladder infections or **cystitis** (sis-TIE-tis). Complete destruction or transsection of the sacral cord produces a condition called an *automatic bladder*. Totally cut off from spinal innervation, the bladder musculature acquires some automatic action and periodic but unpredictable voiding occurs. The term **overactive bladder** refers to the need for frequent urination. The amounts voided are generally small, and feelings of extreme urgency and pain are common. The condition is called *interstitial* (IN-tur-STISH-ul) *cystitis* and is treated with drugs to decrease nervous stimulation and with physical distention of the bladder with fluids to increase capacity.

Quick

1. Through what tube does urine leave the kidney?
2. What structural characteristics of the bladder allow it to expand to hold urine?
3. Through what structure does urine pass from the bladder to the outside of the body?
4. What is incontinence?

Science Applications

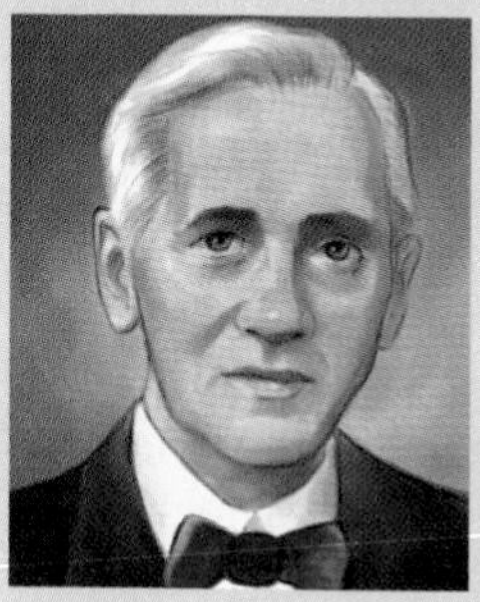

Science Applications
Fighting infection

Alexander Fleming (1881-1955).

Unfortunately, the structure of the urinary tract puts it at risk for infection by bacteria and other microorganisms. Because it is open to the external environment, bacteria can enter easily. In women, the short length of the urethra and its location close to the anus may further increase the risk of bacteria getting to the urinary bladder. Another risk factor is poor technique by health care workers when they insert catheters (tubes) into the urethras of patients who need help voiding their bladders of urine.

A breakthrough in the treatment of urinary tract infections (UTIs) came in 1928 in the laboratory of Scots researcher Alexander Fleming. Some mold spores accidentally contaminated one of the dishes in which Fleming was growing bacteria. He marveled at the fact that no bacteria could grow near the mold growth. He isolated a substance from the mold responsible for this antibacterial effect and named it *penicillin*. Although Fleming had earlier discovered another natural antibiotic (lysozyme) that effectively attacked bacteria that did not often cause disease, Fleming showed that penicillin was effective against a variety of bacteria that cause serious infections in humans. Penicillin became the first "miracle drug" and rapidly became the tool of choice in fighting bacteria. In 1943, another breakthrough came when laboratory worker Mary Hunt brought a moldy cantaloupe to work and researchers found that the new type of mold produced enough penicillin to make commercial production of the antibiotic possible.

Although forms of penicillin and other antibiotics derived from natural sources are still the weapon of choice in battling many infections, the infectious bacteria are evolving into strains that resist common antibiotics. UTIs and other types of infections now require more powerful antibiotics and other special techniques to stop them. Some scientists fear that the era of simple antibiotic therapy may be nearing an end.

Many professions are involved in the fight against infection. Medical supply technicians ensure that devices such as urethral catheters are sterile (free of microorganisms) before they are packaged and sent to hospitals and clinics. Physicians, nurses, and others who deal directly with patients learn proper "sterile technique" to assure that infections are not introduced by medical procedures. To help in this effort, most organizations designate an infection control manager—a health professional with the responsibility to prevent **nosocomial** (no-zo-KOAM-ee-al) **infections** (infections that begin in the hospital). Community health experts including epidemiologists and health service officers from the U.S. government's Centers for Disease Control and Prevention (CDC) also help prevent the spread of infection in local communities and worldwide. Of course, pharmacology researchers and others continue in the quest to find newer and better treatments for UTIs and other infections that threaten human health.

OUTLINE SUMMARY

KIDNEYS

A. Location—under back muscles, behind parietal peritoneum, just above waistline; right kidney usually a little lower than left (Figure 17-1)

B. Internal structure (Figure 17-2)
  1. Cortex—outer layer of kidney substance
  2. Medulla—inner portion of kidney
  3. Pyramids—triangular divisions of medulla
  4. Papilla—narrow, innermost end of pyramid
  5. Pelvis—expansion of upper end of ureter; lies inside kidney
  6. Calyces—divisions of renal pelvis

C. Microscopic structure—nephrons are microscopic units of kidneys; consist of (Figure 17-3):
  1. Renal corpuscle—Bowman's capsule with its glomerulus
     a. Bowman's capsule—the cup-shaped top
     b. Glomerulus—network of blood capillaries surrounded by Bowman's capsule
  2. Renal tubule
     a. Proximal convoluted tubule—first segment
     b. Loop of Henle—extension of proximal tubule; consists of descending limb, loop, and ascending limb
     c. Distal convoluted tubule—extension of ascending limb of loop of Henle
     d. Collecting tubule—straight extension of distal tubule

D. Functions
  1. Excretes toxins and nitrogenous wastes
  2. Regulates levels of many chemicals in blood
  3. Maintains water balance
  4. Helps regulate blood pressure via secretion of renin

FORMATION OF URINE (FIGURE 17-5)

A. Occurs by a series of three processes that take place in successive parts of nephron
  1. Filtration—goes on continually in renal corpuscles; glomerular blood pressure causes water and dissolved substances to filter out of glomeruli into Bowman's capsule; normal glomerular filtration rate 125 ml per minute
  2. Reabsorption—movement of substances out of renal tubules into blood in peritubular capillaries; water, nutrients, and ions are reabsorbed; water is reabsorbed by osmosis from proximal tubules
  3. Secretion—movement of substances into urine in the distal and collecting tubules from blood in peritubular capillaries; hydrogen ions, potassium ions, and certain drugs are secreted by active transport; ammonia is secreted by diffusion

B. Control of urine volume—mainly by posterior pituitary hormone's ADH, which decreases it

URETERS

A. Structure—narrow, long tubes with expanded upper end (renal pelvis) located inside kidney and lined with mucous membrane

B. Function—drain urine from renal pelvis to urinary bladder

URINARY BLADDER

A. Structure (Figure 17-8)
  1. Elastic muscular organ, capable of great expansion
  2. Lined with mucous membrane arranged in rugae, as is stomach mucosa

B. Functions
  1. Storage of urine before voiding
  2. Voiding

OUTLINE SUMMARY—*cont'd*

URETHRA

A. Structure
   1. Narrow tube from urinary bladder to exterior
   2. Lined with mucous membrane
   3. Opening of urethra to the exterior called *urinary meatus*

B. Functions
   1. Passage of urine from bladder to exterior of the body
   2. Passage of male reproductive fluid (semen) from the body

MICTURITION

A. Passage of urine from body (also called *urination* or *voiding*)

B. Regulatory sphincters
   1. Internal urethral sphincter (involuntary)
   2. External urethral sphincter (voluntary)

C. Bladder wall permits storage of urine with little increase in pressure

D. Emptying reflex
   1. Initiated by stretch reflex in bladder wall
   2. Bladder wall contracts
   3. Internal sphincter relaxes
   4. External sphincter relaxes, and urination occurs

E. Urinary retention—urine produced but not voided

F. Urinary suppression—no urine produced but bladder is normal

G. Incontinence—urine is voided involuntarily
   1. May be caused by spinal injury or stroke
   2. Retention of urine may cause cystitis

H. Cystitis—bladder infection

I. Overactive bladder—need for frequent urination
   1. Called interstitial cystitis
   2. Amounts voided are small
   3. Extreme urgency and pain are common

NEW WORDS

anuria
atrial natriuretic hormone (ANH)
Bowman's capsule
calyx
cystitis
glomerulus
glycosuria
incontinence
lithotripsy
lithotriptor
micturition
oliguria
overactive bladder
papilla
polyuria
pyramid
renal colic
trigone
uremia
urination
voiding

REVIEW QUESTIONS

1. Describe the location of the kidneys.
2. Name and describe the internal structures of the kidneys.
3. Define *filtration*, *reabsorption*, and *secretion* as they apply to kidney function.
4. Briefly explain the formation of urine.
5. Name several substances eliminated or regulated by the kidney.
6. Explain the function of the juxtaglomerular apparatus.
7. Describe the structure of the ureters.
8. Describe the structure of the bladder. What is the trigone?
9. Describe the structure of the urethra.
10. Briefly describe the process of micturition.
11. Differentiate between retention and suppression of urine.
12. What is incontinence? What can cause incontinence?

CRITICAL THINKING

13. Explain the salt and water balance maintained by aldosterone and ADH.
14. Why is proper blood pressure necessary for proper kidney function?
15. If a person were doing strenuous work on a hot day and perspiring heavily, would there be a great deal of ADH in the blood or very little? Explain your answer.

CHAPTER TEST

1. The kidneys receive about 20 % of the total amount of blood pumped by the heart each minute.
2. The renal corpuscle is made up of two structures: Bowman's capsule and glomerulus
3. The two parts of the renal tubules that extend into the medulla of the kidney are the loop of Henle and the collecting loop.
4. The two parts of the renal tubules that are in the cortex of the kidney are the proximal and the distal convoluted tubule
5. The process of reabsorption is the movement of substances out of the renal tubules and into the blood capillaries.
6. The process of filtration causes substances in the blood to be pushed into Bowman's capsule as a result of blood pressure in the glomerulus.
7. The process of secretion is the movement of substances from the blood into the distal tubule or the collecting tube.
8. The hormone antidiuretic is released from the posterior pituitary gland and reduces the amount of water lost in the urine.
9. The hormone atrial natriuretic is made by the heart and stimulates the tubules to secrete sodium.
10. The hormone aldosterone is made in the adrenal cortex and causes the tubules to absorb sodium.
11. The involuntary muscle internal urethral sphincter is at the exit of the bladder.
12. Suppression is a condition in which the bladder is able to empty itself but no urine is being produced by the kidneys.
13. Incontinence is a condition in which a person voids urine involuntarily.
14. Retention is a condition in which the bladder is full and the kidney is producing urine but the bladder is unable to empty itself.

CHAPTER TEST—*cont'd*

Match the statement in Column B with the correct term in Column A.

COLUMN A	COLUMN B
15. __G__ Cortex	**a.** the inner layer of the kidney
16. __A__ Medulla	**b.** the expansion of the ureter in the kidney
17. __K__ Pyramids	**c.** the cup-shaped part of the nephron that catches the filtrate
18. __J__ Pelvis	**d.** the tube leading from the bladder to outside the body
19. __B__ Urethra	**e.** the network of capillaries in Bowman's capsule
20. __F__ Bladder	**f.** the saclike structure used to hold urine until it is voided
21. __D__ Ureter	**g.** the outer part of the kidney
22. __H__ Trigone	**h.** an area of the bladder that has openings for the two ureters and the urethra
23. __C__ Bowman's capsule	**i.** the part of the renal tubules that is located between the proximal and distal tubules
24. __E__ Glomerulus	**j.** the tube connecting the kidney and bladder
25. __I__ Loop of Henle	**k.** the triangular divisions in the medulla of the kidney

STUDY TIPS

Before studying Chapter 17, review the synopsis of the urinary system in Chapter 4. The function of the urinary system is to maintain the homeostasis of the blood plasma. The names, locations, and functions of the organs and internal structures of the kidney can be learned using flash cards. The names and locations of the microscopic structures of the nephron can also be learned using flash cards. Notice the directional terms *proximal* and *distal*; these names refer to how far away these structures are from Bowman's capsule. The formation of urine uses three processes: filtration, resorption, and secretion. Filtration was discussed in Chapter 3. *Resorption* means taking material out of the urine and returning it to the blood. *Secretion* means taking material out of the blood and putting it into the urine. Urine volume is controlled by three hormones, each produced in a different organ and regulating volume in a different way. Remember that the body cannot directly move water, it must move solute and pull the water by diffusion. Use flash cards with the name of the hormone, where it is made, its mechanism of action, and its effect on urine volume.

In your study group, use the flash cards and photocopies of the figures of the organs of the urinary system, the internal structures of the kidney, and the microscopic structure of the nephron. Discuss how the kidney forms urine, and discuss the hormones involved in the regulation of urine volume. Make sure you know if the functioning of the hormone will increase or decrease urine volume. Go over the process of micturition. Go over the questions at the back of the chapter and discuss possible test questions.

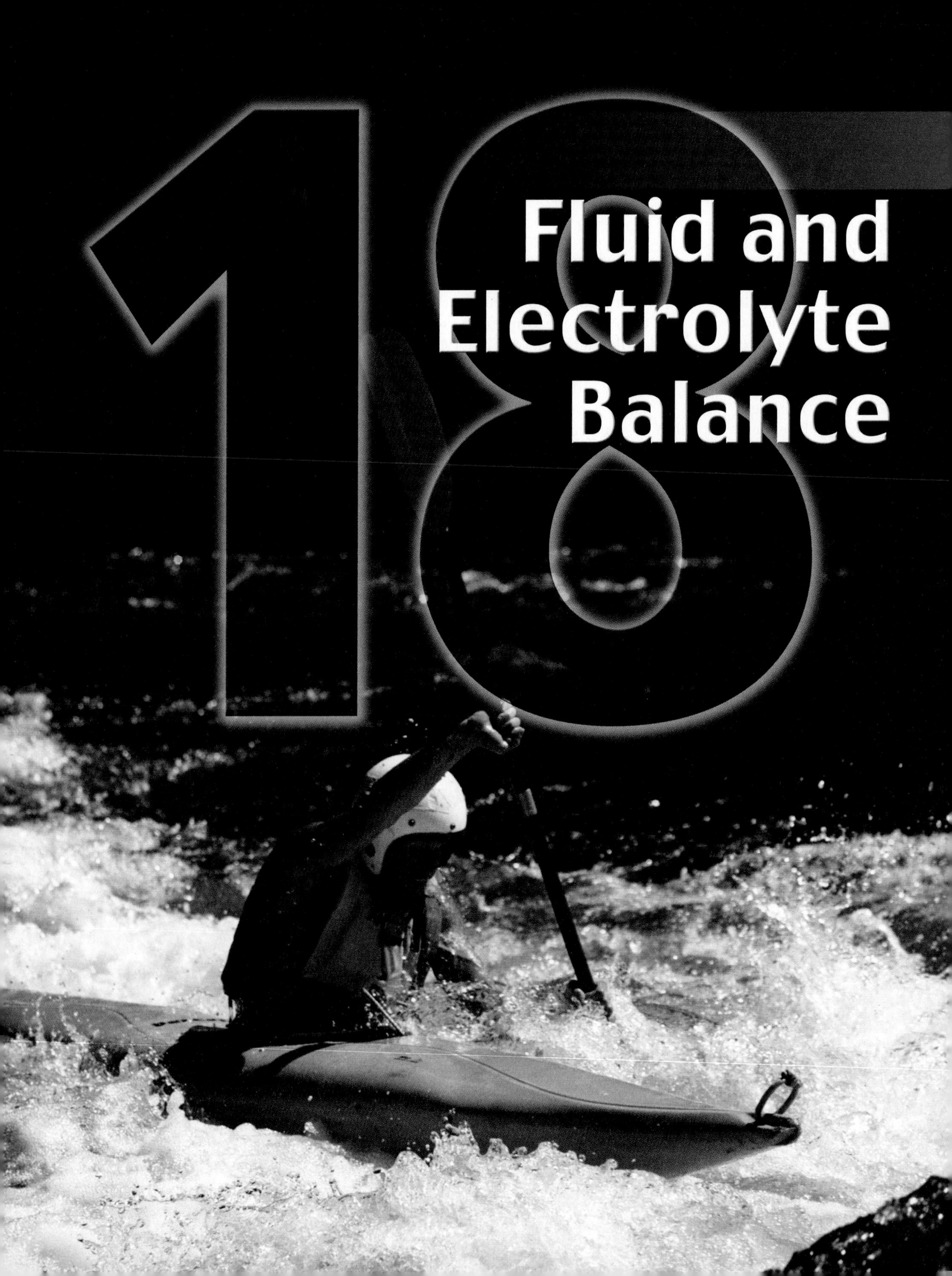

18 Fluid and Electrolyte Balance

Outline

Objectives

AFTER YOU HAVE COMPLETED THIS CHAPTER, YOU SHOULD BE ABLE TO:

1. List, describe, and compare the body fluid compartments and their subdivisions.
2. Discuss avenues by which water enters and leaves the body and the mechanisms that maintain fluid balance.
3. Discuss the nature and importance of electrolytes in body fluids and explain the aldosterone mechanism of extracellular fluid volume control.
4. Explain the interaction between capillary blood pressure and blood proteins.
5. Give examples of common fluid imbalances.

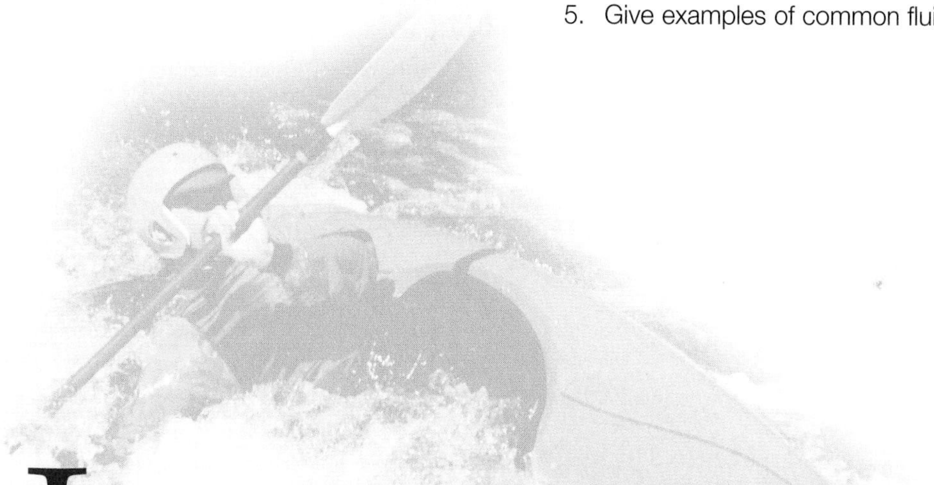

H*ave you ever* wondered why you sometimes excrete great volumes of urine and sometimes excrete almost none at all? Why sometimes you feel so thirsty that you can hardly get enough to drink and other times you want no liquids at all? These conditions and many more relate to one of the body's most important functions—that of maintaining its **fluid** and **electrolyte** balance.

The phrase *fluid balance* implies homeostasis, or relative constancy of body fluid levels—a condition required for healthy survival. It means that both the total volume and distribution of water in the body remain normal and relatively constant. Body "input" of water must be balanced by "output." If water in excess of requirements enters the body, it must be eliminated, and, if excess losses occur, prompt replacement is critical. Because fluid balance refers to normal homeostasis, fluid imbalance means that the total volume of water in the body or the amounts in one or more of its fluid compartments have increased or decreased beyond normal limits. Electrolytes are substances such as salts that dissolve or break apart in water solution. Health and sometimes even survival itself depend on maintaining proper balance of water and the electrolytes within it.

In this chapter you will find a discussion of body fluids and electrolytes, their normal values, the mechanisms that operate to keep them normal, and some of the more common types of fluid and electrolyte imbalances.

BODY FLUIDS

Of the hundreds of compounds present in your body, the most abundant is water. Medical reference tables often refer to "average" fluid volumes based on healthy nonobese young adults. In such tables males weighing 70 kg (154 pounds) will average about 60% of their body weight, nearly 40 L, as water (Figure 18-1); females about 50%. The reason fluid volume values in reference tables are based on nonobese individuals is because of the fact that adipose or fat tissue contains the least amount of water of any body tissue. The more fat present in the body, the less the total water content per pound of body weight. Therefore, regardless of age, obese individuals, with their high body fat content, have less body water per kilogram of weight than slender people. Although a nonobese male body typically consists of about 60% water, an obese male may consist of only 50% water or even less. The female body contains slightly less water per pound of weight because it contains slightly more fat than the male body. Note in Figure 18-2 that age as well as sex influences the amount of water in the body. Infants have more water compared with body weight than adults of either sex. In a newborn, water may account for up to 80% of total body weight. This is the reason fluid imbalances in infants caused by diarrhea, for example, can be so serious. The percentage of body water decreases rapidly during the first 10 years of life and by adolescence, adult values are reached and gender differences, which account for about a 10% variation in body fluid volumes between the sexes, appear. In elderly individuals, the amount of water per pound of body weight decreases. One reason is that old age is often accompanied by a decrease in muscle mass (65% water) and an increase in fat (20% water).

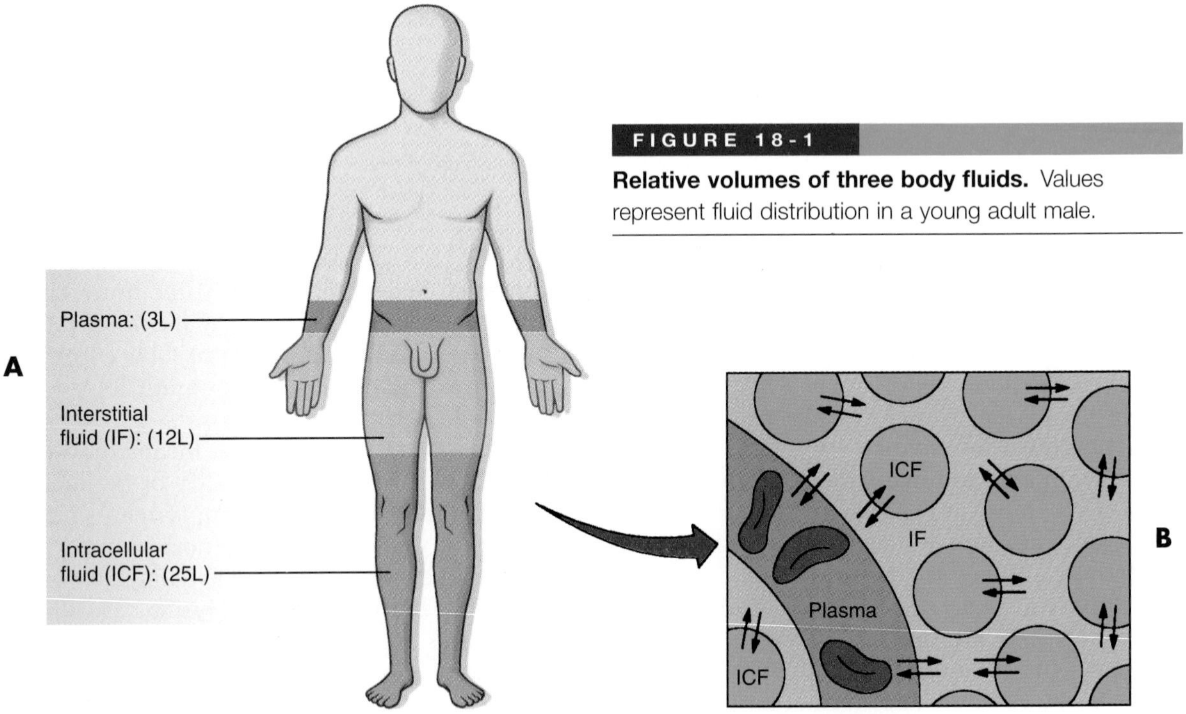

FIGURE 18-1

Relative volumes of three body fluids. Values represent fluid distribution in a young adult male.

BODY FLUID COMPARTMENTS

Total body water can be subdivided into two major **fluid compartments** called the *extracellular* and the *intracellular* fluid compartments. **Extracellular fluid (ECF)** consists mainly of the liquid fraction of whole blood called the *plasma*, found in the blood vessels, and the *interstitial fluid* (IF) that surrounds the cells. In addition, the lymph, cerebrospinal fluid, humors of the eye, and the specialized joint fluids are also considered as extracellular fluid. The term **intracellular fluid (ICF)** refers to the largest volume of water by far. It is located inside cells. Figure 18-2 illustrates the typical proportion of body weight represented by water in the newborn and in adults by gender. Table 18-1 lists the differing volumes of each body fluid compartment as a percentage of body weight in both the newborn and adults of both sexes.

Quick Check

1. What are the two main fluid compartments of the body?
2. What is meant by the term *fluid balance*?

TABLE 18-1

Volumes of Body Fluid Compartments*

BODY FLUID	INFANT	ADULT MALE	ADULT FEMALE
EXTRACELLULAR FLUID			
Plasma	4	4	4
Interstitial Fluid	26	16	11
Intracellular Fluid	45	40	35
TOTAL	75	60	50

*Percentage of body weight.

FIGURE 18-2

Proportion of body weight represented by water.

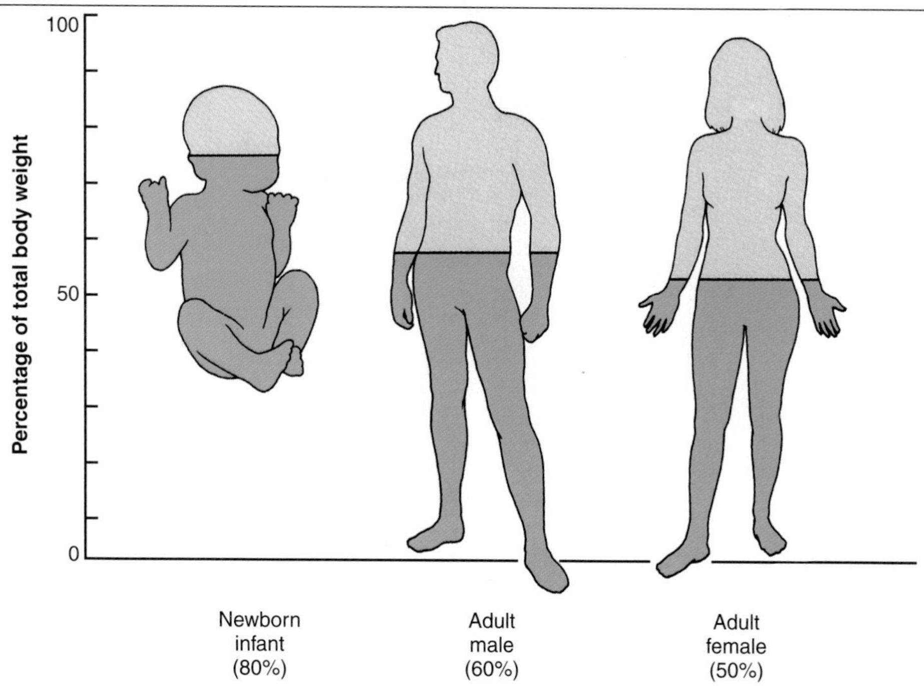

MECHANISMS THAT MAINTAIN FLUID BALANCE

Under normal conditions, homeostasis of the total volume of water in the body is maintained or restored primarily by devices that adjust output (urine volume) to intake and secondarily by mechanisms that adjust fluid intake. There is no question about which of the two mechanisms is more important; the body's chief mechanism, by far, for maintaining fluid balance is to adjust its fluid output so that it equals its fluid intake.

Obviously, as long as output and intake are equal, the total amount of water in the body does not change. Figure 18-3 shows the three sources of fluid intake: the liquids we drink, the water in the foods we eat, and the water formed by catabolism of foods. Table 18-2 gives their normal volumes. However, these can vary a great deal and still be considered normal. Table 18-2 also indicates that fluid output from the body occurs through four organs: the kidneys, lungs, skin, and intestines. The fluid output that changes the most is that from the kidneys. The body main-

FIGURE 18-3

Sources of fluid intake and output.

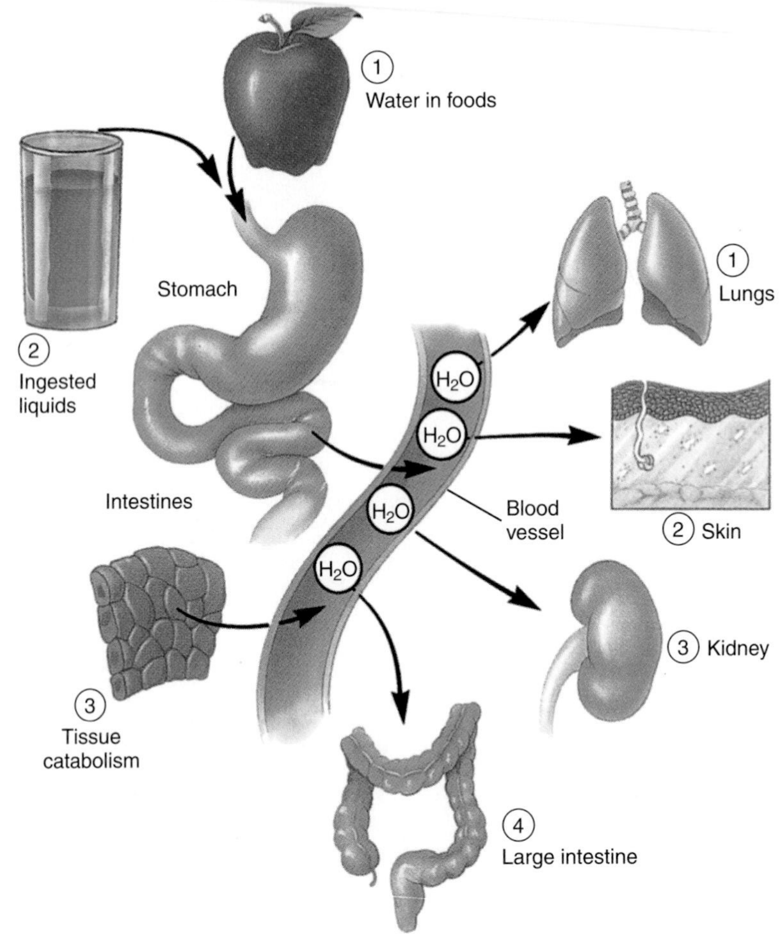

tains fluid balance mainly by changing the volume of urine excreted to match changes in the volume of fluid intake. Everyone knows this from experience. The more liquid one drinks, the more urine one excretes. Conversely, the less the fluid intake, the less the urine volume. How changes in urine volume come about was discussed on pp. 443-444. This would be a good time to review these paragraphs.

It is important to remember from your study of the urinary system that the rate of water and salt resorption by the renal tubules is the most important factor in determining urine volume. Urine volume is regulated chiefly by hormones secreted by the posterior lobe of the pituitary gland (antidiuretic hormone or ADH) and the adrenal cortex (aldosterone). Atrial natriuretic hormone (ANH) from the atrial wall of the heart also affects urine volume. See pp. 443-444 for a review of the hormonal control of urine volume.

Several factors act as mechanisms for controlling plasma, IF, and ICF volumes. We shall limit our discussion to naming only three of these factors, stating their effects on fluid volumes, and giving some specific examples of them. Three of the main factors are:

1. The concentration of electrolytes in ECF
2. The capillary blood pressure
3. The concentration of proteins in blood

Regulation of Fluid Intake

Physiologists disagree about the details of the mechanism for controlling and regulating fluid intake to compensate for factors that would lead to dehydration. In general it appears to operate in this way: when dehydration starts to develop—that is, when fluid loss from the body exceeds fluid intake—salivary secretion decreases, producing a "dry-mouth feeling" and the sensation of thirst. The individual then drinks water, thereby increasing fluid intake and compensating for previous fluid losses. This tends to restore fluid balance (Figure 18-4). If an individual takes nothing by mouth for days, can his or her fluid output decrease to zero? The answer—no—becomes obvious after reviewing the information in Table 18-2. Despite every effort of homeostatic mechanisms to

TABLE 18-2

Typical Normal Values for Each Portal of Water Entry and Exit (24 Hours)

INTAKE	AMOUNT*	OUTPUT	AMOUNT*
Water in foods	700 ml	Lungs (water in expired air)	350 ml
Ingested liquids	1,500 ml	Skin	
Water formed by catabolism	200 ml	By diffusion	350 ml
		By sweat	100 ml
		Kidneys (urine)	1,400 ml
		Intestines (in feces)	200 ml
TOTALS	2,400 ml		2,400 ml

*Amounts vary widely.

compensate for zero intake, some output (loss) of fluid occurs as long as life continues. Water is continually lost from the body through expired air and diffusion through skin.

Although the body adjusts fluid intake, factors that adjust fluid output, such as electrolytes and blood proteins, are far more important.

Quick Check

1. Which does the body primarily adjust, fluid *intake* or fluid *output*?
2. What are the chief ways that fluid leaves the body?

Importance of Electrolytes in Body Fluids

The bonds that hold together the molecules of certain organic substances such as glucose are such that they do not permit the compound to break up or **dissociate** in water solution. Such compounds are called **nonelectrolytes**. Compounds such as ordinary table salt or sodium chloride (NaCl) that have molecular bonds that permit them to break up or dissociate in water solution into separate particles (Na^+ and Cl^-) are electrolytes. The dissociated particles of an electrolyte are ions and carry an electrical charge.

Important positively charged ions include sodium (Na^+), calcium (Ca^{++}), potassium (K^+), and magnesium (Mg^{++}). Important negatively charged ions include chloride (Cl^-), bicarbonate (HCO_3^-), phosphate ($HPO_4^=$), and many proteins. Table 18-3 shows that, although blood plasma contains a number of important electrolytes, by far the most abundant one is sodium chloride (ordinary table salt, Na^+Cl^-).

A variety of electrolytes have important nutrient or regulatory roles in the body. Many ions are major or important "trace" elements in the body (see Chapter 2). Iron, for example, is required for hemoglobin production, and iodine must be available

FIGURE 18-4

Homeostasis of the total volume of body water. A basic mechanism for adjusting intake to compensate for excess output of body fluid is diagrammed.

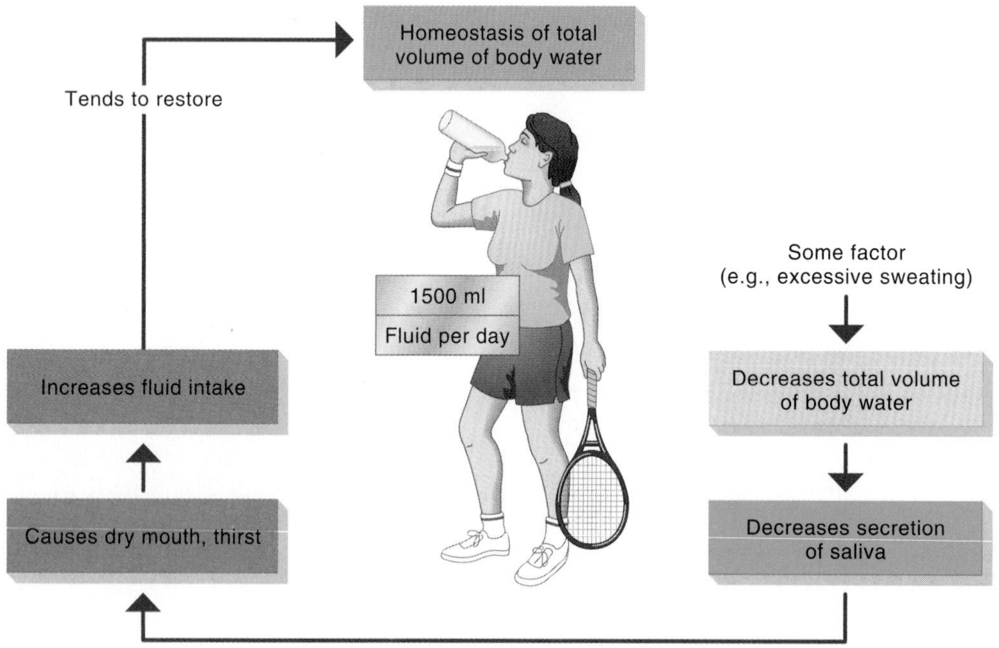

for synthesis of thyroid hormones. Electrolytes are also required for many cellular activities such as nerve conduction and muscle contraction.

In addition, electrolytes influence the movement of water among the three fluid compartments of the body. To remember how ECF electrolyte concentration affects fluid volumes, remember this one short sentence: where sodium goes, water soon follows. If, for example, the concentration of sodium in blood increases, the volume of blood soon increases. Conversely, if blood sodium concentration decreases, blood volume soon decreases.

Figure 18-5 traces one mechanism that tends to maintain fluid homeostasis. Aldosterone, secreted by the adrenal cortex, increases Na^+ reabsorption by the kidney tubules. Water reabsorption also increases, causing an increase in ECF volume. Begin in the upper right of the diagram and follow, in sequence, each of the informational steps. In summary:

1. Overall fluid balance requires that fluid output equal fluid intake.
2. The type of fluid output that changes most is urine volume.
3. Renal tubule regulation of salt and water is the most important factor in determining urine volume.
4. Aldosterone controls sodium reabsorption in the kidney.
5. The presence of sodium causes water to move (where sodium goes, water soon follows).

The flow chart diagram in Figure 18-5 explains, in a concise and brief way, the aldosterone mechanism that helps to restore normal ECF volume when it decreases below normal. Can you construct a similar diagram to show the effect of ADH secretion on ECF volume?

Although wide variations are possible, the average daily diet contains about 100 milliequivalents of sodium. The milliequivalent (mEq) (see Table 18-3) is a unit of measurement related to reactivity. In a healthy individual, sodium excretion from the body by the kidney is about the same as intake. The kidney acts as the chief regulator of sodium levels in body fluids. It is important to know that many electrolytes such as sodium not only pass into and out of the body but also move back and forth between a number of body fluids during each 24-hour period. Figure 18-6 shows the large volumes of sodium-containing internal secretions produced each day. During a 24-hour period, more than 8 L of fluid containing 1000 to 1300 mEq of sodium are poured into the digestive system as part of saliva, gastric secretions, bile, pancreatic juice, and IF secretions. This sodium, along with most of that contained in the diet, is almost completely reabsorbed in the large intestine.

Health & Well-Being

Making Weight

Some sports require athletes to "make weight" or weigh in within certain limits just before a competition. Some athletes add muscle mass until they are over their weight limit and then fast or take diuretics just before weigh-in to lose weight. Their theory is that the increased muscle mass improves their competitive edge. Unfortunately, dehydration and loss of glycogen always result from these techniques. Because water and glycogen cannot possibly be replaced in time for the competition, such an athlete is at a physiological disadvantage. Performance and thus the competitive edge is much greater if an athlete can make weight without resorting to "quick loss" methods.

TABLE 18-3

Common Electrolytes Found in Blood Plasma

POSITIVELY CHARGED IONS	NEGATIVELY CHARGED IONS
142 mEq Na^+	102 mEq Cl^-
4 mEq K^+	26 mEq HCO_3^-
5 mEq Ca^{++}	17 mEq protein
2 mEq Mg^{++}	6 mEq other
	2 mEq $HPO_4^=$
153 mEq/L plasma	153 mEq/L plasma

FIGURE 18-5

Aldosterone mechanism. Aldosterone restores normal extracellular fluid (ECF) volume when such levels decrease below normal. Excess aldosterone, however, leads to excess ECF volume—that is, excess blood volume (hypervolemia) and excess interstitial fluid volume (edema)—and also to an excess of the total Na^+ content of the body.

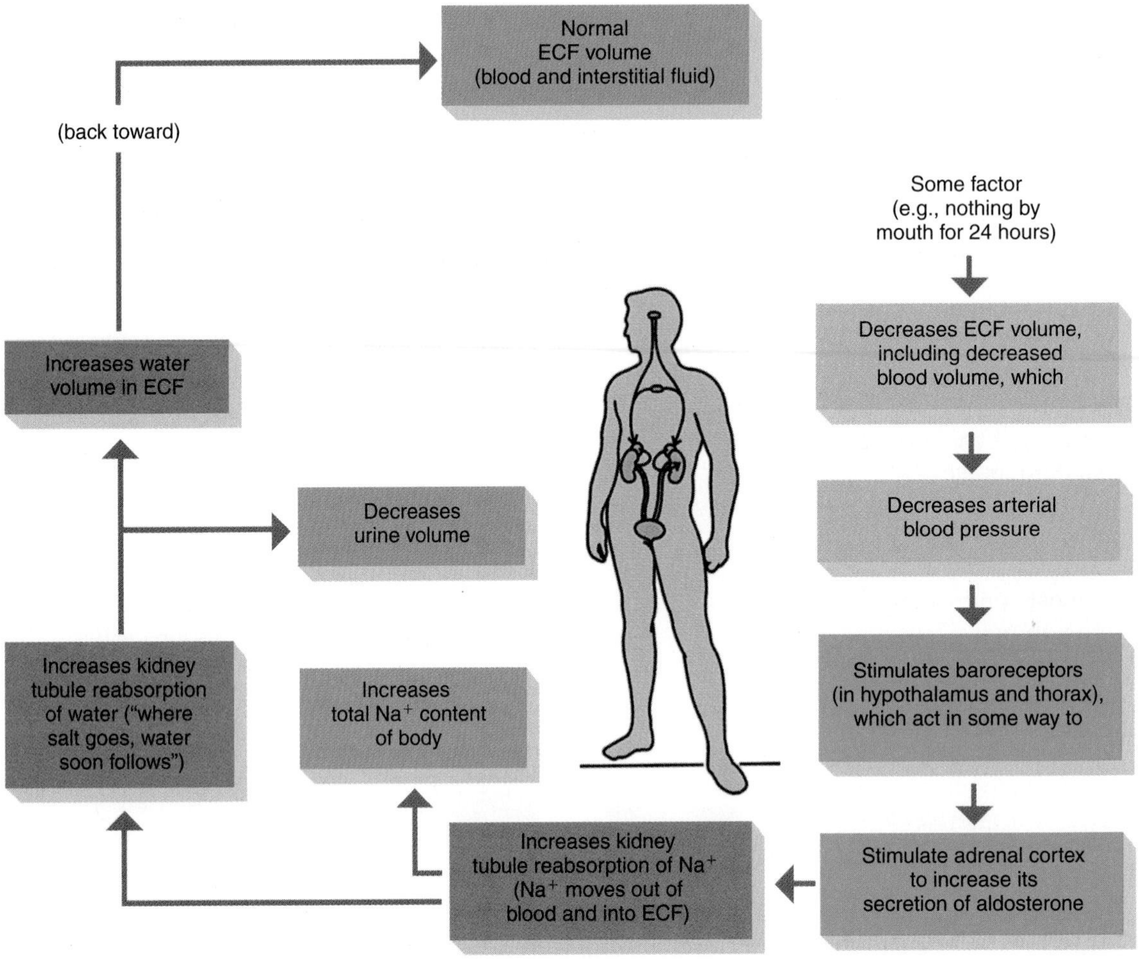

Very little sodium is lost in the feces. Precise regulation and control of sodium levels are required for survival.

Quick

1. What is the difference between an *electrolyte* and a *nonelectrolyte*?
2. What are some of the major roles of ions in the body?
3. What hormones regulate ions in the body?

Capillary Blood Pressure and Blood Proteins

Capillary blood pressure is a "water-pushing" force. It pushes fluid out of the blood in capillaries into the IF. Therefore if capillary blood pressure increases, more fluid is pushed—filtered—out of blood into the IF. The effect of an increase in capillary blood pressure, then, is to transfer fluid from

FIGURE 18-6

Sodium-containing internal secretions. The total volume of these secretions may reach 8000 ml or more in 24 hours.

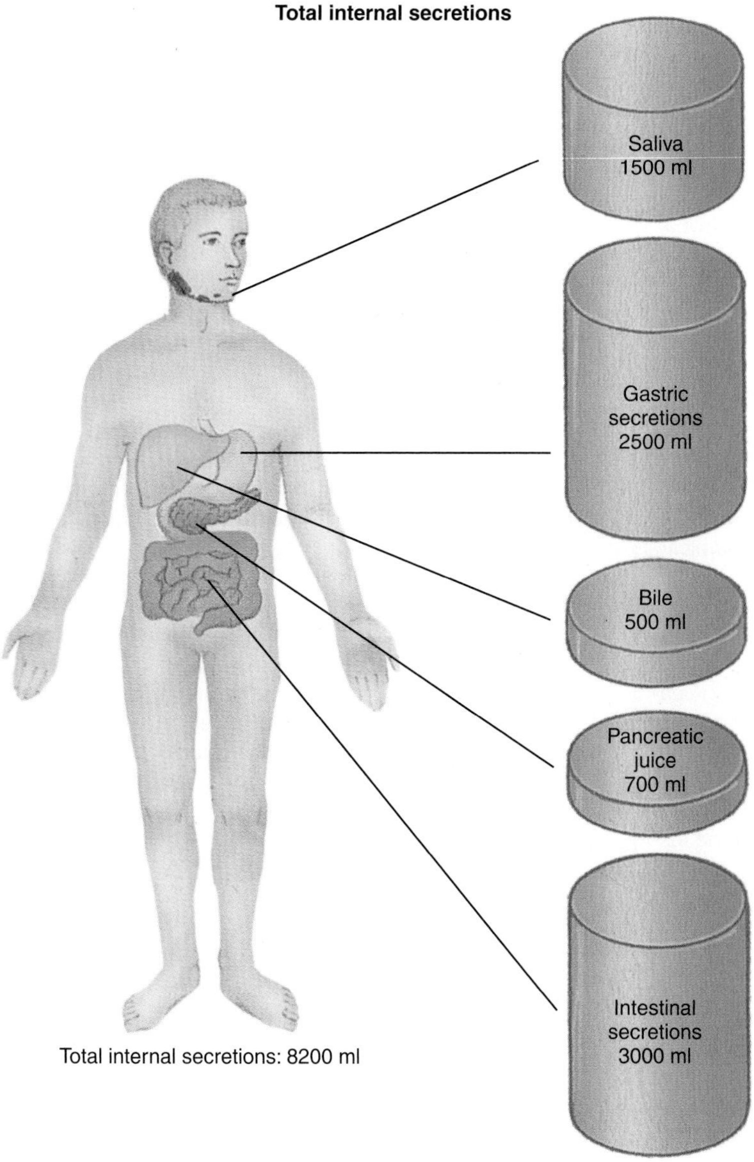

blood to IF. In turn, this fluid shift, as it is called, changes blood and IF volumes. It decreases blood volume by increasing IF volume. If, on the other hand, capillary blood pressure decreases, less fluid filters out of blood into IF.

Water continually moves in both directions through the membranous walls of capillaries (see Figure 18-1). The amount that moves out of capillary blood into IF depends largely on capillary blood pressure, a water-pushing force. The amount

Clinical Application

Diuretics

The word **diuretic** is from the Greek word *diouretikos*, meaning "causing urine." By definition a diuretic drug is a substance that promotes or stimulates the production of urine.

As a group, diuretics are among the most commonly used drugs in medicine. They are used because of their role in influencing water and electrolyte balance, especially sodium, in the body. Diuretics have their effect on tubular function in the nephron, and the differing types of diuretics are often classified according to their major site of action. Examples would include (1) *proximal tubule diuretics* such as acetazolamide (Diamox), (2) *loop of Henle diuretics* such as ethacrynic acid (Edecrin) or furosemide (Lasix), and (3) *distal tubule diuretics* such as chlorothiazide (Diuril).

Classification can also be made according to the effect the drug has on the level or concentration of sodium (Na^+), chloride (Cl^-), potassium (K^+), and bicarbonate (HCO_3^-) ions in the tubular fluid.

Nursing implications for caregivers monitoring patients receiving diuretics both in hospitals and home health care environments include keeping a careful record of fluid intake and output and assessing the patient for signs and symptoms of electrolyte and water imbalance. For example, diuretic-induced dehydration resulting in a loss of only 6% of initial body weight will cause tingling in the extremities, stumbling gait, headache, fever, and an increase in both pulse and respiratory rates.

Clinical Application

Edema

Edema may be defined as the presence of abnormally large amounts of fluid in the intercellular tissue spaces of the body. The condition is a classic example of fluid imbalance and may be caused by disturbances in any factor that governs the interchange between blood plasma and IF compartments. Examples include the following: (1) **Retention of electrolytes (especially Na^+)** in the extracellular fluid as a result of increased aldosterone secretion or after serious kidney disease. (2) **An increase in capillary blood pressure.** Normally, fluid is drawn from the tissue spaces into the venous end of a tissue capillary because of the low venous pressure and the relatively high water-pulling force of the plasma proteins. This balance is upset by anything that increases the capillary hydrostatic pressure. The generalized venous congestion of heart failure is the most common cause of widespread edema. In patients with this condition, blood cannot flow freely through the capillary beds, and therefore the pressure will increase until venous return of blood improves. (3) **A decrease in the concentration of plasma proteins** caused by "leakage" into the interstitial spaces of proteins normally retained in the blood. This may occur as a result of increased capillary permeability caused by infection, burns, or shock.

that moves in the opposite direction (that is, into blood from IF) depends largely on the concentration of proteins in blood plasma. Plasma proteins act as a water-pulling or water-holding force. They hold water in the blood and pull it into the blood from IF. If, for example, the concentration of proteins in blood decreases appreciably—as it does in some abnormal conditions such as dietary deficiency—less water moves into blood from IF. As a result, blood volume decreases and IF volume increases. Of the three main body fluids, IF volume varies the most. Plasma volume usually fluctuates only slightly and briefly. If a pronounced change in its volume occurs, adequate circulation cannot be maintained.

FLUID IMBALANCES

Fluid imbalances are common ailments. They take several forms and stem from a variety of causes, but they all share a common characteristic—that of abnormally low or abnormally high volumes of one or more body fluids.

Dehydration is the fluid imbalance seen most often. In this potentially dangerous condition, IF volume decreases first, but eventually, if treatment has not been given, ICF and plasma volumes also decrease below normal levels. Either too small a fluid intake or too large a fluid output causes dehydration. Prolonged diarrhea or vomiting may result in dehydration because of the loss of body fluids. This is particularly true in infants, in whom the total fluid volume is much smaller than it is in adults. Loss of skin elasticity is a clinical sign of dehydration (Figure 18-7).

Overhydration can also occur but is much less common than dehydration. The grave danger of giving intravenous fluids too rapidly or in too-large amounts is overhydration, which can put too heavy a burden on the heart.

Quick Check

1. How does an increase in capillary blood pressure cause fluid to move into the IF?
2. How do plasma proteins affect fluid balance?
3. What conditions might produce dehydration?

FIGURE 18-7

Testing for dehydration. Loss of skin elasticity is a sign of dehydration. Skin that does not return quickly to its normal shape after being pinched indicates interstitial water loss.

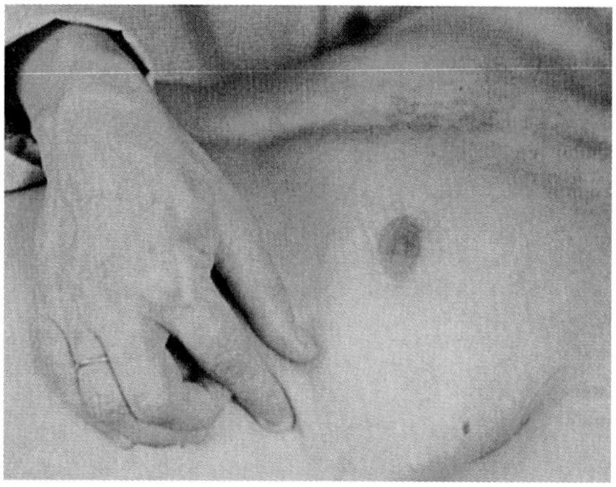

Science Applications

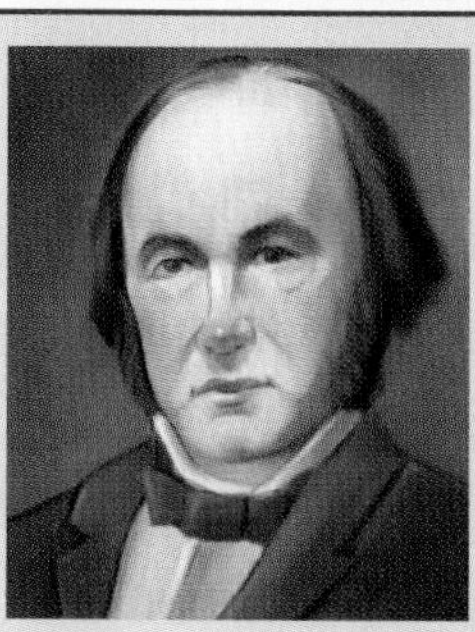

The Constancy of the Body

Claude Bernard (1813-1877).

In 1834, a young Claude Bernard left his boring job as an apprentice apothecary (druggist) in Lyon, France, to make his fortune as a playwright in Paris. His plays were not appreciated in Paris, but he took a medical course and found that many of the doctors appreciated his research skills. Bernard went on to become one of the most important figures in human physiology. He made groundbreaking discoveries in the functions of the pancreas and the liver, discovered the existence of muscles that control blood vessel dilation, and wrote a manual on experimental medicine that set the standard for research practice for a century. However, one of the most fundamental contributions he made to human physiology is the idea that the body is made up of cells living in an internal fluid environment.

Bernard stated that the internal fluid environment of the body is maintained in a relatively constant state—and that's what ensures the survival of the cells and therefore also ensures the survival of the whole body. Recall from Chapter 1 that we now call this concept *homeostasis* (see pp. 14-16). It was Bernard who showed that the actions of hormones and other control mechanisms maintain constant conditions in the body's internal fluid environment. And it was Bernard who showed that nearly every function of the body somehow relates to the success of keeping body fluids constant.

Today, nearly every health care professional uses concepts based on Bernard's original idea to help keep patients alive and healthy. Those who use these ideas most directly are the nurses, health technicians, IV (intravenous) therapists, and others who care for patients on an hour-by-hour basis. It is these professionals who must constantly assess the fluid balance of patients and possibly administer therapies to bring their fluids back into balance. Maintaining a healthy fluid and electrolyte balance is one of the key elements to successful patient care in the modern hospital and clinic.

OUTLINE SUMMARY

BODY FLUIDS

A. Water is most abundant body compound
   1. References to "average" body water volume based on a healthy, nonobese, 70-kg male
   2. Water is 60% of body weight in males; 50% in females (Table 18-1)
   3. Volume averages 40 L in a 70-kg male (Figure 18-1)

B. Variation in total body water is related to:
   1. Total body weight of individual
   2. Fat content of body—the more fat the less water (adipose tissue is low in water content)
   3. Sex—female body about 10% less than male body (Figure 18-2)
   4. Age—in a newborn infant, water may account for 80% of total body weight. In the elderly, water per pound of weight decreases (muscle tissue—high in water—replaced by fat which is lower in water)

BODY FLUID COMPARTMENTS

A. Two major fluid compartments (Table 18-1)
   1. Extracellular fluid (ECF)
      a. Types:
         1) Plasma
         2) Interstitial fluid (IF)
         3) Miscellaneous—lymph; joint fluids; cerebrospinal fluid; eye humors
      b. Called internal environment of body
      c. Surrounds cells and transports substances to and from them
   2. Intracellular fluid (ICF)
      a. Largest fluid compartment
      b. Located inside cells
      c. Serves as solvent to facilitate intracellular chemical reactions

MECHANISMS THAT MAINTAIN FLUID BALANCE

A. Fluid output, mainly urine volume, adjusts to fluid intake; antidiuretic hormone (ADH) from posterior pituitary gland acts to increase kidney tubule reabsorption of sodium and water from tubular urine into blood, thereby tending to increase ECF (and total body fluid) by decreasing urine volume (Figure 18-5)

B. ECF electrolyte concentration (mainly Na^+ concentration) influences ECF volume; an increase in ECF Na^+ tends to increase ECF volume by increasing movement of water out of ICF and by increasing ADH secretion, which decreases urine volume, and this, in turn, increases ECF volume

C. Capillary blood pressure pushes water out of blood, into IF; blood protein concentration pulls water into blood from IF; hence, these two forces regulate plasma and IF volume under usual conditions

D. Importance of electrolytes in body fluids
   1. Nonelectrolytes—organic substances that do not break up or dissociate when placed in water solution (for example, glucose)
   2. Electrolytes—compounds that break up or dissociate in water solution into separate particles called ions (for example, ordinary table salt or sodium chloride)
   3. Ions—the dissociated particles of an electrolyte that carry an electrical charge (for example, sodium ion [Na^+])
   4. Positively charged ions (for example, potassium [K^+] and sodium [Na^+])
   5. Negatively charged particles (ions) (for example, chloride [Cl^-] and bicarbonate [HCO_3^-])

OUTLINE SUMMARY—*cont'd*

6. Electrolyte composition of blood plasma—Table 18-3
7. Sodium—most abundant and important positively charged ion of plasma
   a. Normal plasma level—142 mEq/L
   b. Average daily intake (diet)—100 mEq
   c. Chief method of regulation—kidney
   d. Aldosterone increases Na^+ reabsorption in kidney tubules (Figure 18-5)
   e. Sodium-containing internal secretions—Figure 18-6

E. Capillary blood pressure and blood proteins

FLUID IMBALANCES

A. Dehydration—total volume of body fluids less than normal; IF volume shrinks first, and then if treatment is not given, ICF volume and plasma volume decrease; dehydration occurs when fluid output exceeds intake for an extended period
B. Overhydration—total volume of body fluids greater than normal; overhydration occurs when fluid intake exceeds output; various factors may cause this (for example, giving excessive amounts of intravenous fluids or giving them too rapidly may increase intake above output)

NEW WORDS

dehydration
dissociate
diuretic
edema
electrolyte
extracellular fluid (ECF)
interstitial fluid (IF)
intracellular fluid (ICF)
ions
overhydration

REVIEW QUESTIONS

1. Name and give the location of the three main fluid compartments of the body. Which of these make up extracellular fluid?
2. What factors influence the percent of water in the body? Explain the effect of each factor.
3. List the three sources of water for the body.
4. List the four organs from which fluid output occurs.
5. Differentiate between an electrolyte and a nonelectrolyte.
6. Name three important negative ions.
7. Name three important positive ions.
8. Explain why the body is unable to reduce its fluid output to zero no matter how dehydrated it is.
9. Explain how aldosterone influences water movement between the kidney tubules and the blood.
10. Explain the role of capillary blood pressure in water movement between the plasma and interstitial fluid.
11. Explain the role of plasma proteins in water movement between the plasma and interstitial fluid.
12. Define dehydration and give a possible cause.
13. Define overhydration and give a possible cause.

CRITICAL THINKING

14. Name the three hormones that regulate the urine volume. State where each is made and the specific effect on urine volume.
15. Atrial natriuretic hormone has the opposite effect of aldosterone. Explain its effect on water movement between the kidney tubules and the blood.

CHAPTER TEST

1. The extracellular fluid compartment is composed of __________ and __________.
2. The largest volume of water is in this fluid compartment: __________.

Fill in "more" or "less" in the blanks in questions 3, 4, and 5.

3. In general, an obese person has __________ water per pound of body weight than a slim person.
4. In general, a man has __________ water per pound of body weight than a woman.
5. In general, an infant has __________ water per pound of body weight than an adult.
6. The body's chief mechanism for maintaining fluid balance is to adjust its __________.
7. The body has three sources of fluid intake; the liquids we drink, the water in the food we eat, and __________.
8. The four organs from which fluid output occurs are the __________, __________, __________, and __________.
9. Urine volume is regulated by three hormones: ADH released from the pituitary gland, __________ released from the adrenal cortex, and __________ released from the heart.

CHAPTER TEST—*cont'd*

10. When electrolytes dissociate in water, they form charged particles called __________.
11. The most abundant negatively charged particle in the blood is __________.
12. The most abundant positively charged particle in the blood is __________.
13. When the blood level of aldosterone increases:
    a. sodium is moved from the blood to the kidney tubules
    b. sodium is moved from the kidney tubules to the blood
    c. more urine is formed
    d. ANH is released
14. Aldosterone causes:
    a. an increase in intracellular fluid
    b. a decrease in intracellular fluid
    c. an increase in extracellular fluid
    d. a decrease in extracellular fluid
15. Increased capillary pressure:
    a. moves fluid from the intracellular to the extracellular compartment
    b. moves fluid from the plasma to the interstitial fluid
    c. moves fluid from the interstitial fluid to the plasma
    d. has no effect on fluid movement
16. Blood plasma proteins act to:
    a. move interstitial fluid into the plasma
    b. move plasma into the interstitial fluid
    c. move extracellular fluid into the intracellular fluid
    d. move interstitial fluid into the extracellular fluid

STUDY TIPS

Chapter 18 expands on some of the material from Chapter 17. The terms in the chapter can be learned with flash cards. Remember that plasma and interstitial fluid make up the extracellular fluid. Electrolytes are charged particles or ions. One of the functions of ions is to control water movement. The body cannot directly move water; it must move the electrolytes and the water will follow. Figure 18-5 will help explain this. The capillary blood pressure and blood protein mechanism regulates the movement of water between the blood and interstitial fluid. Blood pressure determines the amount of plasma that is pushed into the interstitial fluid. Plasma proteins determine the amount of water that gets pulled back into the blood.

In your study group, go over the flash cards with the terms. Discuss how electrolytes function in regulating body water. Go over the aldosterone mechanism figure (Figure 18-5). The text suggests drawing your own similar figure using the ADH mechanism. Discuss the plasma protein and capillary blood pressure mechanism for regulating the balance between blood plasma and interstitial fluid. Go over the questions in the back of the chapter and discuss possible test questions.

10 Acid–Base Balance

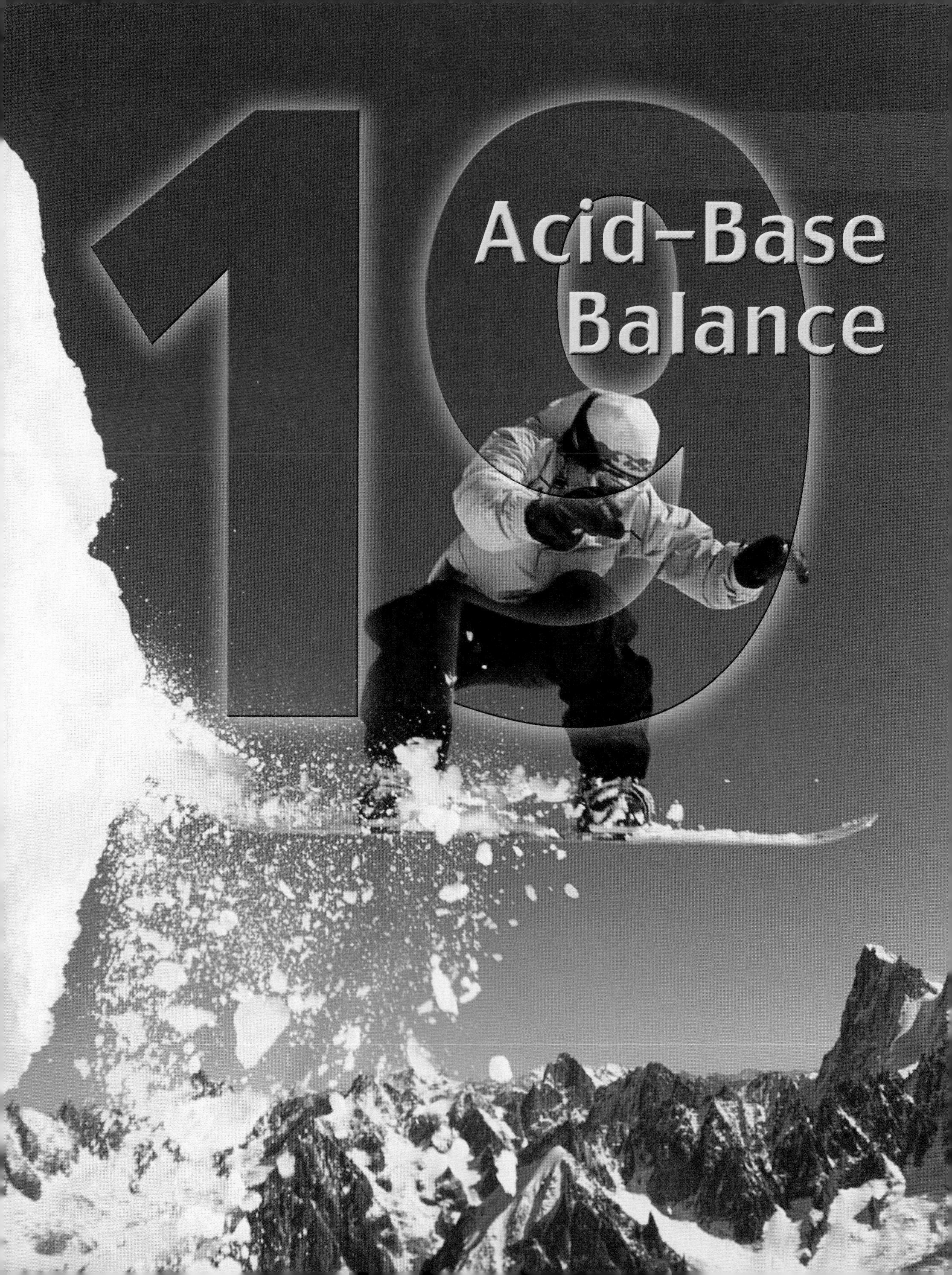

• Outline

• Objectives

AFTER YOU HAVE COMPLETED THIS CHAPTER, YOU SHOULD BE ABLE TO:

1. Discuss the concept of pH and define the term *acid-base balance*.
2. Define the terms *buffer* and *buffer pair* and contrast strong and weak acids and bases.
3. Contrast the respiratory and urinary mechanisms of pH control.
4. Discuss compensatory mechanisms that may help return blood pH to near-normal levels in cases of pH imbalances.
5. Compare and contrast metabolic and respiratory types of pH imbalances.

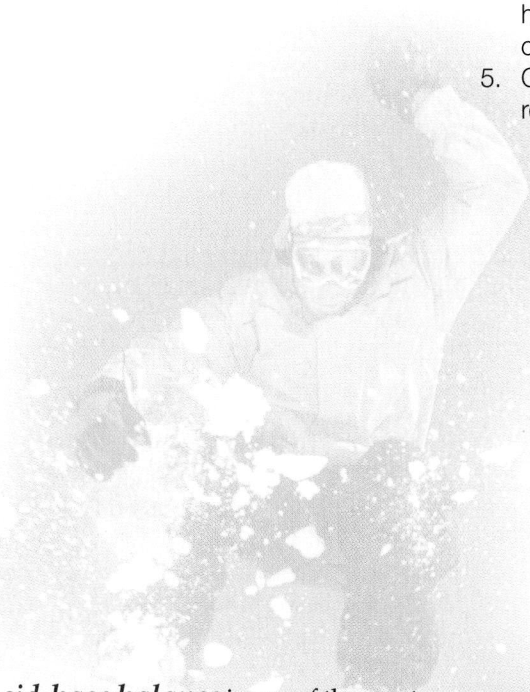

Acid-base balance is one of the most important of the body's homeostatic mechanisms. Maintaining acid-base balance means keeping the concentration of hydrogen ions in body fluids relatively constant. Effective functioning of many important body proteins, such as cellular enzymes and hemoglobin, is closely dependent on maintaining precise regulation of hydrogen ion concentration. This is of vital importance. If the hydrogen ion concentration veers away from normal even slightly, serious illness or even death may occur. Healthy survival depends on the ability of the body to maintain, or quickly restore, the acid-base balance of its fluids if imbalances occur. Acid-base regulation requires a series of coordinated homeostatic mechanisms that involve the blood and other body fluids, the lungs and kidneys. Ultimately all of these mechanisms are based on chemical processes. Recall that many important chemical principles related to the life process were covered in Chapter 2. You may wish to refer back to those principles of biochemistry as you study in this chapter how the body so precisely regulates its acid-base balance.

FIGURE 19-1

The pH range. The overall pH range is expressed numerically on what is called a *logarithmic scale* of 1 to 14. This means that a change of 1 pH unit represents a tenfold difference in actual concentration of hydrogen ions. Note that, as the concentration of H^+ ions increases, the solution becomes increasingly acidic and the pH value decreases. As OH^- concentration increases, the pH value also increases, and the solution becomes more and more basic or alkaline. A pH of 7 is neutral; a pH of 1 is very acidic, and a pH of 13 is very basic.

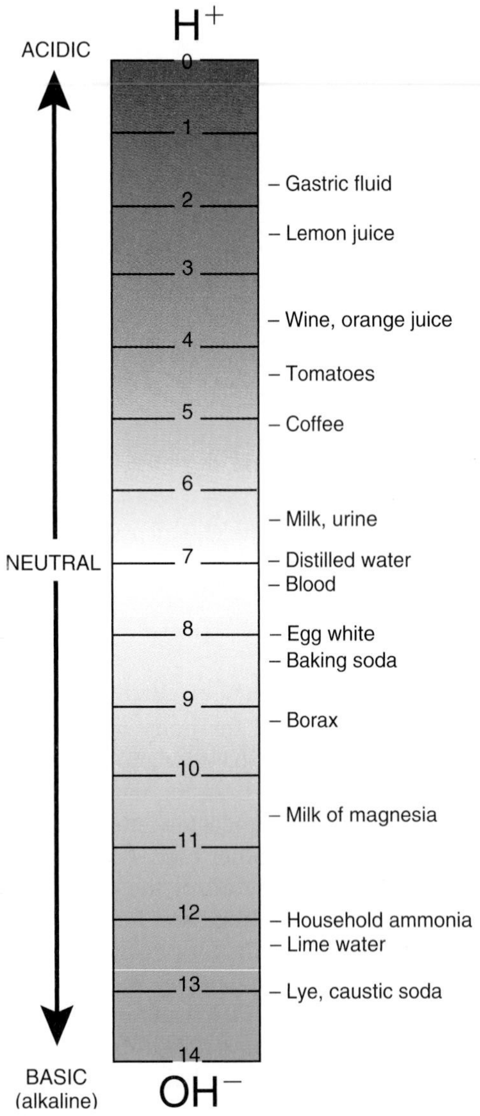

pH OF BODY FLUIDS

Water and all water solutions contain **hydrogen ions (H^+)** and **hydroxide ions (OH^-).** The term *pH* followed by a number indicates a solution's hydrogen ion concentration. More specifically, pH 7.0 means that a solution contains an equal concentration of hydrogen and hydroxide ions. Therefore pH 7.0 also means that a fluid is neutral in reaction (that is, neither acid nor alkaline) (Figure 19-1). The pH of pure water, for example, is 7.0. A pH higher than 7.0 indicates an alkaline or basic solution (that is, one with a lower concentration of hydrogen than hydroxide ions). The more alkaline a solution, the higher is its pH. A pH lower than 7.0 indicates an acid solution (that is, one with a higher hydrogen ion concentration than hydroxide ion concentration). The higher the hydrogen ion concentration, the lower the pH and the more acid a solution is. With a pH of about 1.6, gastric juice is the most acid substance in the body. Saliva has a pH of 7.7, on the alkaline side. Normally, the pH of arterial blood is about 7.45, and the pH of venous blood is about 7.35. By applying the information given in the last few sentences, you can deduce the answers to the following questions. Is arterial blood slightly acid or slightly alkaline? Is venous blood slightly acid or slightly alkaline? Which is a more accurate statement? Venous blood is more acid than arterial blood, or, Venous blood is less alkaline than arterial blood.

Arterial and venous blood are both slightly alkaline because both have a pH slightly higher than 7.0. Venous blood, however, is less alkaline than arterial blood because venous blood's pH of about 7.35 is slightly lower than arterial blood's pH of 7.45.

Quick

1. Of what is pH a measurement?
2. What is meant by saying the pH of a solution is "neutral?"
3. What does it mean when a solution's pH increases?

MECHANISMS THAT CONTROL pH OF BODY FLUIDS

The body has three mechanisms for regulating the pH of its fluids. They are (1) the buffer mechanism, (2) the respiratory mechanism, and (3) the urinary mechanism. Together, they constitute the complex pH homeostatic mechanism—the machinery that normally keeps blood slightly alkaline with a pH that stays remarkably constant. Its usual limits are very narrow, about 7.35 to 7.45.

The slightly lower pH of venous blood compared with arterial blood results primarily from carbon dioxide (CO_2) entering venous blood as a waste product of cellular metabolism. CO_2 is formed during the cellular breakdown of the nutrient glucose in the presence of oxygen. The process is called **aerobic** (air-OH-bik) or **cellular respiration.** As carbon dioxide enters the blood, some of it combines with water (H_2O) and is converted into carbonic acid by **carbonic anhydrase,** an enzyme found in red blood cells. The following chemical equation represents this reaction. If you need to review chemical formulas and equations, please refer to Chapter 2.

$$CO_2 + H_2O \xrightarrow{\textbf{carbonic anhydrase}} H_2CO_3$$

The lungs remove the equivalent of more than 30 L of carbonic acid each day from the venous blood by elimination of CO_2. This almost unbelievable quantity of acid is so well buffered that a liter of venous blood contains only about 1/100,000,000 g more H^+ than does 1 L of arterial blood. What incredible constancy! The pH homeostatic mechanism does indeed control effectively—astonishingly so.

Buffers

Buffers are chemical substances that prevent a sharp change in the pH of a fluid when an acid or base is added to it. Strong acids and bases, if added to blood, would "dissociate" almost completely and release large quantities of H or OH ions. The result would be drastic changes in blood pH. Survival itself depends on protecting the body from such drastic pH changes.

More acids than bases are usually added to body fluids. This is because catabolism, a process that goes on continually in every cell of the body, produces acids that enter blood as it flows through tissue capillaries. In addition to the acids produced by cellular breakdown of nutrients such as glucose and fats, some H^+ may be absorbed directly through the digestive tract. Almost immediately, one of the salts present in blood—a buffer, that is—reacts with these relatively strong acids to change them to weaker acids. The weaker acids decrease blood pH only slightly, whereas the stronger acids formed by catabolism would have decreased it greatly if they were not buffered.

Buffers consist of two kinds of substances and are therefore often called **buffer pairs.** One of the main blood buffer pairs is ordinary baking soda (sodium bicarbonate or $NaHCO_3$) and carbonic acid (H_2CO_3).

Let us consider, as a specific example of buffer action, how the $NaHCO_3$–H_2CO_3 system works with a strong acid or base.

Addition of a strong acid, such as hydrochloric acid (HCl), to the $NaHCO_3$–H_2CO_3 buffer system would initiate the reaction shown in Figure 19-2. Note how this reaction between HCl and $NaHCO_3$ applies the principle of buffering. As a result of the buffering action of $NaHCO_3$, the weak acid, $H \bullet HCO_3$, replaces the very strong acid, HCl, and therefore the H^+ concentration of the blood increases much less than it would have if HCl were not buffered.

If, on the other hand, a strong base, such as sodium hydroxide (NaOH), were added to the same buffer system, the reaction shown in Figure 19-3 would take place. The H^+ of H_2CO_3 ($H \bullet HCO_3$), the weak acid of the buffer pair, combines with the OH^- of the strong base NaOH to form H_2O. Note what this accomplishes. It decreases the number of OH^- added to the solution, and this in turn prevents the drastic rise in pH that would occur without buffering.

Figure 19-2 shows how a buffer system works with a strong acid. Although useful in demonstrating the principles of buffer action, HCl or similar strong acids are never introduced directly into body fluids under normal circumstances. Instead, the $NaCO_3$ buffer system is most often called on to buffer a number of weaker acids produced during catabolism. Lactic acid is a good example. As a weak acid, it does not "dissociate" as completely as HCl. Incomplete dissociation of lactic acid results in fewer hydrogen ions being added to the blood and a less drastic lowering of blood pH than would occur if HCl were added in an equal amount. Without buffering, however, lactic acid

FIGURE 19-2

Buffering action of sodium bicarbonate. Buffering of acid HCl by $NaHCO_3$. As a result of the buffer action, the strong acid (HCl) is replaced by a weaker acid (H • HCO_3). Note that HCl as a strong acid "dissociates" almost completely and releases more H^+ than H_2CO_3. Buffering decreases the number of H^+ in the system.

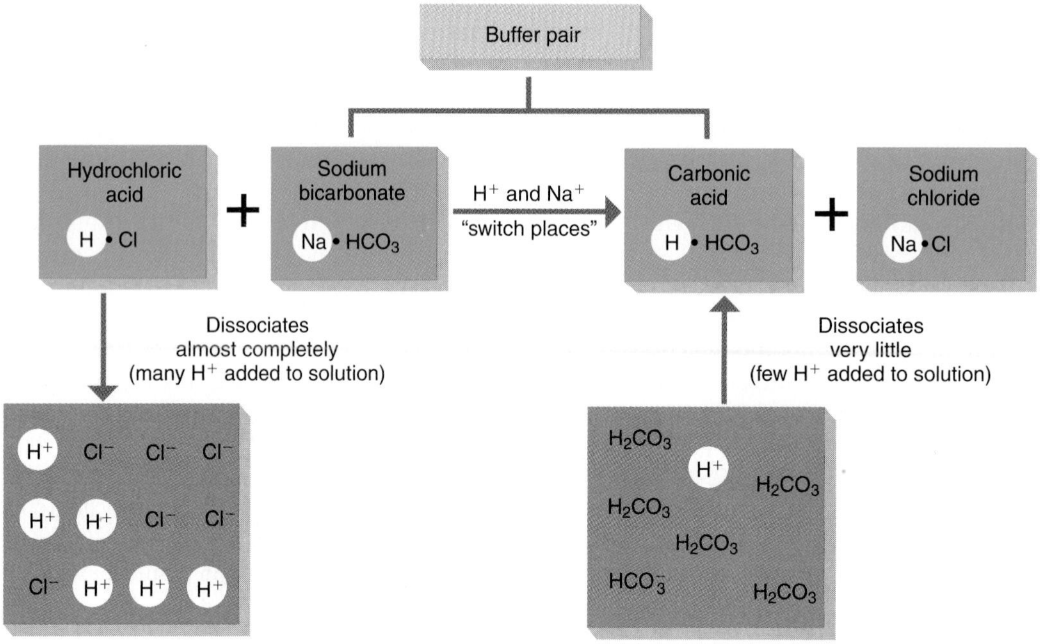

buildup results in significant H^+ accumulation over time. The resulting decrease of pH can produce serious acidosis. Ordinary baking soda (sodium bicarbonate or $NaHCO_3$) is one of the main buffers of the normally occurring "fixed" acids in blood. Lactic acid is one of the most abundant of the "fixed" acids (acids that do not break down to form a gas). Figure 19-4 shows the compounds formed by buffering of lactic acid (a "fixed" acid), produced by normal catabolism of glucose in the absence of oxygen. The following changes in blood result from buffering of fixed acids in tissue capillaries:

1. The amount of H_2CO_3 in blood increases slightly because an acid (such as lactic acid) is converted to H_2CO_3.
2. The amount of bicarbonate in blood (mainly $NaHCO_3$) decreases because bicarbonate ions become part of the newly formed H_2CO_3. Normal arterial blood with a pH of 7.45 contains 20 times more $NaHCO_3$ than H_2CO_3. If this ratio decreases, blood pH decreases below 7.45.
3. The H^+ concentration of blood increases slightly. H_2CO_3 adds hydrogen ions to blood, but it adds fewer of them than lactic acid would have because it is a weaker acid than lactic acid. In other words the buffering mechanisms do not totally prevent blood hydrogen ion concentration from increasing. It simply minimizes the increase.
4. Blood pH decreases slightly because of the small increase in blood concentration.

H_2CO_3 is the most abundant acid in body fluids because it is formed by the buffering of fixed acids and also because CO_2 forms it by combining with H_2O. Large amounts of CO_2, an end product of catabolism, continually pour into tissue capillary blood from cells. Much of the H_2CO_3 formed in blood diffuses into red blood cells where it is

FIGURE 19-3

Buffering action of carbonic acid. Buffering of base NaOH by H_2CO_3. As a result of buffer action, the strong base (NaOH) is replaced by $NaHCO_3$ and H_2O. As a strong base, NaOH "dissociates" almost completely and releases large quantities of OH^-. Dissociation of H_2O is minimal. Buffering decreases the number of OH^- in the system.

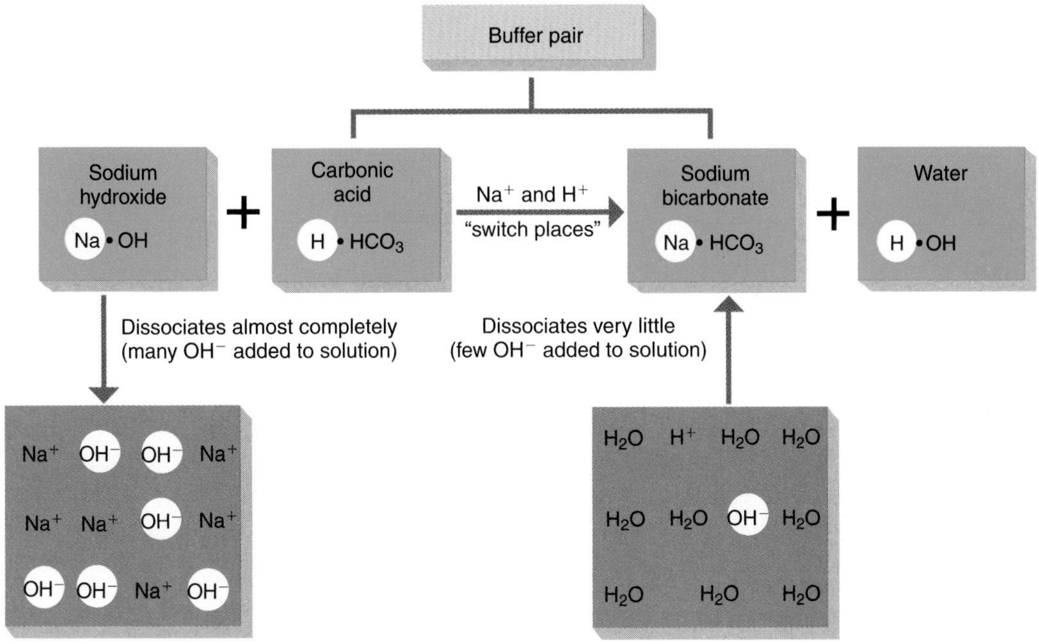

buffered by the potassium salt of hemoglobin. H_2CO_3 breaks down to form the gas, CO_2, and H_2O. This takes place in the blood as it moves through the lung capillaries. Read the next several paragraphs to find out how this affects blood pH.

Quick Check

1. What three mechanisms does the body have for regulating pH of body fluids?
2. What are buffers?

Respiratory Mechanism of pH Control

Respirations play a vital part in regulating H^+ concentrations and controlling body pH. With every expiration, CO_2 and H_2O leave the body in the expired air. The CO_2 has diffused out of the ve-

Health & Well-Being

Bicarbonate Loading

The buildup of lactic acid in the blood, released as a waste product from working muscle cells that burn glucose for energy in the absence of oxygen, a process called **anaerobic** (AN-err-OH-bik) **respiration,** has been blamed for the soreness and fatigue that sometimes accompanies strenuous exercise over time. Some athletes have adopted a technique called **bicarbonate loading,** ingesting large amounts of sodium bicarbonate ($NaHCO_3$) to counteract the effects of lactic acid buildup. Their theory is that fatigue is avoided because the $NaHCO_3$, a base, buffers the lactic acid. Unfortunately, the diarrhea that often results can trigger fluid and electrolyte imbalances. Long-term $NaHCO_3$ abuse can lead to disruption of acid-base balance.

FIGURE 19-4

Lactic acid buffered by sodium bicarbonate. Lactic acid (H • lactate) and other "fixed" acids are buffered by $NaHCO_3$ in the blood. Carbonic acid (H • HCO_3 or H_2CO_3, a weaker acid than lactic acid) replaces lactic acid. As a result, fewer H^+ are added to blood than would be if lactic acid were not buffered.

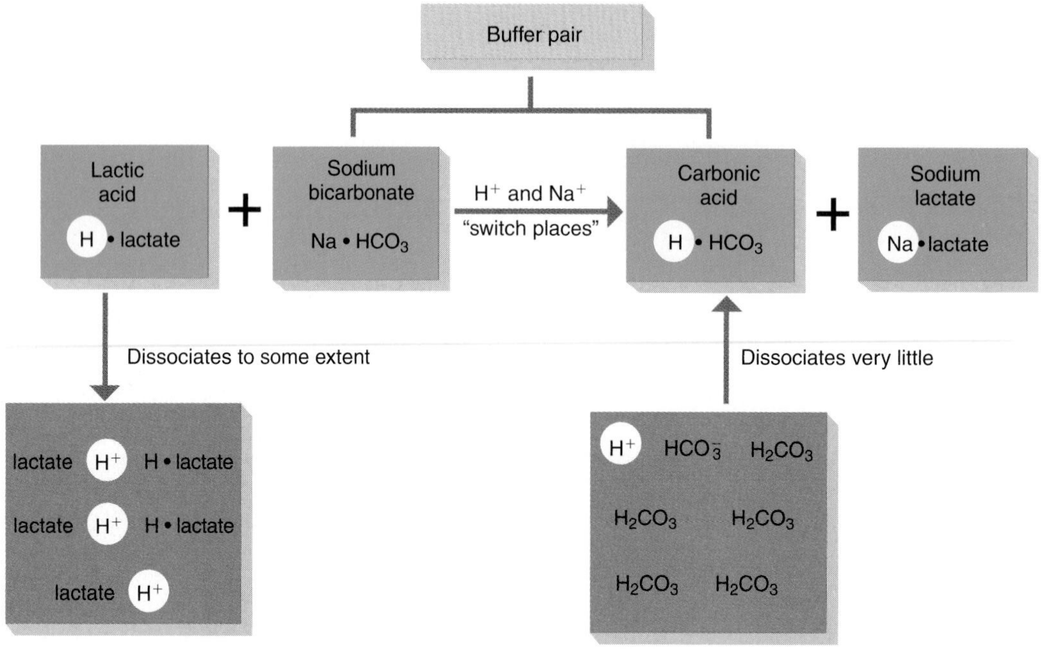

Clinical Application

Diabetic Ketoacidosis

An important part of home care for diabetics involves monitoring the level of glucose in the blood and, especially for patients taking insulin, carefully watching for the appearance of **ketone bodies** in the urine. Accumulation of these acidic substances in the blood results from the excessive metabolism of fats most often in uncontrolled type 1 diabetics. These individuals have trouble metabolizing carbohydrates and instead burn fat as a primary energy source. The accumulation of ketone bodies results in a condition called **diabetic ketoacidosis** that causes the blood to become dangerously acidic. As blood levels of ketones increase they "spill over" into the urine and can be detected by use of appropriate reagent strips.

nous blood as it moves through the lung capillaries. Less CO_2 therefore remains in the arterial blood leaving the lung capillaries, so less of it is available for combining with water to form H_2CO_3. Hence the arterial blood contains less H_2CO_3 and fewer hydrogen ions and has a higher pH (7.45) than does the venous blood (pH 7.35).

Let us consider now how a change in respirations can change blood pH. Suppose you were to pinch your nose shut and hold your breath for a full minute or a little longer. Obviously, no CO_2 would leave your body by way of the expired air during that time, and the blood's CO_2 content would necessarily increase. This would increase the amount of H_2CO_3 and the hydrogen-ion concentration of blood, which in turn would decrease blood pH. Here then are two useful facts to remember. Anything that causes an appreciable decrease in respirations will in time produce **acido-**

FIGURE 19-5

Acidification of urine and conservation of base by distal renal tubule secretion of H^+ ions.

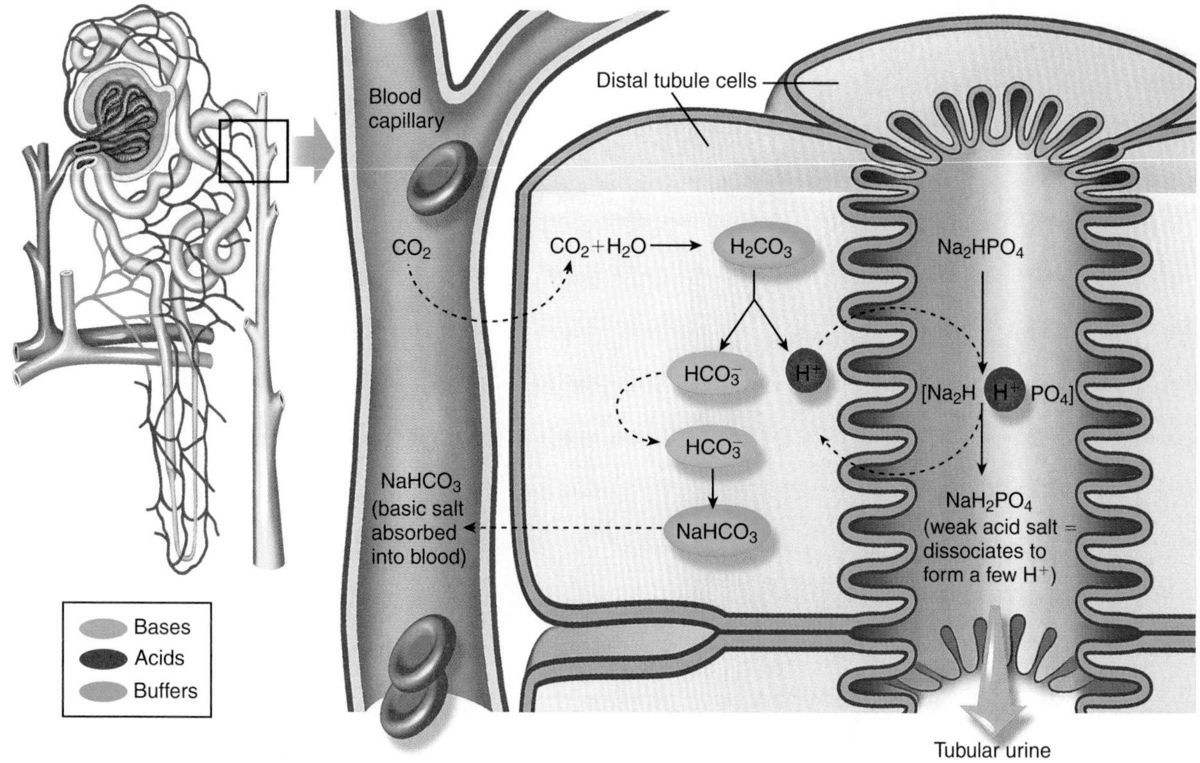

sis. Conversely, anything that causes an excessive increase in respirations will in time produce **alkalosis.** Thus the respiratory control centers in the brain (see p. 379), by increasing or decreasing the rate and depth of respirations, can affect concentrations of CO_2 and H^+ in body fluids.

Urinary Mechanism of pH Control

Most people know that the kidneys are vital organs and that life soon ebbs away if they stop functioning. One reason is that the kidneys are the body's most effective regulators of blood pH. They can eliminate much larger amounts of acid than can the lungs and, if it becomes necessary, they can also excrete excess base. The lungs cannot. In short, the kidneys are the body's last and best defense against wide variations in blood pH. If they fail, homeostasis of pH—acid-base balance—fails.

Because more acids than bases usually enter blood, more acids than bases are usually excreted by the kidneys. In other words, most of the time the kidneys acidify urine; that is, they excrete enough acid to give urine an acid pH frequently as low as 4.8. (How does this compare with normal blood pH?) The distal tubules of the kidneys rid the blood of excess acid and at the same time conserve the base present in it by the two mechanisms illustrated by Figures 19-5 and 19-6. To understand these figures fully, you need to have some grasp of basic chemistry. If necessary, refer to Chapter 2 before proceeding. Then look at Figure 19-5 and find the CO_2 leaving the blood (as it flows through a kidney capillary) and entering

FIGURE 19-6

Acidification of urine by tubule secretion of ammonia (NH_3). An amino acid (glutamine) moves into the tubule cell and loses an amino group (NH_2) to form ammonia, which is secreted into urine. In exchange, the tubule cell reabsorbs a basic salt (mainly $NaHCO_3$) into blood from urine.

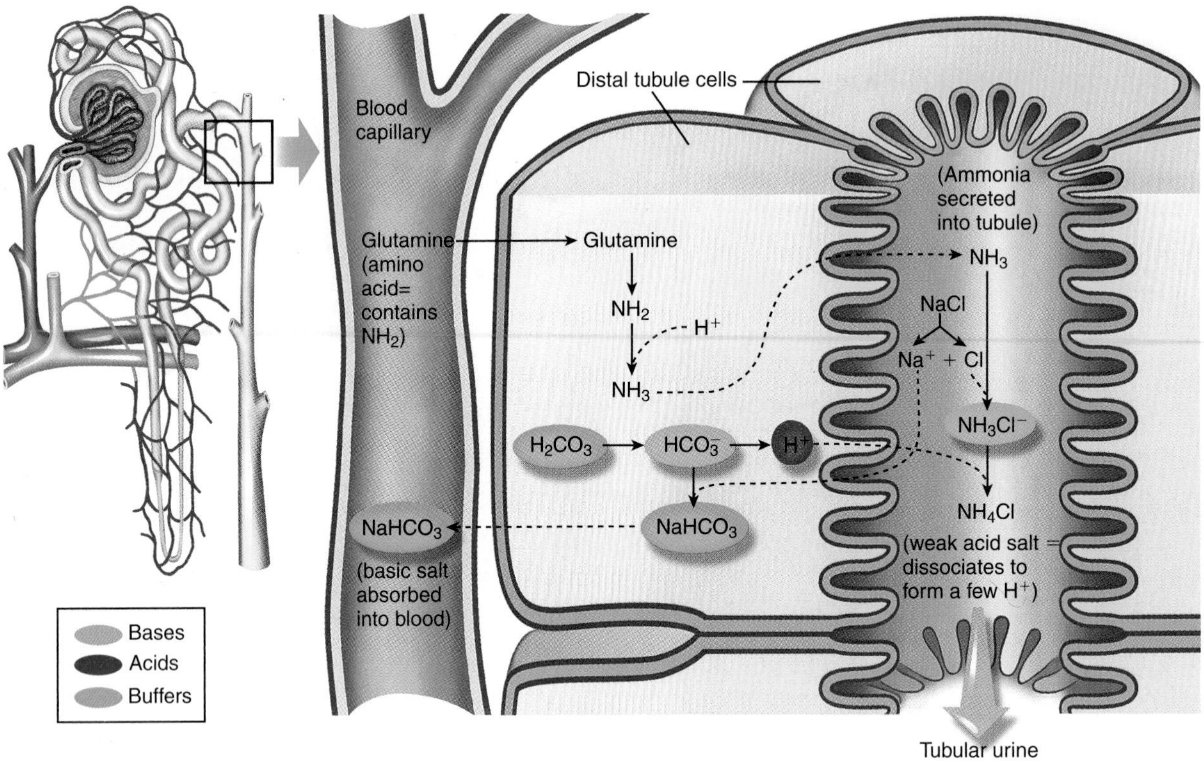

one of the cells that helps form the wall of a distal kidney tubule. Note that in this cell the CO_2 combines with water to form H_2CO_3. This occurs rapidly because the cell contains carbonic anhydrase, an enzyme that accelerates this reaction. As soon as H_2CO_3 forms, some of it dissociates to yield hydrogen ions and bicarbonate ions. Note what happens to these ions. Hydrogen ions diffuse out of the tubule cell into the urine trickling down the tubule. There, it replaces one of the sodium ions (Na^+) in a salt (Na_2HPO_4) to form another salt (NaH_2PO_4), which leaves the body in the urine. Notice next that the Na^+ displaced from Na_2HPO_4 by the H^+ moves out of the tubular urine into a tubular cell. Here it combines with a bicarbonate (HCO_3^-) ion to form sodium bicarbonate, which then is resorbed into the blood. What this complex of reactions has accomplished is to add hydrogen ions to the urine—that is, acidify it—and to conserve $NaHCO_3$ by reabsorbing it into the blood.

Figure 19-6 illustrates another method of acidifying urine, as explained in the legend.

Quick Check

1. How can breathing affect the pH of the blood?
2. By what mechanism can the kidney change the pH of the blood?

pH IMBALANCES

Acidosis and **alkalosis** are the two kinds of pH or acid-base imbalance. In acidosis the blood pH falls as H^+ ion concentration increases or because of a loss of bases. Only rarely does it fall as low as 7.0 (neutrality), and almost never does it become even slightly acid, because death usually intervenes before the pH drops this much. In alkalosis, which develops less often than acidosis, the blood pH is higher than normal because of a loss of acids or an accumulation of bases.

From a clinical standpoint, disturbances in acid-base balance can be considered dependent on the relative quantities (ratio) of H_2CO_3 and $NaHCO_3$ in the blood. Components of this important buffer pair must be maintained at the proper ratio (20 times more $NaHCO_3$ than H_2CO_3) if acid-base balance is to remain normal. It is fortunate that the body can regulate both chemicals in the $NaHCO_3$–H_2CO_3 buffer system. Blood levels of $NaHCO_3$ can be regulated by the kidneys and H_2CO_3 levels by the respiratory system (lungs).

Metabolic and Respiratory Disturbances

Two types of disturbances, metabolic and respiratory, can alter the proper ratio of these components. Metabolic disturbances affect the bicarbonate ($NaHCO_3$) element of the buffer pair, and respiratory disturbances affect the H_2CO_3 element, as follows:

1. **Metabolic disturbances**
   - **a.** *Metabolic acidosis* (bicarbonate deficit). Patients in metabolic acidosis with a bicarbonate deficit often suffer from renal disease, uncontrolled diabetes, prolonged diarrhea, or have ingested toxic chemicals such as antifreeze (ethylene glycol) or wood alcohol (methanol).
   - **b.** *Metabolic alkalosis* (bicarbonate excess). The bicarbonate excess in metabolic alkalosis can result from diuretic therapy, loss of acid-containing gastric fluid caused by vomiting or suction, or from certain diseases such as Cushing syndrome.
2. **Respiratory disturbances**
   - **a.** *Respiratory acidosis* (H_2CO_3 excess). The increase in H_2CO_3 characteristic of respiratory acidosis is caused most frequently by slow breathing, which results in excess CO_2 in arterial blood. Causes include depression of the respiratory center by drugs or anesthesia or by pulmonary diseases such as emphysema and pneumonia.
   - **b.** *Respiratory alkalosis* (H_2CO_3 deficit). Hyperventilation leads to a H_2CO_3 deficit caused by excessive loss of CO_2 in expired air. The result is respiratory alkalosis. Anxiety (hyperventilation syndrome), overventilation of patients on ventilators, or hepatic coma can all reduce H_2CO_3 and CO_2 to dangerously low levels.

Clinical Application

Lactic Acidosis and Metformin

Metformin hydrochloride (Glucophage) is one of the most widely used and effective of the oral antidiabetic drugs. It is used with diet and exercise to lower blood glucose levels in type 2 diabetes mellitus. A rare but very serious complication of metformin therapy is lactic acidosis. It is characterized by elevated blood lactate levels, electrolyte disturbances, and decreased blood pH. It is reported in only about 1 in 33,000 patients taking metformin over the course of a year. However, when it does occur, it can be fatal in nearly 50% of cases. Symptoms include a variety of gastrointestinal and respiratory complaints and feelings of weakness and muscle pain. Patients with kidney and liver disease are known to be at higher risk of developing lactic acidosis while taking the drug.

FIGURE 19-7

The vomit reflex. Severe vomiting results in significant loss of HCl and often leads to metabolic alkalosis.

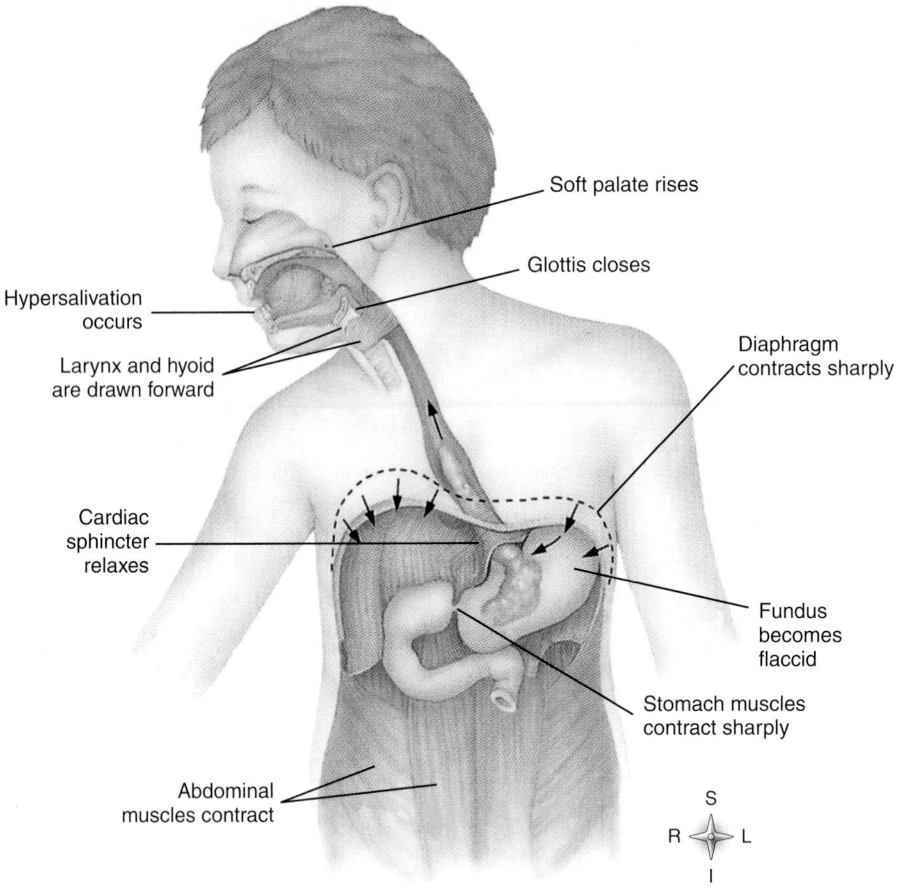
Soft palate rises
Glottis closes
Hypersalivation occurs
Larynx and hyoid are drawn forward
Diaphragm contracts sharply
Cardiac sphincter relaxes
Fundus becomes flaccid
Stomach muscles contract sharply
Abdominal muscles contract
S
R
L
I

Vomiting

Vomiting, sometimes referred to as *emesis* (EM-e-sis), is the forcible emptying or expulsion of gastric and occasionally intestinal contents through the mouth (Figure 19-7). It can occur as a result of many stimuli, including foul odors or tastes, irritation of the stomach or intestinal mucosa, and some vomitive (emetic) drugs such as ipecac. A "vomiting center" in the brain regulates the many coordinated (but primarily involuntary) steps involved. Severe vomiting such as the pernicious vomiting of pregnancy or the repeated vomiting associated with pyloric obstruction in infants can be life-threatening. One of the most frequent and serious complications of vomiting is metabolic alkalosis. The bicarbonate excess of metabolic alkalosis results because of the massive loss of chloride from the stomach as HCl. The loss of chloride causes a compensatory increase of bicarbonate in the extracellular fluid. The result is metabolic alkalosis. Therapy includes intravenous administration of chloride-containing solutions such as **normal saline.** The chloride ions of the solution replace bicarbonate ions and thus help relieve the bicarbonate excess responsible for the imbalance.

The *ratio* of $NaHCO_3$ to H_2CO_3 levels in the blood is the key to acid-base balance. If the normal ratio (20:1 $NaHCO_3/H_2CO_3$) can be maintained, the acid-base balance and pH remain normal despite changes in the absolute amounts of either component of the buffer pair in the blood.

As a clinical example, in a person suffering from untreated diabetes, abnormally large amounts of acids enter the blood. The normal 20:1 ratio is altered as the $NaHCO_3$ component of the buffer pair reacts with the acids. Blood levels of $NaHCO_3$ decrease rapidly in these patients. The result is a lower ratio of $NaHCO_3$ to H_2CO_3 (perhaps 10:1) and lower blood pH. The condition is called **uncompensated metabolic acidosis.** The body attempts to correct or *compensate* for the acidosis by altering the *ratio* of $NaHCO_3$ to H_2CO_3. Acidosis in a diabetic patient is often accompanied by rapid breathing or hyperventilation. This compensatory action of the respiratory system results in a "blow-off" of CO_2. Decreased blood levels of CO_2 result in lower H_2CO_3 levels. A new compensated ratio of $NaHCO_3$ to H_2CO_3 (perhaps 10:0.5) may result. In such individuals the blood pH returns to normal or near-normal levels. The condition is called **compensated metabolic acidosis.**

Quick

1. What is acidosis? What is alkalosis?
2. What factors may cause a metabolic disturbance in pH?
3. What situations may cause a respiratory disturbance in pH?
4. How does vomiting sometimes create an acid-base imbalance?

Science Applications

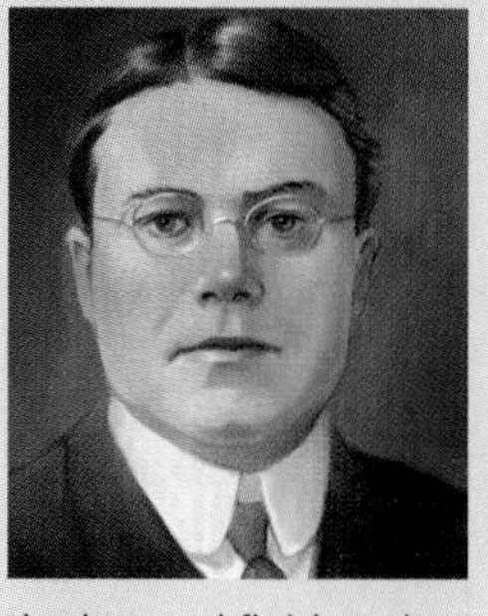

The Body in Balance

Walter Bradford Cannon (1871-1945).

Keeping the pH of the body stable is but one aspect of maintaining health. The American physiologist Walter Cannon gave us a name for the principle of balance, or constancy, of the internal fluid environment of the body—*homeostasis.* In 1932, his popular book *The Wisdom of the Body* finally gave a name to the concept first explained by Claude Bernard seven decades earlier (see p. 465). However, Cannon did more than name the concept. In his book, Cannon explained the incredibly complex set of mechanisms that allow our bodies to adjust to tremendous internal and external fluctuations that would otherwise kill us. Much of Cannon's thought came from his groundbreaking discoveries in how the body copes with stress. In examining the fight-or-flight response, the effects of emotional stimuli, the mechanisms of cardiovascular shock, and in developing the "case study" approach to learning about human health and disease, Walter Cannon developed a clear understanding of the interactive nature of the organs of the body. It was Cannon that led scientists to look at their work in this new framework that explains the "big picture" of human body function.

Cannon's explanation of homeostasis revolutionized the way we look at the body—and how we look at patient care. As with fluid and electrolyte balance, knowledge of the mechanisms of acid-base balance is critical in direct patient care. Therefore, many physicians, nurses, intravenous therapists, first responders (for example, emergency medical technicians and paramedics), and others need a basic knowledge of how the body maintains a constancy of pH in the blood.

OUTLINE SUMMARY

pH OF BODY FLUIDS

A. Definition of pH—a number that indicates the hydrogen ion (H^+) concentration of a fluid; pH 7.0 indicates neutrality, pH higher than 7.0 indicates alkalinity, and pH less than 7.0 indicates acidity—see Figure 19-1
B. Normal arterial blood pH—about 7.45
C. Normal venous blood pH—about 7.35

MECHANISMS THAT CONTROL pH OF BODY FLUIDS

A. Buffers
   1. Definition—substances that prevent a sharp change in the pH of a fluid when an acid or base is added to it—see Figures 19-2 and 19-3
   2. "Fixed" acids are buffered mainly by sodium bicarbonate ($NaHCO_3$)
   3. Changes in blood produced by buffering of "fixed" acids in the tissue capillaries
      a. Amount of carbonic acid (H_2CO_3) in blood increases slightly
      b. Amount of $NaHCO_3$ in blood decreases; ratio of amount of $NaHCO_3$ to the amount of H_2CO_3 does not normally change; normal ratio is 20:1
      c. H^+ concentration of blood increases slightly
      d. Blood pH decreases slightly below arterial level
B. Respiratory mechanism of pH control—respirations remove some CO_2 from blood as blood flows through lung capillaries, the amount of H_2CO_3 in blood is decreased and thereby its H+ concentration is decreased, and this in turn increases blood pH from its venous to its arterial level
C. Urinary mechanism of pH control—the body's most effective regulator of blood pH, kidneys usually acidify urine by the distal tubules secreting hydrogen ions and ammonia (NH_3) into the urine from blood in exchange for $NaHCO_3$ being reabsorbed into the blood

pH IMBALANCES

A. Acidosis and alkalosis are the two kinds of pH or acid-base imbalances
B. Disturbances in acid-base balance depend on relative quantities of $NaHCO_3$ and H_2CO_3 in the blood
C. Body can regulate both of the components of the $NaHCO_3$–H_2CO_3 buffer system
   1. Blood levels of $NaHCO_3$ regulated by kidneys
   2. H_2CO_3 levels regulated by lungs
D. Two basic types of pH disturbances—metabolic and respiratory—can alter the normal 20:1 ratio of $NaHCO_3$ to H_2CO_3 in blood
   1. Metabolic disturbances affect the $NaHCO_3$ levels in blood
   2. Respiratory disturbances affect the H_2CO_3 levels in blood
E. Types of pH or acid-base imbalances
   1. Metabolic disturbances
      a. Metabolic acidosis—bicarbonate ($NaHCO_3$) deficit
      b. Metabolic alkalosis—bicarbonate ($NaHCO_3$) excess; complication of severe vomiting
   2. Respiratory disturbances
      a. Respiratory acidosis (H_2CO_3 excess)
      b. Respiratory alkalosis (H_2CO_3 deficit)
F. In uncompensated metabolic acidosis, the normal ratio of $NaHCO_3$ to H_2CO_3 is changed; in compensated metabolic acidosis, the ratio remains at 20:1, but the total amount of $NaHCO_3$ and H_2CO_3 changes

NEW WORDS

acid solution	alkaline solution	base	carbonic anhydrase
acidosis (metabolic and respiratory)	alkalosis (metabolic and respiratory)	buffer	emesis
		buffer pairs	pH

REVIEW QUESTIONS

1. Explain the relationship between pH and the relative concentration of hydrogen and hydroxide ions in a solution.
2. Write out the chemical reaction that converts carbon dioxide and water to carbonic acid. What enzyme catalyzes this reaction?
3. What are buffers?
4. Explain how a buffer pair would react if more hydrogen ions were added to the blood.
5. Explain how a buffer pair would react if more hydroxide ions were added to the blood.
6. Explain the four changes that occur in the blood as the result of buffering fixed acids.
7. Explain the respiratory mechanism of pH control.
8. Explain how changes in the respiration rate affect blood pH.
9. Explain how the chemical reaction that occurs in the distal tubule of the kidney using NaH_2PO_4 removes hydrogen ions from the blood.
10. Define *acidosis* and *alkalosis*.
11. Explain metabolic disturbances of the buffer pair.
12. Explain respiratory disturbances of the buffer pair.

CRITICAL THINKING

13. Explain how excessive vomiting causes metabolic alkalosis and explain why normal saline can be used to correct it.
14. What is the proper ratio of $NaHCO_3$ and H_2CO_3 in a buffer pair? Explain how the body can use this ratio to correct uncompensated metabolic acidosis.

CHAPTER TEST

1. The enzyme that converts carbon dioxide and water into carbonic acid is __________.
2. __________ are chemical substances that prevent sharp changes in pH when an acid or base is added to it.
3. If a strong acid such as HCl were added to the buffer pair $NaHCO_3$ and H_2CO_3, the $NaHCO_3$ would become __________.
4. If a strong base such as NaOH were added to the buffer pair in question 3, the H_2CO_3 would become __________.
5. The part of the nephron that is important in regulation of blood pH is the __________.
6. When Na_2HPO_4 is used by the kidney to remove hydrogen ions from the blood, the end product that leaves the body in the urine is __________.
7. When ammonia is used by the kidney to remove hydrogen ions from the blood, the end product that leaves the body in the urine is __________.
8. The kidney is more effective in pH regulation than the lung because it can remove __________, which the lung cannot do.
9. The condition in which the blood pH is higher than normal is called __________.
10. The condition in which the blood pH is lower than normal is called __________.
11. For the buffer pair to function properly, the concentration of $NaHCO_3$ must be __________ times greater than the concentration of H_2CO_3.
12. Metabolic disturbances usually have an effect on the __________ part of the buffer pair.
13. Respiratory disturbances usually have an effect on the __________ part of the buffer pair.
14. Severe vomiting is a metabolic disturbance that can cause metabolic __________.
15. An acid solution has:
    - **a.** a pH greater than 7.0
    - **b.** a pH less than 7.0
    - **c.** more hydroxide ions than hydrogen ions
    - **d.** both a and c
16. An alkaline solution has:
    - **a.** a pH greater than 7.0
    - **b.** a pH less than 7.0
    - **c.** more hydrogen ions than hydroxide ions
    - **d.** both b and c
17. Which of the following statements is true?
    - **a.** A solution with a pH of 5 has more hydrogen ions than a solution with a pH of 2
    - **b.** A solution with a pH of 9 is a base
    - **c.** The pH value increases as the number of hydrogen ions increase
    - **d.** Both a and c are true
18. Arterial blood has a pH of 7.45, and venous blood has a pH of 7.35; therefore:
    - **a.** arterial blood is slightly more acid than venous blood
    - **b.** arterial blood is slightly more alkaline than venous blood
    - **c.** venous blood is slightly more alkaline than arterial blood
    - **d.** both a and c

CHAPTER TEST—*cont'd*

For questions 19 through 24, fill in the blank with either increases or decreases.

19. When a fixed acid is buffered in the blood, the amount of $NaHCO_3$ in the blood _________.

20. When a fixed acid is buffered in the blood, the amount of hydrogen ions in the blood _________.

21. When a fixed acid is buffered in the blood, the amount of H_2CO_3 in the blood _________.

22. When a fixed acid is buffered in the blood, the pH of the blood _________.

23. Anything that causes an excessive increase in the respiration rate _________ the pH of the blood.

24. Anything that causes an appreciable decrease in the respiration rate _________the pH of the blood.

STUDY TIPS

It would help you understand Chapter 19 if you remember a little bit of basic chemistry. The pH scale, acids, and bases are covered at the beginning of the chapter. If you need more of an explanation than that, look in Chapter 2 or any high school chemistry text. All you really need to understand is the relationship between the concentration of hydrogen ions or hydroxide ions and pH. Buffer systems can be seen as hydrogen or hydroxide ion sponges. They remove these ions so they have less of an effect on the pH of a solution, in this case, blood. In the $NaHCO_3$–H_2Co_3 buffer system, the sodium bicarbonate can absorb hydrogen ions by having the hydrogen replace the sodium. The carbonic acid can give up one of its hydrogen atoms, which will react with a hydroxide ion to form water. In both cases the pH of the solution will change very little. Blood carries carbon dioxide as carbonic acid. When the lung exhales carbon dioxide, there is less carbonic acid in the blood, and the pH of the blood rises. The kidneys use a similar buffer system to secrete hydrogen ions. The buffer system in the blood usually works well but it can be overwhelmed. Acidosis is a condition in which the blood becomes too acidic and alkalosis is a condition in which the blood becomes too basic.

If you have difficulty with the chemistry in this chapter, discuss it in your study group. Someone in the group may have a stronger background in chemistry. Discuss the pH system. Carefully go over the diagrams of the blood and kidney buffer systems. Review the types of acidosis and alkalosis and what causes each of them. Go over the test questions at the end of the chapter and discuss possible test questions.

20 The Reproductive Systems

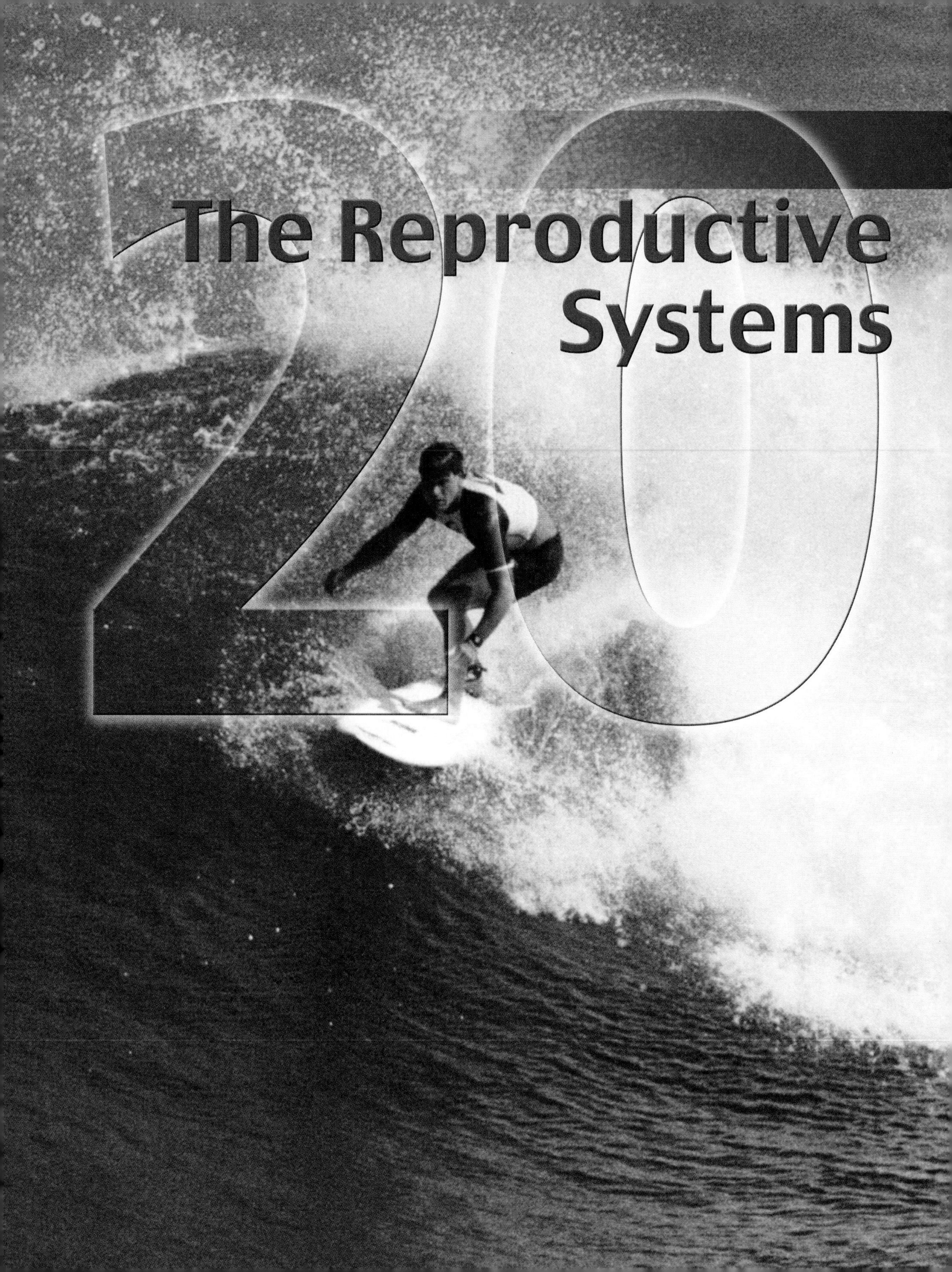

Outline

Objectives

AFTER YOU HAVE COMPLETED THIS CHAPTER, YOU SHOULD BE ABLE TO:

1. List the essential and accessory organs of the male and female reproductive systems and give the general function of each.
2. Describe the gross and microscopic structure of the gonads in both sexes and explain the developmental steps in spermatogenesis and oogenesis.
3. Discuss the primary functions of the sex hormones and identify the cell type or structure responsible for their secretion.
4. Identify and describe the structures that constitute the external genitals in both sexes.
5. Identify and discuss the phases of the endometrial or menstrual cycle and correlate each phase with its occurrence in a typical 28-day cycle.

T*he offspring of* many one-celled plants and bacteria come from a single parent. These organisms are said to be *asexual* because they do not produce specialized reproductive or sex cells called **gametes** (GAM-eets). In humans, gametes, called **ova** and **sperm,** come together during the process of fertilization to produce a cell called the **zygote** (ZYE-gote), which ultimately develops into the new individual. The zygote, which contains an intermingling of genetic messages from the sex cells of both parents, ultimately permits development of new human life. Reproduction in humans therefore is said to be *sexual.* As with all sexually produced offspring, new human life results from the equal contribution of not one but two parent cells—the female ovum and male sperm.

This chapter deals with the structure and function of the reproductive system in men and women. We are truly "fearfully and wonderfully made." Almost any one of the body's organ systems might have inspired this statement, but of them all, perhaps the reproductive systems best deserve such praise. Their ultimate function is to transmit our genes into a new generation, ensuring that our genetic information continues after we are gone. Their awesome achievement is the creation of one of nature's most complex and beautiful structures—the human body. After study of the reproductive system in both sexes, Chapter 21 will go on to cover the topic of human development—a process extending from fertilization until death.

COMMON STRUCTURAL AND FUNCTIONAL CHARACTERISTICS BETWEEN THE SEXES

Although the organs and specific functions of the male and female reproductive systems will be discussed separately, it is important to understand that a common general structure and function can be identified between the systems in both sexes and that both sexes contribute in uniquely important ways to overall reproductive success.

In both men and women, the organs of the reproductive system are adapted for the specific sequence of functions that permit development of sperm or ova followed by successful fertilization and then the normal development and birth of a baby. In addition, production of hormones that permits development of secondary sex characteristics, such as breast development in women and beard growth in men, occurs as a result of normal reproductive system activity.

As you study the specifics of each system, keep in mind that the male organs function to produce, store, and ultimately introduce mature sperm into the female reproductive tract and that the female system is designed to produce ova, receive the sperm, and permit fertilization. In addition, the highly developed and specialized reproductive system in women permits the fertilized ovum to develop and mature until birth. The complex and cyclic control of reproductive functions in both men and women are particularly crucial to overall reproductive success in humans. The production of sex hormones is required not only for development of the secondary sexual characteristics but also for normal reproductive functions in both sexes. This chapter will end with a table comparing reproductive structures and functions in women and men.

Quick Check

1. What are gametes?
2. What is the ultimate function of the reproductive systems?

MALE REPRODUCTIVE SYSTEM

Structural Plan

So many organs make up the male reproductive system that we need to look first at the structural plan of the system as a whole. Reproductive organs can be classified as **essential** or **accessory.**

Essential Organs

The essential organs of reproduction in men and women are called the **gonads.** The gonads of men consist of a pair of main sex glands called the **testes** (TES-teez). The testes produce the male sex cells or **spermatozoa** (sper-ma-toe-ZO-ah).

Accessory Organs

The accessory organs of reproduction in men consist of the following structures:

1. A series of passageways or ducts that carry the sperm from the testes to the exterior
2. Additional sex glands that provide secretions that protect and nurture sperm
3. The external reproductive organs called the external genitals

Table 20-1 lists the names of the essential and accessory organs of reproduction in men, and Figure 20-1 shows the location of most of them. The

TABLE 20-1

Male Reproductive Organs

ESSENTIAL ORGANS	ACCESSORY ORGANS
Gonads: testes (right testis and left testis)	Ducts: epididymis (two), vas deferens (two), ejaculatory duct (two), and urethra
	Supportive sex glands: seminal vesicle (two), bulbourethral or Cowper's gland (two), and prostate gland
	External genitals: scrotum and penis

table and the illustration are included very early in the chapter to provide a preliminary but important overview. Refer back to this table and illustration frequently as you learn about each organ in the pages that follow.

Testes

Structure and Location

The paired **testes** are the gonads of men. They are located in the pouchlike **scrotum** (SKRO-tum), which is suspended outside of the body cavity below the penis (see Figure 20-1). This exposed location provides an environment about 1° C (3°F) cooler than normal body temperature, an important requirement for the normal production and survival of sperm. Each testis is a small, oval gland about 3.8 cm (1.5 inches) long and 2.5 cm (1 inch) wide. The testis is shaped like an egg that has been flattened slightly from side to side. Note in Figure 20-2 that each testis is surrounded by a tough, whitish membrane called the **tunica** (TOO-ni-kah) **albuginea** (al-byoo-JIN-ee-ah). This membrane covers the testicle and then enters the gland to form the many septa that divide it into sections or lobules. As you can see in Figure 20-2, each lobule consists of a narrow but long and coiled **seminiferous** (se-mi-NIF-er-us) **tubule.** These coiled structures form the bulk of the testicular tissue mass. Small, specialized cells lying near the septa that separate the lobules can be seen in Figure 20-3. These are the **interstitial cells** of the testes that secrete the male sex hormone **testosterone** (tes-TOS-te-rone).

Each seminiferous tubule is a long duct with a central lumen or passageway (see Figure 20-3). Sperm develop in the walls of the tubule and are then released into the lumen and begin their journey to the exterior of the body.

FIGURE 20-1

Organization of the male reproductive organs.

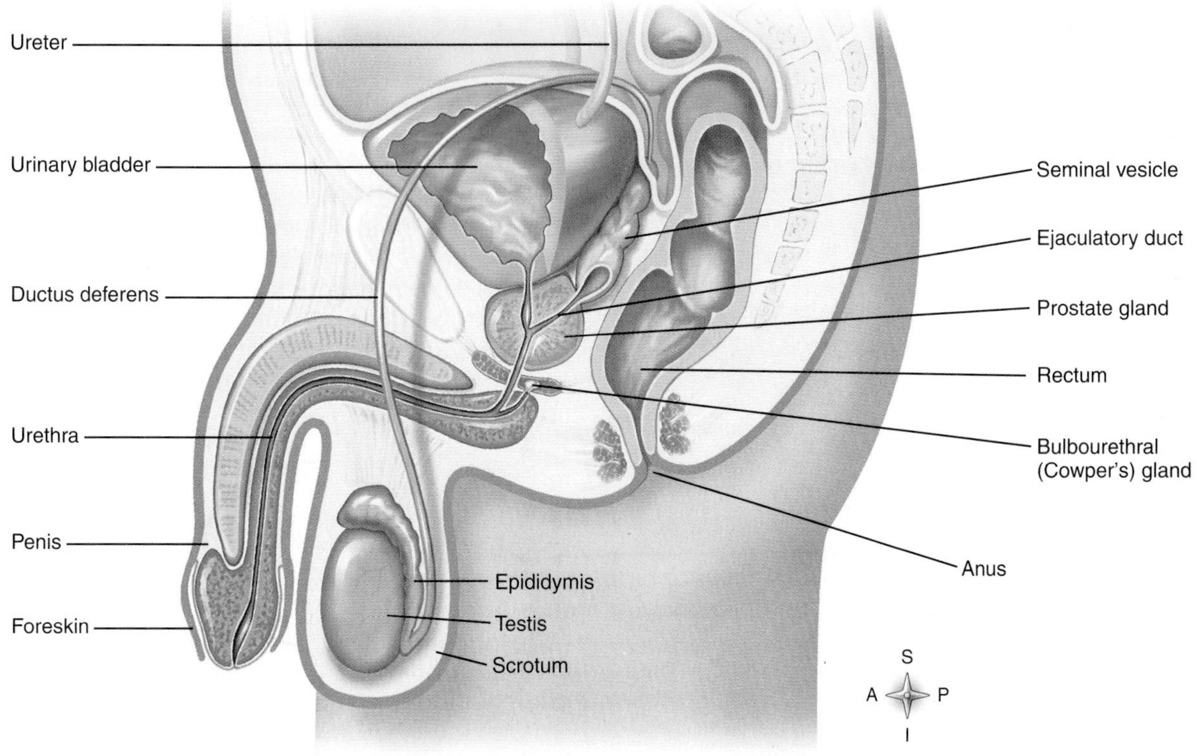

FIGURE 20-2

Tubules of the testis and epididymis. The ducts and tubules are exaggerated in size. In the photograph, the testicle is the darker sphere in the center.

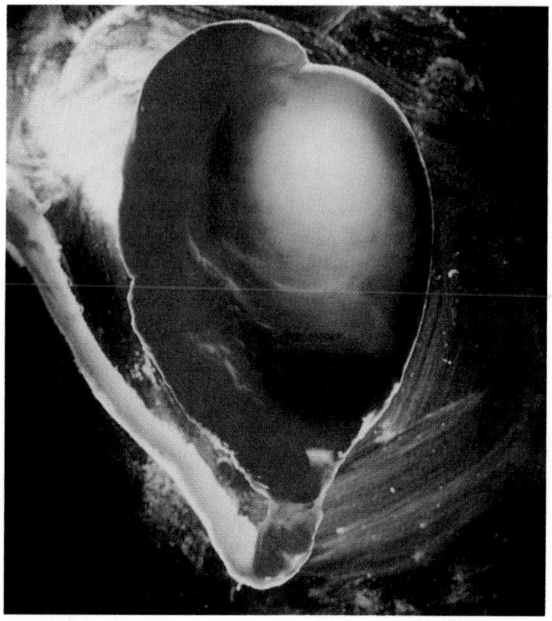

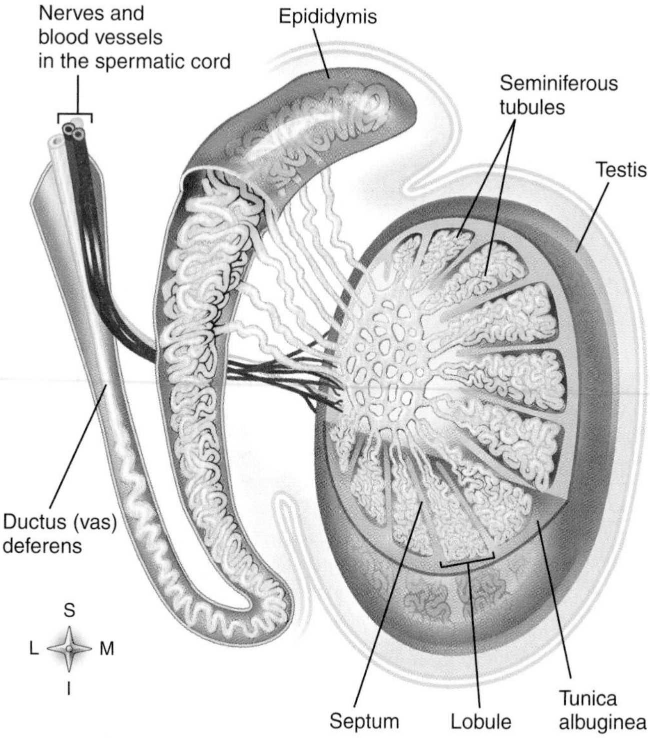

FIGURE 20-3

Testis tissue. Several seminiferous tubules surrounded by septa containing interstitial cells are shown.

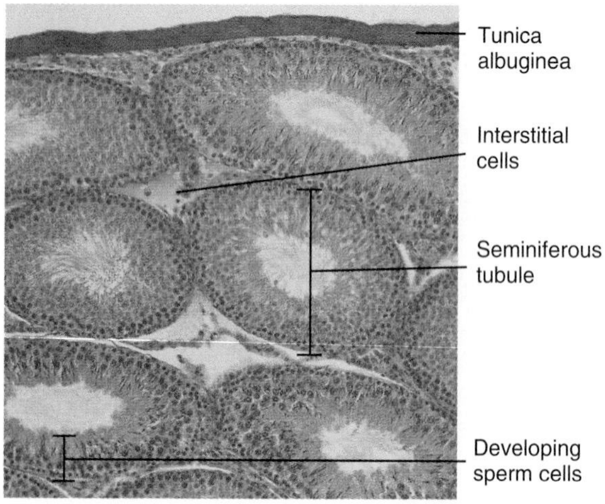

Testis Functions

Spermatogenesis. Sperm production is called **spermatogenesis** (sper-ma-toe-JEN-e-sis). From puberty on, the seminiferous tubules continuously form spermatozoa or sperm. Although the number of sperm produced each day diminish with increasing age, most men continue to produce significant numbers throughout life.

The testes prepare for sperm production before puberty by increasing the numbers of sperm precursor (stem) cells called **spermatogonia** (sper-ma-toe-GO-nee-ah). These cells are located near the outer edge of each seminiferous tubule (Figure 20-4, *A*). Before puberty, spermatogonia increase in number by the process of mitotic cell division, which was described in Chapter 3. Recall that mitosis results in the division of a "parent" cell into two "daughter" cells, each identical to the parent and each containing a complete

FIGURE 20-4

Spermatogenesis. A, Cross section of tubule shows progressive meiotic cell types in the wall of a seminiferous tubule. **B,** Diagram of meiotic events and cell types leading to sperm formation.

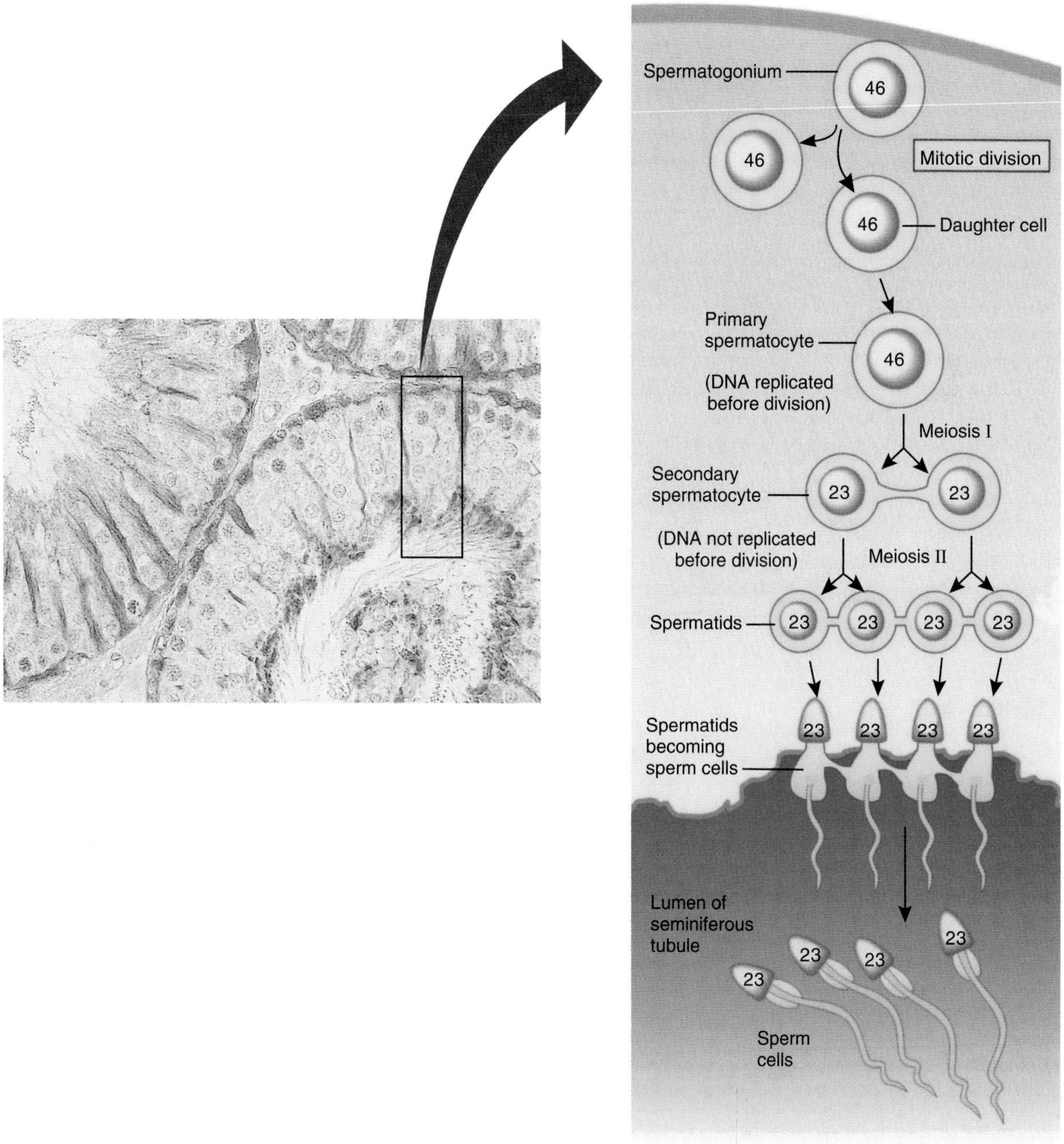

copy of the genetic material represented in the normal number of 46 chromosomes.

When a boy enters puberty, circulating levels of follicle-stimulating hormone (FSH) cause a spermatogonium to undergo a unique type of cell division. When the spermatogonium undergoes cell division and mitosis under the influence of FSH, it produces two daughter cells. One of these cells remains as a spermatogonium and the other forms another, more specialized cell called a **primary spermatocyte** (SPER-ma-toe-site). These primary spermatocytes then undergo a specialized type of division called meiosis (my-O-sis), which ultimately results in sperm formation. Note in Figure 20-4, *B*, that during meiosis two cell divisions occur (not one as in mitosis) and that four daughter cells (not two as in mitosis) are formed. The daughter cells are called **spermatids** (SPER-ma-tids). Unlike the two daughter cells that result from mitosis, the four spermatids, which will develop into spermatozoa, have only half the genetic material and half of the chromosomes (23 instead of 46) of other body cells.

In women, meiosis results in a single ovum, which also has 23 chromosomes. This will be discussed in more detail later in the chapter.

Look again at the diagram of meiosis in Figure 20-4, *B*. It shows that each primary spermatocyte ultimately produces four sperm cells. Note that, in the portion of a seminiferous tubule shown in Figure 20-4, *B*, spermatogonia are found at the outer surface of the tubule; primary and secondary spermatocytes lie deeper in the tubule wall, and mature but immotile sperm are seen about to enter the lumen of the tube and begin their journey through the reproductive ducts to the exterior of the body.

Spermatozoa. Spermatozoa are among the smallest and most highly specialized cells in the body (Figure 20-5, *A*). All of the characteristics that a baby will inherit from its father at fertilization are contained in the condensed nuclear (genetic) material found in each sperm head. However, this genetic information from the father can fuse with genetic material contained in the mother's ovum only if successful fertilization occurs. Ejaculation of sperm into the female vagina during sexual intercourse is only one step in the long journey that these sex cells must make before they can meet and fertilize an ovum. To accomplish their task, these specialized packages of genetic information are equipped with tails for motility and are designed to penetrate the outer membrane of the ovum when contact occurs with it.

The structure of a mature sperm is diagrammed in Figure 20-5, *B*. Note the sperm head containing the nucleus with its genetic material from the father. The nucleus is covered by the **acrosome** (AK-ro-sohm)—a specialized structure containing enzymes that enable the sperm to break down the covering of the ovum and permit entry if contact occurs. In addition to the head with its covering acrosome, each sperm has a midpiece and an elongated tail. Mitochondria in the midpiece break down adenosine triphosphate (ATP) to provide energy for the tail movements required to propel the sperm and allow them to "swim" for relatively long distances through the female reproductive ducts.

Production of testosterone. In addition to spermatogenesis, the other function of the testes is to secrete the male hormone, testosterone. This function is carried on by the interstitial cells of the testes, not by their seminiferous tubules. Testosterone serves the following general functions:

1. It masculinizes. The various characteristics that we think of as "male" develop because of testosterone's influence. For instance, when a young boy's voice changes, it is testosterone that brings this about.
2. It promotes and maintains the development of the male accessory organs (prostate gland, seminal vesicles, and so on).
3. It has a stimulating effect on protein anabolism. Testosterone thus is responsible for the greater muscular development and strength of the male.

A good way to remember testosterone's functions is to think of it as "the masculinizing hormone" and the "anabolic hormone."

Quick Check

1. What is the name of the male gonads?
2. In what specific structures of the gonad are the sperm produced?
3. What hormone is produced in the male gonad?

FIGURE 20-5

Human sperm. A, Micrograph shows the heads and long, slender tails of several spermatozoa. **B,** Illustration shows the components of a mature sperm cell and an enlargement of a sperm head and midpiece.

A

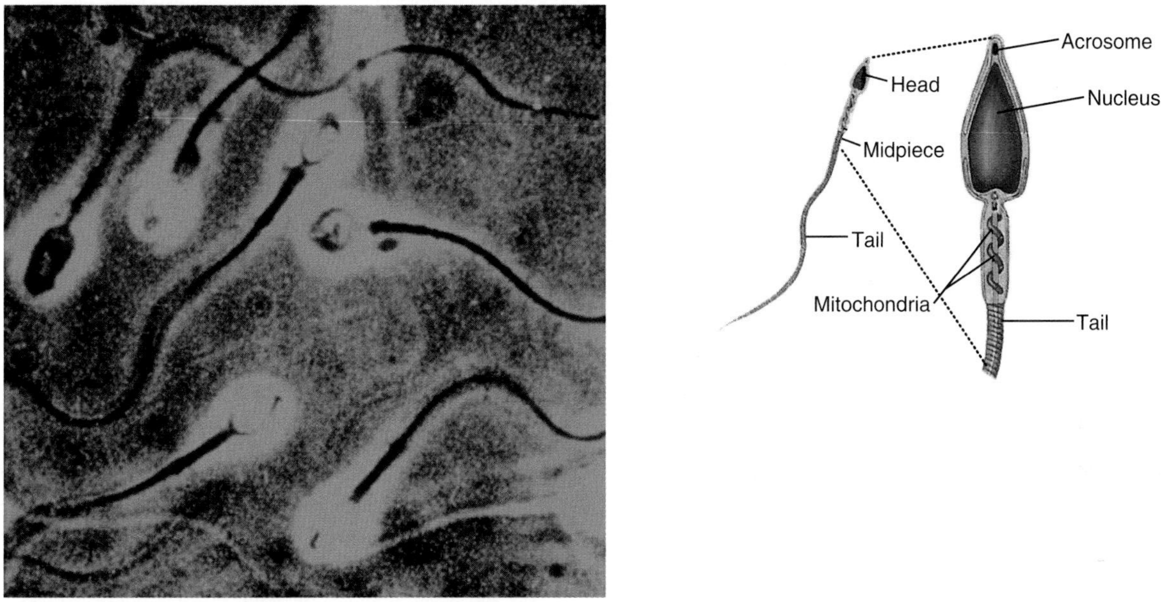

B

Reproductive Ducts

The ducts through which sperm must pass after exiting from the testes until they reach the exterior of the body are important components of the accessory reproductive structures. The other two components included in the listing of accessory organs of reproduction in the male—the supportive sex glands and external genitals—will be discussed separately.

Sperm are formed within the walls of the seminiferous tubules of the testes. When they exit from these tubules within the testis, they enter and then pass, in sequence, through the epididymis, ductus (vas) deferens, ejaculatory duct, and the urethra on their journey out of the body.

Epididymis

Each **epididymis** (ep-i-DID-i-mis) consists of a single and very tightly coiled tube about 6 m (20 feet) in length. It is a comma-shaped structure (see Figure 20-2) that lies along the top and behind the testes inside the scrotum. Sperm mature and develop their ability to move or swim as they are temporarily stored in the epididymis.

Clinical Application

Cryptorchidism

Early in fetal life the testes are located in the abdominal cavity but normally descend into the scrotum about 2 months before birth. Occasionally a baby is born with undescended testes, a condition called **cryptorchidism** (krip-TOR-ki-dizm), which is readily observed by palpation of the scrotum at delivery. The word cryptorchidism is from the Greek words *kryptikos* (hidden) and *orchis* (testis). Failure of the testes to descend may be caused by hormonal imbalances in the developing fetus or by a physical deficiency or obstruction. Regardless of cause, in the cryptorchid infant the testes remain "hidden" in the abdominal cavity. Because the higher temperature inside the body cavity inhibits spermatogenesis, measures must be taken to bring the testes down into the scrotum to prevent permanent sterility. Early treatment of this condition by surgery or by injection of testosterone, which stimulates the testes to descend, may result in normal testicular and sexual development.

Ductus (Vas) Deferens

The **ductus** (DUK-tus) **deferens** (DEF-er-enz) or vas deferens is the tube that permits sperm to exit from the epididymis and pass from the scrotal sac upward into the abdominal cavity. Each ductus deferens is a thick, smooth, very muscular, and movable tube that can easily be felt or "palpated" through the thin skin of the scrotal wall. It passes through the inguinal canal into the abdominal cavity as part of the *spermatic cord,* a connective tissue sheath that also encloses blood vessels and nerves.

Ejaculatory Duct and Urethra

Once in the abdominal cavity, the ductus deferens extends over the top and down the posterior surface of the bladder, where it joins the duct from the seminal vesicle to form the **ejaculatory** (ee-JAK-yoo-lah-toe-ree) **duct.** Note in Figure 20-1 that the ejaculatory duct passes through the substance of the prostate gland and permits sperm to empty into the **urethra,** which eventually passes through the penis and opens to the exterior at the external urethral orifice.

Accessory or Supportive Sex Glands

The term **semen** (SEE-men) or **seminal fluid** is used to describe the mixture of sex cells or sperm produced by the testes and the secretions of the accessory or supportive sex glands. The accessory glands, which contribute more than 95% of the secretions to the gelatinous fluid part of the semen, include the two seminal vesicles, one prostate gland, and two bulbourethral (Cowper's) glands. In addition to the production of sperm, the seminiferous tubules of the testes contribute somewhat less than 5% of the seminal fluid volume. Usually 3 to 5 ml (about 1 teaspoon) of semen is ejaculated at one time, and each milliliter normally contains about 100 million sperm. Semen is alkaline and protects sperm from the acidic environment of the female reproductive tract.

Seminal Vesicles

The paired **seminal vesicles** are pouchlike glands that contribute about 60% of the seminal fluid volume. Their secretions are yellowish, thick, and rich in the sugar fructose. This fraction of the seminal fluid helps provide a source of energy for the highly motile sperm.

Prostate Gland

The **prostate gland** lies just below the bladder and is shaped like a doughnut. The urethra passes through the center of the prostate before traversing the penis to end at the external urinary orifice. The prostate secretes a thin, milk-colored fluid that constitutes about 30% of the total seminal fluid volume. This fraction of the ejaculate helps to activate the sperm and maintain their motility.

Bulbourethral Glands

Each of the two **bulbourethral** (BUL-bo-yoo-REE-thral) **glands** (also called *Cowper's glands*) resemble peas in size and shape. They are located just below the prostate gland and empty their secretions into the penile portion of the urethra. Because the bulbourethral secretion is often released just before most of the rest of the semen is ejaculated, it is

Clinical Application

Prostatic Hypertrophy

A noncancerous condition called **benign** (bee-nine) **prostatic hypertrophy** (hye-PER-tro-fee) is a common problem in older men. The condition is characterized by an enlargement or hypertrophy of the prostate gland. That the urethra passes through the center of the prostate after exiting from the bladder is a matter of considerable clinical significance in this condition. As the prostate enlarges, it squeezes the urethra, frequently closing it so completely that urination becomes very difficult or even impossible. In such cases, surgical removal of part or all of the gland, a procedure called **prostatectomy** (pros-ta-TEC-toe-me), is sometimes performed. Other options, especially for treatment of cancerous prostatic growths, include systemic chemotherapy, cryotherapy (freezing) of prostatic tissue, microwave therapy, hormonal therapy, the placing of radioactive "seeds" directly into the gland, and various types of external-beam x-ray radiation treatments.

FIGURE 20-6

The penis. A, In this sagittal section of the penis viewed from above, the urethra is exposed throughout its length and can be seen exiting from the bladder and passing through the prostate gland before entering the penis to end at the external urethral orifice. **B,** Photograph of a cross section of the shaft of the penis showing the three columns of erectile or cavernous tissue. Note the urethra within the substance of the corpus spongiosum.

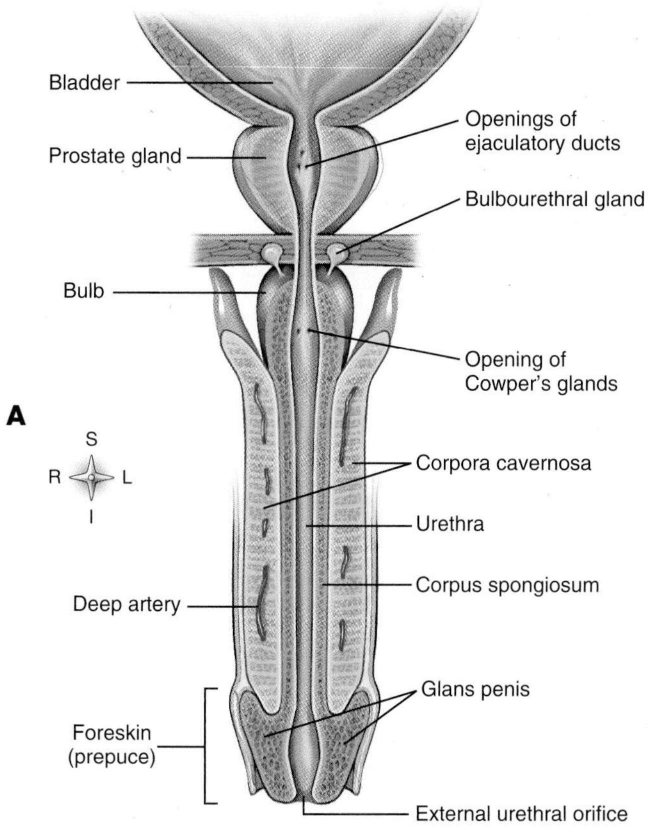

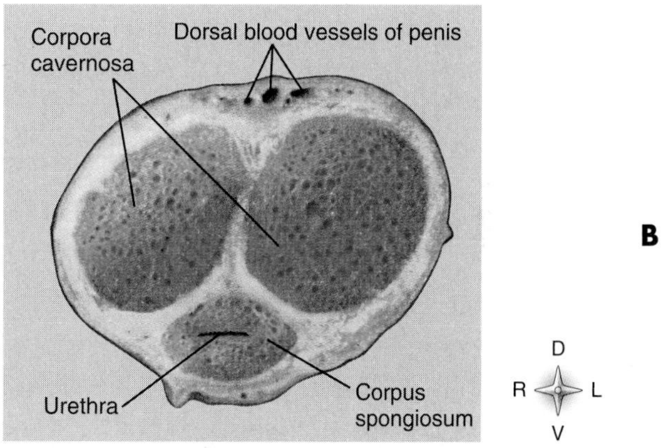

sometimes called the "pre-ejaculate." The mucus-like secretions of these glands lubricate the terminal portion of the urethra and contribute less than 5% of the seminal fluid volume.

External Genitals

The **penis** (PEE-nis) and **scrotum** constitute the external reproductive organs or **genitalia** (jen-i-TAL-ee-ah) of men. The penis (Figure 20-6) is the organ that, when made stiff and erect by the filling of its spongy or erectile tissue components with blood during sexual arousal, can enter and deposit sperm in the vagina during intercourse. The penis has three separate columns of erectile tissue in its shaft: one **corpus** (KOR-pus) **spongiosum** (spun-jee-O-sum), which surrounds the urethra, and two **corpora** (KOR-por-ah) **cavernosa** (kav-er-NO-sa), which lie above. The spongy nature of erectile tissue is apparent in Figure 20-6. At the distal end of the shaft of the penis is the enlarged **glans,** which is covered with highly sensitive skin. Over the sensitive skin of the glans is a doubly folded extension of the skin on the penis's shaft that forms a loose-fitting retractable collar called the **fore-**

skin or **prepuce** (PRE-pus). If the foreskin fits too tightly about the glans, a **circumcision** or surgical removal of the foreskin is usually performed to prevent irritation. The external urethral orifice is the opening of the urethra at the tip of the glans.

The scrotum is a skin-covered pouch suspended from the groin. Internally, it is divided into two sacs by a septum; each sac contains a testis, epididymis, the lower part of the ductus deferens, and the beginning of the spermatic cords.

Quick

1. What duct leads from the epididymis?
2. Which organs produce the fluid in semen?
3. What job do erectile tissues do?

TABLE 20-2

Female Reproductive Organs

ESSENTIAL ORGANS	ACCESSORY ORGANS
Gonads: ovaries (right ovary and left ovary)	Ducts: uterine tubes (two), uterus, vagina
	Accessory sex glands: Bartholin's glands (two), breasts (two)
	External genitals: vulva

FEMALE REPRODUCTIVE SYSTEM

Structural Plan

The structural plan of the reproductive system in both sexes is similar in that organs are characterized as **essential** or **accessory.**

Essential Organs

The essential organs of reproduction in women, the **gonads,** are the paired **ovaries.** The female sex cells or **ova** are produced here.

Accessory Organs

The accessory organs of reproduction in women consist of the following structures:

1. A series of ducts or modified duct structures that extend from near the ovaries to the exterior
2. Additional sex glands, including the mammary glands, which have an important reproductive function only in women
3. The external reproductive organs or external genitals

Table 20-2 lists the names of the essential and accessory organs of reproduction, and Figure 20-7 shows the location of most of them. Refer back to this table and illustration as you read about each structure in the pages that follow.

Ovaries

Structure and Location

The paired ovaries are the gonads of women. They have a puckered, uneven surface; each weighs about 3 g. The ovaries resemble large almonds in size and shape and are attached to ligaments in the pelvic cavity on each side of the uterus.

Embedded in a connective tissue matrix just below the outer layer of each ovary in a newborn baby girl are about 1 million **ovarian follicles;** each contains an **oocyte,** an immature stage of the female sex cell. By the time a girl reaches puberty, however, further development has resulted in the formation of a reduced number (about 400,000) of what are now called **primary follicles.** Each primary follicle has a layer of **granulosa cells** around the oocyte. During the reproductive lifetime of most women, only about 350 to 500 of these primary follicles fully develop into **mature follicles,** which ovulate and release an ovum for potential fertilization. Follicles that do not mature degenerate and are reabsorbed into the ovarian tissue. A mature ovum in its sac is sometimes called a **Graafian** (GRAHF-ee-an) **follicle,** in honor of the Dutch anatomist who discovered the follicle some 300 years ago.

The progression of development from primary follicle to ovulation is shown in Figure 20-8. As the thickness of the granulosa cell layer around the

FIGURE 20-7

Organization of the female reproductive organs.

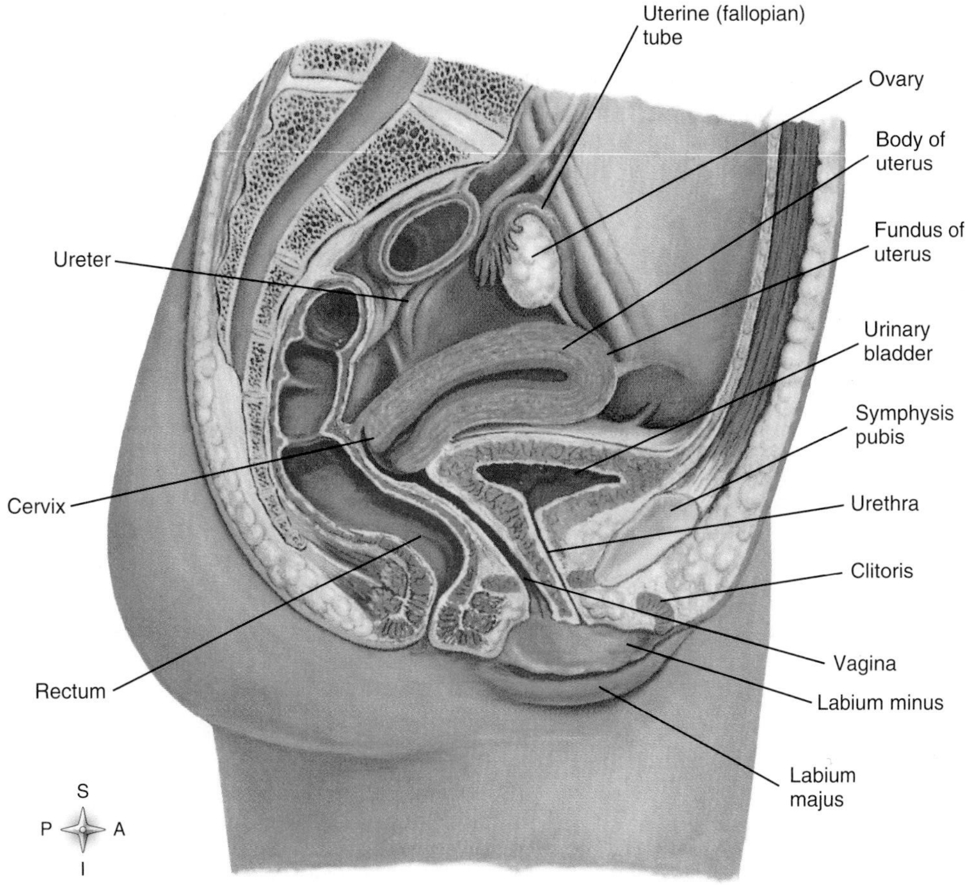

oocyte increases, a hollow chamber called an *antrum* (AN-trum) appears, and a **secondary follicle** is formed. Development continues, and, after ovulation, the ruptured follicle is transformed into a hormone-secreting glandular structure called the **corpus** (KOR-pus) **luteum** (LOO-tee-um), which is described later. Corpus luteum is from the Latin word meaning "yellow body," an appropriate name to describe the yellow appearance of this glandular structure.

Ovary Functions

Oogenesis. The production of female gametes or sex cells is called **oogenesis** (o-o-JEN-e-sis). The specialized type of cell division that results in sperm formation, meiosis, is also responsible for development of ova. During the developmental phases experienced by the female sex cell from its earliest stage to just after fertilization, two meiotic divisions occur. As a result of meiosis in the female sex cell, the number of chromosomes is reduced equally in each daughter cell to half the number (23) found in other body cells (46). However, the amount of cytoplasm is divided unequally. The result is formation of one large ovum and small daughter cells called *polar bodies* that degenerate.

The ovum, with its large supply of cytoplasm, is one of the body's largest cells and is uniquely designed to provide nutrients for rapid development of the embryo until implantation in the uterus oc-

FIGURE 20-8

Diagram of ovary and oogenesis. Cross section of mammalian ovary shows successive stages of ovarian (Graafian) follicle and ovum development. Begin with the first stage (primary follicle) and follow around clockwise to the final state (degenerating corpus luteum).

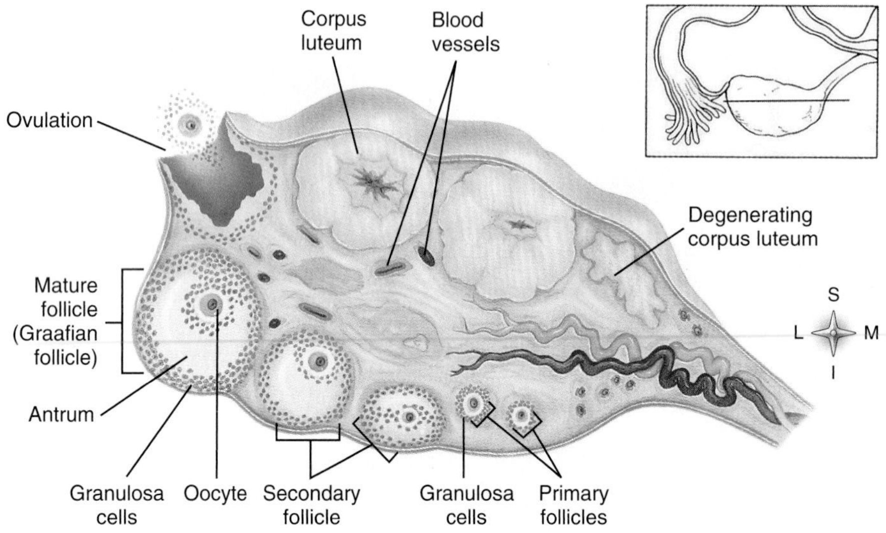

curs. At fertilization, the sex cells from both parents fuse, and the normal chromosome number (46) is achieved.

Production of estrogen and progesterone. The second major function of the ovary, in addition to oogenesis, is secretion of the sex hormones, **estrogen** and **progesterone.** Hormone production in the ovary begins at puberty with the cyclic development and maturation of the ovum. The granulosa cells around the oocyte in the growing and mature follicle secrete estrogen. The corpus luteum, which develops after ovulation, chiefly secretes progesterone but also some estrogen.

Estrogen is the sex hormone that causes the development and maintenance of the female *secondary sex characteristics* and stimulates growth of the epithelial cells lining the uterus. Some of the actions of estrogen include the following:

1. Development and maturation of female reproductive organs, including the external genitals
2. Appearance of pubic hair and breast development
3. Development of female body contours by deposition of fat below the skin surface and in the breasts and hip region
4. Initiation of the first menstrual cycle

Progesterone is produced by the corpus luteum, which is a glandular structure that develops from a follicle that has just released an ovum. If stimulated by the appropriate anterior pituitary hormone, the corpus luteum produces progesterone for about 11 days after ovulation. Progesterone stimulates proliferation and vascularization of the epithelial lining of the uterus and acts with estrogen to initiate the menstrual cycle in girls entering puberty.

Quick Check

1. What is the name of the female gonads?
2. Where are the female glands located?
3. What is oogenesis?
4. What hormones are produced by the female gonads?

FIGURE 20-9

The uterus. Sectioned view shows muscle layers of the uterus and its relationship to the ovaries and vagina.

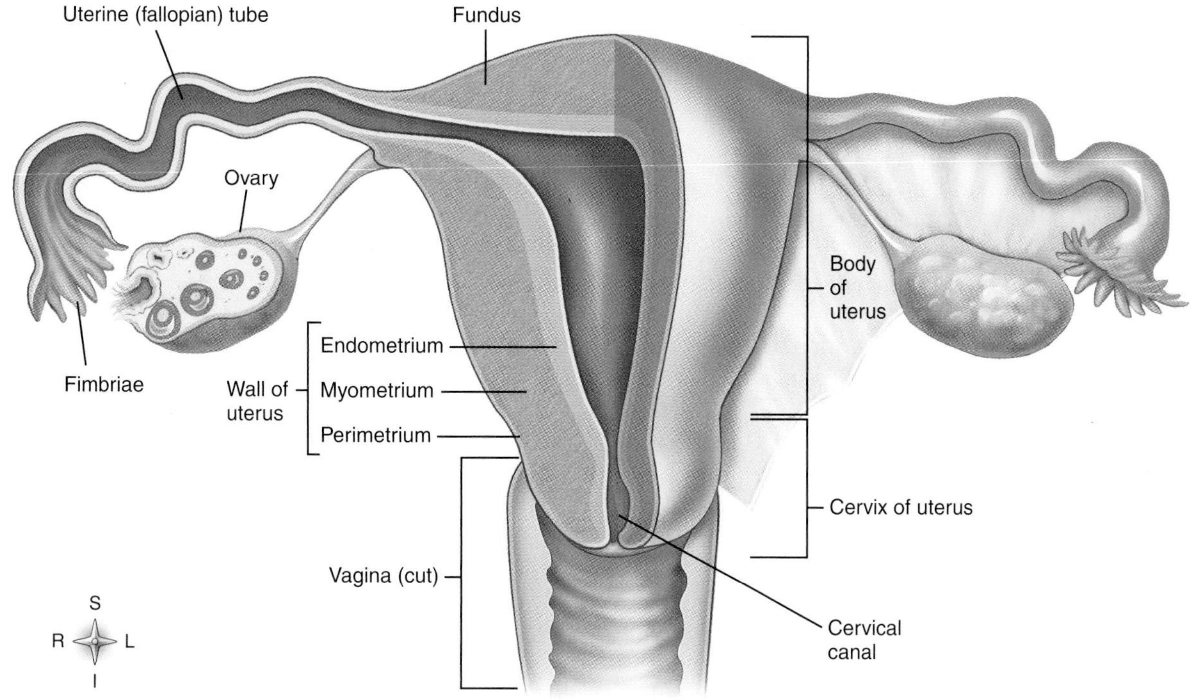

Reproductive Ducts

Uterine Tubes

The two **uterine tubes,** also called **fallopian** (fal-LO-pee-an) **tubes** or **oviducts** (O-vi-dukts), serve as ducts for the ovaries, even though they are not attached to them. The outer end of each tube terminates in an expanded, funnel-shaped structure that has fringelike projections called **fimbriae** (FIM-bree-ee) along its edge. This part of the tube curves over the top of each ovary (Figure 20-9) and opens into the abdominal cavity. The inner end of each uterine tube attaches to the uterus, and the cavity inside the tube opens into the cavity in the uterus. Each tube is about 10 cm (4 inches) in length.

After ovulation the discharged ovum first enters the abdominal cavity and then enters the uterine tube assisted by the wavelike movement of the fimbriae and the beating of the cilia on their surface. After it is in the tube, the ovum begins its journey to the uterus. Some ova never find their way into the oviduct and remain in the abdominal cavity where they are reabsorbed. In Chapter 21 the details of fertilization, which normally occurs in the outer one third of the uterine tube, will be discussed.

The mucosal lining of the uterine tubes is directly continuous with the lining of the abdominal cavity on one end and with the lining of the uterus and vagina on the other. This is of great clinical significance because infections of the vagina or uterus such as gonorrhea may pass into the abdominal cavity, where they may become life threatening.

Uterus

The **uterus** (YOO-ter-us) is a small organ—only about the size of a pear—but it is extremely strong. It is almost all muscle or **myometrium** (my-o-ME-tree-um), with only a small cavity inside. During pregnancy the uterus grows many times larger so that it becomes big enough to hold a baby and a considerable amount of fluid. The uterus is composed of two parts: an upper portion, the **body,** and a lower narrow section, the **cervix.** Just above the level where the uterine tubes attach to the body of the uterus, it rounds out to form a bulging prominence called the **fundus** (see Figure 20-9). Except during pregnancy, the uterus lies in the pelvic cavity just behind the urinary bladder. By the end of pregnancy, it becomes large enough to extend up to the top of the abdominal cavity. It then pushes the liver against the underside of the diaphragm—a fact that explains such a comment as "I can't seem to take a deep breath since I've gotten so big," made by many women late in their pregnancies.

The uterus functions in three processes—menstruation, pregnancy, and labor. The corpus luteum stops secreting progesterone and decreases its secretion of estrogens about 11 days after ovulation. About 3 days later, when the progesterone and estrogen concentrations in the blood are at their lowest, menstruation starts. Small pieces of the mucous membrane lining of the uterus, or the **endometrium** (en-doe-ME-tree-um) pull loose, leaving torn blood vessels underneath. Blood and bits of endometrium trickle out of the uterus into the vagina and out of the body. Immediately after menstruation the endometrium starts to repair itself. It again grows thick and becomes lavishly supplied with blood in preparation for pregnancy. If fertilization does not take place, the uterus again sheds the lining made ready for a pregnancy that did not occur. Because these changes in the uterine lining continue to repeat themselves, they are spoken of as the **menstrual cycle** (see p. 502).

If fertilization occurs, pregnancy begins, and the endometrium remains intact. The events of pregnancy are discussed in Chapter 21.

Menstruation first occurs at puberty, often around the age of 12 years. Normally it repeats itself about every 28 days or 13 times a year for some 30 to 40 years before it ceases at **menopause** (MEN-o-pawz), when a woman is somewhere around the age of 50 years.

Vagina

The **vagina** (vah-JYE-nah) is a distensible tube about 10 cm (4 inches) long made mainly of smooth muscle and lined with mucous membrane. It lies in the pelvic cavity between the urinary bladder and the rectum (see Figure 20-7). As the part of the female reproductive tract that opens to the exterior, the vagina is the organ that sperm enter during their journey to meet an ovum, and it is also the organ from which a baby emerges to meet its new world.

Clinical Application

Ectopic Pregnancy

The term **ectopic** (ek-TOP-ic) **pregnancy** is used to describe a pregnancy resulting from the implantation of a fertilized ovum in any location other than the uterus. Occasionally, because the outer ends of the uterine tubes open into the pelvic cavity and are not actually connected to the ovaries, an ovum does not enter an oviduct but becomes fertilized and remains in the abdominal cavity. Although rare, if implantation occurs on the surface of an abdominal organ or on one of the mesenteries, development may continue to term. In such cases delivery by caesarean section is required. Most ectopic pregnancies involve implantation in the uterine tube and are therefore called *tubal pregnancies*. They result in fetal death and, if not treated, tubal rupture.

Accessory or Supportive Sex Glands

Bartholin's Glands

One of the small **Bartholin's** (BAR-toe-linz) or **greater vestibular** (ves-TIB-yoo-lar) **glands** lies to the right of the vaginal outlet, and one lies to the left of it. Secretion of a mucuslike lubricating fluid is their function. Their ducts open into the space between the labia minora and the vaginal orifice called the **vestibule** (see Figure 20-11).

Breasts

The **breasts** lie over the pectoral muscles and are attached to them by connective tissue ligaments (of Cooper). Breast size is determined more by the amount of fat around the glandular (milk-secreting) tissue than by the amount of glandular tissue itself. Hence the size of the breast has little to do with its ability to secrete adequate amounts of milk after the birth of a baby.

Each breast consists of 15 to 20 divisions or lobes that are arranged radially (Figure 20-10). Each lobe consists of several lobules, and each lobule consists of milk-secreting glandular cells. The milk-secreting cells are arranged in grapelike clusters called *alveoli*. Small **lactiferous** (lak-TIF-er-us) **ducts** drain the alveoli and converge toward the nipple like the spokes of a wheel. Only one lactiferous duct leads from each lobe to an opening in the nipple. The colored area around the nipple is the **areola** (ah-REE-o-lah).

Knowledge of the lymphatic drainage of the breast is important because cancerous cells from breast tumors often spread to other areas of the body through the lymphatic system. This lymphatic drainage is discussed in Chapter 13 (see also Figure 13-5).

Quick Check

1. What is another name for the uterine tubes?
2. What three major functions does the uterus perform?
3. What substance is conducted through lactiferous ducts?

FIGURE 20-10

Lateral view of the breast. Sagittal section of a lactating breast. Notice how the glandular structures are anchored to the overlying skin and to the pectoral muscles by the suspensory ligaments of Cooper. Each lobule of glandular tissue is drained by a lactiferous duct that eventually opens through the nipple.

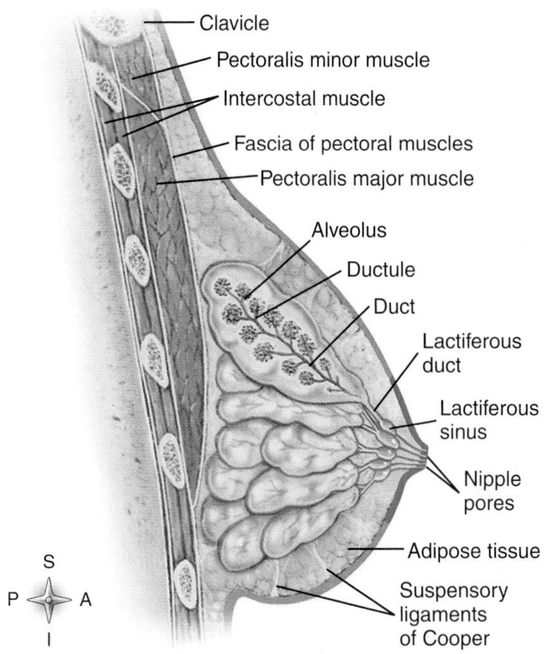

External Genitals

The **external genitalia** or **vulva** (VUL-vah) of women consist of the following:

1. Mons pubis
2. Clitoris
3. Orifice of urethra
4. Labia minora (singular, *labium minus*) (small lips)
5. Hymen
6. Orifice, duct of Bartholin's gland
7. Orifice of vagina
8. Labia majora (singular, *labium majus*) (large lips)

The **mons pubis** is a skin-covered pad of fat over the symphysis pubis. Hair appears on this structure at puberty and persists throughout life. Extending downward from the elevated mons pubis are the **labia** (LAY-bee-ah) **majora** (ma-JO-rah) or "large lips." These elongated folds, which are composed mainly of fat and numerous glands, are covered with pigmented skin and hair on the outer surface and are smooth and free from hair on the inner surface. The **labia minora** or "small lips" are located within the labia majora and are covered with modified skin. These two lips join anteriorly at the midline. The area between the labia minora is the vestibule (Figure 20-11). Several genital structures are located in the vestibule. The **clitoris** (KLIT-o-ris), which is composed of erectile tissue, is located just behind the anterior junction of the labia minora. Situated between the clitoris above and the vaginal opening below is the orifice of the urethra. The vaginal orifice is sometimes partially closed by a membranous **hymen**

FIGURE 20-11

External genitals of the female.

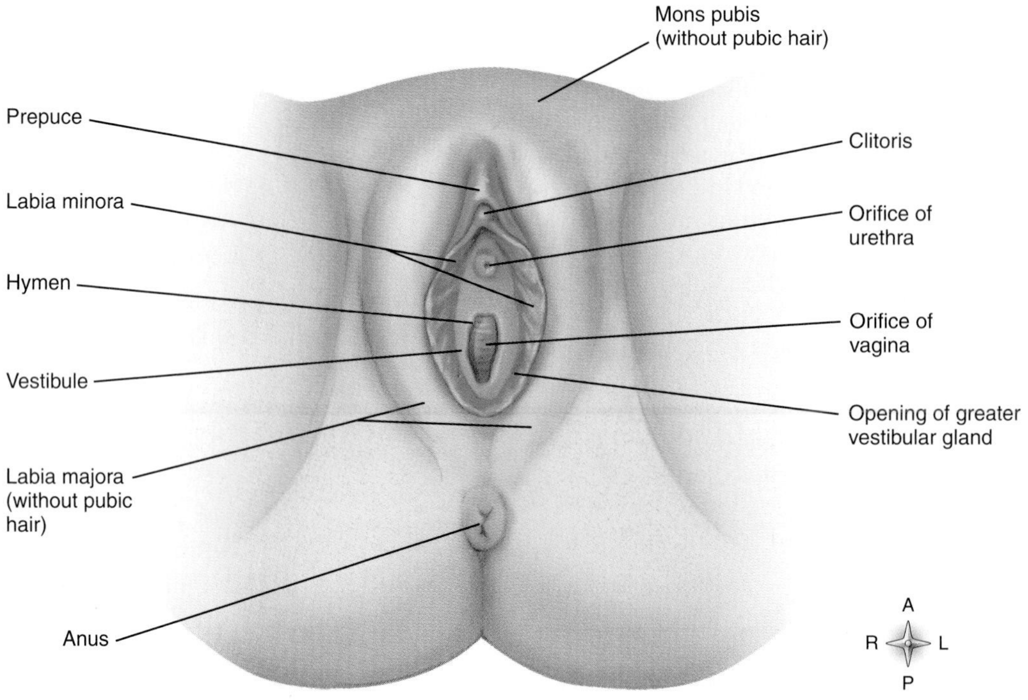

(HYE-men). The ducts of Bartholin's glands open on either side of the vaginal orifice inside the labia minora.

The term **perineum** (pair-i-NEE-um) is used to describe the area between the vaginal opening and anus. This area is sometimes cut in a surgical procedure called an **episiotomy** (e-piz-ee-OT-o-me) to prevent tearing of tissue during childbirth.

Menstrual Cycle

Phases and Events

The menstrual cycle consists of many changes in the uterus, ovaries, vagina, and breasts and in the anterior pituitary gland's secretion of hormones (Figure 20-12). In the majority of women, these changes occur with almost precise regularity throughout their reproductive years. The first indication of changes comes with the first menstrual period. The first **menses** (MEN-seez) or menstrual flow is referred to as the **menarche** (me-NAR-kee).

A typical menstrual cycle covers a period of about 28 days. The length of the cycle varies among women. Some women, for example, may have a regular cycle that covers about 24 days. The length of the cycle also varies within one woman. Some women, for example, may have irregular cycles that range from 21 to 28 days, whereas others may be 2 to 3 months long. Each cycle consists of three phases. The three periods of time in each cycle are called the **menses,** the **proliferative phase,** and the **secretory phase.** Refer often to Figure 20-13 as you read about the events occurring during each phase of the cycle in the pituitary gland, the ovary, and in the uterus. Be sure that you do not overlook the event that occurs around day 14 of a 28-day cycle.

FIGURE 20-12

The 28-day menstrual cycle.

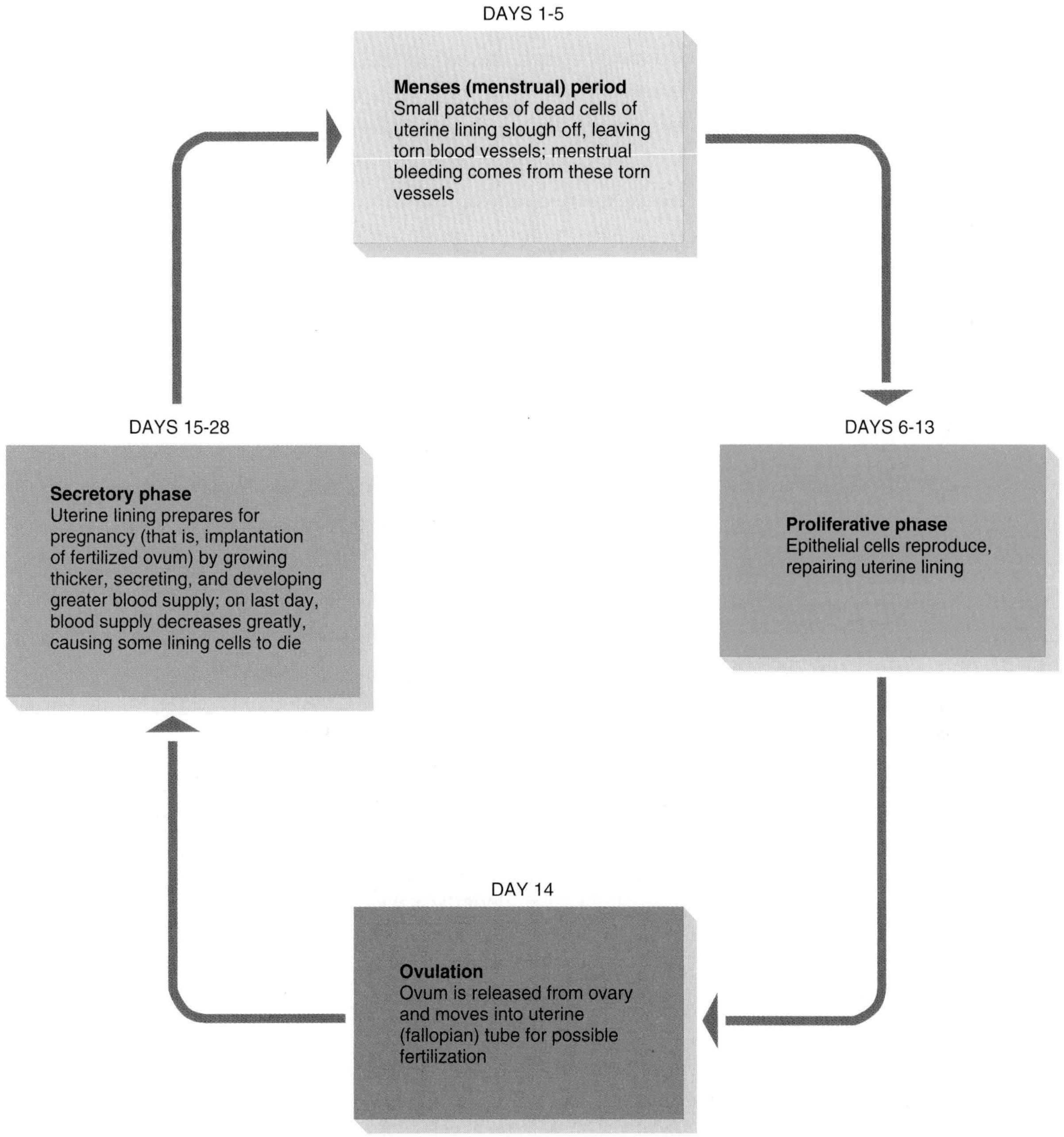

DAYS 1-5
Menses (menstrual) period
Small patches of dead cells of uterine lining slough off, leaving torn blood vessels; menstrual bleeding comes from these torn vessels
DAYS 6-13
Proliferative phase
Epithelial cells reproduce, repairing uterine lining
DAY 14
Ovulation
Ovum is released from ovary and moves into uterine (fallopian) tube for possible fertilization
DAYS 15-28
Secretory phase
Uterine lining prepares for pregnancy (that is, implantation of fertilized ovum) by growing thicker, secreting, and developing greater blood supply; on last day, blood supply decreases greatly, causing some lining cells to die

FIGURE 20-13

The human menstrual cycle. Diagram illustrates the interrelationship of pituitary, ovarian, and uterine functions throughout a usual 28-day cycle. A sharp increase in luteinizing hormone (LH) levels causes ovulation, whereas menstruation (sloughing off of the endometrial lining) is initiated by lower levels of progesterone.

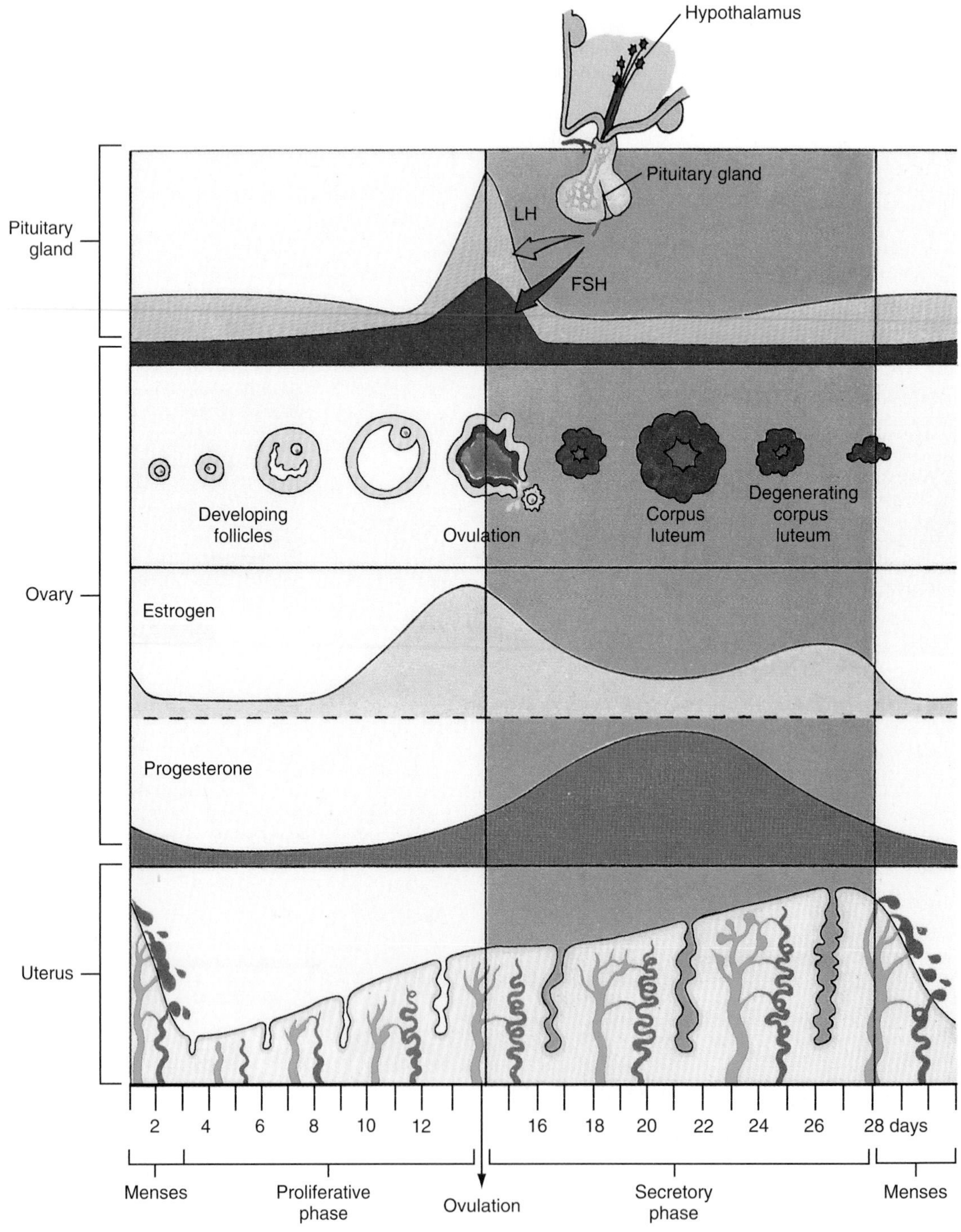

The menses is a period of 4 or 5 days characterized by menstrual bleeding. The first day of menstrual flow is considered day 1 of the menstrual cycle. The proliferative phase begins after the menstrual flow ends and lasts until ovulation. During this period the follicles mature, the uterine lining thickens (proliferates), and estrogen secretion increases to its highest level. The secretory phase of the menstrual cycle begins at ovulation and lasts until the next menses begins. It is during this phase of the menstrual cycle that the uterine lining reaches its greatest thickness and the ovary secretes its highest levels of progesterone.

As a general rule, during the 30 or 40 years that a woman has periods, only one ovum matures each month. However, there are exceptions to this rule. Some months, more than one matures, and some months, no ovum matures. Ovulation occurs 14 days before the next menses begins. In a 28-day cycle, this means that ovulation occurs around day 14 of the cycle, as shown in Figure 20-12. (Recall that the first day of the menses is considered the first day of the cycle.) In a 30-day cycle, however, ovulation would not occur on the 14th cycle day, but the 16th. And in a 25-day cycle, ovulation would occur the 11th cycle day.

The time of ovulation has great practical importance. An ovum lives only a short time after it is ejected from its follicle, and sperm live only a short time after they enter the female body. Fertilization of an ovum by a sperm therefore can occur only around the time of ovulation. In other words, a woman's fertile period lasts only a few days each month.

Control of Menstrual Cycle Changes

The anterior pituitary gland plays a critical role in regulating the cyclic changes that characterize the functions of the female reproductive system (see Chapter 10). From day 1 to about day 7 of the menstrual cycle, the anterior pituitary gland secretes increasing amounts of FSH. A high blood concentration of FSH stimulates several immature ovarian follicles to start growing and secreting estrogens (see Figure 20-13). As the estrogen content of blood increases, it stimulates the anterior pituitary gland to secrete another hormone, luteinizing hormone (LH). LH causes maturing of a follicle and its ovum, ovulation (rupturing of mature follicle with ejection of ovum), and luteinization (formation of a yellow body, the corpus luteum, from the ruptured follicle).

Which hormone—FSH or LH—would you call the "ovulating hormone"? Do you think ovulation could occur if the blood concentration of FSH remained low throughout the menstrual cycle? If you answered LH to the first question and no to the second, you answered both questions correctly. Ovulation cannot occur if the blood level of FSH stays low because a high concentration of this hormone is essential to stimulation of ovarian follicle growth and maturation. With a low level of FSH, no follicles start to grow, and therefore none become ripe enough to ovulate. Ovulation is caused by the combined actions of FSH and LH. Birth control pills that contain estrogen substances suppress FSH secretion. This indirectly prevents ovulation.

Clinical Application

Hysterectomy

The word hysterectomy (his-te-REK-toe-me) comes from the combination of two Greek words: *hystera*, meaning "uterus," and *ektome*, meaning "to cut out." By definition it is the surgical removal of the uterus. *Hysterectomy* is a term that is often misused, however, by incorrectly expanding its definition to include the removal of the ovaries or other reproductive structures. Only the uterus is removed in a hysterectomy. If the total uterus, including the cervix, is removed, the terms *total hysterectomy* or *panhysterectomy* may be used. If the cervical portion of the uterus is left in place and only the body of the organ is removed, the term *subtotal hysterectomy* is appropriate. The actual removal of the uterus may be performed through an incision made in the abdominal wall—*abdominal hysterectomy*—or through the vagina—*vaginal hysterectomy*. The term **oophorectomy** (o-off-o-REK-toe-me) is used to describe removal of the ovaries. Although the two surgical procedures may take place during the same operation—for a woman with uterine or ovarian cancer, for example—the terms used to describe them should not be used interchangeably.

Health & Well-Being

Amenorrhea in Female Athletes

Failure to have a menstrual period is called **amenorrhea.** Amenorrhea occurs in some female athletes, probably resulting from a body fat composition that is too low to sustain normal reproductive function. Although it keeps the hematocrit (red blood cell level) higher than during menstruation, it is not considered a desirable condition. Besides infertility, amenorrhea may cause other problems. For example, the low blood levels of estrogen associated with long-term amenorrhea may cause osteoporosis (loss of bone mass).

TABLE 20-3

Analogous Features of the Reproductive Systems

FEATURES	FEMALE	MALE
Essential organs	Ovaries	Testes
Sex cells	Ova (eggs)	Sperm
Hormones	Estrogen and progesterone	Testosterone
Hormone-producing cells	Granulosa cells and corpus luteum	Interstitial cells
Duct systems	Uterine (fallopian) tubes, uterus, and vagina	Ductus (vas) deferens, urethra, and epididymis
External genitals	Clitoris and vulva	Penis and scrotum

Ovulation occurs, as we have said, because of the combined actions of the two anterior pituitary hormones, FSH and LH. The next question is: what causes menstruation? A brief answer is this: a sudden, sharp decrease in estrogen and progesterone secretion toward the end of the secretory phase causes the uterine lining to break down and another menstrual period to begin.

SUMMARY OF MALE AND FEMALE REPRODUCTIVE SYSTEMS

The reproductive systems in both sexes are centered around the production of highly specialized reproductive cells or gametes (sperm and ova), as well as mechanisms to ensure union of these two cells; the fusion of these cells enables transfer of parental genetic information to the next generation. Table 20-3 compares several analogous components of the reproductive systems in both sexes. You can see that men and women have similar structures to accomplish complementary functions. In addition, the female reproductive system permits development and birth of the offspring—and this will be the first subject of the last chapter in this book.

Quick

1. Which female structure is made of erectile tissue?
2. What is another term for *menses*?
3. Which hormone reaches a high peak just before ovulation?

Science Applications

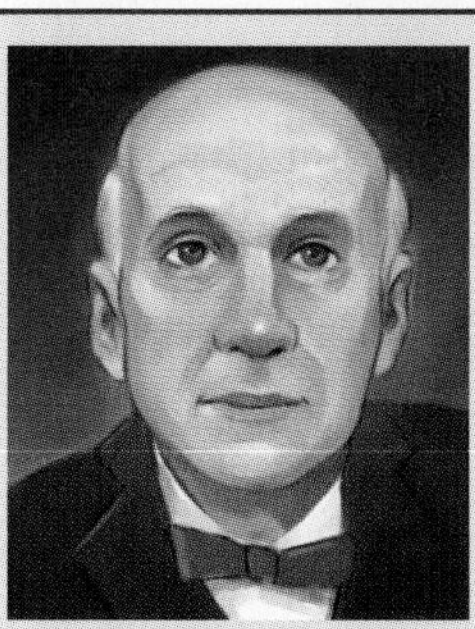

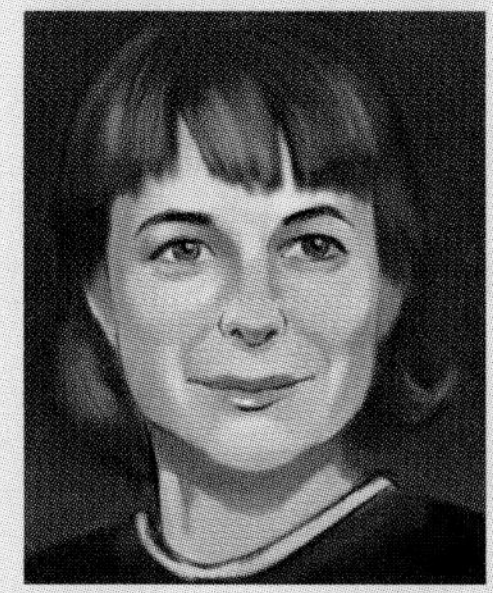

Reproductive Sciences

William Masters (1915-2001) and Virginia Johnson (b. 1925).

The study of human reproduction, and especially sexual function, has many cultural implications. So it is no wonder that American researchers William Masters and Virginia Johnson encountered a great deal of controversy during their decades of pioneering work in the field of human sex and reproduction. After teaming up at Washington University in St. Louis in 1957, they were the first to study human sexual physiology in the laboratory. In 1966, their book *Human Sexual Response* clearly explained the physiology of sex for the first time. Besides making discoveries in the physiology of human sex and reproduction, they also developed therapies for treating sex-related conditions and trained therapists from around the world.

William Masters was a gynecologist (physician specializing in women's health) and Virginia Johnson was a psychologist. This partnership shows the importance of human reproduction in two major fields of study: medicine and psychology. Today, there are many opportunities to apply knowledge of reproductive science in a variety of professions. For example, many psychologists and counselors use biological principles in dealing with clients that seek help with reproductive or sexual issues. Social workers and legal professionals also find that such knowledge can be applied in their professions. Even politicians, religious leaders, social activists, and journalists must be aware of the latest findings in reproductive science to form informed opinions and make reasonable judgments about applying such knowledge in our society.

Of course, the half-century since Masters and Johnson began their work has seen an increase in the number of health professionals working in fields related to human sex and reproduction. For example, urologists (who often deal with men's health issues) and gynecologists are physicians who directly apply reproductive science in their work. Many nurses, therapists, and health technicians join them in providing clients with the help they need. In addition, many community health workers find themselves dealing with their clients' issues related to sexual activity, pregnancy, and fertility.

OUTLINE SUMMARY

COMMON STRUCTURAL AND FUNCTIONAL CHARACTERISTICS BETWEEN THE SEXES

A. Common general structure and function can be identified between the systems in both sexes
B. Systems adapted for development of sperm or ova followed by successful fertilization, development, and birth of offspring
C. Sex hormones in both sexes important in development of secondary sexual characteristics and normal reproductive system activity

MALE REPRODUCTIVE SYSTEM

A. Structural plan—organs classified as essential or accessory
- **1.** Essential organs of reproduction are the gonads (testes), which produce sex cells (sperm)
- **2.** Accessory organs of reproduction
  - **a.** Ducts—passageways that carry sperm from testes to exterior
  - **b.** Sex glands—produce protective and nutrient solution for sperm
  - **c.** External genitals

B. Testes—the gonads of men
- **1.** Structure and location (Figure 20-2)
  - **a.** Testes in scrotum—lower temperature
  - **b.** Covered by tunica albuginea, which divides testis into lobules containing seminiferous tubules
  - **c.** Interstitial cells produce testosterone
- **2.** Functions
  - **a.** Spermatogenesis is process of sperm production (Figure 20-4)
    - **(1)** Sperm precursor cells called *spermatogonia*
    - **(2)** Meiosis produces primary spermatocyte, which forms four spermatids with 23 chromosomes
    - **(3)** Spermatozoa—highly specialized cell
      - **(a)** Head contains genetic material
      - **(b)** Acrosome contains enzymes to assist sperm in penetration of ovum
      - **(c)** Mitochondria in midpiece provide energy for movement
  - **b.** Production of testosterone by interstitial cells
    - **(1)** Testosterone "masculinizes" and promotes development of male accessory organs
    - **(2)** Stimulates protein anabolism and development of muscle strength

C. Reproductive ducts—ducts through which sperm pass after exiting testes until they exit from the body
- **1.** Epididymis—single, coiled tube about 6 m in length; lies along the top and behind the testis in the scrotum
  - **a.** Sperm mature and develop the capacity for motility as they pass through epididymis
- **2.** Ductus (vas) deferens—receives sperm from the epididymis and transports them from scrotal sac through the abdominal cavity
  - **a.** Passes through inguinal canal
  - **b.** Joins duct of seminal vesicle to form the ejaculatory duct

D. Accessory or supportive sex glands—semen: mixture of sperm and secretions of accessory sex glands. Averages 3 to 5 ml per ejaculation, with each milliliter containing about 100 million sperm
- **1.** Seminal vesicles
  - **a.** Pouchlike glands that produce about 60% of seminal fluid volume
  - **b.** Secretion is yellowish, thick, and rich in fructose to provide energy needed by sperm for motility
- **2.** Prostate gland
  - **a.** Shaped like a doughnut and located below bladder
  - **b.** Urethra passes through the gland
  - **c.** Secretion represents 30% of seminal fluid volume—is thin and milk-colored
  - **d.** Activates sperm and is needed for ongoing sperm motility
- **3.** Bulbourethral (Cowper's) glands
  - **a.** Resemble peas in size and shape
  - **b.** Secrete mucuslike fluid constituting less than 5% of seminal fluid volume

OUTLINE SUMMARY—*cont'd*

E. External genitals
  1. Penis and scrotum called *genitalia*
  2. Penis has three columns of erectile tissue—two dorsal columns called *corpora cavernosa* and one ventral column surrounding urethra called *corpus spongiosum*
  3. Glans penis covered by foreskin
  4. Surgical removal of foreskin called *circumcision*

FEMALE REPRODUCTIVE SYSTEM

A. Structural plan—organs classified as essential or accessory
  1. Essential organs are gonads (ovaries), which produce sex cells (ova)
  2. Accessory organs of reproduction
    a. Ducts or modified ducts—including oviducts, uterus, and vagina
    b. Sex glands—including the breasts
    c. External genitals

B. Ovaries
  1. Structure and location
    a. Paired glands weighing about 3 g each
    b. Resemble large almonds
    c. Attached to ligaments in pelvic cavity on each side of uterus
    d. Microscopic structure (Figure 20-8)
      (1) Ovarian follicles—contain an oocyte, which is an immature sex cell (about 1 million at birth)
      (2) Primary follicles—about 400,000 at puberty are covered with granulosa cells
      (3) About 350 to 500 mature follicles ovulate during the reproductive lifetime of most women—sometimes called *Graafian follicles*
      (4) Secondary follicles have a hollow chamber called the *antrum*
      (5) Corpus luteum forms after ovulation
  2. Functions
    a. Oogenesis—this meiotic cell division produces daughter cells with equal chromosome numbers (23) but unequal cytoplasm. Ovum is large; polar bodies are small and degenerate
    b. Production of estrogen and progesterone
      (1) Granulosa cells surrounding the oocyte in the mature and growing follicles produce estrogen
      (2) Corpus luteum produces progesterone
      (3) Estrogen causes development and maintenance of secondary sex characteristics
      (4) Progesterone stimulates secretory activity of uterine epithelium and assists estrogen in initiating menses

C. Reproductive ducts
  1. Uterine (fallopian) tubes
    a. Extend about 10 cm from uterus into abdominal cavity
    b. Expanded distal end surrounded by fimbriae
    c. Mucosal lining of tube is directly continuous with lining of abdominal cavity
  2. Uterus—composed of body, fundus, and cervix (Figure 20-9)
    a. Lies in pelvic cavity just behind urinary bladder
    b. Myometrium is muscle layer
    c. Endometrium lost in menstruation
    d. Menopause—end of repetitive menstrual cycles (about 45-50 years of age)
  3. Vagina
    a. Distensible tube about 10 cm long
    b. Located between urinary bladder and rectum in the pelvis
    c. Receives penis during sexual intercourse and is birth canal for normal delivery of baby at end of term of pregnancy
    d. Accessory or supportive sex glands

D. Accessory or Supportive Sex Glands
  1. Bartholin's (greater vestibular) glands
    a. Secrete mucuslike lubricating fluid
    b. Ducts open between labia minora

Continued

OUTLINE SUMMARY—*cont'd*

2. Breasts (Figure 20-10)
   a. Located over pectoral muscles of thorax
   b. Size determined by fat quantity more than amount of glandular (milk-secreting) tissue
   c. Lactiferous ducts drain at nipple, which is surrounded by pigmented areola
   d. Lymphatic drainage important in spread of cancer cells to other body areas

E. External genitals (Figure 20-11)
1. Include mons pubis, clitoris, orifice of urethra, Bartholin's gland, vagina, labia minora and majora, and hymen
2. Perineum—area between vaginal opening and anus
   a. Surgical cut during childbirth called *episiotomy*

F. Menstrual cycle—involves many changes in the uterus, ovaries, vagina, and breasts (Figures 20-12 and 20-13)
1. Length—about 28 days, varies from month to month among individuals and in the same individual
2. Phases
   a. Menses—about the first 4 or 5 days of the cycle, varies somewhat; characterized by sloughing of bits of endometrium (uterine lining) with bleeding
   b. Proliferative phase—days between the end of menses and secretory phase; varies in length; the shorter the cycle, the shorter the proliferative phase; the longer the cycle, the longer the proliferative phase; examples: in 28-day cycle, proliferative phase ends on day 13, but in 26-day cycle, it ends on the 11th day and in 32-day cycle, it ends on day 17; characterized by repair of endometrium
   c. Secretory phase—days between ovulation and beginning of next menses; secretory about 14 days before next menses; characterized by further thickening of endometrium and secretion by its glands in preparation for implantation of fertilized ovum; combined actions of the anterior pituitary hormones FSH and LH cause ovulation; sudden sharp decrease in estrogens and progesterone bring on menstruation if pregnancy does not occur.

SUMMARY OF MALE AND FEMALE REPRODUCTIVE SYSTEMS

A. In men and women the organs of the reproductive system are adapted for the specific sequence of functions that permit development of sperm or ova after the successful fertilization and then the normal development and birth of offspring
B. The male organs produce, store, and ultimately introduce mature sperm into the female reproductive tract
C. The female system produces ova, receives the sperm, and permits fertilization followed by fetal development and birth, with lactation afterward
D. Production of sex hormones is required for development of secondary sex characteristics and for normal reproductive functions in both sexes

NEW WORDS

areola	estrogen	menses	semen
circumcision	fimbriae	oocyte	seminiferous tubule
clitoris	gametes	ovulation	spermatogenesis
corpus luteum	genitals	perineum	spermatozoa
ejaculation	gonads	polar body	testes
endometrium	Graafian follicle	prepuce	testosterone
epididymis	meiosis	progesterone	vulva
episiotomy	menopause	scrotum	zygote

REVIEW QUESTIONS

1. Describe the structure and location of the testes.
2. Describe the structure of the spermatozoa.
3. List the functions of testosterone.
4. List and briefly describe the reproductive ducts of the male reproductive system.
5. List and briefly describe the glands of the male reproductive system. What does each gland contribute to seminal fluid?
6. Describe the structure and location of the ovaries.
7. Explain the development of an ovarian follicle from the primary follicle to the corpus luteum.
8. List the functions of estrogen.
9. List the functions of progesterone.
10. Describe the structure of the uterine tubes.
11. Describe the structure of the uterus.
12. Describe the structure of the vagina.
13. Describe the structure of the breasts.
14. Explain what occurs during the proliferative phase of the reproductive cycle.
15. Explain what occurs during the secretory phase of the reproductive cycle.
16. Name the four hormones involved in the regulation of the reproductive cycle. Where is each produced, and what is the function of each?

CRITICAL THINKING

17. Differentiate between spermatogenesis and oogenesis. How do these differences relate to the role of the male and female in reproduction?
18. Why are the testes located outside the body cavity in the scrotum?
19. What is unique about the chromosome content of the gametes? Why is this important?

CHAPTER TEST

1. The essential organs of the male reproductive system are the testes.
2. The pouchlike sac where the male gonads are located is called the scrotum
3. The membrane that covers the testicle and also divides the interior into lobes is called the tunica albuginea
4. The seminiferous tube is a long duct in the testicle where sperm develop.
5. The interstitial cells are the cells in the testes that secrete testosterone.
6. The primary spermatocyte develops from a cell called the spermatogonium
7. The primary spermatocyte forms sperm cells by undergoing a specialized type of cell division called Meiosis
8. The sperm cell contains an acrosome which contains an enzyme that can digest the covering of the ovum.
9. The epididymis is a reproductive duct that consists of a tightly coiled tube that lies along the top and behind the testes.
10. The Ductus Deferens is a reproductive duct that permits the sperm to move out of the scrotum upward into the abdominal cavity.
11. The Prostate gland is a gland that secretes a thin, milk-colored fluid that makes up about 20% of the seminal fluid.
12. The seminal vesicles are a pair of glands that produce a thick, yellowish, fructose-rich fluid that makes up about 60% of the seminal fluid.
13. The penis is composed of three columns of erectile tissue: one is called the corpus spongiosum, the other two are called the corpora cavernosa
14. The essential organs of the female reproductive system are the ovaries.
15. Another name for a mature ovarian follicle is a Graafian follicle.
16. The process that produces the female gamete is called oogenesis.
17. Meiosis in the female produces one large ovum and three small daughter cells called Polar bodies, which degenerate.
18. The uterine tubes are the reproductive tubes connecting the ovary and the uterus.
19. The muscle layer of the uterus is called the myometrium
20. The uterus is composed of two parts: the upper part, called the body, and the narrow lower part, called the cervix.
21. The innermost layer of the uterus, which is shed during menstruation, is called the endometrium
22. The vagina is the part of the female reproductive system that opens to the exterior.
23. The Bartholin's glands are glands that secrete a mucuslike lubricating fluid into the vestibule.
24. The milk-secreting glandular cells of the breast are arranged in grapelike structures called alveoli. These drain into lactiferous ducts that converge toward the nipple.

33/33

CHAPTER TEST—*cont'd*

Match the statement in Column B with the correct term in Column A.

COLUMN A

25. H FSH
26. C Menstruation
27. A Corpus luteum
28. B Estrogen
29. D Secretory phase
30. E Progesterone
31. I LH
32. G Proliferative phase
33. F Ovulation

COLUMN B

a. after ovulation, this is what the egg follicle becomes
b. this ovarian hormone reaches its highest concentration in the proliferative phase
c. this is caused by the rapid drop of blood levels of estrogen and progesterone
d. this phase of the reproductive cycle begins after ovulation
e. this ovarian hormone reaches its highest concentration during the secretory phase
f. this term is used to describe the egg being released from the ovary
g. during this phase of the reproductive cycle, the uterine wall begins to thicken
h. this pituitary hormone stimulates the formation of an egg follicle
i. this pituitary hormone can be called the ovulating hormone

STUDY TIPS

Before studying Chapter 20, review the synopsis of the male and female reproductive systems in Chapter 4. Much of the chapter deals with the names, locations, and function of the structures of the male and female reproductive systems. Flash cards will help you learn this material. Meiosis is the process of forming the male and female gametes. Gametes are reproductive cells with half the number of chromosomes as other body cells. Just before meiosis begins, the primary oocyte or spermatocyte doubles its chromosome number to 92. The first division produces cells with 46 chromosomes; the second division produces cells with 23 chromosomes. The role of the male in reproduction is to produce as many sperm cells as possible, so four functional sperm cells are produced during each meiosis. The female's role is the production of one egg cell containing 23 chromosomes. Sixty-nine of the original 92 chromosomes need to be "thrown away." It is the function of the polar bodies to get rid of the extra chromosomes. The responsibility of the female reproductive system is to produce an egg and prepare for a possible pregnancy. If you keep this role in mind, the reproductive cycle may be easier to remember. The reproductive cycle is regulated by four hormones: two from the pituitary gland and two from the ovary. Follicle stimulating hormone does exactly what the name says. *Luteinizing hormone* helps stimulate ovulation which causes the egg follicle to become the corpus *luteum*. Estrogen begins the initial preparation of the uterus. Progesterone prepares the uterus to receive a fertilized egg. Think of progesterone as "pro" (in favor of) "gesterone" (gestation)—it may help you remember what it does.

In your study group, go over the flash cards of the structures and photocopy the figures to help you learn their locations. Discuss the process of meiosis and the differences between spermatogenesis and oogenesis. Discuss the reproductive cycle with emphasis on the hormones involved. Look at the diagram to see the relationship between hormone levels and the effect on the ovary and the uterus. Go over the questions at the end of the chapter and discuss possible test questions.

21 Growth and Development

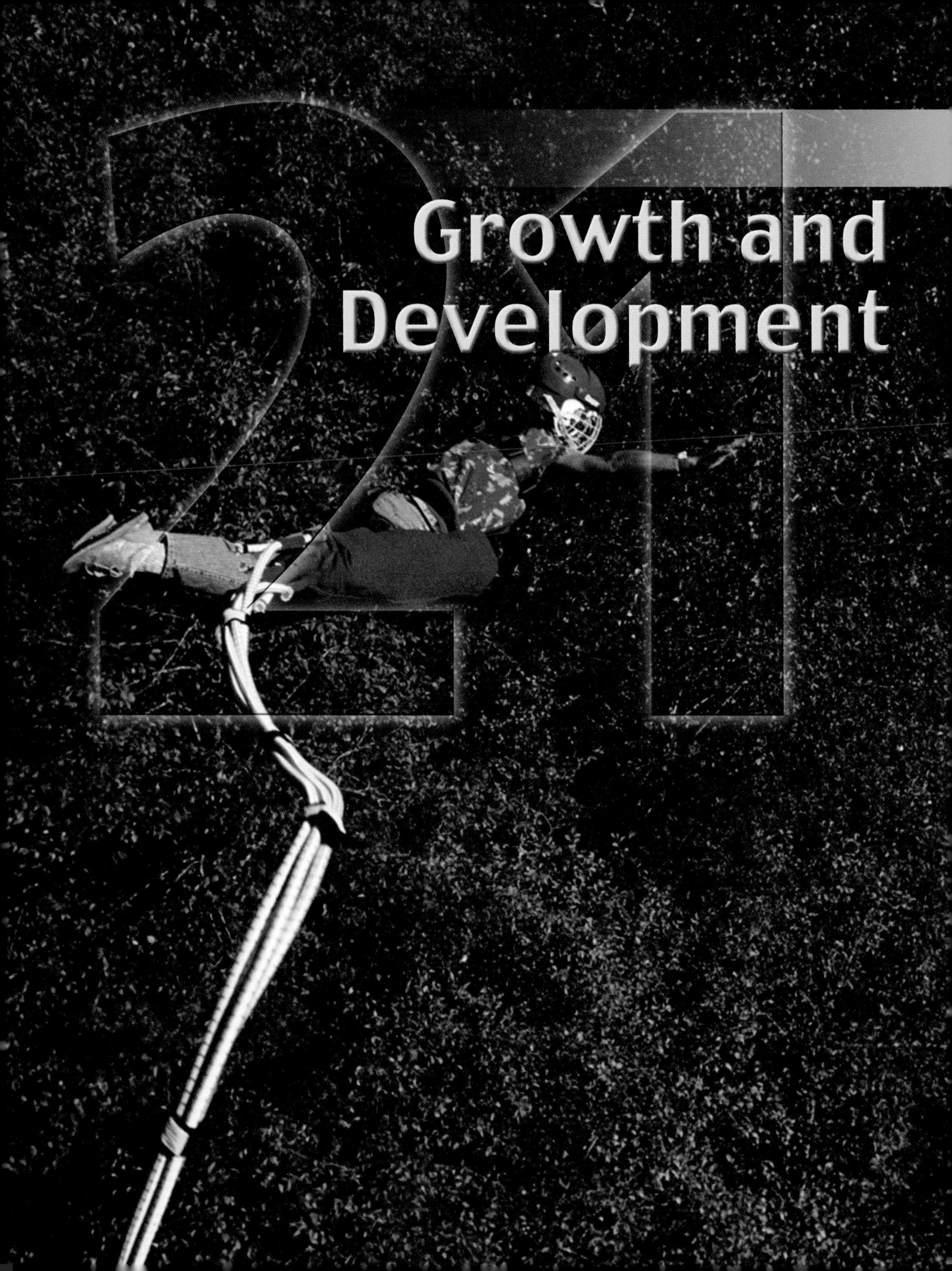

Outline

Objectives

AFTER YOU HAVE COMPLETED THIS CHAPTER, YOU SHOULD BE ABLE TO:

1. Discuss the concept of development as a biological process characterized by continuous modification and change.
2. Discuss the major developmental changes characteristic of the prenatal stage of life from fertilization to birth.
3. Discuss the three stages of labor that characterize a normal vaginal birth.
4. Identify the three primary germ layers and several derivatives in the adult body that develop from each layer.
5. List and discuss the major developmental changes characteristic of the four postnatal periods of life.
6. Discuss the effects of aging on the major body organ systems.

M*any of your* fondest and most vivid memories are probably associated with your birthdays. The day of birth is an important milestone of life. Most people continue to remember their birthday in some special way each year; birthdays serve as pleasant and convenient reference points to mark periods of transition or change in our lives. The actual day of birth marks the end of one phase of life called the **prenatal period** and the beginning of a second called the **postnatal period.** The prenatal period begins at conception and ends at birth; the postnatal period begins at birth and continues until death. Although important periods in our lives such as childhood and adolescence are often remembered as a series of individual and isolated events, they are in reality part of an ongoing and continuous process. In reviewing the many changes that occur during the cycle of life from conception to death, it is often convenient to isolate certain periods such as infancy or adulthood for study. It is important to remember, however, that life is not a series of stop-and-start events or individual and isolated periods of time. Instead, it is a biological process that is characterized by continuous modification and change.

This chapter discusses some of the events and changes that occur in the development of the individual from conception to death. Study of development during the prenatal period is followed by a discussion of the birth process and a review of changes occurring during infancy and adulthood. Finally, some important changes that occur in the individual organ systems of the body as a result of aging are discussed.

PRENATAL PERIOD

The **prenatal stage of development** begins at the time of conception or fertilization (that is, at the moment the female ovum and the male sperm cells unite) (Figure 21-1). The period of prenatal development continues until the birth of the child about 39 weeks later. The science of the development of the individual before birth is called **embryology** (em-bree-OL-o-jee). It is a story of miracles, describing the means by which a new human life is started and the steps by which a single microscopic cell is transformed into a complex human being.

Fertilization to Implantation

After ovulation the discharged ovum first enters the abdominal cavity and then finds its way into a uterine (fallopian) tube. Sperm cells "swim" up the uterine tubes toward the ovum. Look at the relationship of the ovary, the two uterine tubes, and the uterus in Figure 21-2. Recall from Chapter 20 that each uterine tube extends outward from the uterus for about 10 cm. It then ends in the abdominal cavity near the ovary, as you can see in Figure 21-2, in an opening surrounded by fringelike processes, the *fimbriae.* Using the uterus as a point of reference, anatomists divide each uterine tube into three parts. The innermost part of the tube actually extends through the uterine wall, the middle third extends out into the abdominal cavity, and the outermost third of the tube ends near the ovary in the dilated, funnel-shaped opening described above.

Sperm cells that are deposited in the vagina must enter and "swim" through the uterus and then move out of the uterine cavity and through the uterine tube to meet the ovum. Fertilization most often occurs in the outer one third of the oviduct, as shown in Figure 21-2. The fertilized ovum or **zygote** (ZYE-gote) is genetically complete; it represents a new single-celled individual. Time and nourishment are all that is needed for expression of characteristics such as sex, body build, and skin color that were determined at the time of fertilization. As you can see in the figure, the zygote immediately begins mitotic division, and in about 3 days a solid mass of cells called a **morula** (MOR-yoo-lah) is formed (see

FIGURE 21-1

Fertilization. Fertilization is a specific biological event. It occurs when the male and female sex cells fuse. After union between a sperm cell and the ovum has occurred, the cycle of life begins. The scanning electron micrograph shows spermatozoa attaching themselves to the surface of an ovum. Only one will penetrate and fertilize the ovum.

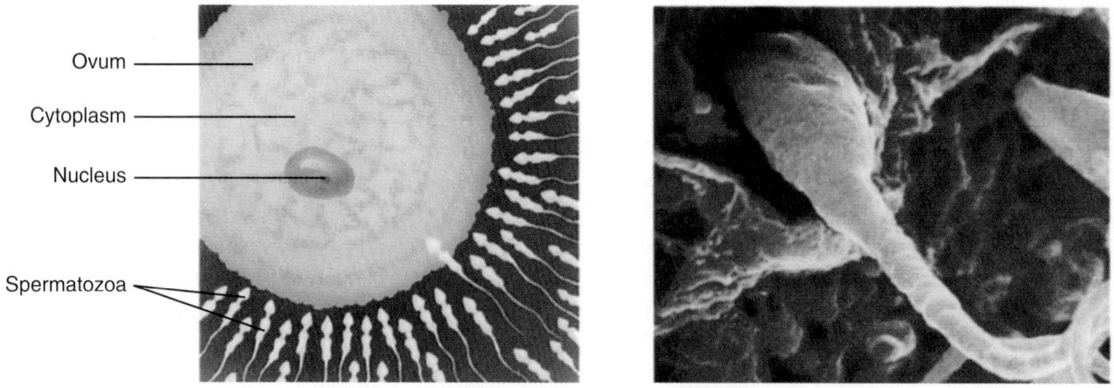

Figure 21-2). The cells of the morula continue to divide, and by the time the developing embryo reaches the uterus, it is a hollow ball of cells called a **blastocyst** (BLAS-toe-sist).

During the 10 days from the time of fertilization to the time when the blastocyst is completely implanted in the uterine lining, no nutrients from the mother are available. The rapid cell division taking place up to the blastocyst stage occurs with no significant increase in total mass compared with the zygote (Figure 21-3). One of the specializations of the ovum is its incredible store of nutrients that help support this embryonic development until implantation has occurred.

Note in Figure 21-4 that the blastocyst consists of an outer layer of cells and an inner cell mass. As the blastocyst develops, it forms a structure with two cavities, the **yolk sac** and **amniotic** (am-nee-OT-ik) **cavity.** The yolk sac is most important in animals, such as birds, that depend heavily on yolk as the sole source of nutrients for the developing embryo. In these animals the yolk sac digests the yolk and provides the resulting nutrients to the embryo. Because uterine flu-

FIGURE 21-2

Fertilization and implantation. At ovulation, an ovum is released from the ovary and begins its journey through the uterine tube. While in the tube, the ovum is fertilized by a sperm to form the single-celled zygote. After a few days of rapid mitotic division, a ball of cells called a *morula* is formed. After the morula develops into a hollow ball called a *blastocyst*, implantation occurs.

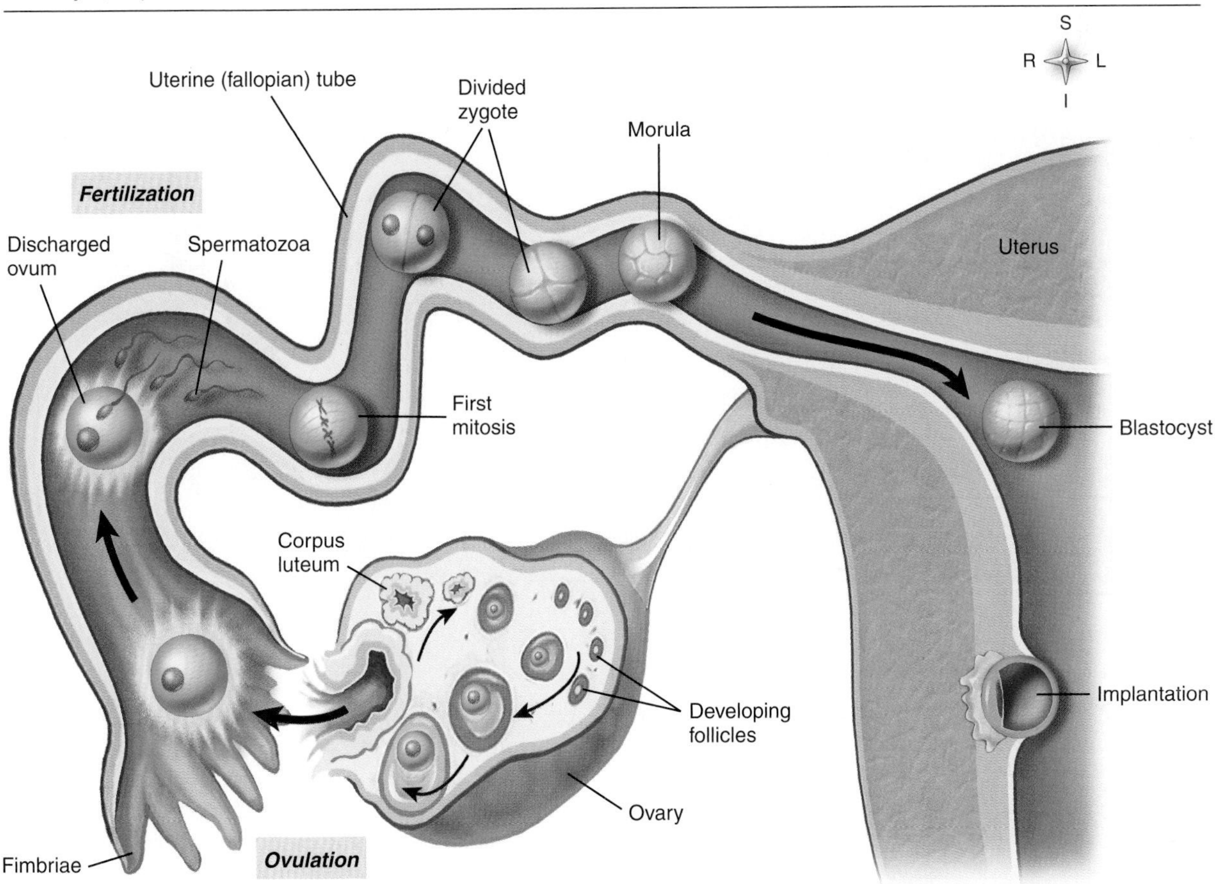

FIGURE 21-3

Early stages of human development. A, Fertilized ovum or zygote. **B** to **D,** Early cell divisions produce more and more cells. The solid mass of cells shown in **D** forms the morula—an early stage in embryonic development.

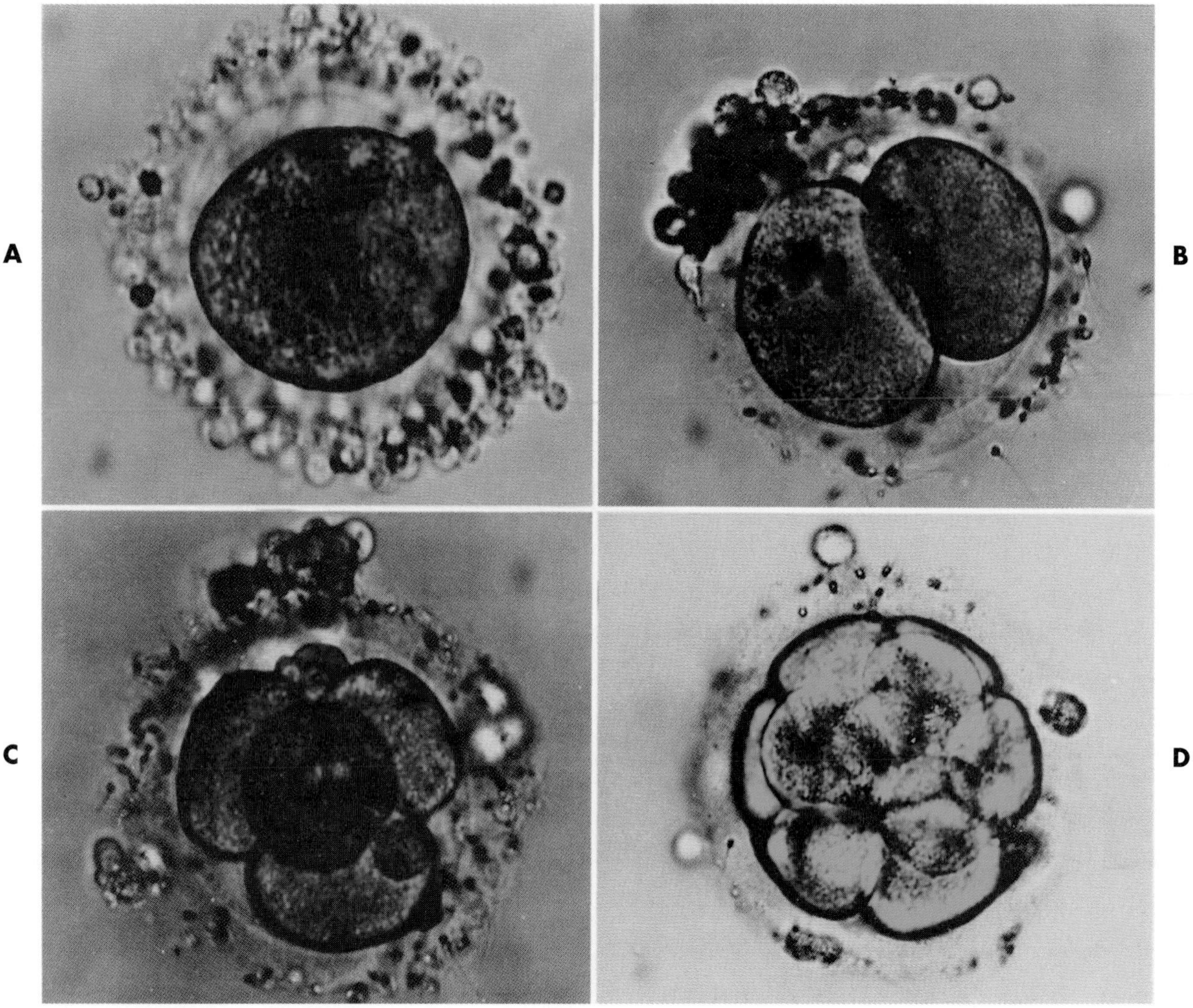

ids provide nutrients to the developing embryo in humans until the placenta develops, the function of the yolk sac is not a nutritive one. Instead, it has other functions, including production of blood cells.

The amniotic cavity becomes a fluid-filled, shock-absorbing sac, sometimes called the *bag of waters*, in which the embryo floats during development. The **chorion** (KO-ree-on), shown in Figures 21-4 and 21-5, develops into an important fetal membrane in the **placenta** (plah-SEN-tah). The *chorionic villi* shown in Figure 21-5 connect the blood vessels of the chorion to the placenta. The placenta (see Figure 21-5) an-

FIGURE 21-4

Implantation and early development. The hollow blastocyst implants itself in the uterine lining about 10 days after ovulation. Until the placenta is functional, nutrients are obtained by diffusion from uterine fluids. Notice the developing chorion and how the blastocyst eventually forms a yolk sac and amniotic cavity.

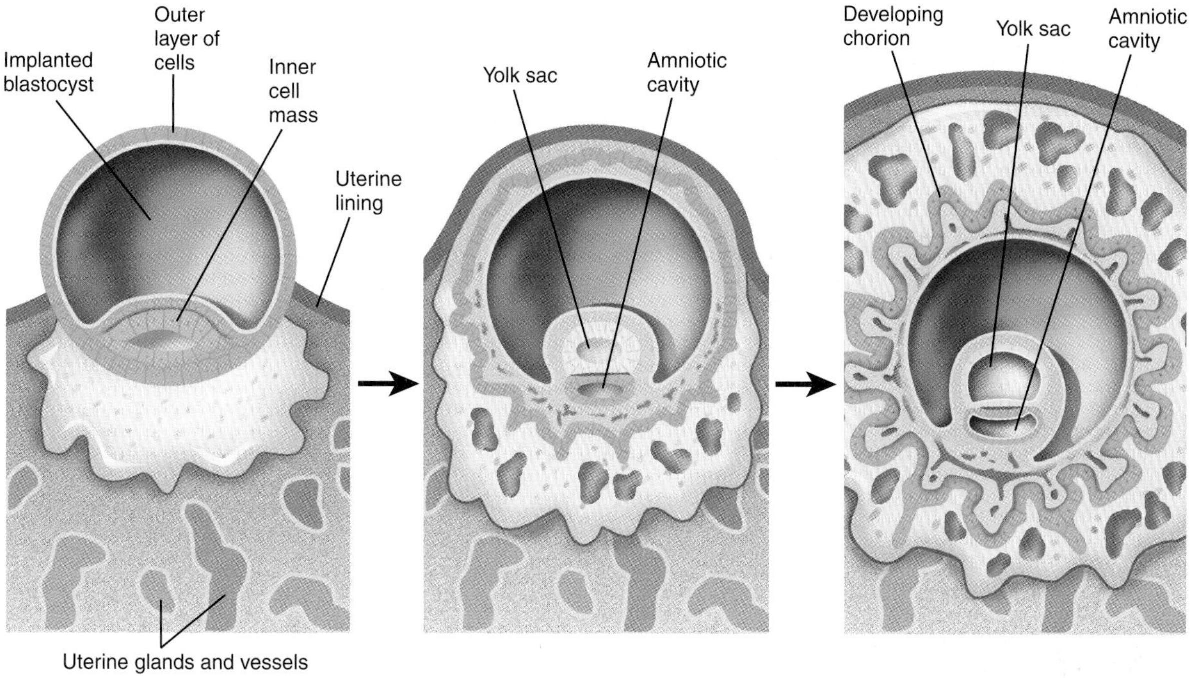

Research, Issues & Trends

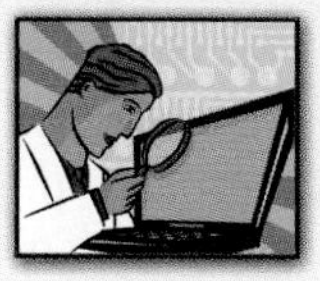

In Vitro Fertilization

The Latin term *in vitro* means, literally, "within a glass." In the case of in vitro fertilization, it refers to the glass laboratory dish where an ovum and sperm are mixed and where fertilization occurs.

In the classic technique, the ovum is obtained from the mother by first inserting a fiberoptic viewing instrument called a **laparoscope** through a very small incision in the woman's abdomen. After it is in the abdominal cavity, the device allows the physician to view the ovary and then puncture and "suck up" an ovum from a mature follicle. Over the years refinements to this technique have been made, and less invasive procedures are currently being used. After about 2.5 days' growth in a temperature-controlled environment, the developing zygote, which by then has reached the 8- or 16-cell stage, is returned by the physician to the mother's uterus. If implantation is successful, growth will continue and the subsequent pregnancy will progress. In the most successful fertility clinics in the United States, a normal term birth will occur in about 30% of in vitro fertilization attempts.

FIGURE 21-5

The placenta: interface between maternal and fetal circulation. A, Relationship of uterus, developing infant, and placenta. **B,** The close placement of the fetal blood supply and the maternal blood in the lacunae of the placenta permits diffusion of nutrients and other substances. It also forms a thin barrier to prevent diffusion of most harmful substances. No mixing of fetal and maternal blood occurs.

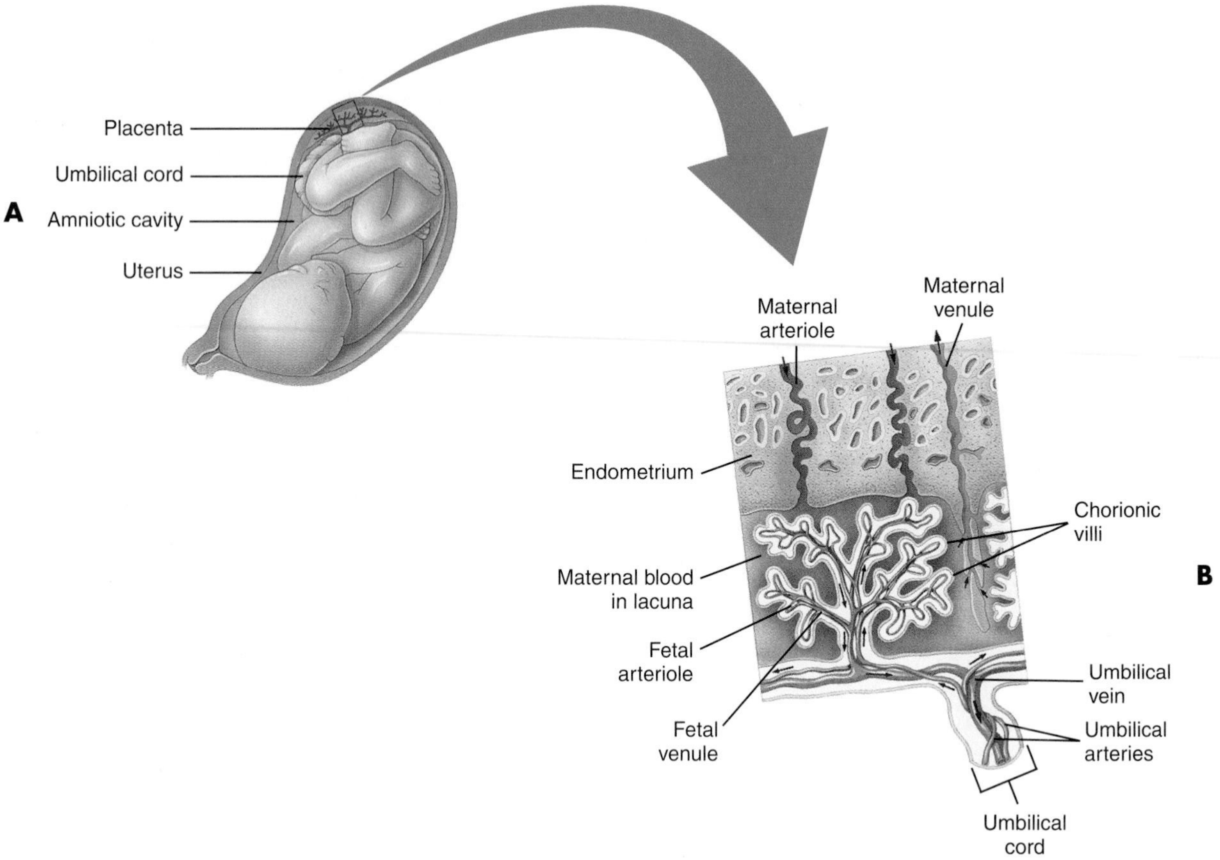

chors the developing fetus to the uterus and provides a "bridge" for the exchange of nutrients and waste products between mother and baby.

The placenta is a unique and highly specialized structure that has a temporary but very important series of functions during pregnancy. It is composed of tissues from mother and child and functions not only as a structural "anchor" and nutritive bridge, but also as an excretory, respiratory, and endocrine organ (see Figure 21-5).

Placental tissue normally separates the maternal blood, which fills the lacunae of the placenta, from the fetal blood so that no intermixing occurs. The very thin layer of placental tissue that separates maternal and fetal blood also serves as an effective "barrier" that can protect the developing baby from many harmful substances that may enter the mother's bloodstream. Unfortunately, toxic substances, such as alcohol and some infectious organisms, may penetrate this protective placental barrier and injure the developing baby. The virus responsible for German measles (rubella), for example, can easily pass through the placenta and cause tragic developmental defects in the fetus.

Research, Issues & Trends

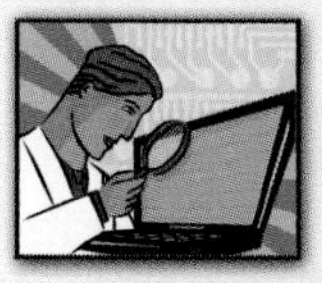

How Long Does Pregnancy Last?

This seems like a silly question to most of us; the answer is 9 months, isn't it? Actually, the length of gestation (the amount of time one is pregnant) is defined in different ways in different situations and can vary from one pregnancy to another. The average gestation in humans is 266 days, starting at the day of conception. But physicians instead usually count from the beginning of the woman's last menstrual period, for an average of 280 days. But these are only averages. What is normal in one case can be different from what is normal in another case. In practice, any pregnancy of less than 37 weeks (259 days) is said to be premature, and any lasting more than 42 weeks (294 days) is said to be postmature. So, as with many statistics regarding human function, what is "normal" can be spoken of only in generalities and averages.

Periods of Development

The length of pregnancy (about 39 weeks)—called the *gestation period*—is divided into three 3-month segments called *trimesters*. A number of terms are used to describe development during these periods known as the first, second, and third trimesters of pregnancy.

During the first trimester or 3 months of pregnancy, many terms are used. *Zygote* describes the ovum just after fertilization by a sperm cell. After about 3 days of constant cell division, the solid mass of cells, identified earlier as the *morula*, enters the uterus. Continued development transforms the morula into the hollow blastocyst, which then implants into the uterine wall.

The embryonic phase of development extends from the third week after fertilization until the end of week 8 of gestation. During this period in the first trimester, the term *embryo* is used to describe the developing individual. The fetal phase is used to indicate the period of development extending from week 9 to week 39. During this period, the term *embryo* is replaced by *fetus*.

By day 35 of gestation (Figure 21-6, *A*), the heart is beating and, although the embryo is only 8 mm (about 3/8 inch) long, the eyes and so-called limb buds, which ultimately form the arms and legs, are clearly visible. Figure 21-6, *C* shows the stage of development of the fetus at the end of the first trimester of gestation. Body size is about 7 to 8 cm (3.2 inches) long. The facial features of the fetus are apparent, the limbs are complete, and gender can be identified. By month 4 (Figure 21-6, *D*) all organ systems are complete and in place.

Formation of the Primary Germ Layers

Early in the first trimester of pregnancy, three layers of specialized cells develop that embryologists call the **primary germ layers** (Table 21-1). Each layer gives rise to definite structures such as the skin, nervous tissue, muscles, or digestive organs. Table 21-1 lists a number of structures derived from each primary germ layer called, respectively, **endoderm** (en-doe-derm) or inside layer, **ectoderm** (ek-toe-derm) or outside layer, and **mesoderm** (mez-o-derm) or middle layer.

Histogenesis and Organogenesis

The process of how the primary germ layers develop into many different kinds of tissues is called **histogenesis** (his-toe-JEN-e-sis). The way that those tissues arrange themselves into organs is called **organogenesis** (or-ga-no-JEN-e-sis). The fascinating story of histogenesis and organogenesis in human development is long and complicated; its telling belongs to the science of embryology. But for

FIGURE 21-6

Human embryos and fetuses. A, At 35 days. **B,** At 49 days. **C,** At the end of the first trimester. **D,** At 4 months.

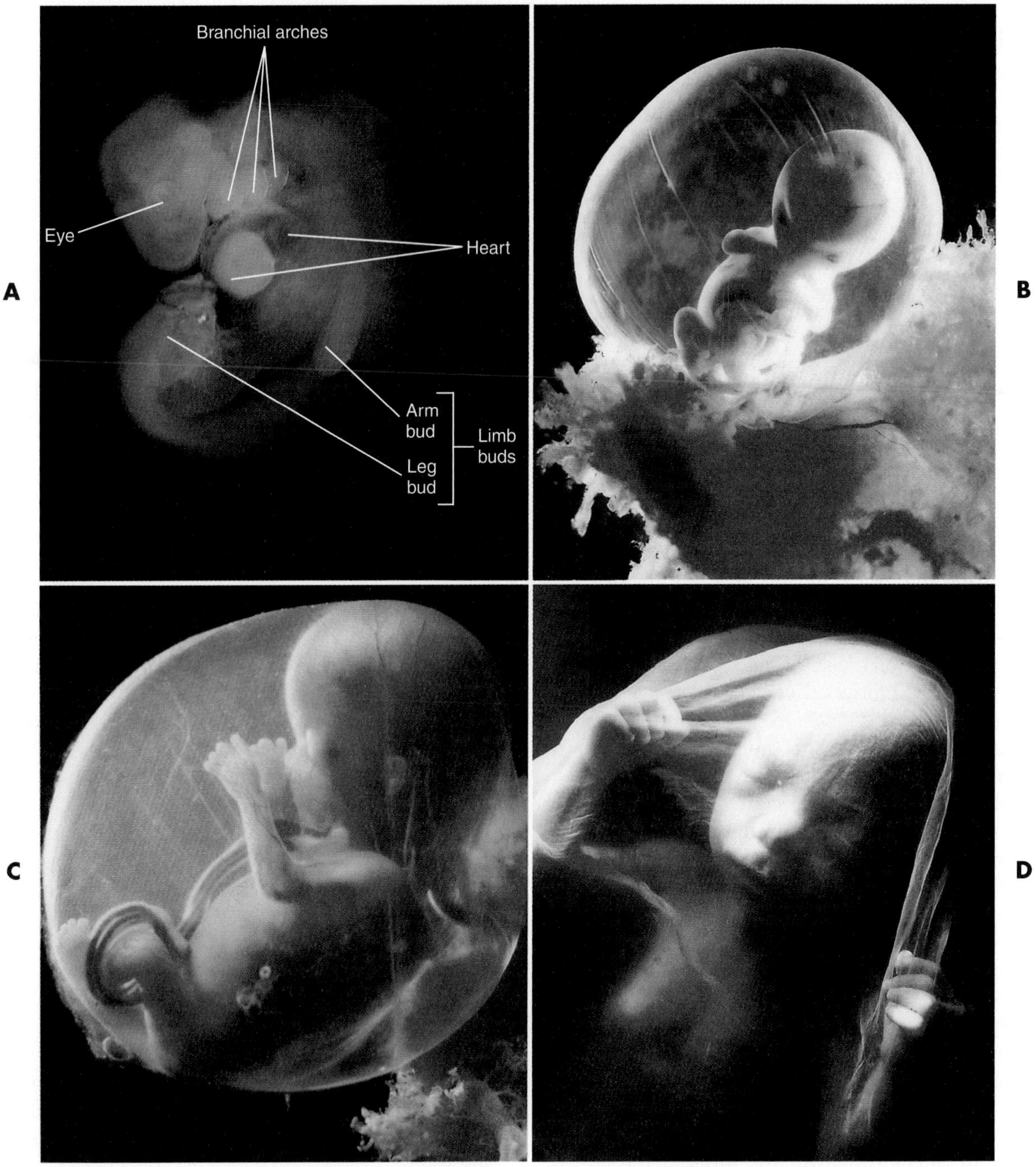

TABLE 21-1

Primary Germ Layer Derivatives

ENDODERM	ECTODERM	MESODERM
Lining of gastrointestinal tract	Epidermis of skin	Dermis of skin
Lining of lungs	Tooth enamel	Circulatory system
Lining of hepatic and pancreatic ducts	Lens and cornea of eye	Many glands
Kidney ducts and bladder	Outer ear	Kidneys
Anterior pituitary gland (adenohypophysis)	Nasal cavity	Gonads
Thymus gland	Facial bones	Muscle
Thyroid gland	Skeletal muscles in head	Bones (except facial)
Parathyroid gland	Brain and spinal cord	
Tonsils	Sensory neurons	
Adrenal medulla		

the beginning student of anatomy and physiology, it seems sufficient to appreciate that life begins when two sex cells unite to form a single-celled zygote and that the new human body evolves by a series of processes consisting of cell differentiation, multiplication, growth, and rearrangement, all of which take place in definite, orderly sequence (Figure 21-7). Development of structure and function go hand in hand, and from 4 months of gestation, when every organ system is complete and in place, until term (about 280 days), fetal development is mainly a matter of growth. Figure 21-8, *A*, shows the normal intrauterine placement of a fetus just before birth in a full-term pregnancy.

Birth Defects

Developmental problems present at birth are often called **birth defects.** Such abnormalities may be structural or functional, perhaps even involving behavior and personality. Birth defects may be caused by genetic factors such as abnormal genes or inheritance of an abnormal number of chromosomes. Birth defects may also be caused by exposure to environmental factors called **teratogens** (TAYR-ah-to-jenz). Teratogens include radiation (for example, x-rays), chemicals (for example, drugs, cigarettes, or alcohol), and infections in the mother (for example, herpes or rubella).

As Figure 21-7 shows, the period during the first trimester when the tissues are beginning to differentiate and the organs are just starting to develop is the time that teratogens are most likely to cause damage. In fact, teratogens can cause spontaneous abortion (miscarriage) if significant damage occurs during the pre-embryonic stage.

Quick

1. What is the postnatal period? The prenatal period?
2. What is a zygote? How is it different from a morula or blastocyst?
3. What are germ layers?
4. What is meant by the term *organogenesis*?

FIGURE 21-7

Critical periods of neonatal development. The red areas show when teratogens are most likely to cause major birth defects and the yellow areas show when minor defects are more likely to arise.

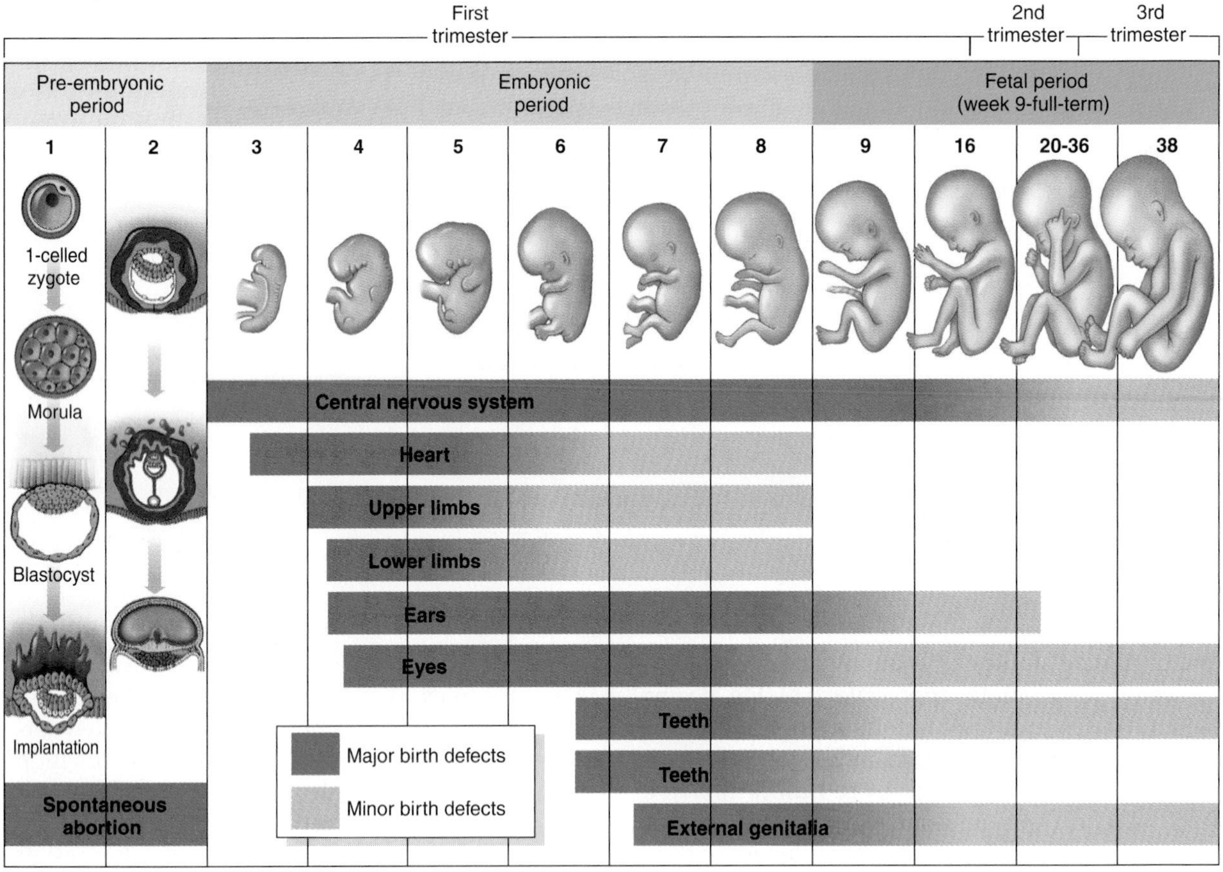

BIRTH OR PARTURITION

The process of birth or **parturition** (par-too-RISH-un) is the point of transition between the prenatal and postnatal periods of life. As pregnancy draws to a close, the uterus becomes "irritable" and, ultimately, muscular contractions begin and cause the cervix to dilate or open, thus permitting the fetus to move from the uterus through the vagina or "birth canal" to the exterior. The process normally begins with the fetus taking a head-down position against the cervix (Figure 21-8, *A*). When contractions occur, the amniotic sac or "bag of waters" ruptures, and labor begins.

Stages of Labor

Labor is the process that results in the birth of a baby. It has three stages (Figure 21-8, *B* to *E*):

1. Stage one—period from onset of uterine contractions until dilation of the cervix is complete
2. Stage two—period from the time of maximal cervical dilation until the baby exits through the vagina
3. Stage three—process of expulsion of the placenta through the vagina

The time required for normal vaginal birth varies widely and may be influenced by many variables,

FIGURE 21-8

Parturition. A, The relation of the fetus to the mother. **B,** The fetus moves into the opening of the birth canal, and the cervix begins to dilate. **C,** Dilation of the cervix is complete. **D,** The fetus is expelled from the uterus. **E,** The placenta is expelled.

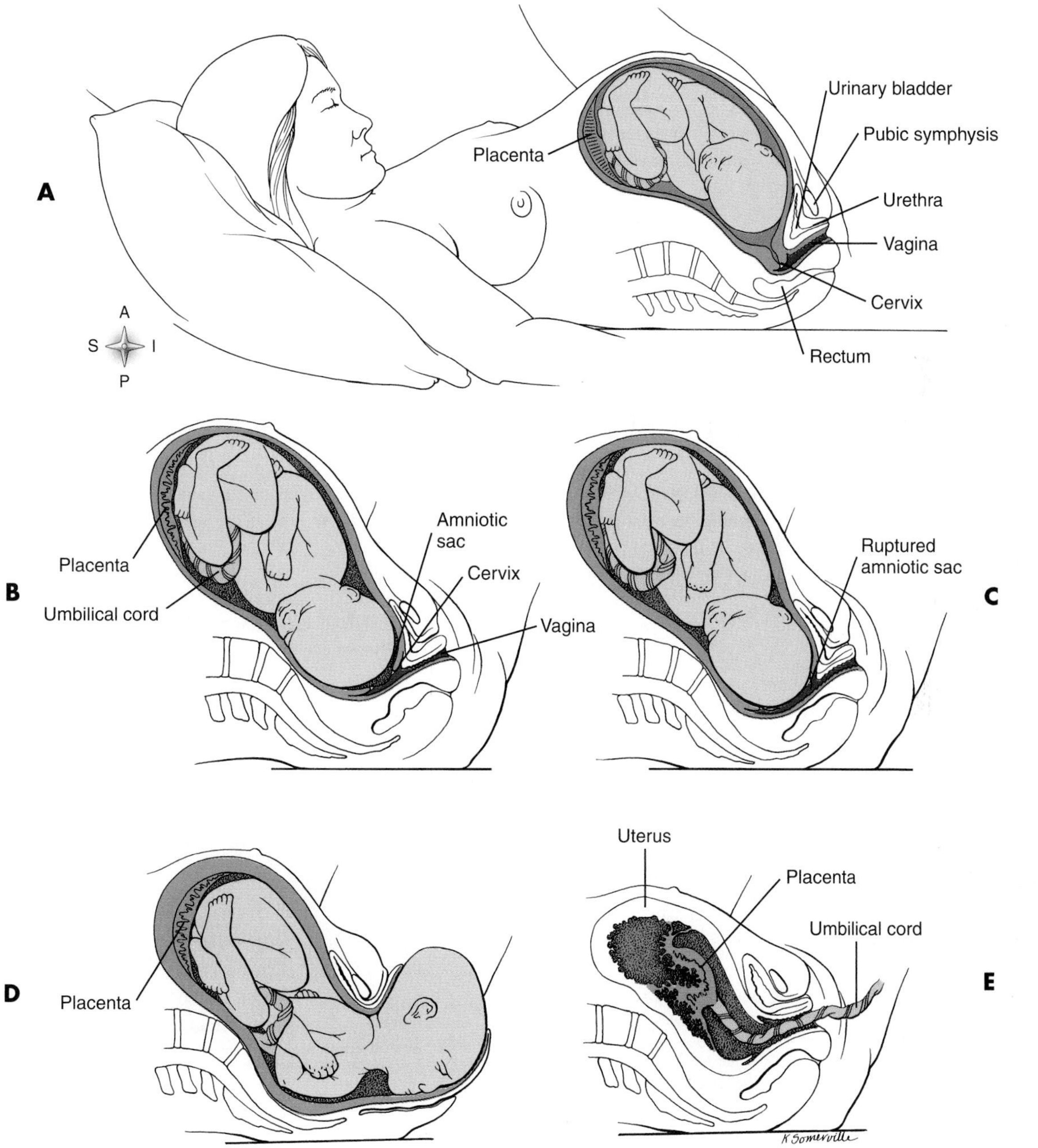

Health & Well-Being

Quickening

Pregnant women usually notice fetal movement for the first time between weeks 16 and 18 of pregnancy. The term **quickening** has been used for generations to describe these first recognizable movements of the fetus. From an occasional "kick" during months 4 and 5 of pregnancy, the frequency of fetal movements steadily increases as gestation progresses. The frequency of fetal movements is an excellent indicator of the unborn baby's health.

Recent studies have shown that simply by recording the number of fetal movements each day after week 28 of pregnancy, a woman can provide her physician with extremely useful information about the health of her unborn child. Ten or more movements during a daily measurement period are considered normal.

Educating pregnant women about fetal movements and how to monitor their frequency is but one example of expanded interest in prenatal home care. Assisting pregnant women with making informed judgments about nutrition, exercise, lifestyle adjustments, and birthing options before they enter the hospital for delivery of their baby is an important and growing part of home health care services.

Research, Issues & Trends

Antenatal Diagnosis and Treatment

Advances in **antenatal** (from the Latin *ante*, "before," *natus*, "birth") **medicine** now permit extensive diagnosis and treatment of disease in the fetus much like any other patient. This new dimension in medicine began with techniques by which Rh^+ babies could be given transfusions before birth.

Current procedures using images provided by ultrasound equipment (Figures *A* and *B*) allow physicians to prepare for and perform, before the birth of a baby, corrective surgical procedures such as bladder repair. These procedures also allow physicians to monitor the progress of other types of treatment on a developing fetus. Figure A shows placement of the ultrasound transducer on the abdominal wall. The resulting image (Figure *B*), called an *ultrasonogram*, shows a 29-week embryo. The image plane is showing the head.

A

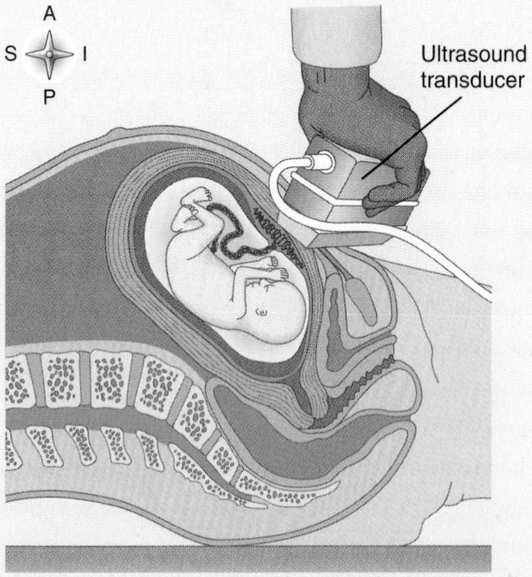

B

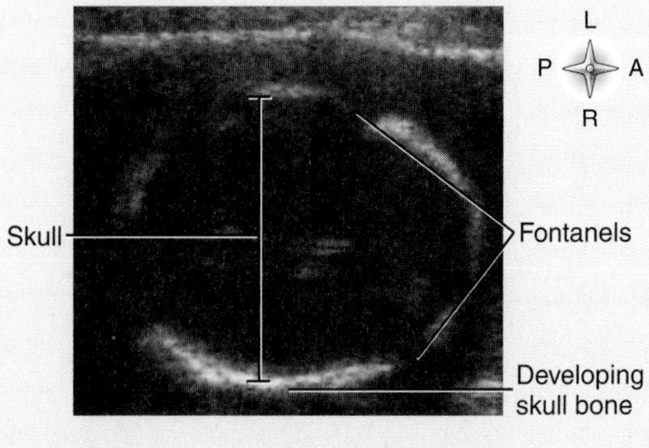

FIGURE 21-9

Changes in the proportions of body parts from birth to maturity. Note the dramatic differences in head size.

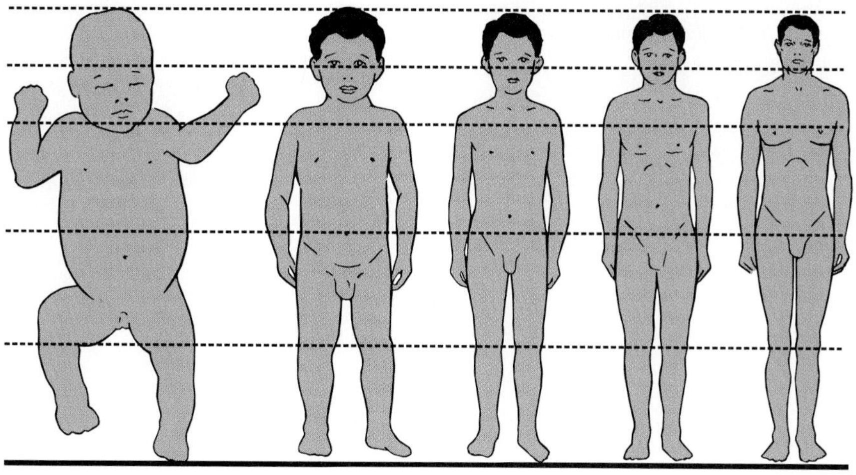

including whether the woman has previously had a child. In most cases, stage one of labor lasts from 6 to 24 hours, and stage two lasts from a few minutes to an hour. Delivery of the placenta (stage three) normally occurs within 15 minutes after the birth of the baby.

Quick Check

1. What is meant by the term *parturition*?
2. What are the three stage of labor?

POSTNATAL PERIOD

The **postnatal period** begins at birth and lasts until death. Although it is often divided into major periods for study, we need to understand and appreciate the fact that growth and development are continuous processes that occur throughout the life cycle. Gradual changes in the physical appearance of the body as a whole and in the relative proportions of the head, trunk, and limbs are quite noticeable between birth and adolescence. Note in Figure 21-9 the obvious changes in the size of bones and in the proportionate sizes between different bones and body areas. The head, for example, becomes proportionately smaller. Whereas the infant head is approximately one fourth the total height of the body, the adult head is only about one eighth the total height. The facial bones also show several changes between infancy and adulthood. In an infant the face is one eighth of the skull surface, but in an adult the face is half of the skull surface. Another change in proportion involves the trunk and lower extremities. The legs become proportionately longer and the trunk proportionately shorter. In addition, the thoracic and abdominal contours change, roughly speaking, from round to elliptical.

Such changes are good examples of the ever-changing and ongoing nature of growth and development. It is unfortunate that many of the changes that occur in the later years of life do not result in increased function. These degenerative changes are certainly important, however, and will be discussed later in this chapter. The following are the most common postnatal periods: (1) **infancy,** (2) **childhood,** (3) **adolescence and adulthood,** and (4) **older adulthood.**

FIGURE 21-10

The neonate infant. The umbilical cord has been cut.

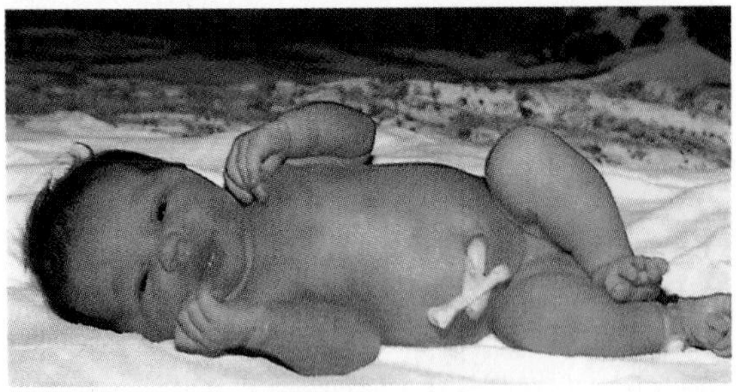

Infancy

The period of infancy begins abruptly at birth and lasts about 18 months. The first 4 weeks of infancy are often referred to as the **neonatal** (nee-o-NAY-tal) **period** (Figure 21-10). Dramatic changes occur at a rapid rate during this short but critical period. **Neonatology** (nee-o-nay-TOL-o-jee) is the medical and nursing specialty concerned with the diagnosis and treatment of disorders of the newborn. Advances in this area have resulted in dramatically reduced infant mortality.

Many of the changes that occur in the cardiovascular and respiratory systems at birth are necessary for survival. Whereas the fetus totally depended on the mother for life support, the newborn infant must become totally self-supporting in terms of blood circulation and respiration immediately after birth. A baby's first breath is deep and forceful. The stimulus to breathe results primarily from the increasing amounts of carbon dioxide (CO_2) that accumulate in the blood after the umbilical cord is cut following delivery.

Many developmental changes occur between the end of the neonatal period and 18 months of age. Birth weight doubles during the first 4 months and then triples by 1 year. The baby also increases in length by 50% by the 12th month. The "baby fat" that accumulated under the skin during the first year begins to decrease, and the plump infant becomes leaner.

Early in infancy the baby has only one spinal curvature (see Figure 6-11). The lumbar curvature appears between 12 and 18 months, and the once-helpless infant becomes a toddler who can stand (Figure 21-11). One of the most striking changes to occur during infancy is the rapid development of the nervous and muscular systems. This permits the infant to follow a moving object with the eyes (2 months); lift the head and raise the chest (3 months); sit when well supported (4 months); crawl (10 months); stand alone (12 months); and run, although a bit stiffly (18 months).

FIGURE 21-11

Normal lumbar curvature of a toddler's spine.

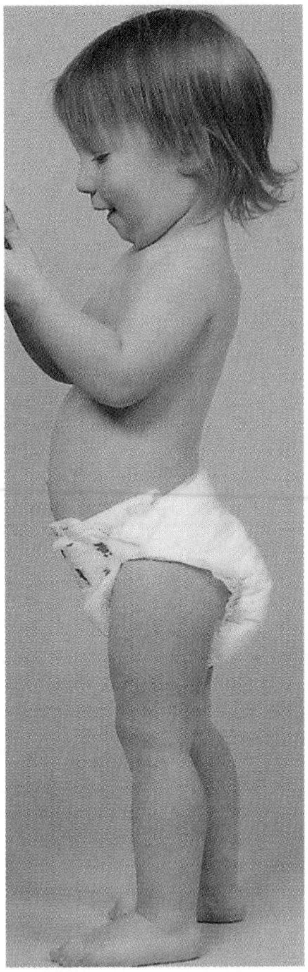

Childhood

Childhood extends from the end of infancy to sexual maturity or puberty—12 to 14 years in girls and 14 to 16 years in boys. Overall, growth during

Research, Issues & Trends

Freezing Umbilical Cord Blood

The concept of development of blood cells from red bone marrow, a process called hemopoiesis, was introduced in Chapter 11. Ultimately, the presence of **"stem cells"** is required for bone marrow to produce blood cells. The fact that umbilical cord blood is rich in these stem cells has great clinical significance.

In the past, if the stem cells in the bone marrow of a child were destroyed as a result of leukemia or by chemotherapy, death would result unless a bone marrow transplant was possible. Infusion of stored umbilical cord blood obtained from the child at the time of birth is an attractive alternative. The blood is rich in stem cells and can be obtained without risk; this procedure is much more cost-effective than a bone marrow transplant.

Removing and freezing umbilical cord blood at the time of birth may become a type of biological insurance against some types of leukemia that may affect a child later in life. Cord blood is readily available at birth and is a better source of stem cells than bone marrow.

After the umbilical cord is cut after birth, the blood that remains in the cord is simply drained into a sterile bag (see photo), frozen, and then stored in liquid nitrogen in one of about a dozen cord-blood centers in the United States.

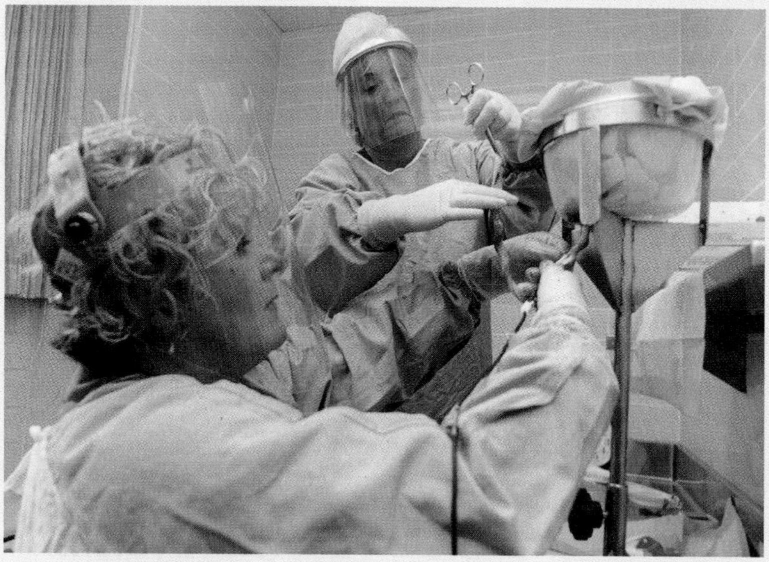

early childhood continues at a rather rapid pace, but month-to-month gains become less consistent. By the age of 6 the child appears more like a preadolescent than an infant or toddler. The child becomes less chubby, the potbelly becomes flatter, and the face loses its babyish look. The nervous and muscular systems continue to develop rapidly during the middle years of childhood; by 10 years of age, the child has developed numerous motor and coordination skills.

The *deciduous teeth,* which began to appear at about 6 months of age, are lost during childhood, beginning at about 6 years of age. The permanent teeth, with the possible exception of the third molars or wisdom teeth, have all erupted by age 14.

Adolescence and Adulthood

The average age range of adolescence varies, but generally the teenage years (13 to 19) are used. The period is marked by rapid and intense physical growth, which ultimately results in sexual maturity. Many of the developmental changes that occur during this period are controlled by the secretion of

Research, Issues & Trends

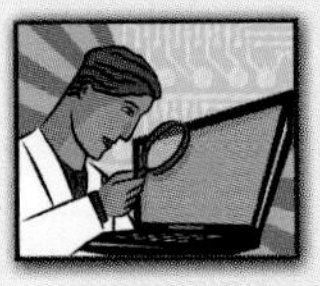

Fetal Alcohol Syndrome

Consumption of alcohol during pregnancy can have tragic effects on a developing fetus. Educational efforts to inform pregnant women about the dangers of alcohol use are now receiving national attention. Even very limited consumption of alcohol during pregnancy poses significant hazards to the developing baby because alcohol can easily cross the placental barrier and enter the fetal bloodstream.

When alcohol enters the fetal blood, the potential result, called **fetal alcohol syndrome (FAS),** can cause tragic congenital abnormalities such as "small head" or **microcephaly** (my-kro-SEF-ah-lee), low birth weight, developmental disabilities such as mental retardation, and even fetal death.

sex hormones and are classified as **secondary sex characteristics.** Breast development is often the first sign of approaching puberty in girls, beginning about age 10. Most girls begin to menstruate at 12 to 13 years of age, which is about 3 years earlier than a century ago. In boys the first sign of puberty is often enlargement of the testicles, which begins between 10 and 13 years of age. Both sexes show a spurt in height during adolescence. In girls the spurt in height begins between the ages of 10 and 12 and is nearly complete by 14 or 15. In boys the period of rapid growth begins between 12 and 13 and is generally complete by 16.

Many developmental changes that began early in childhood are not completed until the early or middle years of **adulthood.** Examples include the maturation of bone, resulting in the full closure of the growth plates, and changes in the size and placement of other body components such as the sinuses. Many body traits do not become apparent for years after birth. Normal balding patterns, for example, are determined at the time of fertilization by heredity but do not appear until maturity. As a general rule, adulthood is characterized by maintenance of existing body tissues. With the passage of years the ongoing effort of maintenance and repair of body tissues become more and more difficult. As a result, degeneration begins. It is the process of aging, and it culminates in death.

Older Adulthood

Most body systems are in peak condition and function at a high level of efficiency during the early years of adulthood. As a person grows older, a gradual but certain decline takes place in the functioning of every major organ system in the body. The study of aging is called *gerontology*. The remainder of this chapter deals with a number of the more common degenerative changes that frequently characterize **senescence** (se-NES-ens) or older adulthood. Many of the biological changes associated with advancing age are shown in Figure 21-12. The illustration highlights the proportion of remaining function in a number of organs in older adulthood when compared with a 21-year-old person.

Quick Check

1. Do the proportions of the human body change during postnatal development?
2. What is the neonatal period of development? Senescence?
3. During which phase of development do the deciduous teeth appear?
4. What biological changes happen during puberty?

EFFECTS OF AGING

Skeletal System

In older adulthood, bones undergo changes in texture, degree of calcification, and shape. Instead of clean-cut margins, older bones develop indistinct and shaggy-appearing margins with spurs—a process called *lipping*. This type of degenerative change restricts movement because of the piling up of bone tissue around the joints. With advancing age, changes in calcification may result in reduction of bone size and in bones that are porous and subject to fracture. The lower cervical and thoracic vertebrae are the site of frequent fractures. The result is curvature of the spine and the shortened stature so typical of late adulthood. Degenerative joint diseases such as **osteoarthritis** (OS-tee-o-ar-THRYE-tis) are also common in elderly adults.

FIGURE 21-12

Some biological changes associated with maturity and aging. Insets show proportion of remaining function in the organs of a person in late adulthood compared with that of a 20 year old.

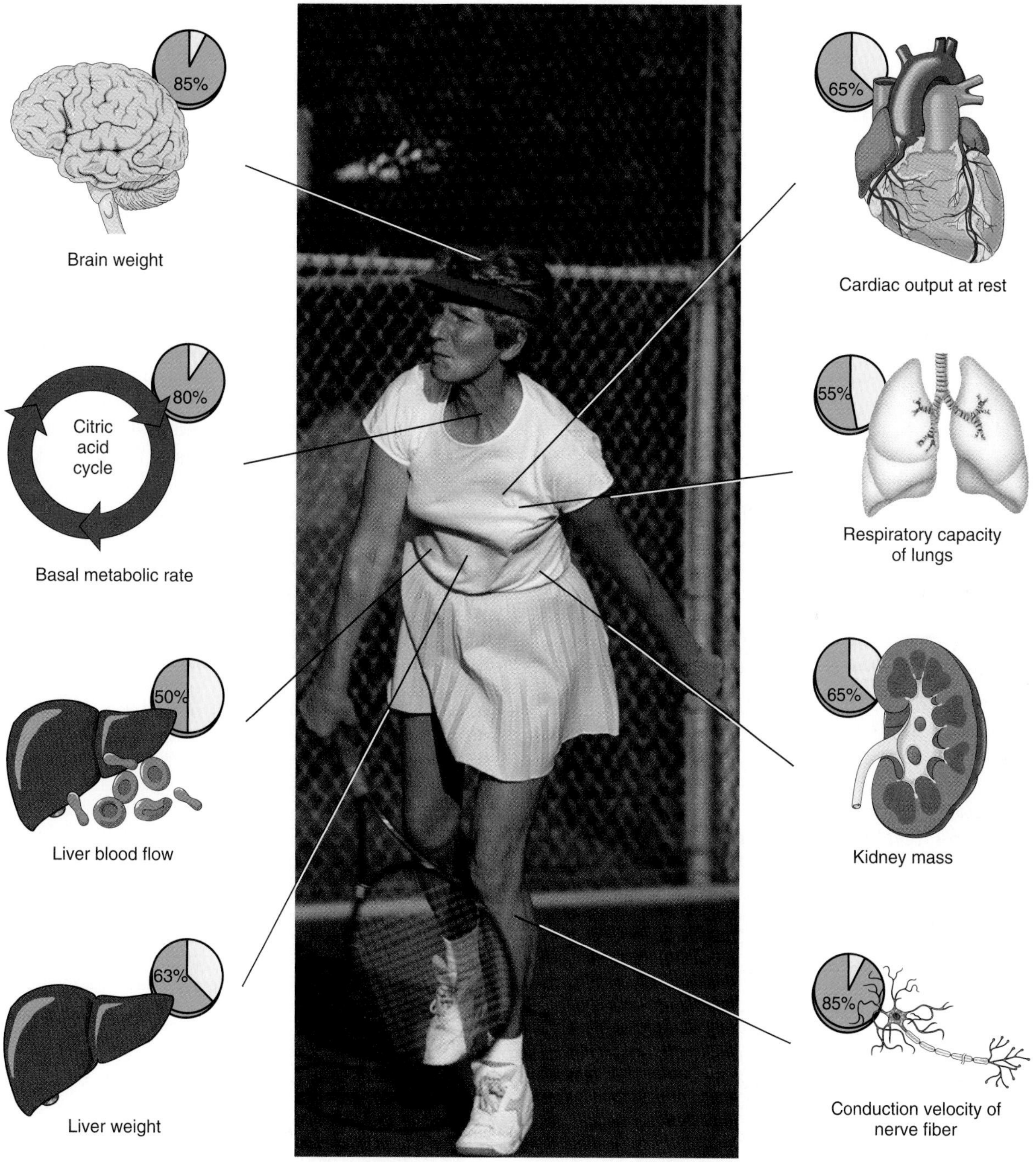

Integumentary System (Skin)

With advancing age the skin becomes dry, thin, and inelastic. It "sags" on the body because of increased wrinkling and skinfolds. Pigmentation changes and the thinning or loss of hair are also common problems associated with the aging process.

Urinary System

The number of nephron units in the kidney decreases by almost 50% between the ages of 30 and 75. Also, because less blood flows through the kidneys as an individual ages, there is a reduction in overall function and excretory capacity or the ability to produce urine. In the bladder, significant age-related problems often occur because of diminished muscle tone. Muscle atrophy (wasting) in the bladder wall results in decreased capacity and inability to empty or void completely.

Respiratory System

In older adulthood the costal cartilages that connect the ribs to the sternum become hardened or calcified. This makes it difficult for the rib cage to expand and contract as it normally does during inspiration and expiration. In time the ribs gradually become "fixed" to the sternum, and chest movements become difficult. When this occurs the rib cage remains in a more expanded position, respiratory efficiency decreases, and a condition called "barrel chest" results. With advancing years a generalized atrophy or wasting of muscle tissue takes place as the contractile muscle cells are replaced by connective tissue. This loss of muscle cells decreases the strength of the muscles associated with inspiration and expiration.

Cardiovascular System

Degenerative heart and blood vessel disease is one of the most common and serious effects of aging. Fatty deposits build up in blood vessel walls and narrow the passageway for the movement of blood, much as the buildup of scale in a water pipe decreases flow and pressure. The resulting condition, called **atherosclerosis** (ath-er-o-skle-RO-sis), often leads to eventual blockage of the coronary arteries and a "heart attack." If fatty accumulations or other substances in blood vessels calcify, actual hardening of the arteries or **arte-**

Science Applications

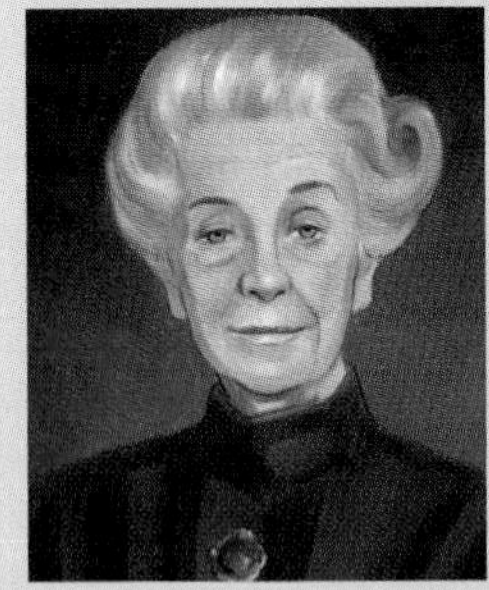

Embryology

Rita Levi-Montalcini (b. 1909).

Rita Levi-Montalcini had just finished a medical degree in her native Italy when in 1938 the Fascist government under Mussolini barred all "non-Aryans" from working in academic and professional careers. Being Jewish, Levi-Montalcini was forced to move to Belgium to work. But when Belgium was about to be invaded by the Nazis, she decided to return home to Italy and work in secret. Her home laboratory was very crude but in it she made some important discoveries about how the nervous system develops during embryonic development. After World War II, she was invited to Washington University in St. Louis to work. There, she discovered the existence of *nerve growth factor (NGF)*, for which she later won the 1986 Nobel Prize. Her discovery of a chemical that regulates the growth of new nerves during early brain development has led to many different paths of investigation. For example, by learning more about growth regulators we now know more about how the nervous system develops and also other tissues, organs, and systems of the body.

Today, many professions make use of the discoveries of embryology—the study of early development. Not only are these discoveries important for health professionals such as obstetricians, obstetric nurses, and others involved in prenatal health care, they are also important in understanding adult medicine as well. In fact, even gerontology (study of aging) and geriatrics (treatment of the aged) have benefited from embryological research. How? By providing insights on how tissue development is regulated in the embryo, scientists can better understand how to possibly stimulate damaged tissue in older adults to repair or regenerate themselves.

riosclerosis (ar-te-ree-o-skle-RO-sis) occurs. Rupture of a hardened vessel in the brain (stroke) is a frequent cause of serious disability or death in the older adult. **Hypertension** or high blood pressure is also more common.

Special Senses

The sense organs, as a group, all show a gradual decline in performance and capacity as a person ages. Most people are farsighted by age 65 because eye lenses become hardened and lose elasticity; the lenses cannot become curved to accommodate for near vision. This hardening of the lens is called **presbyopia** (pres-bee-O-pee-ah), which means "old eye." Many individuals first notice the change at about 40 or 45 years of age, when it becomes difficult to do close-up work or read without holding printed material at arm's length. This explains the increased need, with advancing age, for bifocals or glasses that incorporate two lenses to automatically accommodate for near and distant vision. Loss of transparency of the lens or its covering capsule is another common age-related eye change. If the lens actually becomes cloudy and significantly impairs vision, it is called a **cataract** (KAT-ah-rakt) and must be removed surgically. The incidence of **glaucoma** (glaw-KO-mah), the most serious age-related eye disorder, increases with age. Glaucoma causes an increase in the pressure within the eyeball and, unless treated, often results in blindness.

In many elderly people a very significant loss of hair cells in the organ of Corti (inner ear) causes a serious decline in the ability to hear certain frequencies. In addition, the eardrum and attached ossicles become more fixed and less able to transmit mechanical sound waves. Some degree of hearing impairment is universally present in the older adult.

The sense of taste is also decreased. This loss of appetite may be caused, at least in part, by the replacement of taste buds with connective tissue cells. Only about 40% of the taste buds present at age 30 remain in an individual at age 75.

Quick

1. What are some changes that occur in the skeleton as one ages?
2. How is kidney function affected during old age?
3. What changes in the cardiovascular system occur in older adults?
4. How does one's eyesight change during late adulthood?

Research, Issues & Trends

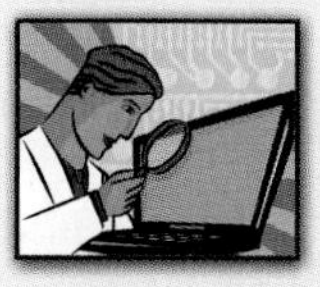

Extending the Human Lifespan

When reviewing the last edition of this textbook, a colleague of ours said that ending with the depressing topic of "degeneration associated with aging" was not appropriate to the overall upbeat tone of our book. At first we thought our ending was better than the most obvious and technically accurate ending: "then you die." But it occurred to us that we could take this opportunity to point out one of the most remarkable and important areas of achievement in modern medical research—extending the length and improving the quality of life.

In the past few decades, the increased availability of better food, safer surroundings, and advanced medical care has extended quality living for many around the world. But even simple changes in lifestyle, regardless of modern medical wonders, can keep the effects of aging from creeping up too soon. Perhaps the three most important "low-tech" methods for improving the quality of life as you age are healthful diet, exercise, and stress management. A healthful diet is not available to some individuals, but it is available to most of us. We are learning more every day about what kind of diet is best, even to the point of being able to manage specific diseases through diet. Exercise performed on a regular basis, even if light or moderate, can keep not only our skeletal and muscular systems more fit but also decreases aging's effects in the nervous system, endocrine system, digestive system, immune system—the list seems endless. And last, even ancient and simple techniques of stress management such as meditation have been shown to help reduce the effects of aging and the diseases that often accompany aging such as heart disease and strokes.

So to end this chapter, and this book, we say: you can stay young if you *eat right*, *exercise*, and *relax*. And keep studying human structure and function so you'll know that you are doing it right!

OUTLINE SUMMARY

A. Prenatal period begins at conception and continues until birth (about 39 weeks)
B. Science of fetal growth and development called *embryology*
C. Fertilization to implantation requires about 10 days
  1. Fertilization normally occurs in outer third of oviduct (Figure 21-2)
  2. Fertilized ovum called a *zygote;* zygote is genetically complete—all that is needed for expression of hereditary traits is time and nourishment
  3. After 3 days of cell division, the zygote has developed into a solid cell mass called a *morula*
  4. Continued cell divisions of the morula produce a hollow ball of cells called a *blastocyst*
  5. Blastocyst implants in the uterine wall about 10 days after fertilization
  6. Blastocyst forms the amniotic cavity and chorion of the placenta (Figure 21-4)
  7. Placenta provides for exchange of nutrients between the mother and fetus
D. Periods of development
  1. Length of pregnancy or gestation period is about 39 weeks
  2. Embryonic phase extends from the third week after fertilization to the end of week 8 of gestation
  3. Fetal phase extends from week 8 to week 39 of gestation
E. Three primary germ layers appear in the developing embryo after implantation of the blastocyst (Table 21-1):
  1. Endoderm—inside layer
  2. Ectoderm—outside layer
  3. Mesoderm—middle layer
  4. All organ systems are formed and functioning by month 4 of gestation (Figure 21-6)
F. Histogenesis and organogenesis
  1. Formation of new organs and tissues occurs from specific development of the primary germ layers
  2. Each primary germ layer gives rise to definite structures such as the skin and muscles
  3. Growth processes include cell differentiation, multiplication, growth, and rearrangement
  4. From 4 months of gestation until delivery, the development of the baby is mainly a matter of growth
G. Birth defects
  1. Any structural or functional abnormality present at birth
  2. May be caused by genetic factors
    a. Abnormal genes
    b. Abnormal number of chromosomes
  3. May be caused by environmental factors
    a. Environmental factors are called teratogens
    b. Include radiation, chemicals, and infections
    c. Especially harmful during the first trimester (Figure 21-7)

BIRTH OR PARTURITION

A. Process of birth called *parturition* (Figure 21-8)
  1. At the end of week 39 of gestation, the uterus becomes "irritable"
  2. Fetus takes head-down position against the cervix
  3. Muscular contractions begin, and labor is initiated
  4. Amniotic sac ("bag of waters") ruptures
  5. Cervix dilates
  6. Fetus moves through vagina to exterior
B. Stages of labor
  1. Stage one—period from onset of uterine contractions until dilation of the cervix is complete
  2. Stage two—period from the time of maximal cervical dilation until the baby exits through the vagina
  3. Stage three—process of expulsion of the placenta through the vagina

OUTLINE SUMMARY—*cont'd*

POSTNATAL PERIOD

A. Postnatal period begins at birth and lasts until death

B. Divisions of postnatal period into isolated time frames can be misleading; life is a continuous process; growth and development are continuous

C. Obvious changes in the physical appearance of the body in—whole and in proportion—occur between birth and maturity (Figure 21-9)

D. Divisions of postnatal period
1. Infancy
2. Childhood
3. Adolescence and adulthood
4. Older adulthood

E. Infancy
1. First 4 weeks called *neonatal period* (Figure 21-10)
2. Neonatology—medical and nursing specialty concerned with the diagnosis and treatment of disorders of the newborn
3. Many cardiovascular changes occur at the time of birth; fetus is totally dependent on mother, whereas the newborn must immediately become totally self-supporting (respiration and circulation)
4. Respiratory changes at birth include a deep and forceful first breath
5. Developmental changes between the neonatal period and 18 months include:
   - **a.** Doubling of birth weight by 4 months and tripling by 1 year
   - **b.** 50% increase in body length by 12 months
   - **c.** Development of normal spinal curvature by 15 months (Figure 21-11)
   - **d.** Ability to raise head by 3 months
   - **e.** Ability to crawl by 10 months
   - **f.** Ability to stand alone by 12 months
   - **g.** Ability to run by 18 months

F. Childhood
1. Extends from end of infancy to puberty—13 years in girls and 15 in boys
2. Overall rate of growth remains rapid but decelerates
3. Continuing development of motor and coordination skills
4. Loss of deciduous or baby teeth and eruption of permanent teeth

G. Adolescence and adulthood
1. Average age range of adolescence varies from 13 to 19 years
2. Period of rapid growth resulting in sexual maturity (adolescence)
3. Appearance of secondary sex characteristics regulated by secretion of sex hormones
4. Growth spurt typical of adolescence; begins in girls at about 10 and in boys at about 12
5. Growth plates fully close in adult; other structures such as the sinuses acquire adult placement
6. Adulthood characterized by maintenance of existing body tissues
7. Degeneration of body tissue begins in adulthood

H. Older adulthood (Figure 21-12)
1. Degenerative changes characterize older adulthood or senescence
2. Every organ system of the body undergoes degenerative changes
3. Senescence culminates in death

EFFECTS OF AGING

A. Skeletal system
1. Aging causes changes in the texture, calcification, and shape of bones
2. Bone spurs develop around joints
3. Bones become porous and fracture easily
4. Degenerative joint diseases such as osteoarthritis are common

B. Integumentary system (skin)
1. With age, skin "sags" and becomes:
   - **a.** Thin
   - **b.** Dry
   - **c.** Wrinkled

Continued

OUTLINE SUMMARY—*cont'd*

   2. Pigmentation problems are common
   3. Frequent thinning or loss of hair occurs
C. Urinary system
   1. Nephron units decrease in number by 50% between ages 30 and 75
   2. Blood flow to kidney and therefore ability to form urine decreases
   3. Bladder problems such as inability to void completely are caused by muscle wasting in the bladder wall
D. Respiratory system
   1. Calcification of costal cartilages causes rib cage to remain in expanded position—barrel chest
   2. Wasting of respiratory muscles decreases respiratory efficiency
   3. Respiratory membrane thickens; movement of oxygen from alveoli to blood is slowed
E. Cardiovascular system
   1. Degenerative heart and blood vessel disease is among the most common and serious effects of aging
   2. Fat deposits in blood vessels (atherosclerosis) decrease blood flow to the heart and may cause complete blockage of the coronary arteries
   3. Hardening of arteries (arteriosclerosis) may result in rupture of blood vessels, especially in the brain (stroke)
   4. Hypertension or high blood pressure is common in older adulthood
F. Special senses
   1. All sense organs show a gradual decline in performance with age
   2. Eye lenses become hard and cannot accommodate for near vision; result is farsightedness in many people by age 45 (presbyopia or "old eye")
   3. Loss of transparency of lens or cornea is common (cataract)
   4. Glaucoma (increase in pressure in eyeball) is often the cause of blindness in older adulthood
   5. Loss of hair cells in inner ear produces frequency deafness in many older people
   6. Decreased transmission of sound waves caused by loss of elasticity of eardrum and fixing of the bony ear ossicles is common in older adulthood
   7. Some degree of hearing impairment is universally present in the aged
   8. Only about 40% of the taste buds present at age 30 remain at age 75

NEW WORDS

amniotic cavity
arteriosclerosis
atherosclerosis
blastocyst
cataract
chorion
ectoderm
embryology
endoderm
fertilization
gerontology
gestation
glaucoma
histogenesis
implantation
mesoderm
morula
neonate
neonatology
organogenesis
osteoarthritis
parturition
placenta
presbyopia
primary germ layers
quickening
senescence
teratogen
yolk sac
zygote

REVIEW QUESTIONS

1. Explain what occurs between ovulation and the implantation of the fertilized egg into the uterus.
2. Explain the function of the chorion and placenta.
3. Name the three primary germ layers, and name three structures that develop from each layer.
4. Define *histogenesis* and *organogenesis.*
5. Describe and give the approximate length of the three stages of labor.
6. What is the stimulus for the baby's first breath?
7. Name three developmental changes that occur during infancy.
8. Briefly explain what occurs during childhood.
9. Briefly explain what occurs during adolescence.
10. Briefly explain what occurs during adulthood.
11. Explain the effects of aging on the skeletal system.
12. Explain the effects of aging on the respiratory system.
13. Explain the effects of aging on the cardiovascular system.
14. Explain the effects of aging on vision.

CRITICAL THINKING

15. Where do the nutrients used by the zygote from fertilization to implantation come from?
16. Explain the evolution of the function of the yolk sac.
17. What hormones are produced by the placenta? What is their function?

CHAPTER TEST

1. The fertilized ovum is called a _________.
2. After about 3 days of mitosis, the fertilized ovum forms a solid mass of cells called the _________.
3. Mitosis continues, and by the time the developing egg reaches the uterus, it has become a solid ball of cells called the _________.
4. The _________ anchors the developing fetus to the uterus and provides a bridge for exchanging of substances between mother and baby.
5. The _________ period lasts about 39 weeks and is divided into trimesters.
6. The three primary germ layers are the _________, _________, and the _________.
7. The process by which the primary germ layers develop into tissues is called _________.
8. The process by which tissues develop into organs is called _________.
9. The process of birth is called _________.
10. The first 4 weeks of infancy is referred to as the _________ period.
11. _________ is a degenerative joint disease that is common in older adults.
12. _________ is another name for "hardening of the arteries."
13. _________ means "old eye" and causes older adults to be farsighted.
14. If the lens of the eye becomes cloudy and impairs vision, the condition is called a _________.
15. _________ causes an increase in pressure within the eyeball.

Continued

CHAPTER TEST—*cont'd*

Match the statement in Column B with the correct term in Column A.

COLUMN A	COLUMN B
16. ______ Infancy	**a.** the deciduous teeth are lost during this period
17. ______ Childhood	**b.** closure of the bone growth plates occurs during this period
18. ______ Adolescence	**c.** this period begins at birth
19. ______ Adulthood	**d.** senescence
20. ______ Older adulthood	**e.** the secondary sex characteristics usually begin to develop during this period

STUDY TIPS

The early developmental stages can be put on flash cards. You might also want to include on the flash card where in the developmental sequence the particular stage is, in other words, what it developed from. Remember to include the functions of the amnion, chorion, and placenta. The term *germ* in *primary germ layer* refers to "germinate." All the structures of the body come from one of these layers. They are named based on their location in the developing embryo. *Endoderm* means inner skin, *mesoderm* means middle skin, and *ectoderm* means outer skin. Use flash cards to match the primary germ layers and the structures that come from each of them. *Genesis* means to create. *Histogenesis* means to create tissues, and *organogenesis* means to create organs. The stages of labor, the important events in the postnatal periods, and the effects of aging on various organ systems can be put on flash cards also.

In your study group, go over the flash cards of the stages of development, making sure you know the proper sequence. Go over the flash cards for the primary germ layers and what organs come from each layer. Review the flash cards for the stages of labor, postnatal periods, and effects of aging. Study the questions at the end of the chapter and discuss possible test questions.

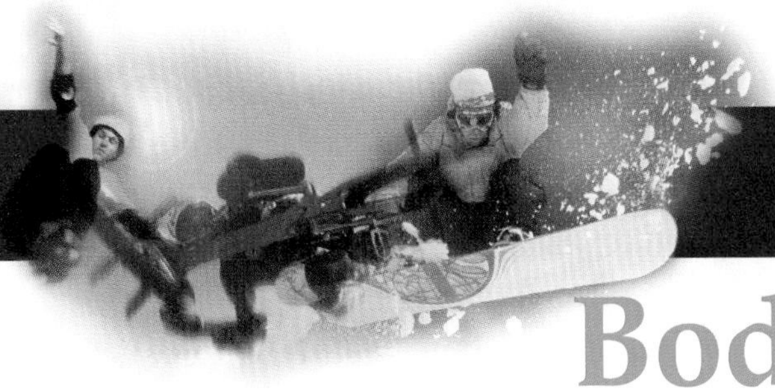

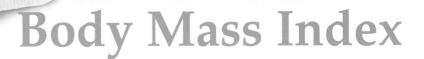

Body Mass Index

Are you a healthy weight? One way that researchers and health professionals use to determine whether you are overweight is called the *body mass index (BMI).* Here is how to calculate your BMI:

1. divide your weight (kg) by your height (m);*
2. multiply your answer from step 1 by itself (that is, square your answer in step 1).

An even easier way is use the diagram shown here. Simply find your weight along the bottom of the graph and go straight up from that point to the horizontal line that is closest to your height. That point is at your BMI. If it is in the 18.5-25 range, you are a healthy weight, according to current research. If it is in the 25-30 range, you are considered to be "overweight" and at a greater than normal risk for health problems such as heart disease and cancer. In the range higher than 30, you are considered to be "obese" and at a very high risk for health problems.

---

* kg is kilograms (to find your weight in kilograms, divide your weight in pounds by 2.2); m is meters (to find your height in meters, divide your height in inches by 39.4)

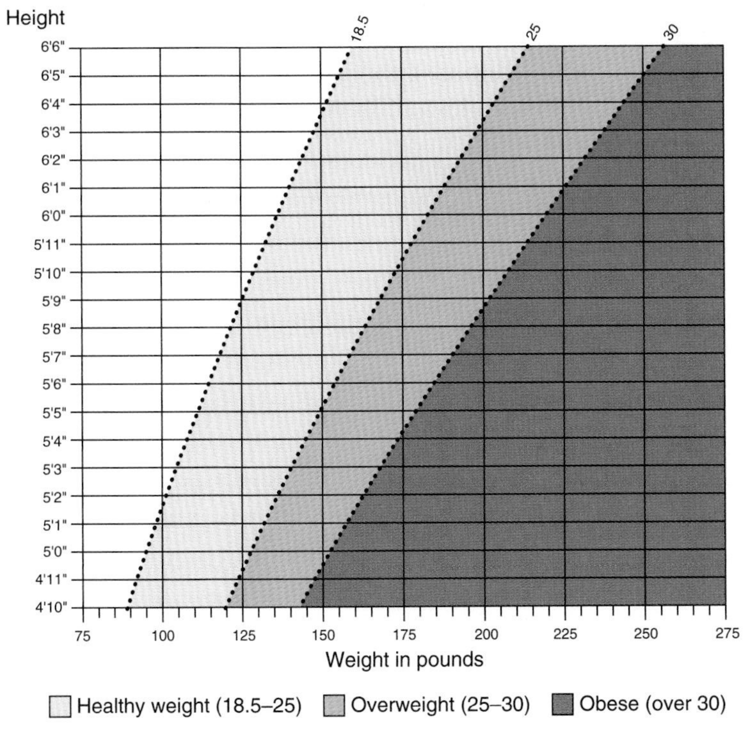

Body mass index chart. (Adapted from the Report of the Dietary Guidelines Advisory Committee on the Dietary Guidelines for Americans, 2000.)

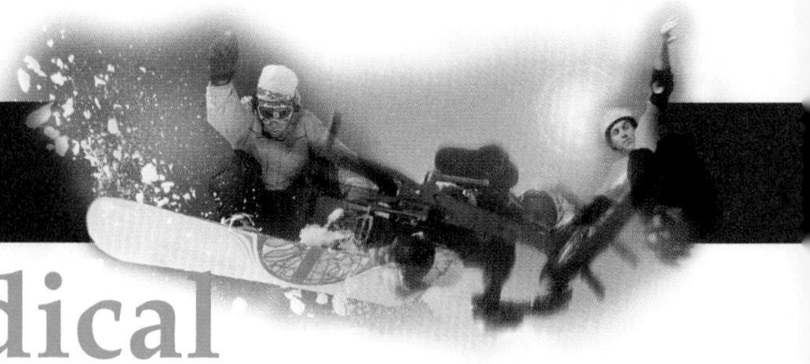

Common Medical Abbreviations, Prefixes, and Suffixes

Abbreviations

aa of each
ā.c̄. before meals
ad lib. as much as desired
alb. albumin
AM before noon
amt. amount
ante before
aq. water
AV. average
Ba barium
b.i.d. twice a day
b.m. bowel movement
BMR basal metabolic rate
BP blood pressure
BRP bathroom privileges
BUN blood urea nitrogen
c̄ with
CBC complete blood cell count
CCU coronary care unit
CHF congestive heart failure
CNS central nervous system
Co cobalt
CVA cerebrovascular accident, stroke
D & C dilation and curettage
d/c discontinue
DOA dead on arrival
Dx diagnosis
ECG electrocardiogram
EDC expected date of confinement
EEG electroencephalogram
EENT ear, eye, nose, throat
EKG electrocardiogram
ER emergency room
FUO fever of undetermined origin
GI gastrointestinal
GP general practitioner
GU genitourinary
h. hour
HCT hematocrit
Hb hemoglobin
H_2O water
h.s. at bedtime
ICU intensive care unit
KUB kidney, ureter, and bladder
MI myocardial infarction
non rep. do not repeat
NPO nothing by mouth
OR operating room
p.c. after meals
per by
PH past history
PI previous illness
PM after noon
p.r.n. as needed
q. every
q.d. every day
q.h. every hour
q.i.d. four times a day
q.n.s. quantity not sufficient
q.o.d. every other day
q.s. quantity required or sufficient
RBC red blood cell
℞ prescription
s̄ without
sp. gr. specific gravity

s̄s one half
stat. at once, immediately
T & A tonsillectomy and adenoidectomy
T.B. tuberculosis
t.i.d. three times a day
TPR temperature, pulse, respiration
TUR transurethral resection
WBC white blood cell

Prefixes

A prefix is a word part used at the *beginning* of a term and describes or alters the meaning of the word part(s) that follow the prefix. For example, *an-* means "without" so *anuria* means "without urine" or the condition of having no urine output.

a- without
ab- away from
ad- to, toward
adeno- glandular
amphi- on both sides
an- without
ante- before, forward
anti- against
bi- two, double, twice
circum- around, about
contra- opposite, against
de- away from, from
di- double
dia- across, through
dis- separate from, apart
dys- difficult
e- out, away
ecto- outside
en- in
endo- in, inside
epi- on
eu- well
ex- from, out of, away from
exo- outside
extra- outside, beyond; in addition
hemi- half
hyper- over, excessive, above
hypo- under, deficient
infra- underneath, below
inter- between, among
intra- within, on the side
intro- into, within
iso- equal, like
para- beside
peri- around, beyond
post- after, behind
pre- before, in front of
pro- before, in front of
re- again
retro- backward, back
semi- half
sub- under, beneath
super- above, over
supra- above, on the upper side
syn- with, together
trans- across, beyond
ultra- excessive

Suffixes

A suffix is a word part used at the *end* of a term and describes or alters the meaning of the word part(s) that come before the suffix. For example, *-ectomy* means "cut out" so *appendectomy* means "appendix cut out" or the procedure of surgically removing the appendix.

-algia pain, painful
-asis condition
-blast young cell
-cele swelling
-centesis puncture for aspiration
-cide killer
-cyte cell
-ectomy cut out
-emia blood
-genesis production, development
-itis inflammation
-kin in motion, action
-logy study of
-megaly enlargement
-odynia pain
-oid resembling
-oma tumor
-osis condition
-opathy disease
-penia abnormal reduction
-pexy fixation
-phagia eating, swallowing
-phasia speaking condition
-phobia fear
-plasty plastic surgery
-plegia paralysis
-poiesis formation
-ptosis downward displacement
-rhaphy suture
-scope instrument for examination
-scopy examination
-stomy creation of an opening
-tomy incision
-uria urine

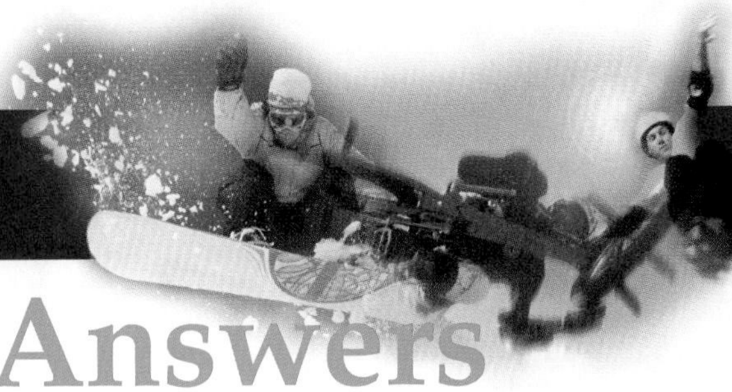

Chapter Test Answers

Chapter 1

1. anatomy
2. physiology
3. chemical, cell, tissue, organ, organ system
4. prone, supine
5. transverse
6. frontal
7. sagittal
8. midsagittal
9. axial
10. appendicular
11. c
12. b
13. d
14. d
15. b
16. e
17. d
18. a
19. c
20. b

Chapter 2

1. matter
2. atoms
3. protons
4. energy
5. compounds
6. covalent
7. ion
8. electrolyte
9. organic
10. solvent
11. dehydration synthesis
12. acids
13. buffers
14. d
15. f
16. g
17. e
18. a
19. c
20. b
21. c
22. a
23. d
24. b
25. c

Chapter 3

1. phospholipid, cholesterol
2. organelle
3. active transport, passive transport
4. pinocytosis
5. DNA, mRNA
6. translation
7. transcription
8. gene
9. genome
10. epithelial, muscle, nerve, connective
11. a
12. c
13. a
14. b
15. c
16. d
17. g
18. c
19. e
20. i
21. b
22. a
23. d
24. f
25. h

Chapter 4

1. gastrointestinal tract
2. skeletal, striated
3. smooth, visceral
4. nerve impulses
5. hair, nails, glands, sense organs
6. thymus
7. urethra
8. testes, ovaries
9. cartilage, ligament
10. f
11. k
12. a
13. i
14. b
15. g
16. c
17. j
18. d
19. e
20. h

Chapter 5

1. cutaneous, serous, mucous
2. basement membrane
3. parietal pleura
4. visceral peritoneum
5. synovial membrane
6. stratum corneum, stratum germinativum
7. keratin
8. dermal papillae
9. eccrine
10. apocrine
11. sebum
12. protection, sensation, temperature regulation
13. c
14. d
15. a
16. b
17. b
18. d
19. a
20. c

Chapter 6

1. articular cartilage
2. medullary cavity
3. trabeculae
4. Haversian systems
5. lacunae
6. osteoclasts
7. osteoblasts
8. endochondral ossification
9. epiphyseal plate
10. axial, appendicular
11. synarthroses, amphiarthroses, diarthroses
12. ligaments
13. c
14. b
15. a
16. d
17. c
18. b
19. a
20. b
21. d
22. d
23. c
24. d
25. c
26. c
27. d
28. b
29. a
30. d
31. a
32. c
33. a
34. b
35. a

Chapter 7

1. muscle fiber
2. heart
3. insertion
4. origin
5. actin
6. myosin
7. sarcomere
8. movement, posture, heat production
9. ATP
10. lactic acid
11. motor unit
12. threshold stimulus
13. isotonic
14. isometric
15. abduction
16. extension
17. supination

18. b
19. d
20. a
21. b
22. d
23. d
24. a
25. c or b
26. c
27. d
28. a
29. c
30. d
31. b

Chapter 8

1. peripheral nervous system
2. central nervous system
3. nerve
4. neurons, glia
5. reflex arc
6. nerve impulse
7. positive, negative
8. sodium
9. synapse
10. neurotransmitters
11. dura mater, arachnoid layer, pia mater
12. 12, 31
13. dermatome
14. parasympathetic nervous system
15. sympathetic nervous system
16. acetylcholine, norepinephrine
17. acetylcholine, acetylcholine
18. cardiac muscle, smooth muscle, glandular epithelial
19. g
20. c
21. e
22. a
23. b
24. f
25. d
26. d
27. a
28. h
29. f
30. b
31. g
32. e
33. c

Chapter 9

1. chemoreceptors, proprioceptors
2. organ of Corti
3. crista ampullaris
4. taste
5. sweet, sour, bitter, salty
6. papillae
7. olfactory receptors
8. e
9. i
10. j
11. b
12. a
13. g
14. c
15. f
16. h
17. d
18. k
19. f
20. g
21. a
22. b
23. e
24. c
25. d

Chapter 10

1. exocrine
2. endocrine, hormones
3. protein, steroid
4. target organ
5. cyclic AMP (cAMP)
6. on the cell membrane, in the nucleus
7. prostaglandins
8. posterior pituitary (neurohypophysis)
9. anterior pituitary (adenohypophysis)
10. posterior pituitary, hypothalamus
11. d
12. b
13. c
14. b
15. b
16. a
17. d
18. f
19. i
20. a

21. e
22. c
23. h
24. g
25. b

Chapter 11

1. plasma
2. albumin, globulin, fibrinogen
3. serum
4. red blood cells (erythrocytes), white blood cells (leukocytes), platelets (thrombocytes)
5. myeloid, lymphatic
6. hemoglobin
7. anemia
8. polycythemia
9. neutrophils
10. B-lymphocytes
11. calcium
12. fibrinogen, fibrin
13. K
14. thrombus
15. embolus
16. antigen
17. A and B, none (no)
18. B, anti-A
19. O
20. AB
21. erythroblastosis fetalis

Chapter 12

1. ventricles
2. atria
3. myocardium
4. interventricular septum
5. endocardium
6. epicardium
7. systole
8. diastole
9. tricuspid (right atrioventricular)
10. stroke volume
11. sinoatrial node
12. Purkinje fibers
13. QRS complex
14. P wave
15. veins
16. arteries
17. capillaries
18. tunica intima
19. tunica adventitia
20. pulmonary circulation
21. foramen ovale, ductus arteriosus
22. blood viscosity, heart rate
23. a. 7
    b. 2
    c. 3
    d. 6
    e. 10
    f. 8
    g. 9
    h. 5
    i. 1
    j. 4

Chapter 13

1. lymph
2. thoracic duct
3. right lymphatic duct
4. cisterna chyli
5. lymph nodes
6. afferent, efferent
7. T-lymphocytes (T-cells), thymosin
8. palatine, pharyngeal, lingual
9. spleen
10. inflammation
11. complement fixation
12. monocytes
13. c
14. b
15. d
16. a
17. B
18. B
19. T
20. B
21. T
22. T
23. B
24. T
25. B

Chapter 14

1. air distributor, gas exchanger
2. nose, pharynx, larynx
3. trachea, bronchial tree, lungs
4. respiratory membrane
5. respiratory mucosa
6. paranasal sinuses

7. lacrimal
8. conchae
9. pharynx
10. larynx
11. trachea
12. primary bronchi, secondary bronchi, bronchioles, alveolar ducts
13. surfactant
14. 3, 2
15. internal respiration
16. external respiration
17. diaphragm
18. oxyhemoglobin
19. bicarbonate, carbaminohemoglobin
20. medulla
21. stretch receptors
22. chemoreceptors
23. tidal
24. tidal, expiratory reserve, inspiratory reserve
25. residual

Chapter 15

1. digestion, absorption
2. muscularis
3. submucosa
4. mucosa
5. serosa
6. uvula, soft palate
7. crown, neck, root
8. parotid, submandibular, sublingual
9. esophagus
10. fundus, body, pylorus
11. duodenum, jejunum, ileum
12. villi
13. lacteal
14. common hepatic duct, cystic duct
15. transverse colon
16. sigmoid colon
17. mesentery, greater omentum
18. absorption
19. e
20. i
21. j
22. k
23. b
24. l
25. f
26. g
27. d
28. c
29. a
30. h

Chapter 16

1. assimilation
2. catabolism
3. anabolism
4. prothrombin, fibrinogen
5. A, D
6. water, fat
7. total metabolic rate
8. basal metabolic rate
9. total metabolic rate
10. convection
11. evaporation
12. fat metabolism
13. protein
14. nonessential amino acids
15. b
16. d
17. c
18. g
19. a
20. e
21. h
22. f

Chapter 17

1. 20
2. Bowman's capsule, glomerulus
3. loop of Henle, collecting tubule
4. proximal convoluted tubule, distal convoluted tubule
5. reabsorption
6. filtration
7. secretion
8. antidiuretic hormone
9. atrial natriuretic hormone
10. aldosterone
11. internal urethral sphincter
12. suppression
13. incontinence
14. retention
15. g
16. a
17. k
18. b
19. d
20. f
21. j
22. h
23. c
24. e
25. i

Chapter 18

1. interstitial fluid, plasma
2. intracellular fluid
3. less
4. more
5. more
6. fluid output
7. water from catabolism
8. kidneys, skin, lungs, intestines
9. aldosterone, atrial natriuretic hormone
10. ions
11. chloride
12. sodium
13. b
14. c
15. b
16. a

Chapter 19

1. carbonic anhydrase
2. buffers
3. H_2CO_3
4. $NaHCO_3$
5. distal tubule
6. NaH_2PO_4
7. NH_4Cl
8. base
9. alkalosis
10. acidosis
11. 20
12. $NaHCO_3$ (bicarbonate)
13. H_2CO_3
14. alkalosis
15. b
16. a
17. b
18. b
19. decreases
20. increases
21. increases
22. decreases
23. increase
24. decrease

Chapter 20

1. testes
2. scrotum
3. tunica albuginea
4. seminiferous tubule
5. interstitial cells
6. spermatogonium
7. meiosis or spermatogenesis
8. acrosome
9. epididymis
10. ductus deferens (vas deferens)
11. prostate gland
12. seminal vesicles
13. corpora cavernosa
14. ovaries
15. Graafian
16. oogenesis
17. polar bodies
18. uterine tubes (oviducts, fallopian tubes)
19. myometrium
20. cervix
21. endometrium
22. vagina
23. Bartholin's
24. alveoli, lactiferous
25. h
26. c
27. a
28. b
29. d
30. e
31. i
32. g
33. f

Chapter 21

1. zygote
2. morula
3. blastocyst
4. placenta
5. gestation
6. ectoderm, mesoderm, endoderm
7. histogenesis
8. organogenesis
9. parturition
10. neonatal
11. osteoarthritis
12. arteriosclerosis
13. presbyopia
14. cataract
15. glaucoma
16. c
17. a
18. e
19. b
20. d

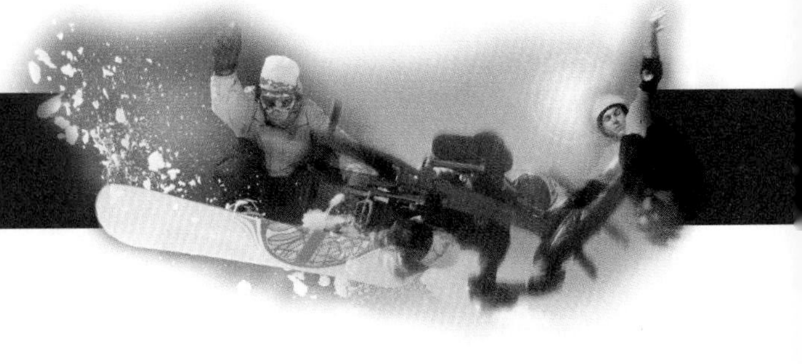

Glossary

A

abdomen (AB-doe-men) body area between the diaphragm and pelvis

abdominal cavity (ab-DOM-i-nal KAV-i-tee) the cavity containing the abdominal organs

abdominal muscles (ab-DOM-i-nal MUS-els) muscles supporting the anterior aspect of the abdomen

abdominal quadrants (ab-DOM-i-nal KWOD-rants) health professionals divide the abdomen (through the navel) into four areas to help locate specific organs

abdominal regions (ab-DOM-i-nal REE-juns) anatomists have divided the abdomen into nine regions to identify the location of organs

abdominopelvic cavity (ab-DOM-i-no-PEL-vik KAV-i-tee) term used to describe the single cavity containing the abdominal and pelvic organs

abduction (ab-DUK-shun) moving away from the midline of the body, opposite motion of adduction

absorption (ab-SORP-shun) passage of a substance through a membrane, such as skin or mucosa, into blood

accessory organ (ak-SES-o-ree OR-gan) an organ that assists other organs in accomplishing their functions

acetabulum (as-e-TAB-yoo-lum) socket in the hip bone (os coxa or innominate bone) into which the head of the femur fits

acetylcholine (as-e-til-KO-lean) chemical neurotransmitter

acid (AS-id) any substance that, when dissolved in water, contributes to an excess of H^- ions (that is, a *low* pH)

acid-base balance (AS-id base BAL-ans) maintaining the concentration of hydrogen ions in body fluids

acidosis (as-i-DOE-sis) condition in which there is an excessive proportion of acid in the blood (and thus an abnormally low blood pH); opposite of alkalosis

acne (AK-nee) a bacterial infection of the skin characterized by red pustules formed when hair follicles become infected

acquired immunity (ah-KWIRED i-MYOO-ni-tee) immunity that is obtained after birth through the use of injections or exposure to a harmful agent

acquired immunodeficiency syndrome (AIDS) (ah-KWIRED i-myoo-no-de-FISH-en-see SIN-drome) disease in which the HIV virus attacks the T cells, thereby compromising the body's immune system

acromegaly (ak-ro-MEG-ah-lee) condition caused by hypersecretion of growth hormone after puberty, resulting in enlargement of facial features (for example, jaw, nose), fingers, and toes

acrosome (AK-ro-sohm) specialized structure on the sperm containing enzymes that break down the covering of the ovum to allow entry

actin (AK-tin) contractile protein found in the thin myofilaments of skeletal muscle

action potential (AK-shun po-TEN-shal) nerve impulse

active transport (AK-tiv TRANS-port) movement of a substance into and out of a living cell requiring the use of cellular energy

Addison's disease (AD-i-sons di-ZEEZ) disease of the adrenal gland resulting in low blood sugar, weight loss, and weakness

adduction (ah-DUK-shun) moving toward the midline of the body, opposite motion of abduction

adenohypophysis (ad-e-no-hye-POF-i-sis) anterior pituitary gland, which has the structure of an endocrine gland

adenoid (AD-e-noyd) literally, glandlike; adenoids, or pharyngeal tonsils, are paired lymphoid structures in the nasopharynx

adenosine diphosphate (ADP) (ah-DEN-o-sen dye-FOS-fate) molecule similar to adenosine triphosphate but containing only two phosphate groups

adenosine triphosphate (ATP) (ah-DEN-o-sen try-FOS-fate) chemical compound that provides energy for use by body cells

adipose (AD-i-pose) fat tissue

adolescence (ad-o-LES-ens) period between puberty and adulthood

adrenal cortex (ah-DREE-nal KOR-teks) outer portion of adrenal gland that secretes hormones called corticoids

adrenal gland (ah-DREE-nal) glands that rest on the top of the kidneys, made up of the cortex and medulla

adrenal medulla (ah-DREE-nal me-DUL-ah) inner portion of adrenal gland that secretes epinephrine and norepinephrine

adrenergic fibers (a-dre-NER-jik FYE-bers) axons whose terminals release norepinephrine and epinephrine

adrenocorticotropic hormone (ACTH) (ah-dree-no-kor-te-ko-TRO-pic HOR-mone) hormone that stimulates the adrenal cortex to secrete larger amounts of hormones

adulthood (ah-DULT-hood) period after adolescence

aerobic respiration (air-O-bik res-pi-RAY-shun) the stage of cellular respiration requiring oxygen

aerobic training (air-O-bik TRAIN-ing) continuous vigorous exercise requiring the body to increase its consumption of oxygen and develop the muscles' ability to sustain activity over a long period

afferent (AF-fer-ent) carrying or conveying toward the center (for example, an afferent neuron carries nerve impulses toward the central nervous system)

agglutinate (ah-GLOO-tin-ate) antibodies causing antigens to clump or stick together

aging process (AJ-ing PROS-es) the gradual degenerative changes that occur after young adulthood as a person ages

AIDS-related complex (ARC) (AIDS ree-LAY-ted KOM-pleks) a more mild form of AIDS that produces fever, weight loss, and swollen lymph nodes

albumin (AL-byoo-min) one of several types of proteins normally found in blood plasma, it helps thicken the blood

aldosterone (AL-doe-ste-rone) hormone that stimulates the kidney to retain sodium ions and water

alimentary canal (al-e-MEN-tar-ee kah-NAL) the digestive tract as a whole

alkaline (AL-kah-lin) base; any substance that, when dissolved in water, contributes to an excess of OH^- ions (thus creating a high pH)

alkalosis (al-kah-LO-sis) condition in which there is an excessive proportion of alkali (base) in the blood, causing an abnormally high blood pH; opposite of acidosis

allergy (AL-er-jee) hypersensitivity of the immune system to relatively harmless environmental antigens

all or none when stimulated, a muscle fiber will contract fully or not at all; whether a contraction occurs depends on whether the stimulus reaches the required threshold

alpha cell (AL-fah sell) pancreatic cell that secretes glucagon

alveolar duct (al-VEE-o-lar dukt) airway that branches from the smallest bronchioles; alveolar sacs arise from alveolar ducts

alveolar sac (al-VEE-o-lar sak) each alveolar duct ends in several sacs that resemble a cluster of grapes

alveolus (al-VEE-o-lus) literally, a small cavity; alveoli of lungs are microscopic saclike dilations of terminal bronchioles

amniotic cavity (am-nee-OT-ik KAV-i-tee) cavity within the blastocyst that will become a fluid-filled sac in which the embryo will float during development

amino acid (ah-MEE-no AS-id) structural units from which proteins are built

amphiarthrosis (am-fee-ar-THRO-sis) slightly movable joint such as the joint joining the two pubic bones

amylase (AM-i-lase) enzyme that digests carbohydrates

anabolic steroid (an-ah-BAHL-ik STARE-oyd) a lipid molecule of the steroid variety that acts as a hormone to stimulate anabolism (specifically protein synthesis) in body tissues such as muscle (example, testosterone)

anabolism (ah-NAB-o-lizm) cells making complex molecules (for example, hormones) from simpler compounds (for example, amino acids), opposite of catabolism

anal canal (AY-nal kah-NAL) terminal portion of the rectum

anaphase (AN-ah-faze) stage of mitosis; duplicate chromosomes move to poles of dividing cell

anaphylactic shock (an-ah-fi-LAK-tik shock) shock resulting from a severe allergic reaction, may be fatal

anatomical position (an-ah-TOM-i-kal po-ZISH-un) the reference position for the body, which gives meaning to directional terms

anatomy (ah-NAT-o-mee) the study of the structure of an organism and the relationships of its parts

androgen (AN-dro-jen) male sex hormone

anemia (ah-NEE-mee-ah) deficient number of red blood cells or deficient hemoglobin

anesthesia (an-es-THEE-zee-ah) loss of sensation

angina pectoris (an-JYE-nah PECK-tor-is) severe chest pain resulting when the myocardium is deprived of sufficient oxygen

angioplasty (AN-jee-o-plas-tee) medical procedure in which vessels occluded by arteriosclerosis ("hardening of arteries") are opened (that is, the channel for blood flow is widened)

angstrom (ANG-strom) unit of length equivalent to 0.0000000001 m (1/10,000,000,000 of a meter or about 1/250,000,000 of an inch)

anion (AN-eye-on) negatively charged particle

anorexia nervosa (an-o-REK-see-ah ner-VO-sah) a behavior involving an irrational fear of being overweight, resulting in severe weight loss from self-starvation

antagonist muscle (an-TAG-o-nist MUS-el) those having opposing actions; for example, muscles that flex the upper arm are antagonists to muscles that extend it

antebrachial (an-tee-BRAY-kee-al) refers to the forearm

antecubital (an-tee-KYOO-bi-tal) refers to the elbow
antenatal medicine (an-tee-NAY-tal MED-i-sin) prenatal medicine
anterior (an-TEER-ee-or) front or ventral; opposite of posterior or dorsal
antibody (AN-ti-bod-ee) substance produced by the body that destroys or inactivates a specific substance (antigen) that has entered the body
antibody-mediated immunity (AN-ti-bod-ee MEE-dee-ate-ed i-MYOO-ni-tee) immunity that is produced when antibodies make antigens unable to harm the body
antidiuretic hormone (ADH) (an-ti-dye-yoo-RET-ik HOR-mone) hormone produced in the posterior pituitary gland to regulate the balance of water in the body by accelerating the reabsorption of water
antigen (AN-ti-jen) substance that, when introduced into the body, causes formation of antibodies against it
antrum (AN-trum) cavity
anuria (ah-NOO-ree-ah) absence of urine
anus (AY-nus) distal end or outlet of the rectum
aorta (ay-OR-tah) main and largest artery in the body
aortic body (ay-OR-tik BOD-ee) small cluster of chemosensitive cells that respond to carbon dioxide and oxygen levels
aortic semilunar valve (ay-OR-tic sem-i-LOO-nar valve) valve between the aorta and left ventricle that prevents blood from flowing back into the ventricle
apex (A-peks) pointed end of a conical structure
apnea (AP-nee-ah) temporary cessation of breathing
apocrine (AP-o-krin) sweat glands located in the axilla and genital regions; these glands enlarge and begin to function at puberty
apoptosis (ap-oh-TOE-sis) programmed cell death by means of several biochemical processes built into each cell; apoptosis clears space for newer cells, as in early embryonic development or in tissue repair
appendicitis (ah-pen-di-SYE-tis) inflammation of the vermiform appendix
appendage (ah-PEN-dij) something that is attached
appendicular (a-pen-DIK-yoo-lar) refers to the upper and lower extremities of the body
appendicular skeleton (a-pen-DIK-yoo-lar SKEL-e-ton) the bones of the upper and lower extremities of the body
aqueous humor (AY-kwee-us HYOO-mor) watery fluid that fills the anterior chamber of the eye, in front of the lens
aqueous (AY-kwee-us) liquid mixture in which water is the solvent; for example, saltwater is an aqueous solution because water is the solvent
arachnoid mater (ah-RAK-noyd MAH-ter) delicate, weblike middle membrane covering the brain, the meninges
areola (ah-REE-o-lah) small space; the pigmented ring around the nipple
areolar (ah-REE-o-lar) a type of connective tissue consisting of fibers and a variety of cells embedded in a loose matrix of soft, sticky gel
arrector pili (ah-REK-tor PYE-lie) smooth muscles of the skin, which are attached to hair follicles; when contraction occurs, the hair stands up, resulting in "goose flesh"
arteriole (ar-TEER-ee-ole) small branch of an artery
artery (AR-ter-ee) vessel carrying blood away from the heart
articular cartilage (ar-TIK-yoo-lar KAR-ti-lij) cartilage covering the joint ends of bones
articulation (ar-tik-yoo-LAY-shun) joint
artificial kidney (ar-ti-FISH-al KID-nee) mechanical device that removes wastes from the blood that would normally be removed by the kidney
artificial pacemaker (ar-ti-FISH-al PAYS-may-ker) an electrical device that is implanted into the heart to treat a heart block
asexual (a-SEKS-yoo-al) one-celled plants and bacteria that do not produce specialized sex cells
assimilation (ah-sim-i-LAY-shun) when food molecules enter the cell and undergo chemical changes
association area (ah-so-shee-AY-shun AIR-ee-ah) region of the cerebral cortex of the brain that functions to put together or associate information from many parts of the brain to help make sense of or analyze the information
astrocyte (AS-tro-site) a glial cell
atherosclerosis (ath-er-o-skle-RO-sis) hardening of the arteries; lipid deposits lining the inside of the arteries
atom (AT-om) smallest particle of a pure substance (element) that still has the chemical properties of that substance; composed of protons, electrons, and neutrons (subatomic particles)
atomic mass (at-AHM-ik mas) combined total number of protons and neutrons in an atom
atomic number (at-AHM-ik NUM-ber) total number of protons in an atom's nucleus; atoms of each element have a characteristic atomic number
atrial natriuretic hormone (ANH) (AY-tree-al na-tree-yoo-RET-ik HOR-mone) hormone secreted by the heart cells that regulates fluid and electrolyte homeostasis
atrioventricular valves (ay-tree-o-ven-TRIK-yoo-lar valvs) two valves that separate the atrial chambers from the ventricles
atrium (AY-tree-um) chamber or cavity; for example, atrium of each side of the heart
atrophy (AT-ro-fee) wasting away of tissue; decrease in size of a part; sometimes referred to as disuse atrophy

auditory tube (AW-di-toe-ree) tube that connects the throat with the middle ear

auricle (AW-ri-kul) part of the ear attached to the side of the head; earlike appendage of each atrium of the heart

autonomic effector (aw-toe-NOM-ik ef-FEK-tor) tissues to which autonomic neurons conduct impulses

autonomic nervous system (ANS) (aw-toe-NOM-ik NER-vus SIS-tem) division of the human nervous system that regulates involuntary actions

autonomic neuron (aw-toe-NOM-ik NOO-ron) motor neurons that make up the autonomic nervous system

AV bundle (A V BUN-dul) fibers in the heart that relay a nerve impulse from the AV node to the ventricles; also known as the bundle of His

avitaminosis (ay-vye-tah-mi-NO-sis) vitamin deficiency

axial (AK-see-al) refers to the head, neck, and torso, or trunk of the body

axial skeleton (AK-see-al SKEL-e-ton) the bones of the head, neck, and torso

axilla (AK-sil-ah) refers to the armpit

axon (AK-son) nerve cell process that transmits impulses away from the cell body

B

B cells (B sells) a lymphocyte; activated B cells develop into plasma cells, which secrete antibodies into the blood

Bartholin's glands (BAR-toe-lins) gland located on either side of the vaginal outlet that secretes mucuslike lubricating fluid; also known as greater vestibular glands

basal ganglia (BAY-sal GANG-glee-ah) see cerebral nuclei

basal metabolic rate (BMR) (BAY-sal met-ah-BOL-ik) number of calories of heat that must be produced per hour by catabolism to keep the body alive, awake, and comfortably warm

base (BAYS) 1. A chemical that, when dissolved in water, reduces the relative concentration of H^+ ions in the whole solution (sometimes by adding OH- ions); 2. In the context of nucleic acids (DNA and RNA), *base* or *nitrogen base* refers to one part of a nucleotide (sugar, phosphate, and base) that is the basic building block of nucleic acid molecules; possible bases include adenine, thymine, guanine, cytosine, and uracil

basement membrane (BASE-ment MEM-brane) the connective tissue layer of the serous membrane that holds and supports the epithelial cells

basophil (BAY-so-fil) white blood cell that stains readily with basic dyes

benign prostatic hypertrophy (be-NINE pros-TAT-ik hye-PER-tro-fee) a noncancerous enlargement of the prostate in older men

benign tumor (be-NINE TOO-mer) a relatively harmless neoplasm

beta cell (BAY-tah sell) pancreatic islet cell that secretes insulin

bicarbonate loading (bye-KAR-bo-nate LOHD-ing) ingesting large amounts of sodium bicarbonate to counteract the effects of lactic acid buildup, thereby reducing fatigue; however, there are potential dangerous side effects

biceps brachii (BYE-seps BRAY-kee-eye) the primary flexor of the forearm

biceps femoris (BYE-seps FEM-o-ris) powerful flexor of the lower leg

bicuspid (bye-KUS-pid) premolars

bicuspid valve (bye-KUS-pid valv) one of the two AV valves, it is located between the left atrium and ventricle and is sometimes called the mitral valve

bile substance that reduces large fat globules into smaller droplets of fat that are more easily broken down

bile duct (dukt) duct that drains bile into the small intestine and is formed by the union of the common hepatic and cystic ducts

biological filtration (bye-o-LOJ-e-kal fil-TRAY-shun) process in which cells alter the contents of the filtered fluid

birth defect (birth DEE-fekt) any abnormality, whether caused by genetic or environmental factors, that exists at birth; see *teratogen*

blackhead (BLACK-hed) when sebum accumulates, darkens, and enlarges some of the ducts of the sebaceous glands; also known as a comedo

bladder (BLAD-der) a sac, usually referring to the urinary bladder

blastocyst (BLAS-toe-sist) postmorula stage of developing embryo; hollow ball of cells

blister (BLIS-ter) a baglike point on the skin caused by some irritant, usually full of fluid

blood-brain barrier (blud brayn BARE-ee-er) two-ply wall formed by the wall of a capillary and the surrounding extensions of a glial cell called an astrocyte; it functions to prevent harmful chemicals from entering vital brain tissue

blood doping (blud DOE-ping) a practice used to improve athletic performance by removing red blood cells weeks before an event and then reinfusing them just before competition to increase the oxygen-carrying capacity of the blood

blood pressure (blud PRESH-ur) pressure of blood in the blood vessels, expressed as systolic pressure/diastolic pressure (for example, 120/80 mm Hg)

blood pressure gradient (blud PRESH-ur GRAY-dee-ent) the difference between two blood pressures in the body

blood types (blud tipes) the different types of blood that are identified by certain antigens in red blood cells (A, B, AB, O, and Rh-negative or Rh-positive)
body (BOD-ee) unified and complex assembly of structurally and functionally interactive components
body composition (BOD-ee com-po-ZISH-un) assessment to identify the percentage of the body that is lean tissue and the percentage that is fat
bolus (BO-lus) a small, rounded mass of masticated food to be swallowed
bone highly specialized connective tissue whose matrix is hard and calcified
bone marrow (MAIR-o) soft material that fills cavities of the bones; red bone marrow is vital to blood cell formation, yellow bone marrow is inactive fatty tissue
bony labyrinth (BONE-ee LAB-i-rinth) the fluid-filled complex maze of three spaces (the vestibule, semicircular canals, and cochlea) in the temporal bone
Bowman's capsule (BO-mens KAP-sul) the cup-shaped top of a nephron that surrounds the glomerulus
brachial (BRAY-kee-al) pertaining to the arm
breast (brest) anterior aspect of the chest; in females, also an accessory sex organ
bronchi (BRONG-ki) the branches of the trachea
bronchiole (BRONG-kee-ole) small branch of a bronchus
buccal (BUK-al) pertaining to the cheek
buffer (BUF-er) compound that combines with an acid or with a base to form a weaker acid or base, thereby lessening the change in hydrogen-ion concentration that would occur without the buffer
buffer pairs (BUF-er) two kinds of chemical substances that prevent a sharp change in the pH of a fluid; for example, sodium bicarbonate ($NaHCO_3$) and carbonic acid (H_2CO_3)
bulbourethral gland (BUL-bo-yoo-REE-thral) small glands located just below the prostate gland whose mucuslike secretions lubricate the terminal portion of the urethra and contribute less than 5% of the seminal fluid volume; also known as Cowper's glands
bundle of His (BUN-dul of his) see *AV bundle*
burn (bern) an injury to tissues resulting from contact with heat, chemicals, electricity, friction, or radiant and electromagnetic energy; classified into three categories, depending on the number of tissue layers involved
bursae (BER-see) small, cushionlike sacs found between moving body parts, making movement easier
bursitis (ber-SYE-tis) inflammation of a bursa

C

calcaneus (kal-KAY-nee-us) heel bone; largest tarsal in the foot
calcitonin (kal-si-TOE-nin) a hormone secreted by the thyroid that decreases calcium in the blood
calorie (c) (KAL-or-ree) heat unit; the amount of heat needed to raise the temperature of 1 g of water 1° C
Calorie (C) (KAL-or-ree) heat unit; kilocalorie; the amount of heat needed to raise the temperature of 1 kilogram of water 1° C
calyx (KAY-liks) cup-shaped division of the renal pelvis
canaliculi (kan-ah-LIK-yoo-lie) an extremely narrow tubular passage or channel in compact bone
canine tooth (KAY-nine) the tooth with the longest crown and the longest root, which is located lateral to the second incisor
capillary (KAP-i-lair-ee) tiny vessels that connect arterioles and venules
capillary blood pressure (KAP-i-lair-ee blud PRESH-ur) the blood pressure found in the capillary vessels
capsule (KAP-sul) found in diarthrotic joints, holds the bones of joints together while allowing movement and is made of fibrous connective tissue lined with a smooth, slippery synovial membrane
carbaminohemoglobin (kar-bam-ee-no-hee-mo-GLO-bin) the compound formed by the union of carbon dioxide with hemoglobin
carbohydrate (kar-bo-HYE-drate) organic compounds containing carbon, hydrogen, and oxygen in certain specific proportions (C,H,O in a 1:2:1 ratio); for example, sugars, starches, and cellulose
carbohydrate loading (kar-bo-HYE-drate LOHD-ing) the method used by athletes to increase the stores of muscle glycogen, allowing more sustained aerobic exercise
carbonic anhydrase (kar-BON-ik an-HYE-drays) the enzyme that converts carbon dioxide into carbonic acid
cardiac (KAR-dee-ak) refers to the heart
cardiac cycle (KAR-dee-ak SYE-kul) each complete heartbeat, including contraction and relaxation of the atria and ventricles
cardiac muscle (KAR-dee-ak MUS-el) the specialized muscle that makes up the heart
cardiac output (KAR-dee-ak OUT-put) volume of blood pumped by one ventricle per minute
cardiac sphincter (KAR-dee-ak SFINGK-ter) a ring of muscle between the stomach and esophagus that prevents food from re-entering the esophagus when the stomach contracts
cardiac vein (KAR-dee-ak vane) any vein that carries blood from the myocardial capillary beds to the coronary sinus
cardiopulmonary resuscitation (CPR) (kar-dee-o-PUL-mo-nair-ree ree-sus-i-TAY-shun) combined external cardiac (heart) massage and artificial respiration
cardiovascular (kar-dee-o-VAS-kyoo-lar) pertaining to the heart and blood vessels
caries (KARE-eez) decay of teeth or of bone

carotid body (kah-ROT-id BOD-ee) chemoreceptor located in the carotid artery that detects changes in oxygen, carbon dioxide, and blood acid levels

carpal (KAR-pal) pertaining to the wrist

cartilage (KAR-ti-lij) a specialized, fibrous connective tissue that has the consistency of a firm plastic or gristle-like gel

catabolism (kah-TAB-o-lizm) breakdown of food compounds or cytoplasm into simpler compounds; opposite of anabolism, the other phase of metabolism

catalyst (KAT-ah-list) chemical that speeds up reactions without being changed itself

cataract (KAT-ah-rakt) opacity of the lens of the eye

catecholamines (kat-e-kol-AM-eens) norepinephrine and epinephrine

catheterization (kath-e-ter-i-ZAY-shun) passage of a flexible tube (catheter) into the bladder through the urethra for the withdrawal of urine (urinary catheterization)

cation (KAT-eye-on) positively charged particle

cavity (KAV-i-tee) hollow place or space in a tooth; dental caries

cecum (SEE-kum) blind pouch; the pouch at the proximal end of the large intestine

cell (sell) the basic biological and structural unit of the body consisting of a nucleus surrounded by cytoplasm and enclosed by a membrane

cell body (sell BOD-ee) the main part of a neuron from which the dendrites and axons extend

cell-mediated immunity (sell MEE-dee-ate-ed i-MYOO-ni-tee) resistance to disease organisms resulting from the actions of cells; chiefly sensitized T cells

cellular respiration (SELL-yoo-lar res-pi-RAY-shun) enzymes in the mitochondrial wall and matrix using oxygen to break down glucose and other nutrients to release energy needed for cellular work

centimeter (SEN-ti-mee-ter) 1/100 of a meter; approximately 2.5 cm equal 1 inch

central nervous system (CNS) (SEN-tral NER-vus SIS-tem) the brain and spinal cord

central venous pressure (SEN-tral VEE-nus PRESH-ur) venous blood pressure within the right atrium that influences the pressure in the large peripheral veins

centriole (SEN-tree-ol) one of a pair of tiny cylinders in the centrosome of a cell; believed to be involved with the spindle fibers formed during mitosis

centromere (SEN-tro-meer) a beadlike structure that attaches one chromatid to another during the early stages of mitosis

cephalic (se-FAL-ik) refers to the head

cerebellum (sair-e-BELL-um) the second largest part of the human brain that plays an essential role in the production of normal movements

cerebral cortex (se-REE-bral KOR-teks) a thin layer of gray matter made up of neuron dendrites and cell bodies that compose the surface of the cerebrum

cerebral nuclei (se-REE-bral NOOK-lee-i) islands of gray matter located in the cerebral cortex that are responsible for automatic movements and postures

cerebrospinal fluid (CSF) (se-ree-bro-SPY-nal FLOO-id) fluid that fills the subarachnoid space in the brain and spinal cord and in the cerebral ventricles

cerebrovascular accident (CVA) (se-ree-bro-VAS-kyoo-lar AK-si-dent) a hemorrhage or cessation of blood flow through cerebral blood vessels resulting in destruction of neurons; commonly called a stroke

cerebrum (se-REE-brum) the largest and uppermost part of the human brain that controls consciousness, memory, sensations, emotions, and voluntary movements

cerumen (se-ROO-men) ear wax

ceruminous gland (se-ROO-mi-nus) gland that produces a waxy substance called cerumen (ear wax)

cervical (SER-vi-kal) refers to the neck

cervix (SER-viks) neck; any necklike structure

chemoreceptors (kee-mo-ree-SEP-tors) receptors that respond to chemicals and are responsible for taste and smell

chest thorax

childhood (CHILD-hood) from infancy to puberty

cholecystectomy (kohl-eh-sis-TEK-to-mee) the surgical removal of the gallbladder

cholecystokinin (CCK) (ko-le-sis-toe-KYE-nin) hormone secreted from the intestinal mucosa of the duodenum that stimulates the contraction of the gallbladder, resulting in bile flowing into the duodenum

chondrocyte (KON-dro-site) cartilage cell

chordae tendineae (KOR-dee ten-DIN-ee) stringlike structures that attach the AV valves to the wall of the heart

chorion (KO-ree-on) develops into an important fetal membrane in the placenta

chorionic gonadotropins (ko-ree-ON-ik go-na-doe-TRO-pins) hormones that are secreted as the uterus develops during pregnancy

chorionic villi (ko-ree-ON-ik VIL-eye) connect the blood vessels of the chorion to the placenta

choroid (KO-royd) middle layer of the eyeball that contains a dark pigment to prevent the scattering of incoming light rays

choroid plexus (KO-royd PLEK-sus) a network of brain capillaries that are involved with the production of cerebrospinal fluid

chromatids (KRO-mah-tids) a chromosome strand

cholinergic fiber (ko-lin-ER-jik FYE-ber) axons whose terminals release acetylcholine

chromatin granules (KRO-mah-tin GRAN-yools) staining substance in the nucleus of cells; divides into chromosomes during mitosis

chromosome (KRO-mo-sohm) DNA molecule that has coiled to form a compact mass during mitosis or meiosis; each chromosome is composed of regions called genes, each of which transmits hereditary information

chyme (kime) partially digested food mixture leaving the stomach

cilia (SIL-ee-ah) hairlike projections of cells

circulatory system (SER-kyoo-lah-tor-ee SIS-tem) the system that supplies transportation for cells of the body

circumcision (ser-kum-SIZH-un) surgical removal of the foreskin or prepuce

cisterna chyli (sis-TER-nah KYE-lye) an enlarged pouch on the thoracic duct that serves as a storage area for lymph moving toward its point of entry into the venous system

citric acid cycle (SIT-rik AS-id SYE-kul) the second series of chemical reactions in the process of glucose metabolism; it is an aerobic process

clavicle (KLAV-i-kul) collarbone, connects the upper extremity to the axial skeleton

cleavage furrow (KLEEV-ij FUR-o) appears at the end of anaphase and begins to divide the cell into two daughter cells

clitoris (KLIT-o-ris) erectile tissue located within the vestibule of the vagina

clone (klone) any of a family of many identical cells descended from a single "parent" cell

cochlea (KOKE-lee-ah) snail shell or structure of similar shape

cochlear duct (KOKE-lee-ar dukt) membranous tube within the bony cochlea

collagen (KOL-ah-jen) principle organic constituent of connective tissue

collecting tubule (ko-LEK-ting TOO-byool) a straight part of a renal tubule formed by distal tubules of several nephrons joining together

colloid (KOL-oyd) dissolved particles with diameters of 1 to 100 millimicrons (1 millimicron equals about 1/25,000,000 of an inch)

colon (KO-lon) intestine

colostomy (ko-LAH-sto-me) surgical procedure in which an artificial anus is created on the abdominal wall by cutting the colon and bringing the cut end or ends out to the surface to form an opening called a stoma

columnar (ko-LUM-nar) shape in which cells are higher than they are wide

combining sites (kom-BINE-ing) antigen-binding sites, antigen receptor regions on antibody molecule; shape of each combining site is complementary to shape of a specific antigen

compact bone (kom-PAKT) dense bone

compensated metabolic acidosis (KOM-pen-say-ted met-ah-BOL-ik as-i-DOE-sis) when metabolic acidosis occurs and the body is able to adjust to return the blood pH to near normal levels

complement (KOM-ple-ment) any of several inactive enzymes normally present in blood, which, when activated, kill foreign cells by dissolving them

complementary base pairing (kom-ple-MEN-ta-ree PAIR-ing) bonding purines and pyridines in DNA; adenine always binds with thymine, and cytosine always binds with guanine

complement fixation (KOM-ple-ment fik-SAY-shun) highly specialized antigen-antibody complexes are formed to destroy a foreign cell

compound (KOM-pound) substance whose molecules have more than one kind of element in them

concave (KON-kave) a rounded, somewhat depressed surface

concentric lamella (kon-SEN-trik lah-MEL-ah) ring of calcified matrix surrounding the Haversian canal

conchae (KONG-kee) shell-shaped structure; for example, bony projections into the nasal cavity

conduction (kon-DUK-shun) transfer of heat energy to the skin and then the external environment

cone receptor cell located in the retina that is stimulated by bright light

conjunctiva (kon-junk-TIE-vah) mucous membrane that lines the eyelids and covers the sclera (white portion)

connective tissue (ko-NEK-tiv TISH-yoo) most abundant and widely distributed tissue in the body; has numerous functions

connective tissue membrane (ko-NEK-tiv TISH-yoo MEM-brane) one of the two major types of body membranes; composed exclusively of various types of connective tissue

constipation (kon-sti-PAY-shun) retention of feces

contact dermatitis (KON-takt der-mah-TIE-tis) a local skin inflammation lasting a few hours or days after being exposed to an antigen

continuous ambulatory peritoneal dialysis (CAPD) (kon-TIN-yoo-us AM-byoo-lah-tor-ee pair-i-toe-NEE-al dye-AL-i-sis) an alternative form of treatment for renal failure rather than the more complex and expensive hemodialysis

contractile unit (kon-TRAK-til YOO-nit) the sarcomere, the basic functional unit of skeletal muscle

contractility (kon-TRAK-til-i-tee) the ability to contract a muscle

contraction (kon-TRAK-shun) ability of muscle cells to shorten or contract

convection (kon-VEK-shun) transfer of heat energy to air that is flowing away from the skin

convex (KON-veks) a rounded, somewhat elevated surface

coronal (ko-RO-nal) literally "like a crown"; a coronal plane divides the body or an organ into anterior and posterior regions

coronary artery (KOR-o-nair-ee AR-ter-ee) the first artery to branch off the aorta, supplies blood to the myocardium (heart muscle)

coronary bypass surgery (KOR-o-nair-ee BYE-pass SER-jer-ee) surgery to relieve severely restricted coronary blood flow; veins are taken from other parts of the body to bypass the partial blockage

coronary circulation (KOR-o-nair-ee ser-kyoo-LAY-shun) delivery of oxygen and removal of waste product from the myocardium (heart muscle)

coronary embolism (KOR-o-nair-ee EM-bo-lizm) blocking of a coronary blood vessel by a clot

coronary heart disease (KOR-o-nair-ee hart di-ZEEZ) disease (blockage or other deformity) of the vessels that supply the myocardium (heart muscle); one of the leading causes of death among adults in the United States

coronary sinus (KOR-o-nair-ree SYE-nus) area that receives deoxygenated blood from the coronary veins and empties into the right atrium

coronary thrombosis (KOR-o-nair-ree throm-BO-sis) formation of a blood clot in a coronary blood vessel

corpora cavernosa (KOR-por-ah kav-er-NO-sah) two columns of erectile tissue found in the shaft of the penis

corpus callosum (KOR-pus kal-LO-sum) where the right and left cerebral hemispheres are joined

corpus luteum (KOR-pus LOO-tee-um) a hormone-secreting glandular structure transformed after ovulation from a ruptured follicle; it secretes chiefly progesterone, with some estrogen secreted as well

corpus spongiosum (KOR-pus spun-jee-O-sum) a column of erectile tissue surrounding the urethra in the penis

cortex (KOR-teks) outer part of an internal organ; for example, the outer part of the cerebrum and of the kidneys

corticoids (KOR-ti-koyds) hormones secreted by the three cell layers of the adrenal cortex

cotransport (ko-TRANS-port) active transport process in which two substances are moved together across a cell membrane; for example, sodium and glucose may be transported together across a membrane

covalent (ko-VAY-lent) bond chemical bond formed when atoms share electrons by overlapping their energy levels (electron shells)

coxal bone (KOKS-al) the pelvic bone or hipbone (also known as the os coxae or the innominate bone); formed by fusion of three distinct bones (ilium, ischium, and pubis) during skeletal development

cranial (KRAY-nee-al) toward the head

cranial cavity (KRAY-nee-al KAV-i-tee) space inside the skull that contains the brain

cranial nerve (KRAY-nee-al nerv) any of 12 pairs of nerves that attach to the undersurface of the brain and conduct impulses between the brain and structures in the head, neck, and thorax

craniosacral (kray-nee-o-SAY-kral) pertaining to parasympathetic nerves

cranium (KRAY-nee-um) bony vault made up of eight bones that encases the brain

crenation (kre-NAY-shun) abnormal notching in an erythrocyte resulting from shrinkage after suspension in a hypertonic solution

cretinism (KREE-tin-izm) dwarfism caused by hyposecretion of the thyroid gland

crista ampullaris (KRIS-tah am-pyoo-LAIR-is) a specialized receptor located within the semicircular canals that detects head movements

crown (krown) topmost part of an organ or other structure

crural (KROOR-al) refers to the leg

cryptorchidism (krip-TOR-ki-dizm) undescended testicles

cubital (KYOO-bi-tal) refers to the elbow

cuboid (KYOO-boyd) resembling a cube

cuboidal (KYOO-boyd-al) cell shape resembling a cube

Cushing's syndrome (KOOSH-ings SIN-drome) condition caused by the hypersecretion of glucocorticoids from the adrenal cortex

cuspid (KUS-pid) canine tooth, serves to pierce or tear food being eaten

cutaneous (kyoo-TANE-ee-us) pertaining to the skin

cutaneous membrane (ku-TANE-ee-us MEM-brane) primary organ of the integumentary system; the skin

cuticle (KYOO-ti-kul) skin fold covering the root of the nail

cyanosis (sye-ah-NO-sis) bluish appearance of the skin caused by deficient oxygenation of the blood

cyclic AMP (cAMP) (SIK-lik A M P) one of several second messengers that delivers information inside the cell and thus regulates the cell's activity

cystic duct (SIS-tik dukt) joins with the common hepatic duct to form the common bile duct

cystitis (sis-TI-tis) inflammation of the urinary bladder

cytoplasm (SYE-toe-plazm) the gellike substance of a cell exclusive of the nucleus and other organelles

D

deciduous (de-SID-yoo-us) temporary; shedding at a certain stage of growth; for example, deciduous teeth that are commonly referred to as baby teeth

deep farther away from the body's surface

deglutition (deg-loo-TISH-un) swallowing

dehydration (dee-hye-DRAY-shun) excessive loss of body water; the most common fluid imbalance; an abnormally low volume of one or more body fluids
dehydration synthesis (dee-hye-DRAY-shun SIN-the-sis) chemical reaction in which large molecules are formed by removing water from smaller molecules and joining them together
deltoid (DEL-toyd) triangular; for example, the deltoid muscle
dendrite (DEN-drite) branching or treelike; a nerve cell process that transmits impulses toward the body
dense bone bone where the outer layer is hard and dense
deoxyribonucleic acid (DNA) (dee-ok-see-rye-bo-NOO-klee-ik AS-id) genetic material of the cell that carries the chemical "blueprint" of the body
depolarization (dee-po-lar-i-ZAY-shun) the electrical activity that triggers a contraction of the heart muscle
dermal-epidermal junction (DER-mal-EP-i-der-mal JUNK-shun) junction between the thin epidermal layer of the skin and the dermal layer providing support for the epidermis
dermal papillae (DER-mal pah-PIL-ee) upper region of the dermis that forms part of the dermal-epidermal junction and forms the ridges and grooves of fingerprints
dermatomes (DER-mah-tohms) skin surface areas supplied by a single spinal nerve
dermis (DER-mis) the deeper of the two major layers of the skin, composed of dense fibrous connective tissue interspersed with glands, nerve endings, and blood vessels; sometimes called the true skin
developmental process (de-vel-op-MEN-tal PROSS-es) changes and functions occurring during a human's early years as the body becomes more efficient and more effective
diabetes insipidus (dye-ah-BEE-teez in-SIP-i-dus) condition resulting from hyposecretion of ADH in which large volumes of urine are formed and, if left untreated, may cause serious health problems
diabetes mellitus (dye-ah-BEE-teez mell-EYE-tus) a condition resulting when the pancreatic islets secrete too little insulin, resulting in increased levels of blood glucose
diabetic ketoacidosis see *ketoacidosis*
dialysis (dye-AL-i-sis) separation of smaller (diffusible) particles from larger (nondiffusible) particles through a semipermeable membrane
diaphragm (DYE-ah-fram) membrane or partition that separates one thing from another; the flat muscular sheet that separates the thorax and abdomen and is a major muscle of respiration
diaphysis (dye-AF-i-sis) shaft of a long bone
diarthroses (dye-ar-THRO-sis) freely movable joint
diarrhea (dye-ah-REE-ah) defecation of liquid feces
diastole (dye-AS-toe-lee) relaxation of the heart, interposed between its contractions; opposite of systole
diastolic pressure (dye-ah-STOL-ik PRESH-ur) blood pressure in arteries during diastole (relaxation) of the heart
diencephalon (dye-en-SEF-ah-lon) "between" brain; parts of the brain between the cerebral hemispheres and the mesencephalon or midbrain
differentiate (dif-er-EN-shee-ayt) a process by which daughter cells become different in structure and function (by using different genes from the genome all cells of the body share), as when some of the original cells of early developmental stages differentiate to become muscle cells and other cells become nerve cells, and so on. (*Differentiation* is another form of this term.)
diffusion (di-FYOO-shun) spreading; for example, scattering of dissolved particles
digestion (di-JEST-chun) the breakdown of food materials either mechanically (i.e., chewing) or chemically (i.e., digestive enzymes)
digestive system (di-JEST-tiv SIS-tem) organs that work together to ensure proper digestion and absorption of nutrients
digital (DIJ-i-tal) refers to fingers and toes
discharging chambers (dis-CHARJ-ing CHAM-bers) the two lower chambers of the heart called ventricles
dissection (di-SEK-shun) cutting technique used to separate body parts for study
dissociation (dis-so-see-AY-shun) separation of ions as they dissolve in water
dissociate (di-SO-see-ate) when a compound breaks apart in solution
distal (DIS-tal) toward the end of a structure; opposite of proximal
distal convoluted tubule (DIS-tal KON-vo-loo-ted TOO-byool) the part of the tubule distal to the ascending limb of the loop of Henle in the kidney
disuse atrophy (DIS-yoos AT-ro-fee) when prolonged inactivity results in the muscles getting smaller in size
diuretic (dye-yoo-RET-ik) a substance that promotes or stimulates the production of urine; diuretic drugs are among the most commonly used drugs in medicine
DNA replication (DNA rep-li-KAY-shun) the unique ability of DNA molecules to make copies of themselves
dopamine (DOE-pah-meen) chemical neurotransmitter
dorsal (DOR-sal) referring to the back; opposite of ventral; in humans, the posterior is dorsal
dorsal body cavity (DOR-sal BOD-ee KAV-i-tee) includes the cranial and spinal cavities
dorsiflexion (dor-si-FLEK-shun) when the top of the foot is elevated (brought toward the front of the lower leg) with the toes pointing upward
double helix (HE-lix) shape of DNA molecules; a double spiral

ductless gland (DUKT-less) specialized gland that secretes hormones directly into the blood

ductus arteriosus (DUK-tus ar-teer-ee-O-sus) connects the aorta and the pulmonary artery, allowing most blood to bypass the fetus' developing lungs

ductus deferens (DUK-tus DEF-er-ens) a thick, smooth, muscular tube that allows sperm to exit from the epididymis and pass from the scrotal sac into the abdominal cavity; also known as the vas deferens

ductus venosus (DUK-tus ve-NO-sus) a continuation of the umbilical vein that shunts blood returning from the placenta past the fetus' developing liver directly into the inferior vena cava

duodenal papillae (doo-o-DEE-nal pah-PIL-ee) ducts located in the middle third of the duodenum that empty pancreatic digestive juices and bile from the liver into the small intestine; there are two ducts, the major duodenal papillae and the minor papillae

duodenum (doo-o-DEE-num) the first subdivision of the small intestine where most chemical digestion occurs

dura mater (DOO-rah MAH-ter) literally "strong or hard mother"; outermost layer of the meninges

dust cells (dust sells) macrophages that ingest particulate matter in the small air sacs of the lungs

dwarfism (DWARF-izm) condition of abnormally small stature, sometimes resulting from hyposecretion of growth hormone

dyspnea (DISP-nee-ah) difficult or labored breathing

E

eardrum (EAR-drum) the tympanic membrane that separates the external ear and middle ear

eccrine (EK-rin) small sweat glands distributed over the total body surface

ectoderm (EK-toe-derm) the innermost of the primary germ layers that develops early in the first trimester of pregnancy

ectopic pregnancy (ek-TOP-ik PREG-nan-see) a pregnancy in which the fertilized ovum implants some place other than in the uterus

edema (e-DEE-mah) excessive fluid in the tissues

effector (ef-FEK-tor) responding organ; for example, voluntary and involuntary muscle, the heart, and glands

efferent (EF-fer-ent) carrying from, as neurons that transmit impulses from the central nervous system to the periphery; opposite of afferent

ejaculation (ee-jak-yoo-LAY-shun) sudden discharging of semen from the body

ejaculatory duct (ee-JAK-yoo-lah-toe-ree dukt) duct formed by the joining of the ductus deferens and the duct from the seminal vesicle that allows sperm to enter the urethra

electrocardiogram (ECG) (e-lek-tro-KAR-dee-o-gram) graphic record of the heart's action potentials

electrolyte (e-LEK-tro-lite) substance that ionizes (dissociates to form ions) in solution, rendering the solution capable of conducting an electric current

electrolyte balance (e-LEK-tro-lite BAL-ans) homeostasis of electrolytes

electron (e-LEK-tron) negatively charged particle orbiting the nucleus of an atom

electron transport system (e-LEK-tron TRANS-port SIS-tem) cellular process within mitochondria that transfers energy from high-energy electrons from glycolysis and the citric acid cycle to ATP molecules so that the energy is available to do work in the cell

element (EL-e-ment) pure substance, composed of only one type of atom

embolism (EM-bo-lizm) obstruction of a blood vessel by foreign matter carried in the bloodstream

embolus (EM-bo-lus) a blood clot or other substance (bubble of air) that is moving in the blood and may block a blood vessel

embryo (EM-bree-o) animal in early stages of intrauterine development; in humans, the first 3 months after conception

embryology (em-bree-OL-o-gee) study of the development of an individual from conception to birth

embryonic phase (em-bree-ON-ik faze) the period extending from fertilization until the end of the eighth week of gestation; during this phase the term *embryo* is used

emesis (EM-e-sis) vomiting

emptying reflex (EMP-tee-ing REE-fleks) the reflex that causes the contraction of the bladder wall and relaxation of the internal sphincter to allow urine to enter the urethra, which is followed by urination if the external sphincter is voluntarily relaxed

emulsify (e-MUL-se-fye) in digestion, when bile breaks up fats

endocarditis (en-doe-kar-DYE-tis) inflammation of the lining of the heart

endocardium (en-doe-KAR-dee-um) thin layer of very smooth tissue lining each chamber of the heart

endochondral ossification (en-doe-KON-dral os-i-fi-KAY-shun) the process in which most bones are formed from cartilage models

endocrine (EN-doe-krin) secreting into the blood or tissue fluid rather than into a duct; opposite of exocrine

endocrine glands (EN-doe-krin) ductless glands that are part of the endocrine system and secrete hormones into intercellular spaces

endocrine system (EN-doe-krin SIS-tem) the series of ductless glands that are found in the body

endoderm (EN-doe-derm) the outermost layer of the primary germ layers that develops early in the first trimester of pregnancy

endometrium (en-doe-MEE-tree-um) mucous membrane lining the uterus

endoneurium (en-doe-NOO-ree-um) the thin wrapping of fibrous connective tissue that surrounds each axon in a nerve

endoplasmic reticulum (ER) (en-doe-PLAS-mik re-TIK-yoo-lum) network of tubules and vesicles in cytoplasm

endorphins (en-DOR-fins) chemical in central nervous system that influences pain perception; a natural painkiller

endosteum (en-DOS-tee-um) a fibrous membrane that lines the medullary cavity

endothelium (en-doe-THEE-lee-um) squamous epithelial cells that line the inner surface of the entire circulatory system and the vessels of the lymphatic system

endurance training (en-DOOR-ance TRAIN-ing) continuous vigorous exercise requiring the body to increase its consumption of oxygen and developing the muscles' ability to sustain activity over a prolonged period

energy level limited region surrounding the nucleus of an atom at a certain distance containing electrons; also called a shell

enkephalins (en-KEF-ah-lins) peptide chemical in the central nervous system that acts as a natural painkiller

enzyme (EN-zime) a functional protein acting as a biochemical catalyst allowing chemical reactions to take place in a suitable time frame

eosinophil (ee-o-SIN-o-fils) white blood cell that is readily stained by eosin

epicardium (ep-i-KAR-dee-um) the inner layer of the pericardium that covers the surface of the heart; it is also called the visceral pericardium

epidermis (ep-i-DER-mis) "false" skin; outermost layer of the skin

epididymis (ep-i-DID-i-mis) tightly coiled tube that lies along the top and behind the testes where sperm mature and develop the ability to swim

epiglottis (ep-i-GLOT-is) lidlike cartilage overhanging the entrance to the larynx

epinephrine (ep-i-NEF-rin) adrenaline; secretion of the adrenal medulla

epineurium (ep-i-NOO-ree-um) a tough fibrous sheath that covers the whole nerve

epiphyseal fracture (ep-i-FEEZ-ee-al FRAK-cher) when the epiphyseal plate is separated from the epiphysis or diaphysis; this type of fracture can disrupt the normal growth of the bone

epiphyseal plate (ep-i-FEEZ-ee-al) the cartilage plate that is between the epiphysis and the diaphysis and allows growth to occur; sometimes referred to as a growth plate

epiphyses (e-PIF-i-sees) ends of a long bone

episiotomy (e-piz-ee-OT-o-mee) a surgical procedure used during birth to prevent a laceration of the mother's perineum or the vagina

epithelial membrane (ep-i-THEE-lee-al MEM-brane) membrane composed of epithelial tissue with an underlying layer of specialized connective tissue

epithelial tissue (ep-i-THEE-lee-al TISH-yoo) covers the body and its parts; lines various parts of the body; forms continuous sheets that contain no blood vessels; classified according to shape and arrangement

erythroblastosis fetalis (e-rith-ro-blas-TOE-sis fee-TAL-is) a disease that may develop when an Rh-negative mother has anti-Rh antibodies and gives birth to an Rh-positive baby and the antibodies react with the Rh positive cells of the baby

erythrocytes (e-RITH-ro-sites) red blood cells

esophagus (e-SOF-ah-gus) the muscular, mucus-lined tube that connects the pharynx with the stomach; also known as the foodpipe

essential organs (ee-SEN-shal OR-gans) reproductive organs that must be present for reproduction to occur and are known as gonads

estrogen (ES-tro-jen) sex hormone secreted by the ovary that causes the development and maintenance of the female secondary sex characteristics and stimulates growth of the epithelial cells lining the uterus

eupnea (YOOP-nee-ah) normal respiration

eustachian tube (yoo-STAY-shun toob) tube extending from inside the ear to the throat to equalize air pressure

evaporation (ee-vap-o-RAY-shun) heat being lost from the skin by sweat being vaporized

exhalation (eks-hah-LAY-shun) moving air out of the lungs; also known as expiration

exocrine (EK-so-krin) secreting into a duct; opposite of endocrine

exocrine gland (EK-so-krin) glands that secrete their products into ducts that empty onto a surface or into a cavity; for example, sweat glands

experimental controls (eks-pair-ih-MEN-tal kon-TROLZ) any procedure within a scientific experiment that ensures that the test situation itself is not affecting the outcome of the experiment

experimentation (eks-pair-ih-men-TAY-shun) performing an experiment, which is usually a test of a tentative explanation of nature called a hypothesis

expiration (eks-pi-RAY-shun) moving air out of the lungs; also known as exhalation

expiratory center (eks-PYE-rah-tor-ee SEN-ter) one of the two most important respiratory control centers, located in the medulla

expiratory muscles (eks-PYE-rah-tor-ee MUS-els) muscles that allow more forceful expiration to increase the rate and depth of ventilation; the internal intercostals and the abdominal muscles

expiratory reserve volume (ERV) (eks-PYE-rah-tor-ee re-ZERV VOL-yoom) the amount of air that can be forcibly exhaled after expiring the tidal volume (TV)

extension (ek-STEN-shun) increasing the angle between two bones at a joint

external auditory canal (eks-TER-nal AW-di-toe-ree kah-NAL) a curved tube (approximately 2.5 cm) extending from the auricle into the temporal bone, ending at the tympanic membrane

external ear (eks-TER-nal) the outer part of the ear that is made up of the auricle and the external auditory canal

external genitalia (eks-TER-nal jen-i-TAIL-yah) external reproductive organs

external intercostals (eks-TER-nal in-ter-KOS-tals) inspiratory muscles that enlarge the thorax, causing the lungs to expand and air to rush in

external nares (eks-TER-nal NAY-reez) nostrils

external oblique (eks-TER-nal o-BLEEK) the outermost layer of the anterolateral abdominal wall

external otitis (eks-TER-nal o-TIE-tis) a common infection of the external ear; also known as swimmer's ear

external respiration (eks-TER-nal res-pi-RAY-shun) the exchange of gases between air in the lungs and in the blood

extracellular fluid (ECF) (eks-trah-SELL-yoo-lar FLOO-id) the water found outside of cells located in two compartments between cells (interstitial fluid) and in the blood (plasma)

F

facial (FAY-shal) referring to the face

fallen arch when the tendons and ligaments of the foot weaken, allowing the normally curved arch to flatten out

fallopian tubes (fal-LO-pee-an toobs) the pair of tubes that conduct the ovum from the ovary to the uterus

false ribs (fawls) the eighth, ninth, and tenth pairs of ribs that are attached to the cartilage of the seventh ribs rather than the sternum

fasciculus (fah-SIK-yoo-lus) little bundle

fat one of the three basic food types; primarily a source of energy

fatigue (fah-TEEG) loss of muscle power; weakness

fat tissue (fat TISH-yoo) adipose tissue; specialized to store lipids

feces (FEE-seez) waste material discharged from the intestines

feedback control loop (FEED-bak kon-TROL loop) a highly complex and integrated communication control network, classified as negative or positive; negative feedback loops are the most important and most numerous homeostatic control mechanisms

femoral (FEM-or-al) referring to the thigh

femur (FEE-mur) the thigh bone, which is the longest bone in the body

fertilization (FER-ti-li-ZAY-shun) the moment the female's ovum and the male's sperm cell unite

fetal alcohol syndrome (FAS) (FEE-tal AL-ko-hol SIN-drome) a condition that may cause congenital abnormalities in a baby that results from a woman consuming alcohol during pregnancy

fetal phase (FEE-tal faze) period extending from the eighth to the thirty-ninth week of gestation; during this phase the term *fetus* is used

fetus (FEE-tus) unborn young, especially in the later stages; in human beings, from the third month of the intrauterine period until birth

fibers (FYE-bers) threadlike structures; for example, nerve fibers

fibrin (FYE-brin) insoluble protein in clotted blood

fibrinogen (fye-BRIN-o-jen) soluble blood protein that is converted to insoluble fibrin during clotting

fibrous connective tissue (FYE-brus ko-NEK-tiv TISH-yoo) strong, nonstretchable, white collagen fibers that compose tendons

fibula (FIB-yoo-lah) the slender non–weight-bearing bone located on the lateral aspect of the leg

fight or flight syndrome (fite or flite SIN-drome) the changes produced by increased sympathetic impulses allowing the body to deal with any type of stress

filtration (fil-TRAY-shun) movement of water and solutes through a membrane by a higher hydrostatic pressure on one side

fimbriae (FIM-bree-ee) fringe

flagellum (flah-JEL-um) single projection extending from the cell surface; only example in humans is the "tail" of the male sperm

flat bone one of the four types of bone; the frontal bone is an example of a flat bone

flat feet when the tendons and ligaments of the foot weaken, allowing the normally curved arch to flatten out

flexion (FLEK-shun) act of bending; decreasing the angle between two bones at the joint

floating ribs (FLOW-ting ribs) the eleventh and twelfth pairs of ribs, which are attached only to the thoracic vertebrae

fluid balance (FLOO-id BAL-ans) homeostasis of fluids; the volumes of interstitial fluid, intracellular fluid, and plasma and total volume of water remain relatively constant

fluid compartments (FLOO-id kom-PART-ments) the areas in the body where the fluid is located; for example, interstitial fluid

follicles (FOL-li-kuls) specialized structures required for hair growth

follicle-stimulating hormone (FSH) (FOL-li-kul STIM-yoo-lay-ting HOR-mone) hormone present in males and females; in males, FSH stimulates the production of sperm; in females, FSH stimulates the ovarian follicles to mature and follicle cells to secrete estrogen

fontanels (FON-tah-nels) "soft spots" on the infant's head; unossified areas in the infant skull

foramen (fo-RAY-men) small opening; for example, the vertebral foramen, which allows the spinal cord to pass through the vertebral canal

foramen ovale (fo-RAY-men o-VAL-ee) shunts blood from the right atrium directly into the left atrium, allowing most blood to bypass the baby's developing lungs

foreskin (FORE-skin) a loose-fitting retractable casing located over the glans of the penis; also known as the prepuce

fractal geometry (FRAK-tul jee-OM-e-tree) the study of surfaces with a seemingly infinite area, such as the lining of the small intestine

free nerve endings (free nerv END-ings) specialized receptors in the skin that respond to pain

frenulum (FREN-yoo-lum) the thin membrane that attaches the tongue to the floor of the mouth

frontal (FRON-tal) lengthwise plane running from side to side, dividing the body into anterior and posterior portions

frontal muscle (FRON-tal MUS-el) one of the muscles of facial expression; it moves the eyebrows and furrows the skin of the forehead

frontal sinusitis (FRON-tal sye-nyoo-SYE-tis) inflammation in the frontal sinus

G

G protein a protein molecule usually imbedded in a cell's plasma membrane that plays an important role in getting a signal from a receptor (also in the plasma membrane) to the inside of the cell

ganglia (GANG-lee-ah) a region of gray (unmyelinated) nerve tissue (usually this term is used only for gray matter regions in the PNS)

gastroesophageal reflux disease (gas-tro-ees-AH-fo-jee-al RE-fluks dih SEEZ) also known as GERD, a set of symptoms resulting from a hiatal hernia that allows stomach (gastric) contents to flow back (reflux) into the esophagus; symptoms include heartburn or chest pain and coughing or choking during or just after a meal

gastroesophageal sphincter (gas-tro-ees-AH-fo-jee-al SFINK-ter) a ring of smooth muscle around the opening of the stomach at the lower end of the esophagus that acts as a valve to allow food to enter the stomach but prevents stomach contents from moving back into the esophagus

gene (jean) one of many segments of a chromosome (DNA molecule); each gene contains the genetic code for synthesizing a protein molecule such as an enzyme or hormone

genitalia (jen-i-TAIL-yah) reproductive organs

genome (JEEN-ome) entire set of chromosomes in a cell; the human genome refers to the entire set of human chromosomes

genomics (jen-OME-iks) field of endeavor involving the analysis of the genetic code contained in the human or other species' genome

gestation (jes-TAY-shun) the length of pregnancy, approximately 9 months in humans

gigantism (jye-GAN-tizm) a condition produced by hypersecretion of growth hormone during the early years of life; results in a child who grows to gigantic size

gland secreting structure

glandular epithelium (GLAN-dyoo-lar ep-i-THEE-lee-um) cells that are specialized for secreting activity

glans the distal end of the shaft of the penis

glaucoma (glaw-KO-mah) disorder characterized by elevated pressure in the eye

glia (GLEE-ah) supporting cells of nervous tissue; also called neuroglia

glioma (glee-O-mah) one of the most common types of brain tumors

globulin (GLOB-yoo-lin) a type of plasma protein that includes antibodies

glomerulus (glo-MARE-yoo-lus) compact cluster; for example, capillaries in the kidneys

glottis (GLOT-is) the space between the vocal cords

glucagon (GLOO-kah-gon) hormone secreted by alpha cells of the pancreatic islets

glucocorticoids (GCs) (gloo-ko-KOR-ti-koyds) hormones that influence food metabolism; secreted by the adrenal cortex

gluconeogenesis (gloo-ko-nee-o-JEN-e-sis) formulation of glucose or glycogen from protein or fat compounds

glucose (GLOO-kose) monosaccharide or simple sugar; the principal blood sugar

gluteal (GLOO-tee-al) of or near the buttocks

gluteus maximus (GLOO-tee-us MAX-i-mus) major extensor of the thigh and also supports the torso in an erect position

glycerol (GLIS-er-ol) product of fat digestion

glycogen (GLYE-ko-jen) polysaccharide made up of a chain of glucose (monosaccharide) molecules; animal starch

glycogen loading (GLYE-ko-jen LOHD-ing) see carbohydrate loading

glycogenesis (glye-ko-JEN-e-sis) formation of glycogen from glucose or from other monosaccharides, fructose, or galactose

glycogenolysis (glye-ko-je-NOL-i-sis) hydrolysis of glycogen to glucose-6-phosphate or to glucose

glycolysis (glye-KOL-i-sis) the first series of chemical reactions in glucose metabolism; changes glucose to pyruvic acid in a series of anaerobic reactions

glycosuria (glye-ko-SOO-ree-ah) glucose in the urine; a sign of diabetes mellitus

goblet cells (GOB-let sells) specialized cells found in simple columnar epithelium that produce mucus

goiter (GOY-ter) enlargement of the thyroid gland

Golgi apparatus (GOL-jee ap-ah-RA-tus) small sacs stacked on one another near the nucleus that makes carbohydrate compounds, combines them with protein molecules, and packages the product in a globule

Golgi tendon receptors (GOL-jee TEN-don ree-SEP-tors) sensors that are responsible for proprioception

gonads (GO-nads) sex glands in which reproductive cells are formed

graafian follicle (GRAF-ee-an FOL-li-kul) a mature ovum in its sac

gradient (GRAY-dee-ent) a slope or difference between two levels; for example, blood pressure gradient: a difference between the blood pressure in two different vessels

gram the unit of measure in the metric system on which mass is based (approximately 454 grams equals one pound)

granulosa cell (gran-yoo-LO-sah sell) cell layer surrounding the oocyte

gray matter (MATT-er) tissue comprising cell bodies and unmyelinated axons and dendrites

greater omentum (GRATE-er o-MEN-tum) a pouchlike extension of the visceral peritoneum

growth hormone (HOR-mone) hormone secreted by the anterior pituitary gland that controls the rate of skeletal and visceral growth

gustatory cell (GUS-tah-tor-ee sell) cells of taste

gyrus (JYE-rus) convoluted ridge

H

hair follicle (hair FOL-li-kul) a small tube where hair growth occurs

hair papilla (hair pah-PIL-ah) a small, cap-shaped cluster of cells located at the base of the follicle where hair growth begins

hamstring muscles (HAM-string MUS-els) powerful flexors of the hip made up of the semimembranosus, semitendinosus, and biceps femoris muscles

Haversian canal (ha-VER-shun kah-NAL) the canal in the Haversian system that contains a blood vessel

Haversian system (hah-VER-shun SIS-tem) the circular arrangements of calcified matrix and cells that give bone its characteristic appearance

heart block (hart blok) a blockage of impulse conduction from atria to ventricles so that the heart beats at a slower rate than normal

heartburn (HART-bern) burning sensation characterized by pain and a feeling of fullness beneath the sternum caused by the esophageal mucosa being irritated by stomach acid

Heimlich maneuver (HIME-lik mah-NOO-ver) lifesaving technique used to free the trachea of objects blocking the airway

hematocrit (he-MAT-o-krit) volume percent of blood cells in whole blood

hemodialysis (hee-mo-dye-AL-i-sis) use of dialysis to separate waste products from the blood

hemoglobin (hee-mo-GLO-bin) iron-containing protein in red blood cells

hemopoiesis (hee-mo-poy-EE-sis) blood cell formation

hemopoietic tissue (hee-mo-poy-ET-ik TISH-yoo) specialized connective tissue that is responsible for the formation of blood cells and lymphatic system cells; found in red bone marrow, spleen, tonsils, and lymph nodes

heparin (HEP-ah-rin) substance obtained from the liver; inhibits blood clotting

hepatic colic flexure (he-PAT-ik KOL-ik FLEK-sher) the bend between the ascending colon and the transverse colon

hepatic ducts (he-PAT-ik dukts) drain bile out of the liver

hepatic portal circulation (he-PAT-ik POR-tal ser-kyoo-LAY-shun) the route of blood flow through the liver

hepatic portal vein (he-PAT-ik POR-tal vane) delivers blood directly from the gastrointestinal tract to the liver

hepatitis (hep-ah-TITE-is) inflammation of the liver due to viral or bacterial infection, injury, damage from alcohol, drugs, or other toxins, or other factors

herpes zoster (HER-peez ZOS-ter) "shingles," viral infection that affects the skin of a single dermatome

hiatal hernia (hy-AYT-al HER-nee-ah) a bulging out (hernia) of the stomach through the opening (hiatus) of the diaphragm through which the esophagus normally passes; this condition may prevent the valve between the esophagus and stomach from closing, thus allowing stomach contents to flow back into the esophagus (see *gastroesophageal reflux disease*)

hiccup (HIK-up) involuntary spasmodic contraction of the diaphragm

hip the joint connecting the legs to the trunk

histogenesis (his-toe-JEN-e-sis) formation of tissues from primary germ layers of embryo

homeostasis (ho-mee-o-STAY-sis) relative uniformity of the normal body's internal environment

homeostatic mechanism (ho-mee-o-STAT-ik MEK-ah-nizm) a system that maintains a constant environment enabling body cells to function effectively

hormone (HOR-mone) substance secreted by an endocrine gland

human immunodeficiency virus (HYOO-man i-myoo-no-de-FISH-en-see VYE-rus) the retrovirus that causes acquired immunodeficiency syndrome (AIDS)

humerus (HYOO-mer-us) the second longest bone in the body; the long bone of the arm

humoral immunity (HYOO-mor-al i-MYOO-ni-tee) antibody-mediated immunity

hybridoma (hye-brid-O-ma) fused or hybrid cells that continue to produce the same antibody as the original lymphocyte

hydrocephalus (hye-dro-SEF-ah-lus) abnormal accumulation of cerebrospinal fluid; "water on the brain"

hydrocortisone (hye-dro-KOR-ti-zone) a hormone secreted by the adrenal cortex; cortisol; compound F

hydrogen ion (HYE-dro-jen eye-on) found in water and water solutions; produces an acidic solution; H^+

hydrolysis (hye-DROL-i-sis) chemical reaction in which water is added to a large molecule causing it to break apart into smaller molecules

hydrostatic pressure (hye-dro-STAT-ik PRESH-ur) the force of a fluid pushing against some surface

hydroxide ion (hye-DROK-side EYE-on) found in water and water solutions; produces an alkaline solution; H^-

hymen (HYE-men) Greek for "membrane"; mucous membrane that may partially or entirely occlude the vaginal outlet

hyperacidity (hye-per-a-SID-i-tee) excessive secretion of acid; an important factor in the formation of ulcers

hypercalcemia (hye-per-kal-SEE-mee-ah) a condition in which there is harmful excess of calcium in the blood

hyperglycemia (hye-per-glye-SEE-mee-ah) higher than normal blood glucose concentration

hyperopia (hye-per-O-pee-ah) farsightedness

hypersecretion (hye-per-se-KREE-shun) too much of a substance is being secreted

hypertension (hye-per-TEN-shun) abnormally high blood pressure

hyperthyroidism (hye-per-THYE-royd-izm) oversecretion of thyroid hormones that increases metabolic rate resulting in loss of weight, increased appetite, and nervous irritability

hypertonic (hye-per-TON-ik) a solution containing a higher level of salt (NaCl) than is found in a living red blood cell (above 0.9% NaCl)

hypertrophy (hye-PER-tro-fee) increased size of a part caused by an increase in the size of its cells

hyperventilation (hye-per-ven-ti-LAY-shun) very rapid deep respirations

hypervitaminosis (hye-per-vye-tah-mi-NO-sis) condition caused by excess amounts of vitamins; usually associated with the use of vitamin supplements

hypodermis (hy-poh-DER-mis) the loose, ordinary (areolar) tissue just under the skin and superficial to the muscles; also called *subcutaneous tissue* or *superficial fascia*

hypoglycemia (hye-po-glye-SEE-mee-ah) lower-than-normal blood glucose concentration

hyposecretion (hye-po-se-KREE-shun) too little of a substance is being secreted

hypothalamus (hye-po-THAL-ah-mus) vital neuroendocrine and autonomic control center beneath the thalamus

hypothermia (hye-po-THER-mee-ah) subnormal core body temperature below 37° C

hypothesis (hye-POTH-e-sis) a proposed explanation of an observed phenomenon (plural, hypotheses)

hypothyroidism (hye-po-THYE-royd-izm) undersecretion of thyroid hormones; early in life results in cretinism; later in life results in myxedema

hypotonic (hye-po-TON-ik) a solution containing a lower level of salt (NaCl) than is found in a living red blood cell (below 0.9% NaCl)

hypovitaminosis (hi-po-VITE-ah-min-oh-sis) condition of having too few vitamin molecules in the body for normal function

hypoventilation (hye-po-ven-ti-LAY-shun) slow and shallow respirations

hypoxia (hy-POCK-see-ah) abnormally low concentration of oxygen in the blood or tissue fluids

hysterectomy (his-te-REK-toe-mee) surgical removal of the uterus

I

ileocecal valve (il-ee-o-SEE-kal valv) the sphincterlike structure between the end of the small intestine and the beginning of the large intestine

ileum (IL-ee-um) the distal portion of the small intestine

iliac crest (IL-ee-ak krest) the superior edge of the ilium

iliopsoas (il-ee-op-SO-as) a flexor of the thigh and an important stabilizing muscle for posture

ilium (IL-ee-um) one of the three separate bones that forms the os coxa

immune system (i-MYOON SIS-tem) the body's defense system against disease

immunization (i-myoo-ni-ZAY-shun) deliberate artificial exposure to disease to produce acquired immunity

implantation (im-plan-TAY-shun) when a fertilized ovum implants in the uterus

inborn immunity (IN-born i-MYOO-ni-tee) immunity to disease that is inherited

incontinence (in-KON-ti-nens) when an individual voids urine involuntarily

incus (IN-kus) the anvil, the middle ear bone that is shaped like an anvil

infancy (IN-fan-see) from birth to about 18 months of age

infant respiratory distress syndrome (IN-fant RES-pi-rah-toe-ree di-STRESS SIN-drome) leading cause of death in premature babies, due to a lack of surfactant in the alveolar air sacs

inferior (in-FEER-ee-or) lower; opposite of superior

inferior vena cava (in-FEER-ee-or VEE-nah KAY-vah) one of two large veins carrying blood into the right atrium

inflammatory response (in-FLAM-ah-toe-ree re-SPONS) nonspecific immune process produced in response to injury and resulting in redness, pain, heat, and swelling and promoting movement of white blood cells to the affected area

inguinal (ING-gwi-nal) of the groin

inhalation (in-hah-LAY-shun) inspiration or breathing in; opposite of exhalation or expiration

inherited immunity (in-HAIR-i-ted i-MYOO-ni-tee) inborn immunity

inhibiting hormone (in-HIB-i-ting HOR-mone) hormone produced by the hypothalamus that slows the release of anterior pituitary hormones

inorganic compound (in-or-GAN-ik KOM-pownd) compound whose molecules do not contain carbon-carbon or carbon-hydrogen bonds

insertion (in-SER-shun) attachment of a muscle to the bone that it moves when contraction occurs (as distinguished from its origin)

inspiration (in-spi-RAY-shun) moving air into the lungs; same as inhalation, opposite of exhalation or expiration

inspiratory muscle (in-SPY-rah-tor-ee MUS-el) the muscles that increase the size of the thorax, including the diaphragm and external intercostals, and allow air to rush into the lungs

inspiratory center (in-SPY-rah-tor-ee SEN-ter) one of the two most important control centers located in the medulla; the other is the expiratory center

inspiratory reserve volume (IRV) (in-SPY-rah-tor-ee re-SERV VOL-yoom) the amount of air that can be forcibly inspired over and above a normal respiration

insulin (IN-suh-lin) hormone secreted by the pancreatic islets

integument (in-TEG-yoo-ment) refers to the skin

integumentary system (in-teg-yoo-MEN-tar-ee SIS-tem) the skin; the largest and most important organ in the body

intercalated disks (in-TER-kah-lay-ted disks) cross striations and unique dark bands that are found in cardiac muscle fibers

intercostal muscle (in-ter-KOS-tal MUS-el) the respiratory muscles located between the ribs

interferon (in-ter-FEER-on) small proteins produced by the immune system that inhibit virus multiplication

internal oblique (in-TER-nal o-BLEEK) the middle layer of the anterolateral abdominal walls

internal respiration (in-TER-nal res-pi-RAY-shun) the exchange of gases that occurs between the blood and cells of the body

interneuron (in-ter-NOO-ron) nerves that conduct impulses from sensory neurons to motor neurons

interphase (IN-ter-faze) the phase immediately before the visible stages of cell division when the DNA of each chromosome replicates itself

interstitial cell (in-ter-STISH-al sell) small specialized cells in the testes that secrete the male sex hormone, testosterone

interstitial cell-stimulating hormone (ICSH) (in-ter-STISH-al sell STIM-yoo-lay-ting HOR-mone) the previous name for luteinizing hormone in males; causes testes to develop and secrete testosterone

interstitial fluid (in-ter-STISH-al FLOO-id) fluid located in the microscopic spaces between the cells

intestine (in-TES-tin) the part of the digestive tract that is after the stomach; separated into two segments, the small and the large

intestinal gland (in-TES-ti-nal) thousands of glands found in the mucous membrane of the mucosa of the small intestines; secrete intestinal digestive juices

intracellular fluid (ICF) (in-tra-SELL-yoo-lar FLOO-id) a fluid located within the cells; largest fluid compartment

in vitro (in VEE-tro) refers to the glass laboratory container where a mature ovum is fertilized by a sperm

involuntary muscle (in-VOL-un-tare-ee MUS-el) smooth muscles that are not under conscious control and are found in organs such as the stomach and small intestine

involution (in-vo-LOO-shun) return of an organ to its normal size after an enlargement; also retrograde or degenerative change

ion (EYE-on) electrically charged atom or group of atoms

ion pump (EYE-on) a specialized cellular component that moves ions from an area of low concentration to an area of high concentration

ionic bond (eye-ON-ik) chemical bond formed by the positive-negative attraction between two ions

iron deficiency anemia (EYE-ern de-FISH-en-see ah-NEE-mee-ah) when there are inadequate levels of iron in the diet so that less hemoglobin is produced; results in extreme fatigue

ischium (IS-kee-um) one of three separate bones that forms the os coxa

isometric (eye-so-MET-rik) type of muscle contraction in which muscle does not shorten

isotonic (eye-so-TON-ik) of the same tension or pressure

J

jaundice (JAWN-dis) abnormal yellowing of skin, mucous membranes, and white of eyes

jejunum (je-JOO-num) the middle third of the small intestine

joints (joynts) articulation

K

Kaposi sarcoma (KS) (KAP-oh-see sar-KOH-mah) a malignant neoplasm (cancer) of the skin characterized by purplish spots

keratin (KARE-ah-tin) protein substance found in hair, nails, outer skin cells, and horny tissues

ketoacidosis (kee-toh-as-ih-DOH-sis) a condition of abnormally low blood pH (acidity) caused by the presence of an abnormally large number of ketone bodies or "keto acids" that are produced when fats are converted to forms of glucose to be used for cellular respiration; often occurs in diabetes mellitus, when it is more specifically called *diabetic ketoacidosis* (see also *acidosis*)

kidney (KID-nee) organ that cleanses the blood of waste products continually produced by metabolism

kilocalorie (Kcal) (KIL-o-kal-o-ree) 1000 calories

kinesthesia (kin-es-THEE-zee-ah) "muscle sense"; that is, sense of position and movement of body parts

Krause's end bulb (KROWZ) skin receptor that detects sensations of cold

Kupffer cell (KOOP-fer sell) macrophage found in spaces between liver cells

L

labia majora (LAY-bee-ah ma-JO-rah) "large lips" of the vulva

labia minora (LAY-bee-ah mi-NO-rah) "small lips" of the vulva

labor (LAY-bor) the process that results in the birth of the baby

lacrimal gland (LAK-ri-mal) the glands that produce tears, located in the upper lateral portion of the orbit

lacteal (LAK-tee-al) a lymphatic vessel located in each villus of the intestine; serves to absorb fat materials from the chyme passing through the small intestine

lactiferous duct (lak-TIF-er-us dukt) the duct that drains the grapelike cluster of milk-secreting glands in the breast

lacuna (lah-KOO-nah) space or cavity; for example, lacunae in bone contain bone cells

lambdoidal suture (LAM-doyd-al SOO-chur) the immovable joint formed by the parietal and occipital bones

lamella (lah-MEL-ah) thin layer, as of bone

lanugo (lah-NOO-go) the extremely fine and soft hair found on a newborn infant

laparoscope (LAP-ah-ro-skope) specialized optical viewing tube

laryngopharynx (lah-ring-go-FAIR-inks) the lowest part of the pharynx

larynx (LAIR-inks) the voice box located just below the pharynx; the largest piece of cartilage making up the larynx is the thyroid cartilage, commonly known as the Adam's apple

lateral (LAT-er-al) of or toward the side; opposite of medial

latissimus dorsi (la-TIS-i-mus DOR-si) an extensor of the upper arm

law a scientific law is a theory, or explanation of a scientific principle, with an extraordinarily high degree of confidence of scientists based on experimentation

lens (lenz) the refracting mechanism of the eye that is located directly behind the pupil

leptin (LEHP-tin) hormone, secreted by fat-storing cells, that regulates how hungry or full we feel and how fat is metabolized by the body

leukemia (loo-KEE-mee-ah) blood cancer characterized by an increase in white blood cells

leukocyte (LOO-ko-site) white blood cells

leukocytosis (loo-ko-SYE-toe-sis) abnormally high white blood cell numbers in the blood

leukopenia (loo-ko-PEE-nee-ah) abnormally low white blood cell numbers in the blood

levodopa (LEV-oh-doh-pah) also called L-*dopa* (el DOH-pah), this chemical is manufactured by the brain cells and then converted to the neurotransmitter dopamine; it has been used to treat disorders involving dopamine deficiencies such as Parkinson disease

ligament (LIG-ah-ment) bond or band connecting two objects; in anatomy a band of white fibrous tissue connecting bones

limbic system (LIM-bik) a collection of various small regions of the brain that act together to produce emotion and emotional response; sometimes called "the emotional brain"

lipase (LYE-pase) fat-digesting enzymes

lipid organic molecule usually composed of glycerol and fatty acid units; types include triglycerides, phospholipids, and cholesterol; a fat, wax, or oil

lithotriptor (LITH-o-trip-tor) a specialized ultrasound generator that is used to pulverize kidney stones

liver glycogenolysis (LIV-er glye-ko-je-NOL-i-sis) chemical process by which liver glycogen is converted to glucose

lock-and-key model (lok and kee MAHD-el) concept that explains how molecules react when they fit together in a complementary way in the same manner that a key fits into a lock to cause the lock to open or close; the analogy is often used to explain the action of hormones, enzymes, and other biological molecules

longitudinal arch (lon-ji-TOO-di-nal) two arches, the medial and lateral, that extend lengthwise in the foot

loop of Henle (loop of HEN-lee) extension of the proximal tubule of the kidney

lumbar (LUM-bar) lower back, between the ribs and pelvis

lumbar puncture (LUM-bar PUNK-chur) when some cerebrospinal fluid is withdrawn from the subarachnoid space in the lumbar region of the spinal cord
lumen (LOO-men) the hollow space within a tube
lung organ of respiration; the right lung has three lobes and the left lung has two lobes
lunula (LOO-nyoo-lah) crescent-shaped white area under the proximal nail bed
luteinization (loo-te-ni-ZAY-shun) the formation of a golden body (corpus luteum) in the ruptured follicle
luteinizing hormone (LH) (LOO-te-nye-zing HOR-mone) acts in conjunction with follicle-stimulating hormone (FSH) to stimulate follicle and ovum maturation and release of estrogen and ovulation; known as the ovulating hormone; in males, causes testes to develop and secrete testosterone
lymph (limf) specialized fluid formed in the tissue spaces that returns excess fluid and protein molecules to the blood
lymph node (limf) performs biological filtration of lymph on its way to the circulatory system
lymphatic capillaries (lim-FAT-ik CAP-i-lair-ees) tiny, blind-ended tubes distributed in the tissue spaces
lymphatic duct (lim-FAT-ik dukt) terminal vessel into which lymphatic vessels empty lymph; the duct then empties the lymph into the circulatory system
lymphatic system (lim-FAT-ik SIS-tem) a system that plays a critical role in the functioning of the immune system, moves fluids and large molecules from the tissue spaces and fat-related nutrients from the digestive system to the blood
lymphatic tissue (lim-FAT-ik TISH-yoo) tissue that is responsible for manufacturing lymphocytes and monocytes; found mostly in the lymph nodes, thymus, and spleen
lymphatic vessels (lim-FAT-ik VES-els) vessels that carry lymph to its eventual return to the circulatory system
lymphocytes (LIM-fo-sites) one type of white blood cell
lyse (lize) disintegration of a cell
lysosome (LYE-so-sohm) membranous organelles containing various enzymes that can dissolve most cellular compounds; hence called digestive bags or suicide bags of cells

M

macrophage (MAK-ro-faje) phagocytic cells in the immune system
malignant (mah-LIG-nant) cancerous growth
malleus (MAL-ee-us) hammer; the tiny middle ear bone that is shaped like a hammer
mammary glands (MAM-er-ee) breasts; classified as external accessory sex organs in females
mastication (mas-ti-KAY-shun) chewing
matrix (MAY-triks) the intracellular substance of a tissue; for example, the matrix of bone is calcified, whereas that of blood is liquid
matter any substance that occupies space and has mass
mature follicle (mah-CHUR FOL-li-kul) graafian follicle
maximum oxygen consumption (VO_{2max}) (MAX-i-mum OKS-i-jen kon-SUMP-shun) the maximum amount of oxygen taken up by the lungs, transported to the tissues and used to do work
mechanoreceptor (mek-an-o-ree-SEP-tor) receptors that are mechanical in nature; for example, equilibrium and balance sensors in the ears
medial (MEE-dee-al) of or toward the middle; opposite of lateral
mediastinum (mee-dee-as-TI-num) a subdivision in the midportion of the thoracic cavity
medulla (me-DUL-ah) Latin for "marrow"; hence the inner portion of an organ in contrast to the outer portion or cortex
medulla oblongata (me-DUL-ah ob-long-GAH-tah) the lowest part of the brainstem; an enlarged extension of the spinal cord; the vital centers are located within this area
medullary cavity (MED-yoo-lair-ee KAV-i-tee) hollow area inside the diaphysis of the bone that contains yellow bone marrow
meiosis (my-O-sis) nuclear division in which the number of chromosomes are reduced to half their original number; produces gametes
Meissner's corpuscle (MIZS-ners KOR-pus-ul) a sensory receptor located in the skin close to the surface that detects light touch
melanin (MEL-ah-nin) brown skin pigment
melanocyte (me-LAN-o-site) specialized cells in the pigment layer that produce melanin
melanoma (mel-ah-NO-mah) a malignant neoplasm (cancer) of the pigment-producing cells of the skin (melanocytes); also called *malignant melanoma*
melatonin (mel-ah-TOE-nin) important hormone produced by the pineal gland that is believed to regulate the onset of puberty and the menstrual cycle; also referred to as the third eye because it responds to levels of light and is thought to be involved with the body's internal clock
membrane (MEM-brane) thin layer or sheet
membranous labyrinth (MEM-brah-nus LAB-i-rinth) a membranous sac that follows the shape of the bony labyrinth and is filled with endolymph
memory cell (MEM-o-ree sell) cells that remain in reserve in the lymph nodes until their ability to secrete antibodies is needed
menarche (me-NAR-kee) beginning of the menstrual function

meninges (me-NIN-jeez) fluid-containing membranes surrounding the brain and spinal cord
menopause (MEN-o-pawz) termination of menstrual cycles
menses (MEN-seez) menstrual flow
menstrual cycle (MEN-stroo-al SYE-kul) the cyclical changes in the uterine lining
mesentery (MEZ-en-tair-ee) a large double fold of peritoneal tissue that anchors the loops of the digestive tract to the posterior wall of the abdominal cavity
mesoderm (MEZ-o-derm) the middle layer of the primary germ layers
messenger RNA (mRNA) (MES-en-jer RNA) a duplicate copy of a gene sequence on the DNA that passes from the nucleus to the cytoplasm
metabolic acidosis (met-ah-BOL-ik as-i-DOE-sis) a disturbance affecting the bicarbonate element of the bicarbonate-carbonic acid buffer pair; bicarbonate deficit
metabolic alkalosis (met-ah-BOL-ik al-kah-LO-sis) disturbance affecting the bicarbonate element of the bicarbonate-carbonic acid buffer pair; bicarbonate excess
metabolism (me-TAB-o-lizm) complex process by which food is used by a living organism
metacarpal (met-ah-KAR-pal) the part of the hand between the wrist and fingers
metaphase (MET-ah-faze) second stage of mitosis, during which the nuclear envelope and nucleolus disappear
metatarsal arch (met-ah-TAR-sal arch) the arch that extends across the ball of the foot; also called the transverse arch
meter (MEE-ter) a measure of length in the metric system; equal to about 39.5 inches
microcephaly (my-kro-SEF-ah-lee) a congenital abnormality in which an infant is born with a small head
microglia (my-KROG-lee-ah) one type of connective tissue found in the brain and spinal cord
micron (MY-kron) 1/1000 millimeter; 1/25,000 inch
microvilli (my-kro-VIL-eye) the brushlike border made up of epithelial cells found on each villus in the small intestine; increases the surface area for absorption of nutrients
micturition (mik-too-RISH-un) urination, voiding
midbrain (MID-brain) one of the three parts of the brainstem
middle ear (MID-ul eer) a tiny and very thin epithelium-lined cavity in the temporal bone that houses the ossicles; in the middle ear, sound waves are amplified
midsagittal (mid-SAJ-i-tal) a cut or plane that divides the body or any of its parts into two equal halves
minerals (MIN-er-als) inorganic elements or salts found naturally in the earth that are vital to the proper functioning of the body
mineralocorticoid (MC) (min-er-al-o-KOR-ti-koyd) hormone that influences mineral salt metabolism; secreted by adrenal cortex; aldosterone is the chief mineralocorticoid
mitochondria (my-toe-KON-dree-ah) threadlike structures
mitosis (my-TOE-sis) indirect cell division involving complex changes in the nucleus
mitral valve (MY-tral valv) also known as the bicuspid valve; located between the left atrium and ventricle
molecule (MOL-e-kyool) particle of matter composed of one or more smaller units called atoms
monoclonal antibody (mon-o-KLONE-al AN-ti-bod-ee) specific antibody produced from a population of identical cells
monocyte (MON-o-site) a phagocyte
mons pubis (monz PYOO-bis) skin-covered pad of fat over the symphysis pubis in the female
morula (MOR-yoo-lah) a solid mass of cells formed by the divisions of a fertilized egg
motor neuron (MO-tor NOO-ron) transmits nerve impulses from the brain and spinal cord to muscles and glandular epithelial tissues
motor unit (MO-tor YOO-nit) a single motor neuron with the muscle cells it innervates
mucocutaneous junction (myoo-ko-kyoo-TAY-nee-us JUNK-shun) the transitional area where the skin and mucous membrane meet
mucosa (myoo-KO-sah) mucous membrane
mucous membrane (MYOO-kus MEM-brane) epithelial membranes that line body surfaces opening directly to the exterior and secrete a thick, slippery material called mucus
mucus (MYOO-kus) thick, slippery material that is secreted by the mucous membrane and that keeps the membrane moist
multiple sclerosis (MS) (MUL-ti-pul skle-RO-sis) the most common primary disease of the central nervous system; a myelin disorder
muscle fiber (MUS-el FYE-ber) the specialized contractile cells of muscle tissue that are grouped together and arranged in a highly organized way
muscular system (MUS-kyoo-lar SIS-tem) the muscles of the body
muscularis (mus-kyoo-LAIR-is) two layers of muscle surrounding the digestive tube that produce wavelike, rhythmic contractions, called peristalsis, which move food material
myelin (MY-e-lin) lipoid substance found in the myelin sheath around some nerve fibers
myelinated fiber (MY-e-li-nay-ted FYE-ber) axons outside the central nervous system that are surrounded by a segmented wrapping of myelin
myeloid (MY-e-loyd) pertaining to bone marrow

myocardial infarction (my-o-KAR-dee-al in-FARK-shun) death of cardiac muscle cells resulting from inadequate blood supply as in coronary thrombosis

myocardium (my-o-KAR-dee-um) muscle of the heart

myofilaments (my-o-FIL-ah-ments) ultramicroscopic, threadlike structures found in myofibrils

myometrium (my-o-MEE-tree-um) muscle layer in the uterus

myopia (my-O-pee-ah) nearsightedness

myosin (MY-o-sin) contractile protein found in the thick filaments of skeletal muscle

myxedema (mik-se-DEE-mah) condition caused by deficiency of thyroid hormone in adults

N

nail body (BOD-ee) the visible part of the nail

nail root the part of the nail that is hidden by the cuticle

nanometer (NAN-o-mee-ter) a measure of length in the metric system; one billionth of a meter

nares (NAY-reez) nostrils

nasal cavity (NAY-zal KAV-i-tee) the moist, warm cavities lined by mucosa located just beyond the nostrils; olfactory receptors are located in the mucosa

nasal septum (NAY-zal SEP-tum) a partition that separates the right and left nasal cavities

nasopharynx (nay-zo-FAIR-inks) the uppermost portion of the tube just behind the nasal cavities

neonatology (nee-o-nay-TOL-o-jee) diagnosis and treatment of disorders of the newborn infant

neoplasm (NEE-o-plazm) an abnormal mass of proliferating cells that may be either benign or malignant

nephritis (ne-FRY-tis) kidney disease; inflammation of the nephrons

nephron (NEF-ron) anatomical and functional unit of the kidney, consisting of the renal corpuscle and the renal tubule

nerve (nerv) collection of nerve fibers

nerve impulse (nerv IM-puls) signals that carry information along the nerves

nervous tissue (NER-vus TISH-yoo) consists of neurons and glia that provide rapid communication and control of body function

neurilemma (noo-ri-LEM-mah) nerve sheath

neurohypophysis (noo-ro-hye-POF-i-sis) posterior pituitary gland

neuromuscular junction (noo-ro-MUS-kyoo-lar JUNK-shun) the point of contact between the nerve endings and muscle fibers

neuron (NOO-ron) nerve cell, including its processes (axons and dendrites)

neurotransmitter (noo-ro-trans-MIT-ter) chemicals by which neurons communicate

neutrophil (NOO-tro-fil) white blood cell that stains readily with neutral dyes

neutron (NOO-tron) electrically neutral particle within the nucleus of an atom

Nobel prize (no-BELL pryz) international award created by the late Alfred Nobel and awarded each year to up three recipients in each of several categories such as chemistry, physics, and medicine or physiology (each Nobel laureate [prizewinner] receives a diploma, a medal, and a cash prize at a ceremony in Stockholm, Sweden)

nodes of Ranvier (nodes of rahn-vee-AY) indentations that are found between adjacent Schwann cells

nonsteroid hormone (nahn-STAYR-oyd HOR-mohn) general type of hormone that does have the lipid steroid structure (derived from cholesterol) but is instead a protein or protein derivative; also sometimes called *protein hormone*

norepinephrine (nor-ep-i-NEF-rin) hormone secreted by adrenal medulla; released by sympathetic nervous system

nose (noze) respiratory organ

nosocomial infection (no-zo-KOAM-ee-al in-FEK-shun) infection that begins in the hospital or clinic

nuclear envelope (NOO-klee-ar EN-vel-ope) membrane that surrounds the cell nucleus

nucleic acids (noo-KLEE-ik AS-ids) the two nucleic acids are ribonucleic acid, found in the cytoplasm, and deoxyribonucleic acid, found in the nucleus; made up of units called nucleotides that each include a phosphate, a five-carbon sugar, and a nitrogen base

nucleolus (noo-KLEE-o-lus) critical to protein formation because it "programs" the formation of ribosomes in the nucleus

nucleoplasm (NOO-klee-o-plazm) a special type of cytoplasm found in the nucleus

nucleus (NOO-klee-us) spherical structure within a cell; a group of neuron cell bodies in the brain or spinal cord; central core of the atom, made up of protons and (sometimes) neutrons

nutrition (noo-TRI-shun) food, vitamins, and minerals that are ingested and assimilated into the body

O

old age see *senescence*

olecranon fossa (o-LEK-rah-non FOS-ah) a large depression on the posterior surface of the humerus

olecranon process (o-LEK-rah-non PROSS-es) the large bony process of the ulna; commonly referred to as the tip of the elbow

olfaction (ol-FAK-shun) sense of smell

olfactory receptor (ol-FAK-tor-ee ree-SEP-tor) chemical receptors responsible for the sense of smell; located in the epithelial tissue in the upper part of the nasal cavity

oligodendrocyte (ol-ih-go-DEN-droh-site) a cell that holds nerve fibers together and produces the myelin sheath around axons in the central nervous system
oliguria (ol-i-GOO-ree-ah) scanty amounts of urine
oocyte (O-o-site) immature stage of the female sex cell
oogenesis (o-o-JEN-e-sis) production of female gametes
oophorectomy (o-off-o-REK-toe-mee) surgical procedure to remove the ovaries
opposition (op-o-ZISH-un) moving the thumb to touch the tips of the fingers; the movement used to hold a pencil to write
optic disc (OP-tic disk) the area in the retina where the optic nerve fibers exit and there are no rods or cones; also known as a blind spot
oral cavity (OR-al KAV-i-tee) mouth
orbicularis oculi (or-bik-yoo-LAIR-is OK-yoo-lie) facial muscle that causes a squint
orbicularis oris (or-bik-yoo-LAIR-is O-ris) facial muscle that puckers the lips
organ (OR-gan) group of several tissue types that performs a special function
organelle (or-gah-NELL) cell organ; for example, the ribosome
organism (OR-gah-nizm) an individual, living thing
organ of Corti (OR-gan of KOR-tee) the organ of hearing located in the cochlea and filled with endolymph
organic (or-GAN-ik) compound whose large molecules contain carbon and that include C-C bonds and/or C–H bonds
organogenesis (or-ga-no-JEN-e-sis) formation of organs from the primary germ layers of the embryo
origin (OR-i-jin) the attachment of a muscle to the bone that does not move when contraction occurs, as distinguished from insertion
oropharynx (o-ro-FAIR-inks) the portion of the pharynx that is located behind the mouth
osmosis (os-MO-sis) movement of a fluid through a semipermeable membrane
ossicles (OS-si-kls) little bones; found in the ears
osteoblast (OS-tee-o-blast) bone-forming cell
osteoclast (OS-tee-o-klast) bone-absorbing cell
osteocyte (OS-tee-o-site) bone cell
osteoporosis (os-tee-o-po-RO-sis) a bone disease in which there is an excessive loss of calcified matrix and collagenous fibers from bone
otitis media (o-TIE-tis MEE-dee-ah) a middle ear infection
ova (O-vah) female sex cells (singular: ovum)
oval window (O-val WIN-doe) a small, membrane-covered opening that separates the middle and inner ear
ovarian follicles (o-VARE-ee-an FOL-i-kuls) contain oocytes
ovaries (O-var-ees) female gonads that produce ova (sex cells)
overhydration (o-ver-hye-DRAY-shun) too large a fluid input that can put a burden on the heart
oviducts (O-vi-dukts) uterine or fallopian tubes
oxygen concentrator (OK-sih-jen) a device used in health care that increases the proportion of oxygen gas in the air of the room in which it is placed—it is sometimes used in respiratory and other conditions that produce hypoxia (low oxygen concentration in the blood)
oxygen debt (OK-sih-jen det) continued increased metabolism that occurs in a cell to remove excess lactic acid that resulted from exercise
oxygen therapy (OK-sih-jen THAYR-ah-pee) administration of oxygen gas to individuals suffering from hypoxia (low oxygen concentration in the blood)
oxyhemoglobin (ok-see-hee-mo-GLO-bin) hemoglobin combined with oxygen
oxytocin (ok-se-TOE-sin) hormone secreted by the posterior pituitary gland before and after delivering a baby; thought to initiate and maintain labor, it also causes the release of breast milk into ducts for the baby to suck

P

pacemaker (PASE-may-ker) see *sinoatrial node*
pacinian corpuscle (pah-SIN-ee-an KOR-pus-ul) a receptor found deep in the dermis that detects pressure on the skin surface
palate (PAL-let) the roof of the mouth; made up of the hard (anterior portion of the mouth) and soft (posterior portion of the mouth) palates
palmar (PAHL-mar) palm of the hand
pancreas (PAN-kree-as) endocrine gland located in the abdominal cavity; contains pancreatic islets that secrete glucagon and insulin
pancreatic islets (pan-kree-AT-ik eye-LETS) endocrine portion of the pancreas; made up of alpha and beta cells among others
papillae (pah-PIL-ee) small, nipple-shaped elevations
paralysis (pah-RAL-i-sis) loss of the power of motion, especially voluntary motion
paranasal sinus (pair-ah-NAY-sal SYE-nus) four pairs of sinuses that have openings into the nose
parasympathetic nervous system (PNS) (par-ah-sim-pah-THE-tic NER-vus SIS-tem) part of the autonomic nervous system; ganglia are connected to the brainstem and the sacral segments of the spinal cord; controls many visceral effectors under normal conditions
parathyroid glands (pair-ah-THYE-royd) endocrine glands located in the neck on the posterior aspect of the thyroid gland; secrete parathyroid hormone
parathyroid hormone (PTH) (pair-ah-THYE-royd HOR-mone) hormone released by the parathyroid gland that increases the concentration of calcium in the blood

parietal (pah-RYE-i-tal) of the walls of an organ or cavity

parietal pericardium (pah-RYE-i-tal pair-i-KAR-dee-um) pericardium surrounding the heart like a loose-fitting sack to allow the heart enough room to beat

parietal portion (pah-RYE-i-tal POR-shun) serous membrane that lines the walls of a body cavity

Parkinson disease (PARK-in-son) a chronic disease of the nervous system characterized by a set of signs called *parkinsonism* that results from a deficiency of the neurotransmitter dopamine in certain regions of the brain that normally inhibit overstimulation of skeletal muscles; parkinsonism is characterized by muscle rigidity and trembling of the head and extremities, forward tilt of the body, and shuffling manner of walking

parturition (par-too-RISH-un) act of giving birth

patella (pah-TEL-ah) small, shallow pan; the kneecap

pectoral girdle (PEK-toe-ral GIR-dul) shoulder girdle; the scapula and clavicle

pectoralis major (pek-tor-RAL-is MAY-jor) major flexor of the upper arm

pedal (PEED-al) foot

pelvic cavity (PEL-vik KAV-i-tee) the lower portion of the ventral cavity; the distal portion of the abdominopelvic cavity

pelvic girdle (PEL-vik GIR-dul) connects the legs to the trunk

pelvis (PEL-vis) basin or funnel-shaped structure

penis (PEE-nis) forms part of the male genitalia; when sexually aroused, becomes stiff to enable it to enter and deposit sperm in the vagina

pepsinogen (pep-SIN-o-jen) component of gastric juice that is converted into pepsin by hydrochloric acid

peptide bond (PEP-tyde bond) covalent bond linking amino acids within a protein molecule

pericarditis (pair-i-kar-DYE-tis) when the pericardium becomes inflamed

pericardium (pair-i-KAR-dee-um) membrane that surrounds the heart

perilymph (PAIR-i-limf) a watery fluid that fills the bony labyrinth of the ear

perineal (pair-i-NEE-al) area between the anus and genitals; the perineum

perineum (pair-i-NEE-um) see *perineal*

periosteum (pair-i-OS-tee-um) tough, connective tissue covering the bone

peripheral (pe-RIF-er-al) pertaining to an outside surface

peripheral nervous system (PNS) (pe-RIF-er-al NER-vus SIS-tem) the nerves connecting the brain and spinal cord to other parts of the body

peristalsis (pair-i-STAL-sis) wavelike, rhythmic contractions of the stomach and intestines that move food material along the digestive tract

peritoneal space (pair-i-toe-NEE-al) small, fluid-filled space between the visceral and parietal layers that allows the layers to slide over each other freely in the abdominopelvic cavity

peritoneum (pair-i-toe-NEE-um) large, moist, slippery sheet of serous membrane that lines the abdominopelvic cavity (parietal layer) and its organs (visceral layer)

peritonitis (pair-i-toe-NYE-tis) inflammation of the serous membranes in the abdominopelvic cavity; sometimes a serious complication of an infected appendix

permeable membrane (PER-mee-ah-bul MEM-brane) a membrane that allows passage of substances

pernicious anemia (per-NISH-us ah-NEE-mee-ah) deficiency of red blood cells because of a lack of vitamin B_{12}

peroneal muscles (per-o-NEE-al MUS-els) plantar flexors and evertors of the foot; the peroneus longus forms a support arch for the foot

perspiration (per-spi-RAY-shun) transparent, watery liquid released by glands in the skin that eliminates ammonia and uric acid and helps maintain body temperature; also known as sweat

pH (pee-AYCH) mathematical expression of relative $H+$ concentration (acidity); pH value higher than 7 is basic, pH value less than 7 is acidic, pH value equal to 7 is neutral

phagocytes (FAG-o-sites) white blood cells that engulf microbes and digest them

phagocytosis (fag-o-sye-TOE-sis) ingestion and digestion of articles by a cell

phalanges (fah-LAN-jeez) the bones that make up the fingers and toes

pharynx (FAIR-inks) organ of the digestive and respiratory system; commonly called the throat

phospholipid (fos-fo-LIP-id) phosphate-containing fat molecule

photopigments (fo-toe-PIG-ments) chemicals in retinal cells that are sensitive to light

phrenic nerve (FREN-ik nerv) the nerve that stimulates the diaphragm to contract

physiology (fiz-ee-OL-o-jee) the study of body function

pia mater (PEE-ah MAH-ter) the vascular innermost covering (meninx) of the brain and spinal cord

pigment layer (PIG-ment LAY-er) the layer of the epidermis that contains the melanocytes that produce melanin to give skin its color

pineal gland (PI-nee-al) endocrine gland located in the third ventricle of the brain; produces melatonin

pinocytosis (pin-o-sye-TOE-sis) the active transport mechanism used to transfer fluids or dissolved substances into cells

pituitary gland (pi-TOO-i-tair-ee) endocrine gland located in the skull, made up of the adenohypophysis and the neurohypophysis

placenta (plah-SEN-tah) anchors the developing fetus to the uterus and provides a "bridge" for the exchange of nutrients and waste products between the mother and developing baby

plantar (PLAN-tar) pertaining to the sole of the foot

plantar flexion (PLAN-tar FLEK-shun) the bottom of the foot is directed downward; this motion allows a person to stand on his or her tiptoes

plasma (PLAZ-mah) the liquid part of the blood

plasma cells (PLAZ-mah sells) cells that secrete copious amounts of antibody into the blood

plasma membrane (PLAZ-mah MEM-brane) membrane that separates the contents of a cell from the tissue fluid; encloses the cytoplasm and forms the outer boundary of the cell

plasma protein (PLAZ-mah PRO-teen) any of several proteins normally found in the plasma; includes albumins, globulins, and fibrinogen

platelet plug (PLAYT-let) a temporary accumulation of platelets (thrombocytes) at the site of an injury; it precedes the formation of a blood clot

pleura (PLOOR-ah) the serous membrane in the thoracic cavity

pleural cavity (PLOOR-al KAV-i-tee) a subdivision of the thorax

pleural space (PLOOR-al) the space between the visceral and parietal pleuras filled with just enough fluid to allow them to glide effortlessly with each breath

pleurisy (PLOOR-i-see) inflammation of the pleura

plica (PLYE-kah) multiple circular folds

pneumocystitis (noo-mo-sis-TYE-tis) a protozoan infection, most likely to invade the body when the immune system has been compromised

pneumothorax (noo-mo-THO-raks) accumulation of air in the pleural space, causing collapse of the lung

polycythemia (pol-ee-sye-THEE-mee-ah) an excessive number of red blood cells

polyuria (pol-ee-YOO-ree-ah) unusually large amounts of urine

pons (ponz) the part of the brainstem between the medulla oblongata and the midbrain

popliteal (pop-li-TEE-al) behind the knee

pore pinpoint-size openings on the skin that are outlets of small ducts from the eccrine sweat glands

posterior (pos-TEER-ee-or) located behind; opposite of anterior

posterior pituitary gland (pos-TEER-ee-or pi-TOO-i-tair-ee) neurohypophysis; hormones produced are ADH and oxytocin

posterior root ganglion (pos-TEER-ee-or GANG-lee-on) ganglion located near the spinal cord; where the neuron cell body of the dendrites of the sensory neuron is located

postganglionic neurons (post-gang-glee-ON-ik NOO-rons) autonomic neurons that conduct nerve impulses from a ganglion to cardiac or smooth muscle or glandular epithelial tissue

postnatal period (POST-nay-tal PEER-ee-od) the period after birth and ending at death

postsynaptic neuron (post-si-NAP-tik NOO-ron) a neuron situated distal to a synapse

posture (POS-chur) position of the body

precapillary sphincter (pree-CAP-pi-lair-ee SFINGK-ter) smooth muscle cells that guard the entrance to the capillary

preganglionic neurons (pree-gang-glee-ON-ik NOO-rons) autonomic neurons that conduct nerve impulses between the spinal cord and a ganglion

prenatal period (PREE-nay-tal PEER-i-od) the period after conception until birth

presbyopia (pres-bee-O-pee-ah) farsightedness of old age

presynaptic neuron (pree-si-NAP-tik NOO-ron) a neuron situated proximal to a synapse

primary follicles (PRYE-mare-ee FOL-i-kuls) the follicles present at puberty; covered with granulosa cells

primary germ layers (PRYE-mare-ee jerm LAY-ers) three layers of specialized cells that give rise to definite structures as the embryo develops

primary spermatocyte (PRY-mar-ee SPER-mah-toe-site) specialized cell that undergoes meiosis to ultimately form sperm

prime mover (prime MOO-ver) the muscle responsible for producing a particular movement

productany substance formed as a result of a chemical reaction

progesterone (pro-JES-ter-ohn) hormone produced by the corpus luteum; stimulates secretion of the uterine lining; with estrogen, helps to initiate the menstrual cycle in girls entering puberty

prolactin (pro-LAK-tin) hormone secreted by the anterior pituitary gland during pregnancy to stimulate the breast development needed for lactation

pronate (PRO-nate) to turn the palm downward

prone used to describe the body lying in a horizontal position facing downward

prophase (PRO-faze) first stage of mitosis during which chromosomes become visible

proprioceptors (pro-pree-o-SEP-tors) receptors located in the muscles, tendons, and joints; allows the body to recognize its position

prostaglandins (PGs) (pross-tah-GLAN-dins) a group of naturally occurring fatty acids that affect many body functions

prostatectomy (pross-tah-TEK-toe-mee) surgical removal of part or all of the prostate gland

prostate gland (PROSS-tate) lies just below the bladder; secretes a fluid that constitutes about 30% of the seminal fluid volume; helps activate sperm and helps them maintain motility

protease (PRO-tee-ase) protein-digesting enzyme

protein (PRO-teen) one of the basic nutrients needed by the body; a nitrogen-containing organic compound composed of a folded strand of amino acids

proteinuria (pro-teen-YOO-ree-ah) presence of abnormally high amounts of plasma protein in the urine; usually an indicator of kidney disease

proteome (PRO-tee-ome) the entire group of proteins encoded by the genome; see genome

proteomics (pro-tee-OME-iks) the endeavor that involves the analysis of the proteins encoded by the genome, with the ultimate goal of understanding the role of each protein in the body

prothrombin (pro-THROM-bin) a protein present in normal blood that is required for blood clotting

prothrombin activator (pro-THROM-bin AK-tiv-ayt-or) a protein formed by clotting factors from damaged tissue cells and platelets; it converts prothrombin into thrombin, a step essential to forming a blood clot

proton (PRO-ton) positively charged particle within the nucleus of an atom

proximal (PROK-si-mal) next or nearest; located nearest the center of the body or the point of attachment of a structure

proximal convoluted tubule (PROK-si-mal kon-vo-LOO-ted TOOB-yool) the first segment of a renal tubule

pseudo (SOO-doe) false

pubis (PYOO-bis) joint in the midline between the two pubic bones

pulmonary artery (PUL-mo-nair-ee AR-ter-ee) artery that carries deoxygenated blood from the right ventricle to the lungs

pulmonary circulation (PUL-mo-nair-ee ser-kyoo-LAY-shun) venous blood flow from the right atrium to the lung and returning to the left atrium

pulmonary semilunar valve (PUL-mo-nair-ee sem-i-LOO-nar valv) valve located at the beginning of the pulmonary artery

pulmonary vein (PUL-mo-nair-ee vane) any vein that carries oxygenated blood from the lungs to the left atrium

pulmonary ventilation (PUL-mo-nair-ee ven-ti-LAY-shun) breathing; process that moves air in and out of the lungs

pupil (PYOO-pil) the opening in the center of the iris that regulates the amount of light entering the eye

Purkinje fibers (pur-KIN-jee FYE-bers) specialized cells located in the walls of the ventricles; relay nerve impulses from the AV node to the ventricles causing them to contract

P wave deflection on an ECG that occurs with depolarization of the atria

pyloric sphincter (pye-LOR-ik SFINGK-ter) sphincter that prevents food from leaving the stomach and entering the duodenum

pylorus (pye-LOR-us) the small narrow section of the stomach that joins the first part of the small intestine

pyramids (PEER-ah-mids) triangular-shaped divisions of the medulla of the kidney

Q

QRS complex (QRS KOM-pleks) deflection on an ECG that occurs as a result of depolarization of the ventricles

quadriceps femoris (KWOD-re-seps fe-MOR-is) extensor of the lower leg

quickening (KWIK-en-ing) when a pregnant woman first feels recognizable movements of the fetus

R

radiation (ray-dee-AY-shun) flow of heat waves away from the blood

radiography (ray-de-OG-rah-fee) imaging technique using x-rays that pass through certain tissues more easily than others, allowing an image of tissues to form on a photographic plate; invented by Wilhelm Röntgen in 1895

radius (RAY-dee-us) one of the two bones in the forearm; located on the thumb side of the forearm

reabsorption (ree-ab-SORP-shun) process of absorbing again that occurs in the kidneys

reactant (ree-AK-tant) any substance entering (and being changed by) a chemical reaction

receiving chambers (ree-SEE-ving CHAME-bers) atria of the heart; receive blood from the superior and inferior vena cava

receptor (ree-SEP-tor) peripheral beginning of a sensory neuron's dendrite

rectum (REK-tum) distal portion of the large intestine

rectus abdominis (REK-tus ab-DOM-i-nis) muscle that runs down the middle of the abdomen; protects the abdominal viscera and flexes the spinal column

reflex (REE-fleks) involuntary action

reflex arc (REE-fleks ark) allows an impulse to travel in only one direction

reflux (REE-fluhks) backflow, as in flow of stomach contents back into esophagus

refraction (ree-FRAK-shun) bending of a ray of light as it passes from a medium of one density to one of a different density

releasing hormones (ree-LEE-sing HOR-mones) hormone produced by the hypothalamus gland that causes the anterior pituitary gland to release its hormones

renal calculi (REE-nal KAL-kyoo-lie) kidney stones

renal colic (REE-nal KOL-ik) pain caused by the passage of a kidney stone

renal corpuscle (REE-nal KOR-pus-ul) the part of the nephron located in the cortex of the kidney

renal pelvis (REE-nal PEL-vis) basinlike upper end of the ureter that is located inside the kidney

renal tubule (REE-nal TOOB-yool) one of the two principal parts of the nephron

repolarization (ree-po-lah-ri-ZAY-shun) begins just before the relaxation phase of cardiac muscle activity

reproductive system (ree-pro-DUK-tiv SIS-tem) produces hormones that permit the development of sexual characteristics and the propagation of the species

residual volume (RV) (re-ZID-yoo-al VOL-yoom) the air that remains in the lungs after the most forceful expiration

respiratory acidosis (RES-pi-rah-tor-ee as-i-DOE-sis) a respiratory disturbance that results in a carbonic acid excess

respiratory alkalosis (RES-pi-rah-tor-ee al-kah-LO-sis) a respiratory disturbance that results in a carbonic acid deficit

respiratory arrest (RES-pi-rah-tor-ee ah-REST) cessation of breathing without resumption

respiratory control centers (RES-pi-rah-tor-ee kon-TROL SEN-ters) centers located in the medulla and pons that stimulate the muscles of respiration

respiratory membrane (RES-pi-rah-tor-ee MEM-brane) the single layer of cells that makes up the wall of the alveoli

respiratory mucosa (RES-pi-rah-tor-ee myoo-KO-sah) mucus-covered membrane that lines the tubes of the respiratory tree

respiratory muscles (RES-pi-rah-tor-ee MUS-els) muscles that are responsible for the changing shape of the thoracic cavity that allows air to move in and out of the lungs

respiratory system (re-SPY-rah-tor-ee SIS-tem) the organs that allow the exchange of oxygen from the air with the carbon dioxide from the blood

respiratory therapist (RES-pih-rah-tor-ee THAYR-ah-pist) health professional who helps patients increase respiratory function or overcome or cope with the effects of respiratory conditions

respiratory tract (RES-pi-rah-tor-ee trakt) the two divisions of the respiratory system are the upper and lower respiratory tracts

reticular formation (re-TIK-yoo-lar for-MAY-shun) located in the medulla where bits of gray and white matter mix intricately

retina (RET-i-nah) innermost layer of the eyeball; contains rods and cones and continues posteriorly with the optic nerve

retroperitoneal (re-tro-pair-i-toe-NEE-al) area outside of the peritoneum

Rh-negative (R H NEG-ah-tiv) red blood cells that do not contain the antigen called Rh factor

RhoGAM (RO-gam) an injection of a special protein given to an Rh-negative woman who is pregnant to prevent her body from forming anti-Rh antibodies, which may harm an Rh-positive baby

Rh-positive (R H POZ-i-tiv) red blood cells that contain an antigen called Rh factor

ribonucleic acid (RNA) (rye-bo-noo-KLEE-ik AS-id) a nucleic acid found in the cytoplasm that is crucial to protein synthesis

ribosomal RNA (rRNA) (rye-bo-SOHM-al R-N-A) a form of RNA that makes up most of the structures (subunits) of the ribosome organelle of the cell

ribosome (RYE-bo-sohm) organelle in the cytoplasm of cells that synthesizes proteins; also known as a protein factory

rods receptors located in the retina that are responsible for night vision

rotation (ro-TAY-shun) movement around a longitudinal axis; for example, shaking your head "no"

rugae (ROO-gee) wrinkles or folds (singular: ruga [ROO-gah])

"rule of nines" a frequently used method to determine the extent of a burn injury; the body is divided into 11 areas of 9% each to help estimate the amount of skin surface burned in an adult

S

sagittal (SAJ-i-tal) longitudinal; like an arrow

salivary amylase (SAL-i-vair-ee AM-i-lase) digestive enzyme found in the saliva that begins the chemical digestion of carbohydrates

saltatory conduction (SAL-tah-tor-ee kon-DUK-shun) when a nerve impulse encounters myelin and "jumps" from one node of Ranvier to the next

sarcomere (SAR-ko-meer) contractile unit of muscle; length of a myofibril between two Z bands

scapula (SKAP-yoo-lah) shoulder blade

Schwann cells (shwon sells) large nucleated cells that form myelin

scientific method (sye-en-TIF-ik METH-od) any logical and systematic approach to discovering principles of nature, often involving testing of tentative explanations called *hypotheses*

sclera (SKLE-rah) white outer coat of the eyeball
scrotum (SKRO-tum) pouchlike sac that contains the testes
sebaceous gland (se-BAY-shus) oil-producing glands found in the skin
sebum (SEE-bum) secretion of sebaceous glands
secondary sexual characteristics (SEK-on-dair-ee SEK-shoo-al kair-ak-ter-IS-tiks) sexual characteristics that appear at the onset of puberty
second messenger (SEK-und MES-en-jer) chemical that provides communication within a hormone's target cell; for example, cyclic AMP
sella turcica (SEL-lah TER-si-kah) small depression of the sphenoid bone that contains the pituitary gland
semen (SEE-men) male reproductive fluid
semicircular canals (sem-i-SIR-kyoo-lar kah-NALS) located in the inner ear; contains a specialized receptor called crista ampullaris that generates a nerve impulse on movement of the head
semilunar valves (sem-i-LOO-nar valvs) valves located between the two ventricular chambers and the large arteries that carry blood away from the heart; valves found in the veins
seminal fluid (SEM-i-nal FLOO-id) semen
seminal vesicle (SEM-i-nal VES-i-kul) paired, pouchlike glands that contribute about 60% of the seminal fluid volume; rich in fructose, which is a source of energy for sperm
seminiferous tubule (se-mi-NIF-er-us TOOB-yool) long, coiled structure that forms the bulk of the testicular mass
senescence (se-NES-enz) older adulthood; aging
sensory neurons (SEN-sor-ee NOO-rons) neurons that transmit impulses to the spinal cord and brain from all parts of the body
serosa (se-RO-sah) outermost covering of the digestive tract; composed of the parietal pleura in the abdominal cavity
serotonin (sair-o-TOE-nin) a neurotransmitter that belongs to a group of compounds called catecholamines
serous membrane (SE-rus MEM-brane) a two-layered epithelial membrane that lines body cavities and covers the surfaces of organs
serum (SEER-um) blood plasma minus its clotting factors, still contains antibodies
shingles (SHING-guls) see *herpes zoster*
sickle cell anemia (SIK-ul sell ah-NEE-mee-ah) severe, possibly fatal, hereditary disease caused by an abnormal type of hemoglobin
sickle cell trait (SIK-ul sell trate) when only one defective gene is inherited and only a small amount of hemoglobin that is less soluble than usual is produced
sigmoid colon (SIG-moyd KO-lon) S-shaped segment of the large intestine that terminates in the rectum
signal transduction (tranz-DUK-shen) a term that refers to the whole process of getting a chemical signal (such as a hormone or neurotransmitter) to the inside of a cell; in a way, signal transduction is really "signal translation" by the cell
sinoatrial (SA) node (sye-no-AY-tree-al) the heart's pacemaker; where the impulse conduction of the heart normally starts; located in the wall of the right atrium near the opening of the superior vena cava
sinus (SYE-nus) a space or cavity inside some of the cranial bones
sinusitis (sye-nyoo-SYE-tis) sinus infections
skeletal muscle (SKEL-e-tal MUS-el) also known as voluntary muscle; muscles under willed or voluntary control
skeletal system (SKEL-e-tal SIS-tem) the bones, cartilage, and ligaments that provide the body with a rigid framework for support and protection
smooth muscle (MUS-el) muscles that are not under conscious control; also known as involuntary or visceral; forms the walls of blood vessels and hollow organs
sodium-potassium pump (SO-dee-um po-TAS-ee-um) a system of coupled ion pumps that actively transports sodium ions out of a cell and potassium ions into the cell at the same time—found in all living cells
solute (SOL-yoot) substance that dissolves into another substance; for example, in saltwater the salt is the solute dissolved in water
solvent (SOL-vent) substance in which other substances are dissolved; for example, in saltwater the water is the solvent for salt
somatic nervous system (so-MA-tik NER-vus SIS-tem) the motor neurons that control the voluntary actions of skeletal muscles
specific immunity (spe-SI-fik i-MYOON-i-tee) the protective mechanisms that provide specific protection against certain types of bacteria or toxins
sperm the male spermatozoon; sex cell
spermatids (SPER-mah-tids) the resulting daughter cells from the primary spermatocyte undergoing meiosis; these cells have only half the genetic material and half the chromosomes of other body cells
spermatogenesis (sper-mah-toe-JEN-e-sis) the production of sperm cells
spermatogonia (sper-mah-toe-GO-nee-ah) sperm precursor cells
spermatozoa (sper-mah-tah-ZO-ah) sperm cells (singular: spermatozoon)
sphincter (SFINGK-ter) ring-shaped muscle
spinal cavity (SPY-nal KAV-i-tee) the space inside the spinal column through which the spinal cord passes
spinal nerves (SPY-nal nervs) nerves that connect the spinal cord to peripheral structures such as the skin and skeletal muscles

spinal tracts (SPY-nal trakts) the white columns of the spinal cord that provide two-way conduction paths to and from the brain; ascending tract carries information to the brain, whereas descending tracts conduct impulses from the brain

spindle fiber (SPIN-dul FYE-ber) a network of tubules formed in the cytoplasm between the centrioles as they are moving away from each other

spirometer (spi-ROM-e-ter) an instrument used to measure the amount of air exchanged in breathing

spleen largest lymphoid organ; filters blood, destroys worn out red blood cells, salvages iron from hemoglobin, and serves as a blood reservoir

splenectomy (splen-NEK-toe-mee) surgical removal of the spleen

splenic flexure (SPLEEN-ik FLEK-shur) where the descending colon turns downward on the left side of the abdomen

spongy bone (SPUN-jee) porous bone in the end of the long bone, may be filled with marrow

squamous (SKWAY-mus) scalelike

squamous suture (SKWAY-mus SOO-chur) the immovable joint between the temporal bone and the sphenoid bone

stapes (STAY-peez) tiny, stirrup-shaped bone in the middle ear

staph (staff) a short form of *Staphylococcus*, a category of bacteria that can infect the skin and other organs, sometimes seriously

Stensen's ducts (STEN-sens dukts) the ducts of the parotid gland as they enter the mouth

sternoclavicular joint (ster-no-klah-VIK-yoo-lar joynt) the direct point of attachment between the bones of the upper extremity and the axial skeleton

sternocleidomastoid (stern-o-klye-doe-MAS-toyd) "strap" muscle located on the anterior aspect of the neck

steroid hormones (STE-royd HOR-mones) lipid-soluble hormones that pass intact through the cell membrane of the target cell and influence cell activity by acting on specific genes

stimulus (STIM-yoo-lus) agent that causes a change in the activity of a structure

stoma (STO-mah) an opening, such as the opening created in a colostomy procedure

stomach (STUM-ak) an expansion of the digestive tract between the esophagus and small intestine

stratum corneum (STRA-tum KOR-nee-um) the tough outer layer of the epidermis; cells are filled with keratin

stratum germinativum (STRA-tum JER-mi-nah-tiv-um) the innermost of the tightly packed epithelial cells of the epidermis; cells in this layer are able to reproduce themselves

strength training (strength TRAIN-ing) contracting muscles against resistance to enhance muscle hypertrophy

striated muscle (STRYE-ay-ted MUS-el) see *skeletal muscle*

stroke volume (stroke VOL-yoom) the amount of blood that is ejected from the ventricles of the heart with each beat

subcutaneous tissue (sub-kyoo-TAY-nee-us TISH-yoo) tissue below the layers of skin; made up of loose connective tissue and fat

submucosa (sub-myoo-KO-sah) connective tissue layer containing blood vessels and nerves in the wall of the digestive tract

sudoriferous gland (soo-doe-RIF-er-us) glands that secrete sweat; also referred to as sweat glands

sulcus (SUL-kus) furrow or groove

superficial (soo-per-FISH-al) near the body surface

superior (soo-PEER-ee-or) higher, opposite of inferior

superior vena cava (soo-PEER-ee-or VEE-nah KAY-vah) one of two large veins returning deoxygenated blood to the right atrium

supinate (SOO-pi-nate) to turn the palm of the hand upward; opposite of pronate

supine (SOO-pine) used to describe the body lying in a horizontal position facing upward

supraclavicular (soo-prah-cla-VIK-yoo-lar) area above the clavicle

surfactant (sur-FAK-tant) a substance covering the surface of the respiratory membrane inside the alveolus, which reduces surface tension and prevents the alveoli from collapsing

suture (SOO-chur) immovable joint

sweat (swet) transparent, watery liquid released by glands in the skin that eliminates ammonia and uric acid and helps maintain body temperature; also known as perspiration

sympathetic nervous system (sim-pah-THEH-tik NER-vus SIS-tem) part of the autonomic nervous system; ganglia are connected to the thoracic and lumbar regions of the spinal cord; functions as an emergency system

sympathetic postganglionic neurons (sim-pah-THE-tik post-gang-glee-ON-ik NOO-rons) dendrites and cell bodies are in sympathetic ganglia and axons travel to a variety of visceral effectors

sympathetic preganglionic neurons (sim-pah-THE-tik pree-gang-glee-ON-ik NOO-rons) dendrites and cell bodies are located in the gray matter of the thoracic and lumbar segments of the spinal cord; leaves the cord through an anterior root of a spinal nerve and terminates in a collateral ganglion

synapse (SIN-aps) junction between adjacent neurons

synaptic cleft (si-NAP-tik kleft) the space between a synaptic knob and the plasma membrane of a postsynaptic neuron

synaptic knob (si-NAP-tik nob) a tiny bulge at the end of a terminal branch of a presynaptic neuron's axon that contains vesicles with neurotransmitters

synarthrosis (sin-ar-THRO-sis) a joint in which fibrous connective tissue joins bones and holds them together tightly; commonly called sutures

synergist (SIN-er-jist) muscle that assists a prime mover

synovial fluid (si-NO-vee-al FLOO-id) the thick, colorless lubricating fluid secreted by the synovial membrane

synovial membrane (si-NO-vee-al MEM-brane) connective tissue membrane lining the spaces between bones and joints that secretes synovial fluid

system (SIS-tem) group of organs arranged so that the group can perform a more complex function than any one organ can perform alone

systemic circulation (sis-TEM-ik ser-kyoo-LAY-shun) blood flow from the left ventricle to all parts of the body and back to the right atrium

systole (SIS-toe-lee) contraction of the heart muscle

T

target organ cell (TAR-get OR-gan sell) organ or cell acted on by a particular hormone and responding to it

tarsals (TAR-sals) seven bones of the heel and back part of the foot; the calcaneus is the largest

taste buds chemical receptors that generate nerve impulses, resulting in the sense of taste

telemetry (tel-EM-et-ree) technology by which data, such as heart activity monitored by an electrocardiograph, can be sent to a remote location through telephone wires, radio waves, or other communication pathway

telophase (TEL-o-faze) last stage of mitosis in which the cell divides

temporal (TEM-po-ral) muscle that assists the masseter in closing the jaw

tendons (TEN-dons) bands or cords of fibrous connective tissue that attach a muscle to a bone or other structure

tendon sheath (TEN-don sheeth) tube-shaped structure lined with synovial membrane that encloses certain tendons

tenosynovitis (ten-o-sin-o-VYE-tis) inflammation of a tendon sheath

teratogen (TAYR-ah-to-jen) any environmental factor that causes a birth defect (abnormality present at birth); common teratogens include radiation (for example, x-rays), chemicals (for example, drugs, cigarettes, or alcohol), and infections in the mother (for example, herpes or rubella)

testes (TES-teez) male gonads that produce the male sex cells or sperm

testosterone (tes-TOS-te-rone) male sex hormone produced by the interstitial cells in the testes; the "masculinizing hormone"

tetanic contraction (te-TAN-ik kon-TRAK-shun) sustained contraction

tetanus (TET-ah-nus) sustained muscular contraction

thalamus (THAL-ah-mus) located just above the hypothalamus; its functions are to help produce sensations and associate sensations with emotions; plays a part in the arousal mechanism

theory (THEE-ree) an explanation of a scientific principle that has been tested experimentally and found to be true; compare to *hypothesis* and *law*

thermoregulation (ther-mo-reg-yoo-LAY-shun) maintaining homeostasis of body temperature

thoracic duct (thor-AS-ik dukt) largest lymphatic vessel in the body

thorax (THOR-aks) chest

threshold stimulus (THRESH-hold STIM-yoo-lus) minimal level of stimulation required to cause a muscle fiber to contract

thrombin (THROM-bin) protein important in blood clotting

thrombocytes (THROM-bo-sites) also called platelets; play a role in blood clotting

thrombosis (throm-BO-sis) formation of a clot in a blood vessel

thrombus (THROM-bus) stationary blood clot

thymosin (THY-mo-sin) hormone produced by the thymus that is vital to the development and functioning of the body's immune system

thymus gland (THY-mus) endocrine gland located in the mediastinum; vital part of the body's immune system

thyroid gland (THY-royd) endocrine gland located in the neck that stores its hormones until needed; thyroid hormones regulate cellular metabolism

thyroid-stimulating hormone (TSH) (THY-royd STIM-yoo-lay-ting HOR-mone) a tropic hormone secreted by the anterior pituitary gland that stimulates the thyroid gland to increase its secretion of thyroid hormone

thyroxine (T_4) (thy-ROK-sin) thyroid hormone that stimulates cellular metabolism

tibia (TIB-ee-ah) shinbone

tibialis anterior (tib-ee-AL-is an-TEER-ee-or) dorsiflexor of the foot

tidal volume (TV) (TIE-dal VOL-yoom) amount of air breathed in and out with each breath

tinea pedis (TIN-ee-ah PED-is) athlete's foot, a fungal infection of the skin characterized by redness and itching

tissue (TISH-yoo) group of similar cells that perform a common function

tissue fluid (TISH-yoo FLOO-id) a dilute saltwater solution that bathes every cell in the body

tissue hormone (TISH-yoo HOR-mone) prostaglandins; produced in a tissue and diffuses only a short distance to act on cells within the tissue

tissue typing (TISH-yoo TIE-ping) a procedure used to identify tissue compatibility before an organ transplant

T-lymphocytes (T LIM-fo-sites) cells that are critical to the function of the immune system; produce cell-mediated immunity

tonic contraction (TON-ik kon-TRAK-shun) special type of skeletal muscle contraction used to maintain posture

tonsillectomy (ton-si-LEK-toe-mee) surgical procedure used to remove the tonsils

tonsillitis (ton-si-LIE-tis) an inflammation of the tonsils

tonsils (TON-sils) masses of lymphoid tissue; protect against bacteria; three types: palatine tonsils, located on each side of the throat; pharyngeal tonsils (adenoids), near the posterior opening of the nasal cavity; and lingual tonsils, near the base of the tongue

total metabolic rate (TMR) (TOE-tal met-ah-BOL-ik) total amount of energy used by the body per day

trabeculae (trah-BEK-yoo-lee) needlelike threads of spongy bone that surround a network of spaces

trachea (TRAY-kee-ah) the windpipe; the tube extending from the larynx to the bronchi

transcription (trans-KRIP-shun) when the double stranded DNA molecules unwind and form mRNA

transitional epithelium (tranz-IH-shen-al ep-ih-THEE-lee-um) type of epithelial tissue that forms membranes capable of stretching without breaking, as in the urinary bladder; cells in this type of tissue can stretch from roughly columnar out to flattened (squamous) and back without damage

translation (trans-LAY-shun) the synthesis of a protein by ribosomes

transverse arch (TRANS-vers) see *metatarsal arch*

transversus abdominis (trans-VER-sus ab-DOM-i-nis) the innermost layer of the anterolateral abdominal wall

trapezium (trah-PEE-zee-um) the carpal bone of the wrist that forms the saddle joint that allows the opposition of the thumb

trapezius (trah-PEE-zee-us) triangular muscle in the back that elevates the shoulder and extends the head backwards

triceps brachii (TRY-seps BRAY-kee-eye) extensor of the elbow

tricuspid valve (try-KUS-pid valv) the valve located between the right atrium and ventricle

trigone (TRY-gon) triangular area on the wall of the urinary bladder

triiodothyronine (T_3) (try-eye-o-doe-THY-ro-nine) thyroid hormone that stimulates cellular metabolism

tropic hormone (TRO-pik HOR-mone) hormone that stimulates another endocrine gland to grow and secrete its hormones

true ribs the first seven pairs of ribs that are attached to the sternum

tumor (TOO-mer) growth of tissues in which cell proliferation is uncontrolled and progressive

tunica adventitia (TOO-ni-kah ad-ven-TISH-ah) the outermost layer found in blood vessels

tunica albuginea (TOO-ni-kah al-byoo-JIN-ee-ah) a tough, whitish membrane that surrounds each testis and enters the gland to divide it into lobules

tunica intima (TOO-ni-kah IN-tih-mah) endothelium that lines the blood vessels

tunica media (TOO-ni-kah MEE-dee-ah) the muscular middle layer found in blood vessels; the tunica media of arteries is more muscular than that of veins

T wave deflection on an electrocardiogram that occurs with repolarization of the ventricles

twitch a quick, jerky response to a single stimulus

tympanic (tim-PAN-ik) drumlike

type 1 diabetes mellitus (tipe won dye-ah-BEE-teez mell-EYE-tus) a condition resulting when the pancreatic islets secrete too little insulin, resulting in increased levels of blood glucose; formerly known as *juvenile-onset diabetes* or *insulin-dependent diabetes mellitus*

type 2 diabetes mellitus (tipe too dye-ah-BEE-teez mell-EYE-tus) a condition resulting when cells of the body become less sensitive to the hormone insulin and perhaps the pancreatic islets secrete too little insulin, resulting in increased levels of blood glucose; formerly known as *maturity-onset diabetes* or *insulin-independent diabetes mellitus*

U

ulcer (UL-ser) a necrotic open sore or lesion

ulna (UL-nah) one of the two forearm bones; located on the little finger side

ultrasonogram (ul-tra-SOHN-o-gram) a technique using sound to produce images

umbilical artery (um-BIL-i-kul AR-ter-ee) two small arteries that carry oxygen-poor blood from the developing fetus to the placenta

umbilical cord (um-BIL-i-kul) flexible structure connecting the fetus with the placenta, which allows the umbilical arteries and vein to pass

umbilical vein (um-BIL-i-kul vane) a large vein carrying oxygen-rich blood from the placenta to the developing fetus

urea (yoo-REE-ah) nitrogen-containing waste product

uremia (yoo-REE-mee-ah) high levels of nitrogen-containing waste products in the blood; also referred to as uremic poisoning

uremic poisoning (yoo-REE-mik POY-zon-ing) see *uremia*

urethra (yoo-REE-thrah) passageway for elimination of urine; in males, also acts as a genital duct that carries sperm to the exterior

urinary meatus (YOOR-i-nair-ee mee-AY-tus) external opening of the urethra
urinary system (YOOR-i-nair-ee SIS-tem) system responsible for excreting liquid waste from the body
urination (yoor-i-NAY-shun) passage of urine from the body; emptying of the bladder
urine (YOOR-in) fluid waste excreted by the kidneys
uterus (YOO-ter-us) hollow, muscular organ where a fertilized egg implants and grows
uvula (YOO-vyoo-lah) cone-shaped process hanging down from the soft palate that helps prevent food and liquid from entering the nasal cavities

V

vagina (vah-JYE-nah) internal tube from the uterus to the vulva
vas deferens (vas DEF-er-enz) see *ductus deferens*
vastus (VAS-tus) wide; of great size
vein (vane) vessel carrying blood toward the heart
ventral (VEN-tral) of or near the belly; in humans, front or anterior; opposite of dorsal or posterior
ventricles (VEN-tri-kuls) small cavities
venule (VEN-yool) small blood vessels that collect blood from the capillaries and join to form veins
vermiform appendix (VERM-i-form ah-PEN-diks) a tubular structure attached to the cecum composed of lymphatic tissue
vertebrae (VER-te-bray) bones that make up the spinal column
vertebral column (ver-TEE-bral KOL-um) the spinal column, made up of a series of separate vertebrae that form a flexible, curved rod
vestibular nerve (ves-TIB-yoo-lar nerv) a division of the vestibulocochlear nerve (the eighth cranial nerve)
vestibule (VES-ti-byool) located in the inner ear; the portion adjacent to the oval window between the semicircular canals and the cochlea
villi (VIL-eye) fingerlike folds covering the plicae of the small intestines
visceral pericardium (VIS-er-al pair-i-KAR-dee-um) the pericardium that covers the heart
visceral portion (VIS-er-al POR-shun) serous membrane that covers the surface of organs found in the body cavity
vital capacity (VC) (VYE-tal kah-PAS-i-tee) largest amount of air that can be moved in and out of the lungs in one inspiration and expiration
vitamins (VYE-tah-mins) organic molecules needed in small quantities to help enzymes operate effectively
vitreous humor (VIT-ree-us HYOO-mor) the jellylike fluid found in the eye, posterior to the lens
voiding (VOYD-ing) emptying of the bladder
volar (VO-lar) palm or sole
voluntary muscle (VOL-un-tair-ee MUS-el) see *skeletal muscle*
vulva (VUL-vah) external genitals of the female

W

wart raised bump that is a benign neoplasm (tumor) of the skin caused by viruses
white matter (wite MATT-er) nerves covered with white myelin
withdrawal reflex (with-DRAW-al REE-fleks) a reflex that moves a body part away from an irritating stimulus

Y

yolk sac (yoke sak) in humans, involved with the production of blood cells in the developing embryo

Z

zona fasciculata (ZO-nah fas-sic-yoo-LAY-tah) middle zone of the adrenal cortex that secretes glucocorticoids
zona glomerulosa (ZO-nah glo-mare-yoo-LO-sah) outer zone of the adrenal cortex that secretes mineralocorticoids
zona reticularis (ZO-nah re-tik-yoo-LAIR-is) inner zone of the adrenal cortex that secretes small amounts of sex hormones
zygomaticus (zye-go-MAT-ik-us) muscle that elevates the corners of the mouth and lips; also known as the smiling muscle
zygote (ZYE-gote) a fertilized ovum

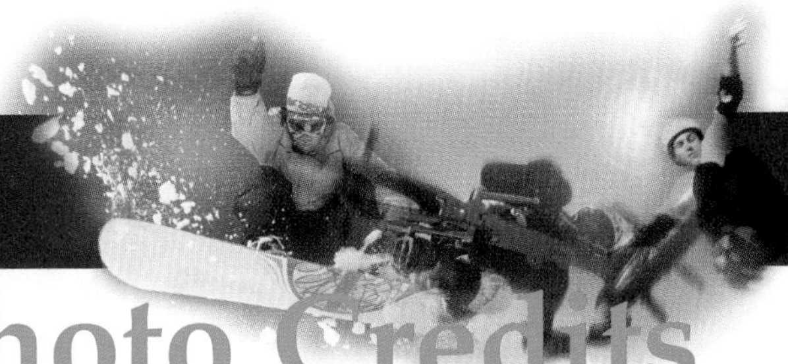

Illustration/Photo Credits

Chapter 1

1-1, 1-3, 1-5, 1-6, 1-7, 1-9, Barbara Cousins; 1-2, 1-8, Terry Cockerham/Synapse Media Production; Science Applications box, Joe Kulka, National Library of Medicine.

Chapter 2

2-1, 2-7, 2-10, 2-11, Network Graphics; 2-2, 2-3, Precision Graphics; 2-5, 2-6, 2-9, Rolin Graphics; 2-8, JB Wooskey and Associates; Science Applications box, Joe Kulka.

Chapter 3

3-1, 3-2, William Ober; 3-3, Lennart Nilsson; 3-4, 3-6, Rolin Graphics; 3-8, 3-9(B), 3-10 (B), 3-11(B), 3-12(B), 3-14(B), Barbara Cousins; 3-9(A), 3-10(A), 3-11(A), 3-12(A), 3-14(A), 3-16, 3-17, 3-18, 3-19, 3-21, 3-22, courtesy Gartner LP, Hiatt JL (from *Color textbook of histology*, 1997, Saunders); 3-13, courtesy Stanley Erlandsen (from *Color atlas of histology*, 1992, Mosby); 3-15, Photo Take; 3-20, Edward Reschke; Science Applications box, Joe Kulka.

Chapter 4

4-2, 4-3, 4-4, 4-5, 4-6, 4-7, 4-8, 4-9, 4-10, 4-11, 4-12, 4-13, Barbara Cousins; Science Applications box, Joe Kulka, (Medical Imaging of the Body) Photo Researchers.

Chapter 5

5-1, 5-2, 5-6, Rolin Graphics; 5-3, Edward Reschke; 5-4, 5-7, Christine Oleksyk; 5-5, David Scharf/Peter Arnold, Inc; 5-8, Barbara Cousins; 5-9, Courtesy of Dr Richard L Judd and Dwight D Ponsell (from *Mosby's first responder*, 2/e, 1988, Mosby); Decubitus Ulcer box, courtesy PA Potter and AG Perry (from *Fundamentals of nursing*, 2001, Mosby); Science Applications box, Joe Kulka.

Chapter 6

6-1, 6-2, 6-7, 6-10, 6-13 (art), 6-14 (art), 6-15 (art), 6-16 (art), 6-19, 6-20, Table 5-7, Barbara Cousins; 6-3, 6-4, courtesy Gartner LP, Hiatt JL (from *Color textbook of histology*, 1997, Saunders); 6-5, Stephen Oh; 6-6, Network Graphics; 6-11, Ron Edwards; 6-12, 6-13 (photo), 6-14 (photo), 6-15 (photo), 6-16 (photo), courtesy B Vidic and FR Suarez (from *Photographic atlas of the human body*, 1984, Mosby); Clinical Application box: Epiphyseal Fracture, JM Booher and GA Thibodeau; Clinical Application box: Palpable Bony Landmarks, Terry Cockerham/Synapse Media Production; Knee Joint Box, Stewart Halpernin (photo), Rolin Graphics (art); Science Applications box, Joe Kulka.

Chapter 7

7-1, Christine Oleksyk; 7-2, Network Graphics; 7-3(A), Barbara Cousins; 7-3(B), courtesy Dr HE Huxley; 7-4, courtesy Stanley Erlandsen (from *Color atlas of histology*, 1992, Mosby); 7-5, 7-9(A,C), Carpal Tunnel Box, Rolin Graphics; 7-6, 7-7, 7-8, John V Hagen; 7-9(B), 7-10(B), 7-11, Terry Cockerham/Synapse Media Production; Intramuscular Injection Box, Barbara Cousins; Science Applications box, Joe Kulka.

Chapter 8

8-2(A, B), 8-13, 8-16, 8-20, Rolin Graphics; 8-2(C), Edward Reschke; 8-3, 8-4, 8-5, 8-6, 8-7, 8-8, 8-12, 8-14, 8-19, Barbara Cousins; 8-9(A), 8-10(A,B),

William Ober; 8-9(B), 8-10(inset), 8-11(photo), courtesy B Vidic and FR Suarez (from *Photographic atlas of the human body*, 1984, Mosby); 8-11(drawing), Parkinson Disease box, George J Wassilchenko; 8-15, 8-17, Network Graphics; 8-18, Raychel Ciemma; Herpes Zoster box (photo), courtesy TP Habif (from *Clinical dermatology*, ed 2, 1990 Mosby); Science Applications box, Joe Kulka.

Chapter 9

9-1, Christine Oleksyk; 9-2, George Wassilchenko; 9-3, Refractive Eye Surgery box, Barbara Cousins; 9-4, Ernest W Beck; 9-5, Table 9-1, Cochlear Implant box, Rolin Graphics; 9-6, Focusing Problems box, Network Graphics; 9-7(D), Photo Researchers; 9-8, Joan Beck; Color Blindness box, courtesy Ishihara (from *Tests for colour blindness*, Tokyo, Japan, 1973, Kanehara Shuppan Co, Ltd); Science Applications box, Joe Kulka.

Chapter 10

10-1, 10-9, 10-11, Barbara Cousins; 10-2, 10-3, Network Graphics; 10-4, 10-8, Rolin Graphics; 10-5, Barbara Cousins; 10-6, Ernest W Beck; 10-10, Graphic Works; 10-12, GA Thibodeau and KT Patton (from *Anatomy & physiology*, ed 5, 2003, Mosby); Thyroid Hormone Abnormalities box (A), HM Seidel et al (from *Mosby's guide to physical examination*, ed 4, 1999, Mosby); Thyroid Hormone Abnormalities box (B), LV Bergman & Associates, Cold Springs, New York; Adrenal Hormone Abnormalities, courtesy Gower Medical Publishers; Science Applications box, Joe Kulka.

Chapter 11

11-1, 11-6(A), Table 11-1, Barbara Cousins; 11-2, Sickle Cell Anemia box, courtesy G Bevelander and JA Ramaley (from *Essentials of histology*, ed 8, Mosby); 11-3, 11-7, Rolin Graphics; 11-4, courtesy Stanley Erlandsen (from *Color atlas of histology*, 1992, Mosby); 11-5, courtesy A Arlan Hinchee; 11-6, GA Thibodeau and KT Patton (from *Anatomy & physiology*, ed 5, 2003, Mosby); 11-8, Molly Babich/John Daugherty; Science Applications box, Joe Kulka.

Chapter 12

12-1, 12-4, 12-7, 12-8, 12-9(A), 12-10, 12-11, 12-15, 12-17, Barbara Cousins; 12-2, Rusty Jones; 12-3 (top), Christine Oleksyk; 12-3(bottom), George J Wassilchenko; 12-5, 12-14, 12-16, Network Graphics; 12-6, Marcia Williams; 12-12, Karen Waldo; 12-13, Rolin Graphics; Science Applications box, Joe Kulka.

Chapter 13

13-1, Barbara Cousins; 13-2, G David Brown; 13-3, Joan Beck; 13-4, courtesy Philip Ballinger and Eugene D Frank (*Merrill's atlas of radiographic positions & radiologic procedures*, vol 1, ed 10, Mosby); 13-5, George J Wassilchenko; 13-6, 13-11, 13-12, Rolin Graphics; 13-8, 13-9, Network Graphics; 13-10, courtesy Emma Shelton; 13-13, courtesy Dr James T Barrett; Science Applications box, Joe Kulka.

Chapter 14

14-1, 14-2, 14-6(A), 14-7(art), Heimlich Maneuver box, Oxygen Therapy box, Barbara Cousins; 14-4, Margaret Garrity; 14-5, George J Wassilchenko; 14-6(C), Custom Medical Stock Photo; 14-7(photo), courtesy Stanley Erlandsen (from *Color atlas of histology*, 1992, Mosby); 14-8, 14-14 (heart and lungs), Network Graphics; 14-9, 14-12, Rolin Graphics; 14-11, Laurie O'Keefe; 14-14(inset and brainstem), William Ober; Lung Volume Reduction Surgery box, courtesy Andrew P Evan, University of Indiana; Science Applications box, Joe Kulka.

Chapter 15

15-4, Photo Researchers, Inc, New York, NY; 15-5, 15-6, 15-7, 15-16, Barbara Cousins; 15-8, Rolin Graphics; 15-10, courtesy Daffner RH (*Introduction to clinical radiation*, 1978, Mosby); 15-12, courtesy B. Vidic and F.R. Suarez (from *Photographic atlas of the human body*, 1984, Mosby); 15-13, 15-14, CNRI Science Photo Library/Photo Researchers; 15-15, Michael P Schenck; Malocclusion box, GA Thibodeau and KT Patton (from *Anatomy & physiology*, ed 5, Mosby); Gallstones and Weight Loss box, courtesy JM Thompson and SF Wilson (from

Health assessment for nursing practice, 1996, Mosby); Science Applications box, Joe Kulka.

Chapter 16

16-1, 16-5, Network Graphics; 16-2, 16-3, 16-4, Rolin Graphics; Science Applications box, Joe Kulka.

Chapter 17

17-1(B), 17-2(B), from P Abrahams, RT Hutchings, SC Marks (*McMinn's color atlas of human anatomy*, ed 4, St Louis, Mosby); 17-2(A), 17-3, from DJ Brundage (*Renal disorders*, St Louis, 1992, Mosby); 17-4, 17-8, Ernest W Beck; 17-5, Rolin Graphics; 17-6, courtesy PA Potter and AG Perry (*Fundamentals of nursing*, ed 4, Mosby); 17-7, courtesy G Bevelander and JA Ramaley (from *Essentials of histology*, ed 8, Mosby); Artificial Kidney box, Patrick Watson; Science Applications box, Joe Kulka.

Chapter 18

18-1, P Abrahams, RT Hutchings, SC Marks (*McMinn's color atlas of human anatomy*, ed 4, St Louis, Mosby); 18-2, Rolin Graphics; 18-3, Joan Beck; 18-4, Network Graphics; 18-7, courtesy O Epstein (*Clinical examination*, ed 3, Mosby, 2003); Science Applications box, Joe Kulka.

Chapter 19

19-5, 19-6, Barbara Cousins; 19-7, Laurie O'Keefe; Science Applications box, Joe Kulka.

Chapter 20

20-1, 20-2(art), 20-4(B), 20-9, 20-11, Barbara Cousins; 20-2(photo), Lennart Nilsson; 20-4(A), courtesy Stanley Erlandsen (from *Color atlas of histology*, 1992, Mosby); 20-5(A), Carolyn B Coulam/John A McIntyre; 20-5(B), William Ober; 20-6(B), courtesy B Vidic and FR Suarez (from *Photographic atlas of the human body*, 1984, Mosby); 20-7, 20-10, George J Wassilchenko; 20-8, Kevin A Somerville/Kathy Mitchell Gray; 20-13, Yvonne Wylie Walston; Science Applications box, Joe Kulka.

Chapter 21

21-1(art), Rolin Graphics; 21-1(photo), 21-6, Lennart Nilsson; 21-2, 21-4, Barbara Cousins; 21-3, courtesy Lucinda L Veek, Jones Institute for Reproductive Medicine; 21-5, Kevin A Somerville; 21-7, courtesy Goodenough et al (*Human biology*, Saunders College Publishing); 21-8, 21-9, Ernest W Beck; 21-10, courtesy Marjorie M Pyle, for Lifecircle, Costa Mesa, California; 21-11, Pat Watson; Science Applications box, Joe Kulka.

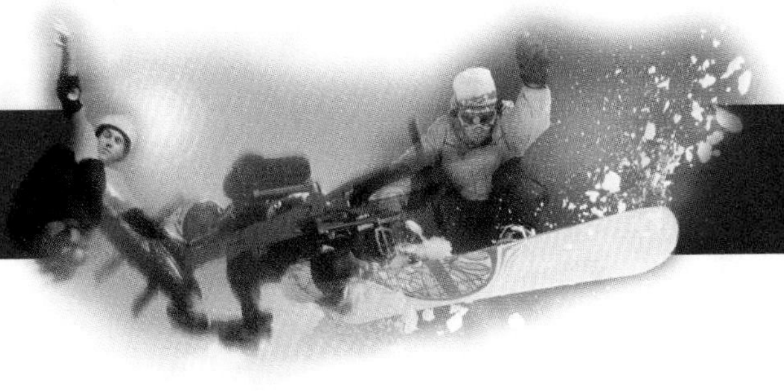

Index

A

Page numbers followed by *b* indicate boxed material; page numbers followed by *f* indicate figures; page numbers followed by *t* indicate tables.

B

C

G

H

I

J

K

L

N

O

S

T